AF866924

Management of Shoulder Instability

Rachel M. Frank • John M. Tokish
Editors

Management of Shoulder Instability

A Case-Based Guide

Springer

Editors
Rachel M. Frank
Orthopedic Surgery
University of Colorado Anschutz Medical Center
Denver, CO, USA

John M. Tokish
Orthopedic Surgery
Mayo Clinic
Scottsdale, AZ, USA

ISBN 978-3-032-18088-9 ISBN 978-3-032-18089-6 (eBook)
https://doi.org/10.1007/978-3-032-18089-6

© The Editor(s) (if applicable) and The Author(s), under exclusive license to Springer Nature Switzerland AG 2026

This work is subject to copyright. All rights are solely and exclusively licensed by the Publisher, whether the whole or part of the material is concerned, specifically the rights of translation, reprinting, reuse of illustrations, recitation, broadcasting, reproduction on microfilms or in any other physical way, and transmission or information storage and retrieval, electronic adaptation, computer software, or by similar or dissimilar methodology now known or hereafter developed.
The use of general descriptive names, registered names, trademarks, service marks, etc. in this publication does not imply, even in the absence of a specific statement, that such names are exempt from the relevant protective laws and regulations and therefore free for general use.
The publisher, the authors and the editors are safe to assume that the advice and information in this book are believed to be true and accurate at the date of publication. Neither the publisher nor the authors or the editors give a warranty, expressed or implied, with respect to the material contained herein or for any errors or omissions that may have been made. The publisher remains neutral with regard to jurisdictional claims in published maps and institutional affiliations.

This Springer imprint is published by the registered company Springer Nature Switzerland AG
The registered company address is: Gewerbestrasse 11, 6330 Cham, Switzerland

If disposing of this product, please recycle the paper.

To the surgeons, scientists, and innovators who push our field forward every single day. Your commitment to meticulous technique, thoughtful innovation, and compassionate care inspires the work within these pages. May this work contribute, in some small way, to advancing the care of shoulder instability for the next generation of clinicians and the patients they serve. This work is for you.

To our mentors, colleagues, and trainees—past and present—whose curiosity, precision, and dedication have shaped the understanding and management of shoulder instability. This work is for you as well.

To the patients who entrust us with their shoulders, and challenge us to continue to get better so that they can get better, we are grateful and remain committed.

Rachel and JT

Preface

Management of Shoulder Instability was conceived with a simple but ambitious goal: to create a comprehensive, contemporary, and surgically focused resource that reflects the rapidly evolving landscape of shoulder instability care. Instability remains one of the most challenging and high-stakes problems in shoulder and sports medicine. Its management demands not only technical precision but also a deep understanding of anatomy, biomechanics, pathology, patient factors, and the spectrum of treatment options, from non-operative strategies to the most advanced reconstructive and salvage procedures.

This textbook brings together *39 chapters* authored by leading surgeons and scientists from around the world. Each chapter was selected and structured to provide practical, technique-driven guidance while grounding recommendations in the best available evidence. Our contributors offer both the foundational principles and the nuanced decision-making that define modern shoulder instability surgery. The breadth of topics, from first-time dislocators to complex revision scenarios, bone loss evaluation, open and arthroscopic stabilization, capsular procedures, graft options, rehabilitation, return-to-play considerations, and emerging technologies, reflects the full spectrum of care required to serve athletes and patients of all backgrounds.

We are proud that this text balances *technical depth and surgical detail* with *clinical relevance*, emphasizing pearls, pitfalls, and real-world application. The authors' collective experience, innovation, and generosity in sharing insights elevate this work far beyond a simple procedural manual.

We are grateful to our colleagues, trainees, and mentors who have shaped our understanding of instability, and to our patients, whose trust drives our continued pursuit of excellence. We also thank our contributing authors for their expertise and commitment, and our editorial and production teams for their dedication in bringing this textbook to life.

It is our hope that this volume serves as a definitive reference for practicing surgeons, fellows, and residents, and inspires the next generation of clinicians and investigators to continue advancing the care of shoulder instability.

Denver, CO, USA — Rachel M. Frank
Scottsdale, AZ, USA — John M. Tokish

Acknowledgments

The creation of *Management of Shoulder Instability* has been a deeply collaborative effort, and we are fortunate to have worked with an extraordinary group of contributors, colleagues, and supporters who made this textbook possible.

First and foremost, we extend our sincere gratitude to the *chapter authors*—a distinguished group of surgeons, researchers, and educators from around the world. Your expertise, generosity of time, and commitment to advancing the care of shoulder instability are reflected in every chapter. This text stands on the strength of your work.

We are also grateful to our *mentors and colleagues* who have shaped our clinical and surgical perspectives over the years. Your influence is woven into the principles and techniques presented throughout this book. To the trainees, students, residents, and fellows—your curiosity, energy, and dedication continue to push our field forward and remind us why education matters.

A special thank you to the *patients* who place their trust in us. Your resilience and partnership inspire the innovation and clinical excellence that drive continued progress in shoulder instability care.

We appreciate the exceptional efforts of the *editorial, production, and publishing teams*, whose professionalism, attention to detail, and unwavering support guided this project from concept to completion. Your behind-the-scenes work ensures that the science, art, and techniques within these pages are communicated clearly and effectively.

To our families, friends, pets, and loved ones, thank you for your patience, encouragement, and understanding throughout the many hours devoted to this project. Your support sustains us, particularly during those late-night and weekend hours.

We dedicate this work to all who strive to improve the care of patients with shoulder instability and advance the field of shoulder surgery for generations to come.

Rachel M. Frank
John M. Tokish

About the Book

Management of Shoulder Instability is a comprehensive, contemporary resource designed for orthopedic surgeons, sports medicine specialists, shoulder and elbow surgeons, fellows, residents, and allied clinicians who manage the full spectrum of shoulder instability. With *39 expertly authored chapters*, this volume integrates foundational principles with advanced surgical concepts to provide a complete, practical guide to evaluating and treating instability in athletes and patients of all ages.

The text emphasizes *surgical technique*, decision-making, and evidence-based management across a broad range of scenarios, from first-time dislocators to complex revision cases, from bone loss evaluation to open and arthroscopic stabilization, from capsular procedures to reconstructive and graft-based solutions. Each chapter offers high-yield pearls, pitfalls, and clinical insights derived from extensive operative experience.

Designed to serve as both a reference and a surgical companion, this book reflects the latest innovations in shoulder preservation, advanced imaging, biomechanics, return-to-play criteria, and post-operative rehabilitation. With contributions from world-renowned experts, *Management of Shoulder Instability* delivers the depth, clarity, and practical relevance essential for those committed to restoring stability and function in the shoulder.

Contents

Editors and Contributors

About the Editors

Rachel M. Frank, MD is Professor of Orthopaedic Surgery at the University of Colorado School of Medicine and Director of the Joint Preservation Program. She is also a team physician for the US Womens National Soccer Team and the Colorado Rapids professional soccer team. A nationally and internationally recognized sports medicine and shoulder surgeon, she specializes in cartilage restoration, complex knee and shoulder surgery, and shoulder instability in athletes. She has authored hundreds of peer-reviewed publications, book chapters, and textbooks, and is a frequently invited lecturer and surgical educator around the world. Her clinical and academic work centers on innovation, high-quality patient care, and advancing the science of joint preservation and sports medicine.

John M. Tokish, MD is Professor of Orthopaedic Surgery at the Mayo Clinic Arizona, former president of the Arthroscopy Association of North America (AANA), and a globally recognized leader in shoulder and sports medicine surgery. A retired military surgeon, he has deep experience in the humbling and rewarding study of shoulder instability; his research has centered on instability, shoulder reconstruction, arthroscopic technique development, and surgical education; and he continues to contribute to the literature and serves in multiple national leadership roles.

Together, Dr. Frank and Dr. Tokish bring complementary expertise and a shared passion for improving shoulder instability care through education, research, and surgical innovation. Their collaborative approach and dedication to elevating the field are reflected throughout this textbook.

Contributors

Jeffrey S. Abrams Department of Orthopedic Surgery, Princeton Orthopedic Associates, Princeton, NJ, USA

Abdulaziz F. Ahmed Department of Orthopaedic Surgery, Division of Sports Medicine, University of Colorado School of Medicine, Aurora, CO, USA

Fares Hamdan Al-Jahdali Orthopaedic Surgery, Department of Surgery, Faculty of Medicine, Dalhousie University, Halifax, NS, Canada

Department of Orthopedics, Prince Mohammed Bin Abdulaziz Hospital, Ministry of National Guard-Health Affairs, Madinah, Saudi Arabia

Mahdi AlSaffar Department of Orthopedics, New Jahra Hospital, Al Jahra, Kuwait

Yasser Al Shehab Department of Orthopedics, King Abdullah bin Abdulaziz University, Riyadh, Saudi Arabia

David W. Altchek Sports Medicine and Shoulder Service, Hospital for Special Surgery, New York, NY, USA

Robert A. Arciero Department of Orthopaedic Surgery, University of Connecticut, Farmington, CT, USA

Justin W. Arner Department of Orthopaedic Surgery, University of Pittsburgh Medical Center, Pittsburgh, PA, USA

Andrew Assenmacher Department of Orthopedic Surgery, ProMedica Health System, Toledo, OH, USA

George S. Athwal McFarlane Hand & Upper Limb Centre, St. Joseph's Health Care, London, ON, Canada

Yousif Atwan Department of Orthopaedic Surgery, Mayo Clinic, Rochester, MN, USA

Douglas W. Bartels Mayo Clinic Health Systems – Eau Claire, Department of Orthopaedic Surgery, Eau Claire, WI, USA

Stanford University School of Medicine, Department of Orthopaedic Surgery, Redwood City, CA, USA

Stephanie A. Boden Department of Orthopedic Surgery, University of Louisville, Louisville, KY, USA

Pascal Boileau ICR-Institut de Chirurgie Réparatrice—Groupe KANTYS, Institute for Sports and Reconstructive Surgery, Nice, France

Desmond Bokor Faculty of Medicine, Health and Human Sciences, Macquarie University, Sydney, NSW, Australia

James P. Bradley Department of Orthopaedic Surgery, University of Pittsburgh Medical Center, Pittsburgh, PA, USA

Jonathan Bravman Department of Orthopedic Surgery, University of Colorado, Aurora, CO, USA

Christopher M. Brusalis Sports Medicine Institute, Hospital for Special Surgery, New York, NY, USA

Colin J. Burgess Department of Orthopaedic Surgery, Orthopaedic Research of Virginia, Richmond, VA, USA

Paul Caldwell Department of Orthopaedic Surgery, Orthopaedic Research of Virginia/Tuckahoe Orthopaedics Associates, Richmond, VA, USA

Camilo Andres Estrada Cely Orthopedics and Traumatology, Hospital Serena del Mar, Cartagena de Indias, Provincia de Cartagena, Bolívar, Colombia

Peter Chalmers Department of Orthopaedic Surgery, University of Utah, Salt Lake City, UT, USA

Joshua Chiang Perelman School of Medicine, University of Pennsylvania, Philadelphia, PA, USA

Wendell Cole Department of Orthopaedic Surgery, New York University, New York, NY, USA

John E. Conway Department of Orthopaedic Surgery, University of Texas Health Science Center at Houston/McGovern Medical School, Houston, TX, USA

Antonio Cusano Department of Orthopaedic Surgery, University of Connecticut, Farmington, CT, USA

Stephen D. Daniels Department of Orthopedic Surgery, University of Colorado, Aurora, CO, USA

Jasan Dannaway Faculty of Medicine, Health and Human Sciences, Macquarie University, Sydney, NSW, Australia

Maria E. Dey Hazra Steadman Philippon Research Institute, Vail, CO, USA

Giovanni Di Giacomo Department of Orthopaedic Surgery, Concordia Hospital, Rome, Italy

James Dove Department of Orthopaedic Surgery, Warren Alpert Medical School of Brown University, Providence, RI, USA

T. Bradley Edwards Fondren Orthopedic Group, Houston, TX, USA

Texas Orthopedic Hospital, Houston, TX, USA

Fondren Orthopedic Research Institute, Houston, TX, USA

Jonathan Erickson Southern California Orthopedic Institute, Van Nuys, CA, USA

Michael J. Foster Steadman Philippon Research Institute, Vail, CO, USA

The Steadman Clinic, Vail, CO, USA

Rachel M. Frank Orthopedic Surgery, University of Colorado Anschutz Medical Center, Denver, CO, USA

Michael T. Freehill Stanford University School of Medicine, Department of Orthopaedic Surgery, Redwood City, CA, USA

Matthew S. Fury Sports Medicine and Shoulder Service, Hospital for Special Surgery, New York, NY, USA

Phob Ganokroj The Steadman Philippon Research Institute, Vail, CO, USA
Faculty of Medicine Siriraj Hospital, Mahidol University, Bangkok, Thailand

Mark Getelman Southern California Orthopedic Institute, Van Nuys, CA, USA

Eddie Gontee Morehouse School of Medicine, Atlanta, Georgia

Bonnie P. Gregory Department of Orthopaedic Surgery, University of Texas Health Science Center at Houston/McGovern Medical School, Houston, TX, USA

B. Gage Griswold Medical College of Georgia, Augusta University, Augusta, GA, USA

Jared A. Hanson Steadman Philippon Research Institute, Vail, CO, USA
University of Colorado School of Medicine, Aurora, CO, USA

Rony-Orijit Dey Hazra Steadman Philippon Research Institute, Vail, CO, USA
Department for Shoulder and Elbow Surgery, Charité Universitätsmedizin Berlin, Center for Musculoskeletal Surgery, Berlin, Germany

Maximilian Hinz Department of Sports Orthopaedics, Technical University of Munich, Munich, Germany

Andreas B. Imhoff Department of Sports Orthopaedics, Technical University of Munich, Munich, Germany

Garrett R. Jackson Department of Orthopaedic Surgery, Rush University Medical Center, Chicago, IL, USA

Daniel J. Kaplan NYU Langone Health, New York University Langone Medical Center, New York, NY, USA

Ann Marie Kelly Orthopaedic Surgery, Dartmouth-Hitchcock Medical Center, Lebanon, NH, USA

John D. A. Kelly IV Orthopaedic Surgery, Sports Medicine, University of Pennsylvania, Philadelphia, PA, USA

Moin Khan Division of Orthopaedic Surgery, Department of Surgery, McMaster University, Hamilton, ON, Canada

Jason Khoury McFarlane Hand & Upper Limb Centre, St. Joseph's Health Care, London, ON, Canada

Joseph T. Labrum IV Department of Orthopaedic Surgery, Mayo Clinic, Rochester, MN, USA

Juan David Lacouture Orthopedics and Traumatology, Hospital Serena del Mar, Cartagena de Indias, Provincia de Cartagena, Bolívar, Colombia

Alex Lencioni Department of Orthopedic Surgery, University of Colorado, Aurora, CO, USA

Daniel Lewis Department of Orthopaedic Surgery, University of Utah, Salt Lake City, UT, USA

Christopher M. Loftis Tennessee Orthopaedic Alliance, Columbia, TN, USA

Tennessee Orthopeaedic Alliance, Center for Research and Education Foundation, Nashville, TN, USA

Marco Maiotti Shoulder and Knee Unit Mediterranea Hospital, Naples, Italy

Shoulder Unit Villa Stuart Hospital, Rome, Italy

Stephen E. Marcaccio Department of Orthopaedic Surgery, Warren Alpert Medical School of Brown University, Providence, RI, USA

Carlo Massoni Shoulder and Knee Unit Mediterranea Hospital, Naples, Italy

Shoulder Unit Villa Stuart Hospital, Rome, Italy

James C. Messina Department of Orthopaedic Surgery, University of Connecticut, Farmington, CT, USA

Peter J. Millett Steadman Philippon Research Institute, Vail, CO, USA

The Steadman Clinic, Vail, CO, USA

Anthony Miniaci Florida Atlantic University, Boca Raton, FL, USA

Baptist Health Orthopedic Care, Boca Raton, FL, USA

Joshua Mizels Department of Orthopaedic Surgery, University of Utah, Salt Lake City, UT, USA

Tucker Morey University of Kansas School of Medicine, Kansas City, KS, USA

Philipp Moroder Department of Shoulder and Elbow Surgery, Schulthess Klinik, Zurich, Switzerland

Patrick Morrissey Department of Orthopaedic Surgery, Warren Alpert Medical School of Brown University, Providence, RI, USA

Mary K. Mulcahey Department of Orthopaedic Surgery and Rehabilitation, Loyola University Medical Center, Maywood, IL, USA

Jordan Nester Oschner Orthopedic Surgery, New Orleans, LA, USA

Clayton W. Nuelle Mizzou Joint Preservation Center, Department of Orthopaedic Surgery, University of Missouri, Columbia, MO, USA

Michael J. O'Brien Department of Orthopaedic Surgery, Tulane University School of Medicine, New Orleans, LA, USA

Nicholas A. Ott Andrews Research and Education Foundation, Andrews Institute, Gulf Breeze, FL, USA

Brett D. Owens Department of Orthopaedic Surgery, Warren Alpert Medical School of Brown University, Providence, RI, USA

Stephen A. Parada Medical College of Georgia, Augusta University, Augusta, GA, USA

Robert L. Parisien Orthopaedic Surgery and Sports Medicine, Mount Sinai Health System, New York, NY, USA

Liam A. Peebles Tulane University School of Medicine, New Orleans, LA, USA

Jonas Pogorzelski Department of Sports Orthopaedics, Technical University of Munich, Munich, Germany

OC Erlangen, Erlangen, Germany

Matthew T. Provencher Department of Orthopaedic Surgery and Sports Medicine, The Steadman Clinic and the Steadman Philippon Research Institute, Vail, CO, USA

Sumit Raniga Faculty of Medicine, Health and Human Sciences, Macquarie University, Sydney, NSW, Australia

Anthony A. Romeo DuPage Medical Group, Westmont, IL, USA

Marco-Christopher Rupp Steadman Philippon Research Institute, Vail, CO, USA

Joan C. Rutledge Steadman Philippon Research Institute, Vail, CO, USA

Zachary Salas Department of Orthopaedic Surgery, Tulane University School of Medicine, New Orleans, LA, USA

Joaquin Sanchez-Sotelo Department of Orthopaedic Surgery, Mayo Clinic, Rochester, MN, USA

Felix H. Savoie III Department of Orthopaedic Surgery, Tulane University School of Medicine, New Orleans, LA, USA

Michael J. Scarcella Cleveland Clinic Sports Medicine, Department of Orthopaedic Surgery, Cleveland, OH, USA

Adam Seidl Department of Orthopedic Surgery, University of Colorado, Aurora, CO, USA

James S. Shaha Pioneer Peak Orthopedics, Palmer, AK, USA

Conor Smith Mizzou Joint Preservation Center, Department of Orthopaedic Surgery, University of Missouri, Columbia, MO, USA

Matthew Smith Mizzou Joint Preservation Center, Department of Orthopaedic Surgery, University of Missouri, Columbia, MO, USA

Giovanni Spagna Department of Shoulder and Elbow Surgery, Schulthess Klinik, Zurich, Switzerland

Paolo Spinello Department of Orthopaedic Surgery, Concordia Hospital, Rome, Italy

Daniel J. Stokes Department of Orthopaedic Surgery, Division of Sports Medicine, University of Colorado School of Medicine, Aurora, CO, USA

Misty Suri Ochsner Andrews Sports Medicine Institute, Department of Orthopedic Surgery, Ochsner Health System, New Orleans, LA, USA

Edward J. Testa Department of Orthopaedic Surgery, Warren Alpert Medical School of Brown University, Providence, RI, USA

John M. Tokish Orthopedic Surgery, Mayo Clinic, Scottsdale, AZ, USA

Arjun Verma Oschner Orthopedic Surgery, New Orleans, LA, USA

Nikhil N. Verma Department of Orthopaedic Surgery, Rush University Medical Center, Chicago, IL, USA

Matthew L. Vopat Department of Orthopedic Surgery and Sports Medicine, University of Kansas Medical Center, Kansas City, KS, USA

John Weldy Department of Orthopaedic Surgery, Tulane University School of Medicine, New Orleans, LA, USA

Ryan J. Whalen Center for Outcomes Based Orthopaedic Research, Steadman Philippon Research Institute, Vail, CO, USA

Ivan Wong Orthopaedic Surgery, Department of Surgery, Faculty of Medicine, Dalhousie University, Halifax, NS, Canada

Part I
General Topics

Shoulder Anatomy and Biomechanics

1

Joshua Mizels, Daniel Lewis, and Peter Chalmers

Introduction

The glenohumeral (GH) joint is a highly complex and mobile joint. Because of the shallow glenoid fossa, the GH joint relies on the delicate balance between dynamic and static stabilizers to ensure congruency of the GH joint throughout range of motion [1–4].

Osseous Anatomy

Proximal Humerus

The anatomy of the proximal humerus consists of the humeral head and proximal humeral shaft [5]. The humeral head articulates with the glenoid fossa of the scapula to form the GH joint [5]. In the coronal plane, the humeral head articular surface has a diameter of curvature that ranges from 46 to 51 mm with an associated surface arc of 145–150° [1]. The diameter of curvature in the axial plane is slightly lower than that in the coronal plane, and as such the humeral head is the ellipsoid at the periphery and spherical closer to the center [1].

J. Mizels (✉) · D. Lewis · P. Chalmers
Department of Orthopaedic Surgery, University of Utah, Salt Lake City, UT, USA
e-mail: josh.mizels@hsc.utah.edu; dan.lewis@hsc.utah.edu; peter.chalmers@hsc.utah.edu

The humeral head is also offset relative to the shaft, but this relationship is highly variable. On average, the center of rotation lies 6–10 mm medial and 0–3 mm posterior to the axis of the humeral shaft [1]. Humeral head retroversion, defined as the angle between the plane of the articular surface and the transepicondylar axis, on average, is between 15 and 26° [1].

The anatomic neck separates the humeral head from the greater and lesser tuberosities. The greater tuberosity is located laterally, while the lesser tuberosity is an anterior structure [5]. The humeral head height, measured from the anatomic neck to the articular surface, averages between 18 and 19 mm [1]. The neck shaft angle, measured between the long axis of the humeral shaft and the anatomic neck, ranges from 130 to 140° [6].

Glenoid

The glenoid is pear shaped when looked at en face, wider in the anterior-posterior dimension inferiorly and narrower superiorly by a ratio of 1–0.8 [1]. The height measured from superior-inferior averages 39 mm, and the anterior-posterior width, on average, measures 23 mm superiorly and 29 mm inferiorly [1]. This is significantly smaller than the dimensions of the humeral head in both the coronal and axial planes.

© The Author(s), under exclusive license to Springer Nature Switzerland AG 2026
R. M. Frank, J. M. Tokish (eds.), *Management of Shoulder Instability*,
https://doi.org/10.1007/978-3-032-18089-6_1

Glenoid version and inclination are also highly variable. Version, the angle between the glenoid articular surface and the long axis of the scapula in the axial plane, can range from 2° of anteversion to 8° of retroversion [1]. Inclination, the same angle in the coronal plane, ranges from 12° of superior inclination to 11° of inferior tilt [1].

Glenoid Labrum

The glenoid labrum is the peripheral fibrocartilage of the GH joint [7]. The cross-sectional anatomy of the labrum is described as having three sides and one free edge [7]. The sides include (1) the superficial side which is free and responds to the humeral head; (2) the articular side which is adherent to the glenoid cavity; and (3) the peripheral side which is adherent to the GH joint capsule [7]. The morphology of the labrum varies throughout the GH joint according to its location. Superiorly, the articular side of the labrum is variable and is often not adherent to the glenoid cavity. Here, it can be free and "meniscus-like" [7]. Inferiorly, the labrum is larger and strongly adherent to the glenoid cavity [7]. This area serves as the scapular attachment for the inferior glenohumeral ligament (IGHL).

The labrum also has normal anatomic variants, and the superior region is the most variable. In younger patients, the labrum can be strongly adherent to the glenoid [7, 8]. However, with time, a recess develops which is physiologic if there is glenoid articular cartilage present at the most peripheral attachment of the labrum [7]. A Buford complex can occur here as well, consisting of a "cord-like" middle glenohumeral ligament (MGHL) and an absent labrum [7, 9].

The labrum has three main functions. First, it acts to increase the contact area between the humeral head and glenoid. Anteroposteriorly, this is an increase by 2 mm and supero-inferiorly this is by 4.5 mm [7]. Next, it helps to create negative intra-articular pressure to resist both shear and traction stresses on the GH joint [7]. Finally, it serves as the attachment for the capsular and glenohumeral ligamentous insertions. Together, the labrum and ligaments form a "complex" to absorb stress [7, 10].

Glenohumeral Ligaments

The glenohumeral ligaments (see Fig. 1.1) consist of the superior glenohumeral ligament (SGHL), middle glenohumeral ligament (MGHL), anteroinferior glenohumeral ligament (AIGHL), posteroinferior glenohumeral ligament (PIGHL), and coracohumeral ligament (CHL). To understand their respective attachment points, the humeral head and glenoid can be looked at as a clockface. On the humeral side, 12 o'clock is the most superior aspect, and 3 o'clock is anterior, irrespective of laterality. On the glenoid side, 12 o'clock is the midpoint of the insertion of the long head of biceps tendon (LHBT), and 3 o'clock is anterior, irrespective of laterality.

The SGHL originates just anterior to the supraglenoid tubercle at the 12:30 to 12:45 position on the glenoid clockface and inserts at the 12:55 to 1:40 position on the humeral clockface, just lateral (4.8–6.7 mm) to the margin of the articular cartilage. The SGHL is taut in adduction and external rotation [11, 12]. The SGHL contributes to biceps stability. The CHL is a key stabilizer of the biceps pulley and serves as an

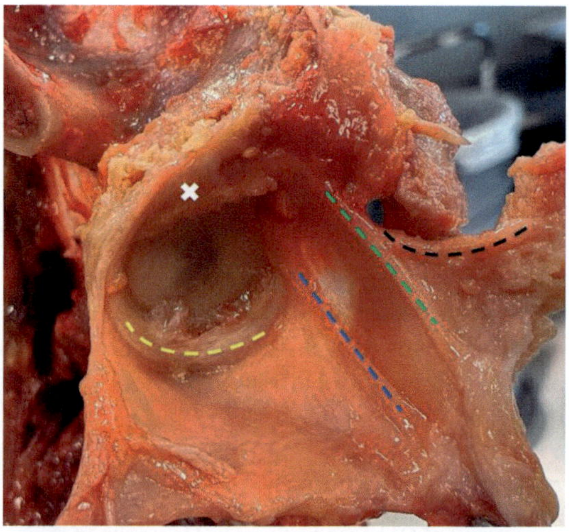

Fig. 1.1 Posterior view of the glenoid and capsulolabral complex. White "X": superior labrum with long head of biceps tendon (LHBT) attachment; black dotted line: coracohumeral ligament (CHL); green dotted line: superior glenohumeral ligament (SGHL); blue dotted line; inferior glenohumeral ligament (IGHL); yellow dotted line: inferior labrum

intra-articular reinforcement of the rotator interval. This allows for a close relationship with the intra-articular portion of the LHBT before its glenoid insertion [11, 13].

The MGHL originates on the glenoid adjacent to the SGHL at the 1:50 to 2:35 clockface position and inserts at the 2:10 to 3:35 positions on the humeral clockface [12]. Laterally, it blends with the subscapularis inserting 9 mm from the margin of the articular cartilage and 10.8 mm medial to the most inferior aspect of the lesser tuberosity [12]. The MGHL is taut in 45° of abduction and external rotation [12].

The AIGHL is the largest of the glenohumeral ligaments [12]. It has a broad origin on the glenoid side, having both bony attachments and being confluent with the labrum. On the glenoid clockface, it attaches from the 3:30 to 4:05 clockface positions and 1.2 mm medial to the most lateral portion of the glenoid labrum [12]. On the humeral clockface, it inserts from the 4:05 to 5:10 position and 8 mm lateral to the margin of the articular cartilage on the surgical neck of the humerus—this may serve as a landmark for arthroscopic repair [12]. The AIGHL acts as a key stabilizer of anterior GH stability.

The PIGHL has both bony and ligamentous attachments at its glenoid origin, from the 7:35 to 8:50 positions on the glenoid clockface [12]. On the humeral clockface, it inserts at the 7:40 to 8:50 position 9 mm lateral to the margin of the articular surface [12]. The PIGHL, with the posterior labrum and joint capsule, contributes to posterior GH stability particularly when the shoulder is in 90° of abduction [12, 14].

Finally, the CHL has a broad origin on the lateral aspect of the coracoid about 14.1 mm posterior to the tip of the coracoid [12]. From its scapular origin, it generally splits into three branches, anterior, posterior, and central [12]. While the anterior limb covers almost the entirety of the subscapularis, the posterior limb inserts on the greater tuberosity as well as the supraspinatus and infraspinatus [12]. The primary central branch inserts at the 11:55 to 12:40 positions on the humeral clockface, just anterior to the humeral head cartilage [12]. The CHL prevents humeral head translation both posteriorly and inferiorly and has been implicated in multidirectional shoulder instability [12, 15].

Rotator Cuff

The rotator cuff (see Figs. 1.2 and 1.3) consists of the subscapularis, supraspinatus, infraspinatus, and teres minor. Each rotator cuff muscle will be discussed separately. The muscles of the rotator cuff are all distinct structures, but the distal portions of their tendons interweave and envelop the deeper glenohumeral joint capsule. There are two bare areas of capsule that are not enveloped in myotendinous tissue: the rotator interval and axillary recess.

Subscapularis

The subscapularis is the largest muscle of the rotator cuff. It originates anteriorly from the scapula on the medial 2/3 of the subscapular fossa and has a "comma-shaped" insertion on lesser tuberosity and medial aspect of the bicipital groove [16, 17]. Its insertion on the lesser tuberosity is trapezoidal in shape tapered from wider proximally to narrowed distally. In an anatomic study, the subscapularis insertion on the humeral head is reported to measure 24–40 mm in length from proximal to distal and 18–20 mm in width [18]. The subscapularis's insertion is purely tendinous at the articular surface and has a musculocapsular attachment inferiorly [16, 19].

Additionally, the tendon of the subscapularis extends past its insertion and fuses with the tendon of the supraspinatus to form a sheath over the bicipital groove, which stabilizes the tendon of the long head of the biceps [17, 19]. The upper portion of the tendon has been shown to be the strongest [16]. The subscapularis has dual innervation from the upper and lower subscapular nerves. The primary action of the subscapularis is internal rotation of the humerus, but it also contributes to abduction, adduction, flexion, and extension depending on arm position [17, 19]. Blood supply to the subscapularis is provided by the subscapular artery [17].

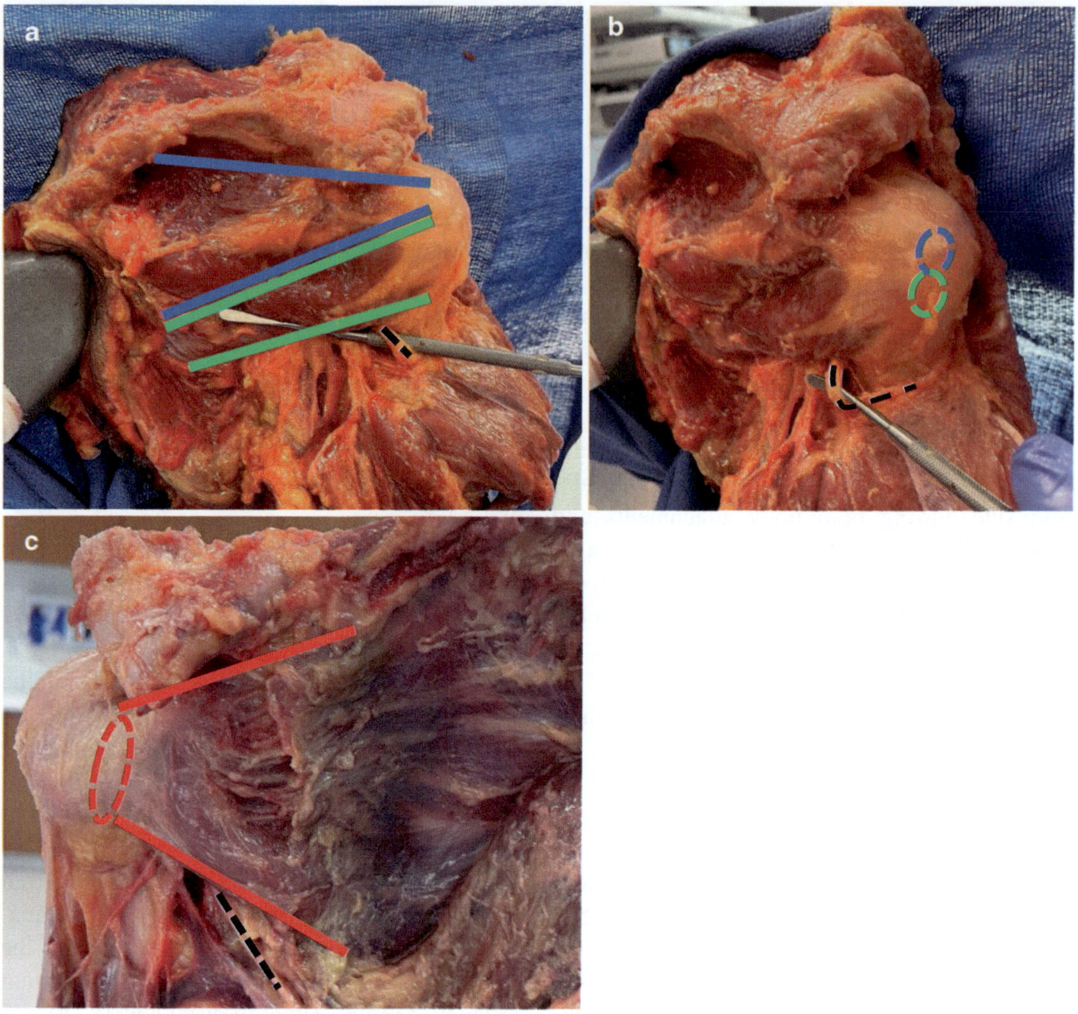

Fig. 1.2 The rotator cuff. (**a**) Posterior, (**b**) lateral, and (**c**) anterior view of shoulder. Blue solid line: infraspinatus; blue dashed line: infraspinatus footprint; green solid line: teres minor; green dashed line: teres minor footprint; red solid line: subscapularis; red dashed line: subscapularis footprint; black dotted line: axillary nerve

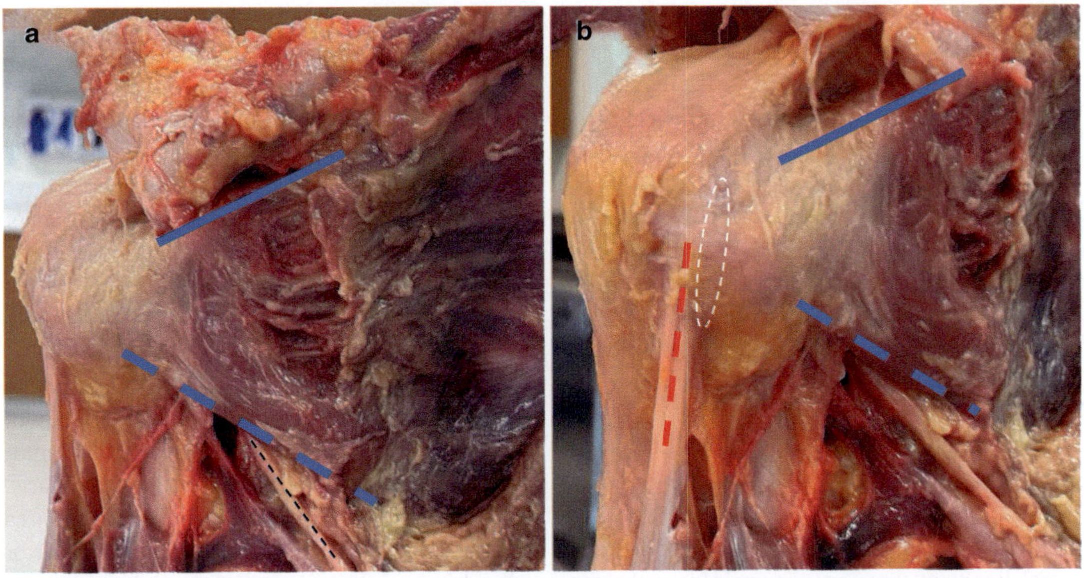

Fig. 1.3 (**a**) Anterior view of shoulder; (**b**) anterior-oblique view of shoulder. Blue solid line: upper border of subscapularis (SS); blue dotted line: inferior border of subscapularis; red dotted line: long head of biceps tendon (LHBT) in the bicipital groove; white dotted ellipse: lesser tuberosity; black dotted line: axillary nerve

Infraspinatus

The infraspinatus is a bipennate muscle that originates from the medial 2/3 of the infraspinatus fossa on the posterior scapula and interdigitates with the supraspinatus as it inserts onto the humerus on the greater tuberosity [16, 17]. It wraps around the posterior aspect of the supraspinatus tendon and has a trapezoidal insertion as it tapers distally for 16 mm [16]. Its footprint is reported from 16 to 29 mm in length and 13 to 19 mm in width [16, 18]. The "bare area" of the humerus represents the interval from the posterior articular surface to the inferior aspect of the infraspinatus insertion [16]. The primary function of the infraspinatus is extension and external rotation of the arm [17]. Innervation is provided by the suprascapular nerve, and blood supply to the infraspinatus is the suprascapular artery [17].

Supraspinatus

The supraspinatus originates from the medial 2/3 supraspinous fossa of the scapula and inserts on the greater tuberosity in the sulcus between the bicipital groove and the bare area of the humerus [16, 17]. Its insertion is tapered, wider proximally at the humeral articular surface [16]. Its insertion has been reported with an average length of 16–28 mm and width of 12–25 mm [16, 18]. As described above, the posterior insertion of the supraspinatus interdigitates with the anterior insertion of the infraspinatus [16, 17]. The area of the tendon just proximal to its insertion is less vascularized, and therefore more prone to tears. The primary function of the supraspinatus is to initiate shoulder abduction as in greater degrees of abduction the deltoid is the primary contributor to abduction [17]. Like the infraspinatus, the supraspinatus is innervated by the suprascapular nerve, and blood supply is provided by the suprascapular artery [17].

Teres Minor

The teres minor arises from the superior 2/3 of the dorsal aspect of the lateral scapular border; it is the smallest muscle of the rotator cuff, yet it has a relatively large insertional footprint about 10 mm inferior to the humeral articular surface

[16, 17]. The length of its insertion is reported as 20–29 mm and with a width of 11–21 mm [18]. The teres minor insertion tapers distally from a tendinous insertion proximally to a musculocapsular insertion distally in a triangular shape [16]. The teres minor functions in conjunction with the infraspinatus to extend and externally rotate the arm, particularly in abduction [17]. Innervation is provided by the axillary nerve. The teres minor has dual blood supply, from both the posterior circumflex humeral artery and circumflex scapular artery [17].

Rotator Cable

The rotator cable is a component of the coracohumeral ligament that serves to reinforce the tendons of the supraspinatus and infraspinatus. Its fibers run perpendicular to the tendon fibers and are intimately associated to the tendon fibers. It forms a crescent-moon-shaped cord of tissue that provides a transverse reinforcement to both the infraspinatus and supraspinatus tendons. The rotator cable runs from the intertubercular groove anteriorly to the posterior aspect of the greater tubercle posteriorly [17].

Rotator Interval

The rotator interval (see Fig. 1.4) is a triangular area formed by the anterior border of the supraspinatus, superior border of the subscapularis, and bordered medially by the glenoid. This area contains the coracohumeral ligament, superior glenohumeral ligament, and long head of the biceps tendon [17].

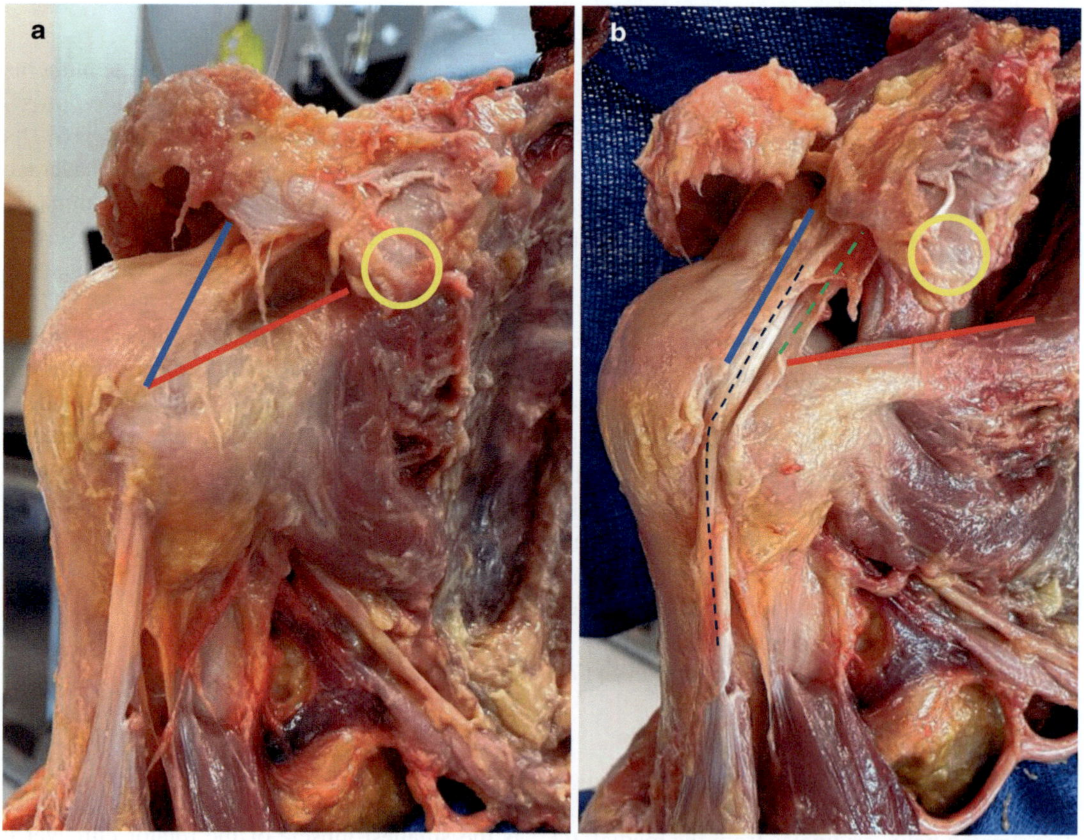

Fig. 1.4 Anterior view of shoulder. (**a**) rotator interval intact. (**b**) rotator interval released. Blue line: anterior margin of supraspinatus; red line: superior margin of subscapularis; yellow circle: coracoid process; black dotted line; long head of biceps tendon (LHBT); green dotted line: coracohumeral ligament (CHL)

Axillary Recess

The axillary recess is a large pouch of capsule on the inferior aspect of the glenohumeral joint that is bounded by the anterior and posterior bands of the inferior glenohumeral ligament [17]. This recess provides the passive abduction of the glenohumeral joint, and thus the size of the recess is determined by the degree of abduction.

The Axillary Nerve

The axillary nerve (see Fig. 1.5) is the most important nerve for shoulder function. The axillary nerve originates from the posterior cord of the brachial plexus [20]. It then courses inferolaterally along the anterior border of the subscapularis muscle and wraps around its inferior border about 1 cm medial to the musculotendinous junction [20, 21]. It then courses posteriorly through the quadrilateral space, passing just 1 cm from the inferior glenoid rim, before bifurcating into two branches [21]. The anterior division is classically located 5–7 cm distal to the lateral edge of the acromion, but this can be variable [21, 22]. The anterior branch courses underneath the deltoid muscle where it innervates all three heads [21]. The posterior branch innervates the teres minor and the skin overlying the deltoid [21].

Biomechanics

The shoulder is the most mobile joint in the human body. This joint is complex because there are 4 separate joints (glenohumeral, acromioclavicular, scapulothoracic, sternoclavicular) with 18 separate muscles acting upon it to allow the upper extremity to reach many positions in space [23]. This discussion will focus on the biomechanics of the GH joint.

The GH joint relies on the balance between static (osseous and capsulolabral structures) and dynamic (*muscular*) stabilizers to ensure stability, and pathology of any of the features can lead to GH instability. The first important static stabilizer is the glenoid labrum, which increases the depth of the relatively flat osseous glenoid and thereby increasing contact with the humeral head

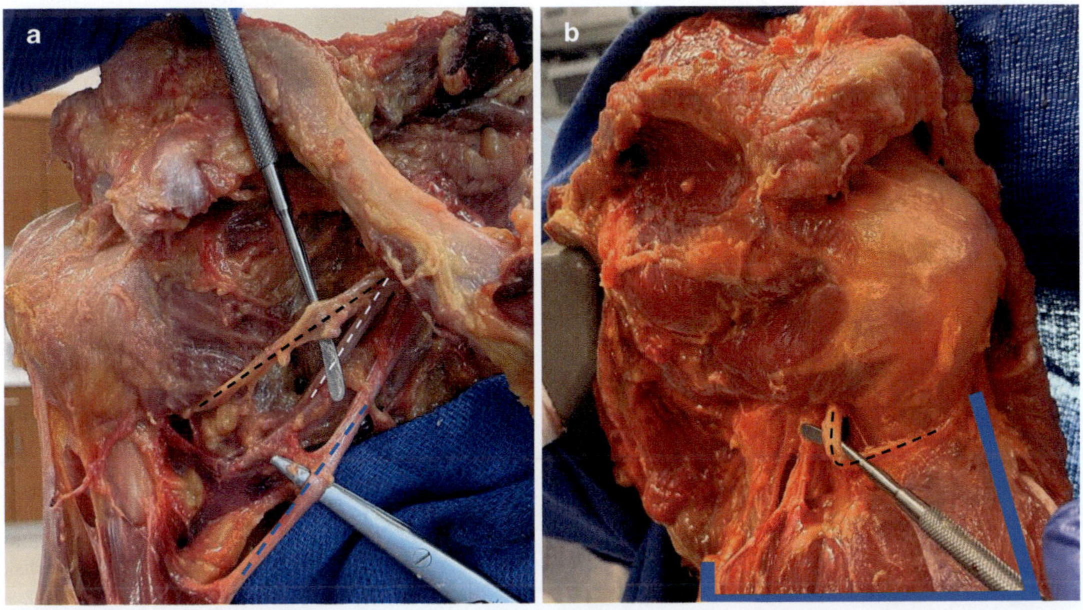

Fig. 1.5 (**a**) Anterior view of shoulder, (**b**) posterior-lateral view of shoulder. Black dotted line: axillary nerve; white dotted line: radial nerve; blue dotted line: musculocutaneous nerve; blue solid line: deltoid muscle reflected, deep surface of muscle visible

[7, 23, 24]. The glenohumeral ligaments, which are the primary static stabilizers, only tighten during end ranges of motion to allow GH mobility [23]. The SGHL is tight during shoulder adduction, MGHL during 45° of abduction, and the IGHL during 90° of abduction and external rotation [11, 23].

During mid ranges of motion, when the GH ligaments are lax, the rotator cuff and other shoulder muscles act as the primary stabilizers of the GH joint. Generally, these muscle forces can either be classified as compressive or translational forces [23, 25]. Compressive forces act to stabilize the GH joint by centering the humeral head within the concave glenoid cavity via the concavity-compression mechanism. Translational forces, which can be directed in either the anterior-posterior or superior-inferior plane, act to destabilize the GH joint unless they are balanced via force coupling [23–27]. The rotator cuff plays a key role in providing compressive forces, and resisting the translational forces of the deltoid and pectoralis major which destabilize the GH joint superiorly and anteriorly, respectively [23, 25, 28]. The rotator cuff external rotators (infraspinatus and teres minor) contribute to anterior joint stability, and the internal rotators (subscapularis) contribute to posterior stability [23]. Both the subscapularis and infraspinatus pull inferiorly on the humerus, countering the superior pull of the deltoid and establishing the coronal muscular balance of the shoulder. Thus, the overall stability of the GH joint has to be evaluated with regards to the balance of various muscles, which can act as agonists, or "force couples" or antagonists [25].

The osseous anatomy plays an important role in GH biomechanics as well. The glenoid track, first described by Itoi et al. [29], represents the change in contact area between the glenoid and humeral head as the glenohumeral joint is taken through range of motion [29, 30]. From the perspective of the posterior humeral head articular surface, its contact point with the glenoid changes from inferomedial to superolateral with progressive arm abduction [29, 30]. This creates the glenoid track that is 83% of the total glenoid width [29, 30]. In the absence of bone loss, the intact glenoid track ensures osseous stability of the glenohumeral joint [29, 30].

However, both unipolar and bipolar bone loss can cause instability of the GH joint. Glenoid bone loss causes the width of the glenoid track to decrease, thus creating instability [30]. In the setting of glenoid bone loss (i.e., Bankart lesion), one must calculate the "effective" glenoid track. This is done by first calculating the physiologic glenoid track (as discussed above, 83% of the width of an intact glenoid) and subtracting out the width of the glenoid defect [30]. In the setting of humeral bone loss (i.e., Hill-Sachs lesion), one must determine whether the lesion is "on track" or "off track," which has replaced the concept or "engaging" versus "non-engaging" lesions [30]. If a Hill-Sachs lesion lies within the "effective" glenoid track, then there is sufficient glenoid support to ensure stability of the GH joint [30]. Conversely, if the Hill-Sachs lesion lies outside of the glenoid track, then there is a lack of glenoid support leading to instability of the GH joint [30]. Determining the degree of bipolar bone loss is important when evaluating and treating shoulder instability.

References

1. Getz CL, Ricchetti ET, Verborgt O, Brolin TJ. Normal and pathoanatomy of the arthritic shoulder: considerations for shoulder arthroplasty. J Am Acad Orthop Surg. 2019;27:e1068–76.
2. Provencher MT, Midtgaard KS, Owens BD, Tokish JM. Diagnosis and management of traumatic anterior shoulder instability. J Am Acad Orthop Surg. 2021;29:e51–61.
3. Frank RM, Romeo AA, Provencher MT. Posterior glenohumeral instability. J Am Acad Orthop Surg. 2017;25:610–23.
4. Streubel PN, Krych AJ, Simone JP, Dahm DL, Sperling JW, Steinmann SP, O'Driscoll SW, Sanchez-Sotelo J. Anterior glenohumeral instability. J Am Acad Orthop Surg. 2014;22:283–94.
5. Kamer L, Noser H, Popp AW, Lenz M, Blauth M. Computational anatomy of the proximal humerus: an ex vivo high-resolution peripheral quantitative computed tomography study. J Orthop Transl. 2016;4:46–56.
6. Robertson DD, Yuan J, Bigliani LU, Flatow EL, Yamaguchi K. Three-dimensional analysis of the proximal part of the humerus: relevance to arthroplasty*. J Bone Joint Surg Am Vol. 2000;82:1594–602.

7. Clavert P. Glenoid labrum pathology. Orthop Traumatol Surg Res. 2015;101:S19–24.
8. Clavert P, Kempf J-F, Wolfram-Gabel R, Kahn J-L. Are there age induced morphologic variations of the superior glenoid labrum? About 100 shoulder arthroscopies. Surg Radiol Anat. 2005;27:385–8.
9. Williams MM, Snyder SJ, Buford D. The Buford complex—the "cord-like" middle glenohumeral ligament and absent anterosuperior labrum complex: a normal anatomic capsulolabral variant. Arthroscopy. 1994;10:241–7.
10. Terry GC, Hammon D, France P, Norwood LA. The stabilizing function of passive shoulder restraints. Am J Sports Med. 1991;19:26–34.
11. Felli L, Biglieni L, Fiore M, Coviello M, Borri R, Cutulo M. Functional study of glenohumeral ligaments. J Orthop Sci. 2012;17:634–7.
12. Dekker TJ, Aman ZS, Peebles LA, Storaci HW, Chahla J, Millett PJ, Provencher MT. Quantitative and qualitative analyses of the Glenohumeral ligaments: an anatomic study. Am J Sports Med. 2020;48:1837–45.
13. Petchprapa CN, Beltran LS, Jazrawi LM, Kwon YW, Babb JS, Recht MP. The rotator interval: a review of anatomy, function, and Normal and abnormal MRI appearance. Am J Roentgenol. 2010;195:567–76.
14. O'Brien SJ, Schwartz RS, Warren RF, Torzilli PA. Capsular restraints to anterior-posterior motion of the abducted shoulder: a biomechanical study. J Shoulder Elb Surg. 1995;4:298–308.
15. Yang H, Tang K, Chen W, Dong S, Jin T, Gong J, Li J, Wang H, Wang J, Xu J. An anatomic and histologic study of the coracohumeral ligament. J Shoulder Elb Surg. 2009;18:305–10.
16. Curtis AS, Burbank KM, Tierney JJ, Scheller AD, Curran AR. The insertional footprint of the rotator cuff: an anatomic study. Arthroscopy. 2006;22:603–609.e1.
17. Ricchetti ET, Entezari V, Derwin KA. Structure and function of the rotator cuff. In: Matsen F, Cordasco FA, Sperling J, Lippitt S, editors. Rockwood and Matsen's the shoulder. 6th ed. Philadelphia: Elsevier; 2021. p. 691–702.
18. DeFranco MJ, Cole BJ. Current perspectives on rotator cuff anatomy. Arthroscopy. 2009;25:305–20.
19. Morag Y, Jamadar DA, Miller B, Dong Q, Jacobson JA. The subscapularis: anatomy, injury, and imaging. Skeletal Radiol. 2011;40:255–69.
20. Hachadorian ME, Mitchell BC, Siow MY, Wang W, Bastrom T, Sullivan TB, Huang BK, Edmonds EW, Kent WT. Identifying the axillary nerve during shoulder surgery: an anatomic study using advanced imaging. JSES Int. 2020;4:987–91.
21. Chalmers PN, van Thiel GS, Trenhaile SW. Surgical exposures of the shoulder. J Am Acad Orthop Surg. 2016;24:250–8.
22. Burkhead WZ, Scheinberg RR, Box G. Surgical anatomy of the axillary nerve. J Shoulder Elb Surg. 1992;1:31–6.
23. Goetti P, Denard PJ, Collin P, Ibrahim M, Hoffmeyer P, Lädermann A. Shoulder biomechanics in normal and selected pathological conditions. EFORT Open Rev. 2020;5:508–18.
24. Vidt ME, Santago AC, Marsh AP, Hegedus EJ, Tuohy CJ, Poehling GG, Freehill MT, Miller ME, Saul KR. Modeling a rotator cuff tear: individualized shoulder muscle forces influence glenohumeral joint contact force predictions. Clin Biomech (Bristol, Avon). 2018;60:20–9.
25. Labriola JE, Lee TQ, Debski RE, McMahon PJ. Stability and instability of the glenohumeral joint: the role of shoulder muscles. J Shoulder Elb Surg. 2005;14:S32–8.
26. Lippitt SB, Vanderhooft JE, Harris SL, Sidles JA, Harryman DT, Matsen FA. Glenohumeral stability from concavity-compression: a quantitative analysis. J Shoulder Elb Surg. 1993;2:27–35.
27. Lippitt S, Matsen F. Mechanisms of glenohumeral joint stability. Clin Orthop Relat Res. 1993;291:20–8.
28. Porcellini G, Caranzano F, Campi F, Pellegrini A, Paladini P. Glenohumeral instability and rotator cuff tear. Sports Med Arthrosc Rev. 2011;19:395–400.
29. Yamamoto N, Itoi E, Abe H, Minagawa H, Seki N, Shimada Y, Okada K. Contact between the glenoid and the humeral head in abduction, external rotation, and horizontal extension: a new concept of glenoid track. J Shoulder Elb Surg. 2007;16:649–56.
30. di Giacomo G, Itoi E, Burkhart SS. Evolving concept of bipolar bone loss and the Hill-Sachs lesion: from "engaging/non-engaging" lesion to "on-track/off-track" lesion. Arthroscopy. 2014;30:90–8.

2 Shoulder Arthroscopy: Patient Positioning and Portal Placement

Mahdi AlSaffar, Yasser Al Shehab, and Moin Khan

Introduction

Advancements in shoulder arthroscopy have resulted in a shift from open surgical procedures toward minimally invasive techniques allowing for a comprehensive assessment of the joint, more anatomic repair of pathology, reduced post-operative pain, and potentially faster recovery. An understanding of proper patient positioning enhances visualization and avoids potential technical errors and complications. The most utilized positions for shoulder arthroscopy are the lateral decubitus and the beach chair positions. Each position has its own advantages and disadvantages when performing open/arthroscopic shoulder stabilization procedures. Most of the debate revolves around the overall ease of performing different shoulder procedures and is highly surgeon-dependent. The choice of position most often relates to a surgeon's training and familiarity. Although further research is required, one can expect similar outcomes between patients treated in either position. Despite some studies suggesting that the lateral decubitus position may be associated with a reduced risk of recurrence [1], high-quality comparative studies are required. Surgeons should proceed with the position that allows them to fully mobilize relevant tissue and perform a robust and appropriate repair. This will depend on the circumstances of the case, the training of the surgeon, and the equipment available.

A thorough understanding of shoulder anatomy is critical regardless of the choice of position to optimize portal placement. Arthroscopy allows for a unique assessment of joint pathology, utilizing multiple portals for visualization as required. This is not always achievable with open surgery. Surface anatomy of the acromion, clavicle, scapular spine, coracoid, and acromioclavicular joint is helpful when planning optimal portal placement. When placing portals, the distance between these bones and neurovascular structures must be considered. Defining the boundaries of these landmarks will support the safe and accurate placement of the portal.

This chapter will review relevant patient positioning and portal placement for shoulder instability procedures.

M. AlSaffar
Department of Orthopedics, New Jahra Hospital, Al Jahra, Kuwait

Y. Al Shehab
Department of Orthopedics, King Abdullah bin Abdulaziz University, Riyadh, Saudi Arabia

M. Khan (✉)
Division of Orthopaedic Surgery, Department of Surgery, McMaster University, Hamilton, ON, Canada
e-mail: Khanmm2@mcmaster.ca

© The Author(s), under exclusive license to Springer Nature Switzerland AG 2026
R. M. Frank, J. M. Tokish (eds.), *Management of Shoulder Instability*,
https://doi.org/10.1007/978-3-032-18089-6_2

Case

A 21-year-old male martial artist presents to your clinic following an anterior shoulder dislocation 3 weeks ago. The injury occurred during a professional sparing match and was reduced on site by a physician. This is his third dislocation. He reports regular feelings of instability particularly with throwing movements and abduction and external rotation. On examination he has full range of motion with a strongly positive apprehension and relocation rest. Screening radiographs do not demonstrate any bony involvement. MRI demonstrates anterior inferior labral tear extending from the 2 o'clock to the 6 o'clock position on the glenoid face. CT scan does not demonstrate any glenoid bony involvement, a small on track hill Sachs lesion is present. He is looking to proceed with surgical stabilization.

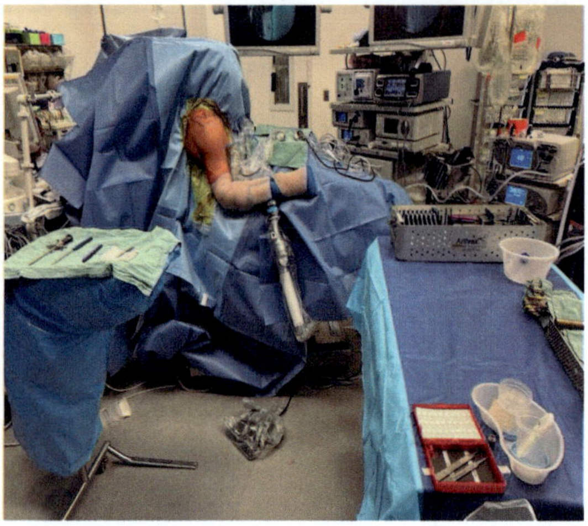

Fig. 2.1 Beach chair setup

Positioning

Beach Chair Position

Beach chair positioning has been in practice since the early 1980s. The first description was given by Skyhar et al. in 1988. In this description, the patient is sitting up at a minimum of 60°. For arthroscopic shoulder stabilization, the patient's affected side is moved off the edge of the table to the medial border of the scapula. A 10-1b (4.5-kg) sandbag is placed under the ipsilateral hip to facilitate rotation of the patient's upper torso at least 30° away from the edge of the table, allowing for improved access to the posterior aspect of the shoulder [2].

The use of the beach chair position was encouraged to resolve concerns for potential nerve injuries that were associated with the lateral decubitus position [3]. Beach chair positioning requires specific bed and arm attachments (Fig. 2.1). The patient is initially positioned supine on the operating table and then raised upright with hip flexion from 45 to 90° depending on the procedure and the surgeon's preference. Thighs and legs are strapped and well-padded to stabilize the patient from shifting sideways and to avoid pressure sores. This orientation allows for visualization of the glenohumeral joint through the arthroscope in "anatomic" positioning, one of the primary advantages of this position. Additionally, patients can be quite comfortable seated in the beach chair position while awake if required or desired by the medical team. Compared to lateral decubitus, there is also a decreased risk of neurovascular injuries from traction, which has a reported incidence of up to 10–30% in the lateral decubitus position [2, 17]. The beach chair is also considered the position of choice for open shoulder stabilization. Surgeons have improved access to the anterior working portal and more control over arm position and rotation.

Disadvantages of this position include the potential for cerebral hypoperfusion and difficulty in visualizing and instrumenting the inferior and posterior aspect of the glenoid and the requirement for specialized beach chair attachments.

Author's Preferred Technique (Sequence of Beach Chair Positioning)

Attach and secure the beach chair attachment centrally on the bed, exposing the side to be operated on
Transfer patient supine onto the bed
While the patient is awake, adjust the patient proximal and distal by asking the patient to move such that the greater trochanter is in line with the hinge of the beach chair. This will facilitate appropriate placement of the patient when raising them to the seated position. Lining up the greater trochanter with the hinge facilitates hip flexion and avoids lumbar spine flexion during elevation
Apply a triangle shaped bolster under the knees, ensuring that it is underneath the bedsheets and over the gel pads to prevent it from sliding on the sheets when the patient is elevated
Secure thighs with straps or blankets—this is particularly useful with large or obese patients where the legs may externally rotate outward as they are raised up
Position the side bolster and tuck in both upper limbs during anesthesia induction
Ensure placement of endotracheal tube away from the operative side, and stabilize the head piece
It is essential at this point (preferably with the patient supine) to re-examine shoulder range of motion and the extent of glenohumeral translation, especially in the anteroposterior direction. Depending on the examination under anesthesia, additional procedures may be added (e.g., posterior/anterior capsular plication)
Elevate the bed to 90°, and readjust the head and neck positions if needed
Position a mayo stand in front of the patient for later use during the procedure
Secure arm holding device to the middle rail of the operating table. This allows for appropriate movement of the operative shoulder
Ensure optimal monitor and tower positions prior to prepping and draping (Fig. 2.2)

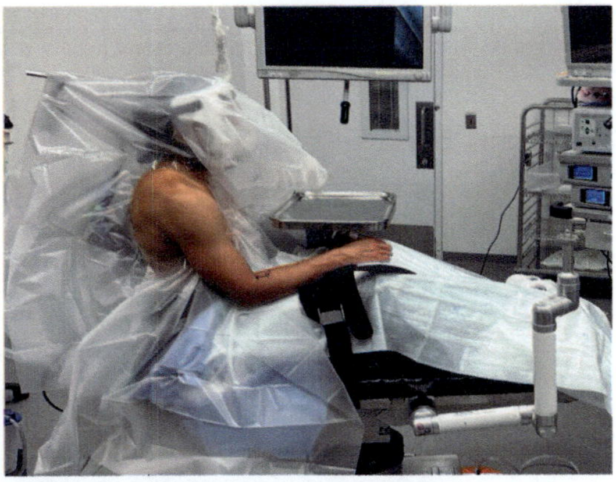

Fig. 2.2 Patient position prior to draping

Lateral Decubitus Position

The first shoulder arthroscopies were completed in the lateral decubitus position. This position takes advantage of lateral and upward traction. Surgeons favoring the lateral decubitus position argue that it provides easier access to the glenohumeral joint, improved intraarticular exposure, and better visualization. Some research suggests a decreased risk of recurrent instability with the lateral decubitus position related to the potentially improved ability to optimize the anchor position. Baron et al. performed a systematic review and reported that surgeons utilizing the lateral decubitus position were more consistent in placing the lower 6 o'clock anchor and were able to place more anchors overall [4]. The patient is generally positioned laterally on the operating table tilted at a 30–45° angle to make the glenoid surface parallel to the floor. Padding between the legs, axilla, knees, and ankles is used to avoid pressure sores. A special pneumatic bean bag (or posts) is applied to maintain the position throughout the procedure. After prepping and draping, the arm is usually suspended with traction in a 45° abduction/30° flexion position.

Author's preferred technique (sequence of lateral decubitus positioning) is as follows:

After induction of general anesthesia, position the patient at a lateral angle of 30–45° to make the glenoid surface parallel to the floor
Ensure enough padding between the thighs and between the bed and axilla, knees, and ankles
Secure the position by either using a pneumatic bean bag or two side posts (one for symphysis pubis, the other for lower lumbar spine). Additional straps are needed on the trunk and hips
Fix the lateral traction tower or arm holding device on the opposite rail of the operative side (care is needed to ensure the optimal position as it is difficult) (Fig. 2.3)

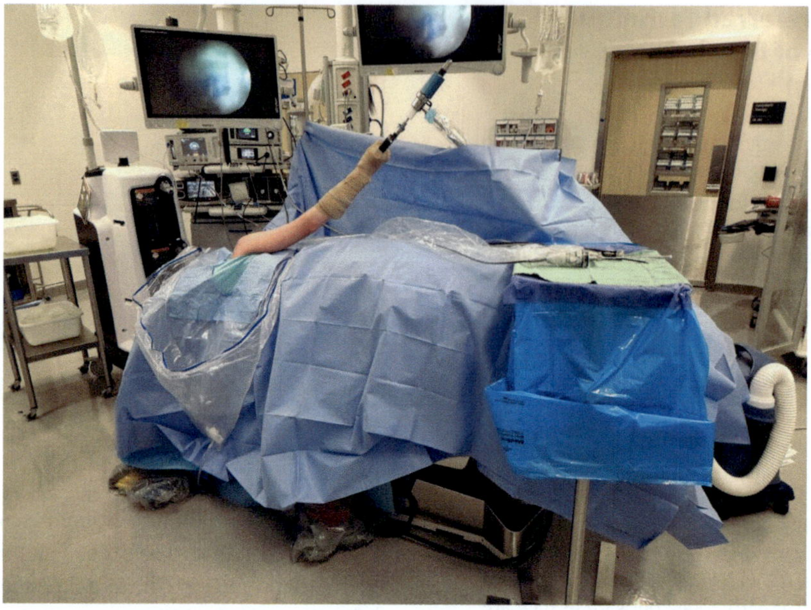

Fig. 2.3 Lateral decubitus position

	Beach chair	Lateral decubitus
Advantages	Anatomic orientation Ability to convert to open procedures Easier access to anterior working portal Suitable for "awake" surgery Allows for increased arm manipulation during procedure	Increased intraarticular visualization Lower risk of cerebral hypoperfusion Easier for placing inferior glenoid anchors
Disadvantages	Risk of cerebral hypoperfusion Requires special bed and arm devices Difficulty in placing inferior glenoid anchors during instability surgery	Increased risk of traction nerve injuries Difficulty working through anterior portal Cannot convert to open

Portal Placement

Relevant Anatomy

Prior to the placement of portals, the surgeon must have a comprehensive understanding of relevant anatomy and structures at risk. The most vulnerable structures during shoulder arthroscopy are the axillary nerve, the cephalic vein, and the suprascapular artery and nerve [5]. Familiarization with the location and movement of these structures is fundamental to preventing a portal placement injury (Fig. 2.4).

The course of the axillary nerve is posterior to the coracoid and inferior to the lateral border of the subscapularis medial to the musculotendinous junction. When the arm is abducted, this nerve may be as close as 3.1 cm from the leading edge of the acromion [6]. At this juncture, the axillary nerve will generally double branch to supply the inferior capsule. It is possible that distending the capsule may decrease the risk of injury to the anteroinferior joint during arthroscopic surgery [7]. As the capsule distends, the distance between the nerve and joint increases. This can be achieved through abduction, external rotation, and traction. Post-capsule, the axillary nerve travels posteriorly within the quadrilateral space and divides into a posterior and anterior trunk. The posterior trunk is comprised of three

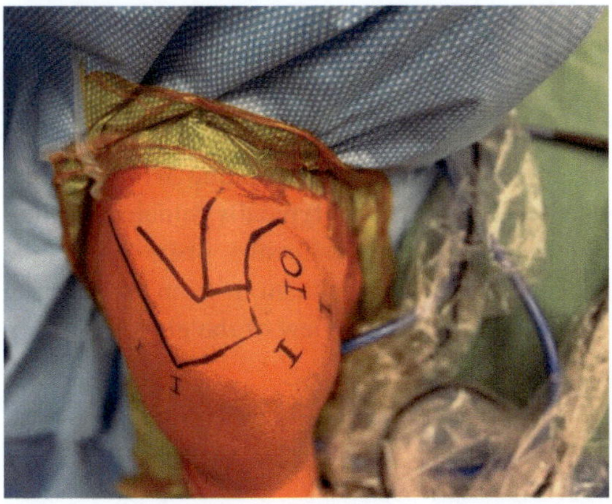

Fig. 2.4 Common portals when managing shoulder instability. Posterior, posterior lateral, high interval, and anterior and anterior inferior portal

components: the superolateral cutaneous branch; the deltoid posterior branch; and the nerve to the teres minor [8]. The anterior branch of the axillary nerve is, on average, 5–7 cm distal to the lateral tip of the acromion. This branch courses around the humerus and innervates the triple heads of the deltoid muscle [6].

The suprascapular nerve is located at the upper trunk of the brachial plexus and courses through the posterior neck triangle. The suprascapular artery travels alongside this nerve until the suprascapular notch. Upon entering the suprascapular notch, the nerve is situated 3 cm medial to the supraglenoid tubercle [9]. The nerve then moves within he notch below the transverse scapular, whereas the artery courses on a different trajectory and travels above the transverse scapular outside the notch. The nerve transfers its motor branch to the supraspinatus within 1 cm of exiting the notch before taking a nonlinear lateral path to the base of the scapular spine. Here, the nerve is approximately 1.8 cm from the midline of the posterior glenoid. It then bends medially to supply the infraspinatus [9].

The cephalic vein in the upper arm traverses through the superficial fascia of the deltopectoral grove interval and extends southward through the coracoclavicular fascia to the axillary vein under the clavicle. The vein is most susceptible to a portal placement injury at the deltopectoral interval. If injured at this juncture, a superficial hematoma will customarily result. In up to 25% of patients, the cephalic vein may be located less than 1 cm from the anterior portal [5].

Common Portals Utilized in Shoulder Instability

Posterior Portal

The glenohumeral joint and subacromial space are standardly viewed through the posterior portal. A typical placement of this portal is 2–3 cm inferior and 1 cm medially from the posterolateral corner of the acromion in the "soft spot" of the posterior shoulder [7]. This area can be found directly over the glenohumeral joint in the interval between the infraspinatus superiorly and the teres minor inferiorly.

For patients with shoulder instability, an alternative posterior portal placement of 3 cm distal to the posterior lateral corner of the acromion and 2 cm lateral to the joint line may be preferred [10]. The benefit of this positioning is that it provides improved access to the posterior labrum and axillary pouch when compared to the standard portal placement [10].

Abduction distraction maneuvers may be helpful in circumstances where glenohumeral space entry proves difficult [11].

Portal placement presents an increased risk to the axillary and suprascapular nerves due to the proximity of these structures to the "soft spot." On average, the axillary nerve is situated 49 mm from the posterior soft spot portal, but it can be as proximate as 30 mm. The suprascapular nerve is as close as 29 mm from the posterior soft spot portal [5].

Anterior Central (Mid-Glenoid) Portal

Once the posterior portal is established, an anterior central portal can be constructed using an "outside-in" or "inside-out" technique. The anterior central portal is standardly located lateral to the tip of the coracoid process (also known as the shoulder's "lighthouse") and inferior to the anterolateral corner of the acromion. Anterior central portal creation occurs through the rotator interval. This interval is bordered medially by the glenoid, superiorly by the anterior border of the supraspinatus, inferiorly by the superior border of the subscapularis, and laterally by the humeral head.

In the "outside-in" approach, a spinal needle is inserted 1–2 cm inferomedial to the anterolateral acromion under direct visualization. To prevent injury to the brachial plexus and axillary vessels during this step, the needle must be maintained lateral to the coracoid [12]. The needle is properly situated when it is slightly above the upper border of the subscapularis and reaches the 6 o'clock position on the glenoid. When performing stabilization procedures, it is necessary to ensure that the trajectory of the portal allows for the placement of inferior anchors.

When developing this portal using an inside-out technique, the scope can be advanced through to the rotator interval. The scope is then removed, and a switching stick is placed in the sheath and advanced through the soft tissues under the skin. A small incision is made over the switching stick, and a cannula can be placed and advanced into the shoulder joint. Both the inside-out or outside-in technique are effective in the development of this portal; however, for the purposes of instability surgery, confirming the trajectory of the portal on the glenoid face with a spinal needle provides an advantage for the outside in technique over the inside out.

It is important to note that the cephalic vein and musculocutaneous nerve are most at risk due to their proximity to the portal. Incising the skin superficially and utilizing a cannula can prevent iatrogenic injury to the cephalic vein. On average, the musculocutaneous nerve is situated 33+/−6.2 mm inferior to the tip of the coracoid [13]. To prevent injury to these structures, care must be taken to avoid an overly inferior portal placement.

High Interval/Anterior Superior Lateral (ASL) Portal

A high-interval portal can be constructed by utilizing an "outside-in" technique with a spinal needle. This portal is typically situated slightly anterior to the supraspinatus fibers above the biceps tendon. Visualization from this portal allows for an on-face view of the glenoid.

Five O'clock Portal

An anteroinferior portal can be constructed 1.5–2 cm distal to the coracoid tip [14]. The primary benefit of this portal is that it permits access to the anterior and anteroinferior glenoid and labrum.

Anteroinferior portals are generally developed at maximum arm abduction using the "inside out technique" where the camera is directed from the posterior portal to the 5 o'clock position of the glenoid. The arthroscope is then removed to permit a switching stick to be inserted through the cannula and pushed through the capsule. The portal exits laterally through the conjoined tendon through the lower aspect of the subscapularis.

Seven O'clock Portal

The 7 o'clock portal is typically utilized for posteroinferior labral fixation and allows for access to the inferior recess of the shoulder [15]. The portal can be constructed by utilizing an "inside-out" or "outside-in" technique. When employing the "inside-out" technique, a switching stick is placed through the anterior portal to the 7 o'clock position on the glenoid. The stick can then be pushed through the capsule and a skin incision is made. When utilizing the "outside-in" technique, an incision is created 2 to 3 cm inferior to the posterior portal.

The structures most at risk with the 7 o'clock portal are the suprascapular nerve and artery, axillary nerve, and posterior circumflex humeral artery. On average, this portal is located 29+/−3 mm from the suprascapular and axillary nerves and 39+/−4 mm from the circumflex artery [15].

Axillary Pouch Portal

For anchor placement on the posteroinferior glenoid rim, the axillary pouch portal is a safer alternative to posteroinferior placement. An axillary pouch portal is also used in cases of humeral aversions of glenohumeral ligament lesions to allow for the placement of a humeral anchor [16].

To create this portal, an "outside-in" technique beginning 2–3 cm inferior to the posterolateral acromion and 2 cm lateral to the posterior viewing portal is utilized. The spinal needle must be angulated medially and inferiorly into the joint. This method may decrease axillary nerve risk when compared to the 7 o'clock portal as it creates distance between the nerve and the portal [16].

Wilmington Portal

This portal is ideal when access to the posterolateral region (10–11 o'clock) of the glenoid is required. The portal is situated approximately 1 cm lateral and 1 cm anterior to the posterolateral edge of the acromion.

Naviaser Portal

The Naviaser portal is advantageous for suture fixation and anchor placement during SLAP repair [18]. This portal is constructed superiorly in the soft spot between the clavicle, acromion, and scapular spine. From this location, a needle is inserted laterally and anteriorly through the capsule. It is permissible to place the needle under the biceps anchor when conducting a SLAP repair.

The structures primarily at risk when utilizing this portal are the scapular nerve and artery due to their 3 cm proximity to the supraglenoid tubercle [9].

Halifax Portal

The far medial portal (Halifax) has been described for use in anatomic glenoid reconstruction and arthroscopic Latarjet procedures to overcome the technical difficulties associated with passing bone grafts to reconstruct the anterior glenoid. Using an "inside-out" technique and while viewing from the anterosuperior portal, a switching stick is passed from the posterior portal directed anteriorly, parallel to the glenoid articular surface, and exiting through the rotator interval just superior to the upper border of the subscapularis tendon and lateral to the conjoint tendon. Introducing a distal tibia allograft using this portal should make lining the articular surfaces easier while avoiding step-off defects. Wong et al. found that the Halifax portal, when established correctly, lies approximately 48 mm from subclavian vessels, 46 mm from the axillary nerve, and 50 mm from the musculocutaneous nerve [19].

References

1. Frank RM, Saccomanno MF, McDonald LS, Moric M, Romeo AA, Provencher MT. Outcomes of arthroscopic anterior shoulder instability in the beach chair versus lateral decubitus position: a systematic review and meta-regression analysis. Arthroscopy. 2014;30(10):1349–65.
2. Skyhar MJ, Altchek DW, Warren RF, Wickiewicz TL, O'Brien SJ. Shoulder arthroscopy with the patient in the beach-chair position. Arthroscopy. 1988;4(4):256–9.
3. Li X, Eichinger JK, Hartshorn T, Zhou H, Matzkin EG, Warner JP. A comparison of the lateral decubitus and beach-chair positions for shoulder surgery: advantages and complications. JAAOS-J Am Acad Orthop Surg. 2015;23(1):18–28.
4. Baron JE, Duchman KR, Hettrich CM, Glass NA, Ortiz SF, MOON Shoulder Group, Baumgarten KM, Bishop JY, Bollier MJ, Bravman JT, Brophy RH. Beach chair versus lateral decubitus position: differences in suture anchor position and number during arthroscopic anterior shoulder stabilization. Am J Sports Med. 2021, 49(8):2020–6.

5. Meyer M, Graveleau N, Hardy P, Landreau P. Anatomic risks of shoulder arthroscopy portals: anatomic cadaveric study of 12 portals. Arthroscopy. 2007;23(5):529–36.
6. Burkhead WZ Jr, Scheinberg RR, Box G. Surgical anatomy of the axillary nerve. J Shoulder Elb Surg. 1992;1(1):31–6.
7. Andrews JR, Carson WG Jr, Ortega K. Arthroscopy of the shoulder: technique and normal anatomy. Am J Sports Med. 1984;12(1):1–7.
8. Ball CM, Steger T, Galatz LM, Yamaguchi K. The posterior branch of the axillary nerve: an anatomic study. JBJS. 2003;85(8):1497–501.
9. Bigliani LU, Dalsey RM, McCann PD, April EW. An anatomical study of the suprascapular nerve. Arthroscopy. 1990;6(4):301–5.
10. Wolf EM, Eakin CL. Arthroscopic capsular plication for posterior shoulder instability. Arthroscopy. 1998;14(2):153–63.
11. O'Brien SJ, Gonzalez DM, Wright JM, Fealy S. The adduction distraction maneuver. Arthroscopy. 1997;13(4):530–2.
12. Matthews LS, Zarins B, Michael RH, Helfet DL. Anterior portal selection for shoulder arthroscopy. Arthroscopy. 1985;1(1):33–9.
13. Lo IK, Burkhart SS, Parten PM. Surgery about the coracoid: neurovascular structures at risk. Arthroscopy. 2004;20(6):591–5.
14. Resch H, Wykypiel HF, Maurer H, Wambacher M. The antero-inferior (transmuscular) approach for arthroscopic repair of the Bankart lesion: an anatomic and clinical study. Arthroscopy. 1996;12(3):309–19.
15. Davidson PA, Rivenburgh DW. The 7-o'clock postero-inferior portal for shoulder arthroscopy. Am J Sports Med. 2002;30(5):693–6.
16. Bhatia DN, de Beer JF. The axillary pouch portal: a new posterior portal for visualization and instrumentation in the inferior glenohumeral recess. Arthroscopy. 2007;23(11):1241-e1.
17. Peruto CM, Ciccotti MG, Cohen SB. Shoulder arthroscopy positioning: lateral decubitus versus beach chair. Arthroscopy. 2009;25(8):891–6.
18. Neviaser TJ. Arthroscopy of the shoulder. Orthop Clin North Am. 1987;18(3):361–72.
19. Moga I, Konstantinidis G, Wong IH. The safety of a far medial arthroscopic portal for anatomic glenoid reconstruction: a cadaveric study. Orthop J Sports Med. 2018;6(9):2325967118795404.

3 Physical Examination and Classification of Shoulder Instability: A Case-Based Guide

Wendell Cole, John Weldy, Eddie Gontee, and Mary K. Mulcahey

Introduction

The shoulder joint allows for the largest range of motion of any joint in the human body. The stability of the shoulder is complex requiring highly synchronized interactions between static and dynamic forces, which ultimately allow function throughout three main degrees of freedom: flexion/extension, abduction/adduction, and internal/external rotation. Primary static stabilization involves the bony anatomy of the shoulder, glenohumeral ligaments, the glenoid labrum, and joint capsule [1]. The primary dynamic stabilizers include the rotator cuff musculature, the deltoid, biceps, latissimus, and pectoralis major. Combined with the negative intra articular pressure created by the interface between the glenoid labrum and the humeral head, these structures create a joint compressive force directing the humeral head into the glenoid surface [1]. Disruption of this relationship leads to recurrent shoulder instability. Understanding the interplay between the dynamic and static shoulder stabilizers provides a framework for the diagnosis, management, and treatment for acute and recurrent shoulder instability.

W. Cole
Department of Orthopaedic Surgery, New York University, New York, NY, USA
e-mail: wcole@tulane.edu

J. Weldy
Department of Orthopaedic Surgery, Tulane University School of Medicine, New Orleans, LA, USA
e-mail: jweldy@tulane.edu

E. Gontee
Morehouse School of Medicine, Atlanta, Georgia
e-mail: egontee@msm.edu

M. K. Mulcahey (✉)
Department of Orthopaedic Surgery and Rehabilitation, Loyola University Medical Center, Maywood, IL, USA

Anterior Shoulder Instability

Case #1: A 17-year-old right-hand-dominant male high school football player presents to the emergency department after sustaining an injury to the right shoulder during a game. He reports reaching out to make a tackle as he was knocked to the ground by an opposing player. He has no previous history of shoulder instability. The patient has an obvious sulcus sign, limited shoulder range of motion, and he is neurovascularly intact. X-rays demonstrate an anterior shoulder dislocation. The patient undergoes conscious sedation, and the shoulder is successfully reduced. He is placed into a sling and told to follow-up with an orthopedic surgeon within 1 week.

Case #2: A 32-year-old left-hand-dominant male presents to clinic complaining of recurrent right shoulder instability. He was involved in a motor vehicle collision 2 years ago, and he

© The Author(s), under exclusive license to Springer Nature Switzerland AG 2026
R. M. Frank, J. M. Tokish (eds.), *Management of Shoulder Instability*,
https://doi.org/10.1007/978-3-032-18089-6_3

was admitted for multiple traumatic injuries including a right shoulder dislocation. The patient reports that his shoulder was reduced in the emergency room, and he was placed into a sling. His shoulder pain improved immediately. He returned to work within a couple weeks of being discharged. The patient notes intermittent symptoms of right shoulder subluxation, which occurs during a variety of activities. He denies any subsequent right shoulder dislocations. On physical exam he is neurovascularly intact, and he has full shoulder range of motion. The patient has a positive apprehension sign and positive load and shift.

Background

Anterior shoulder instability is the most common form of shoulder instability and may present after a traumatic shoulder dislocation, or it may be more subtle such as in cases with an unrecognized injury or a patient with a genetic predisposition [2]. In general, traumatic anterior shoulder dislocation results from a direct collision or a fall on an outstretched hand with the arm abducted and externally rotated [2, 3]. The incidence of traumatic anterior shoulder dislocation ranges from 11.2 to 23.9 in 100,000 injuries, with a predominance among males in their second and third decades participating in contact sports [4–6]. Shoulder instability may be classified into two main categories: traumatic, unidirectional instability, and Bankart lesion (TUBS), which often requires surgery and atraumatic, multidirectional, bilateral instability (AMBRI), that often responds to rehabilitation. In cases of failed rehabilitation/nonoperative measures, these patients may require surgery including a possible inferior capsular shift.

Nonsurgical management has been shown in recent studies to result in increased risk of recurrence and a notable increased risk of glenoid bone loss [7]. The effectiveness of rehabilitation for patients who have sustained a primary traumatic shoulder dislocation is currently debated.

History

When evaluating a patient with a primary anterior shoulder dislocation or chronic shoulder instability, it is important to perform a thorough history and physical examination. This should include a detailed assessment keeping in mind additional risk factors, which may contribute to recurrence. It is necessary to inquire about present and past activity level as well as prior history of trauma including complete dislocation requiring manual reduction. Patients may describe the classic "clunk" or other mechanical symptoms such as popping or clicking, and some may report the ability to relocate the shoulder independently. Others who may have more subtle shoulder instability may present with vague reports of pain or weakness when the arm is placed in certain positions, particularly in an abducted/externally rotated position. A thorough history should also include questions about patient age, sex, dominant hand, activity level, associated injuries, and genetic factors. Several risk factors for recurrent shoulder instability have been defined including male sex, age <20, and younger age at time of primary traumatic anterior shoulder dislocation, participating in contact sports or sports that involve overhead activity [8].

During the initial evaluation, it is also important to consider atraumatic causes of recurrent instability, which may be secondary to generalized ligamentous laxity derived from soft tissue disorders such as Marfan syndrome and Ehlers-Danlos syndrome. Patients with generalized ligamentous laxity are at an increased risk for recurrent instability as well as primary dislocation events [9, 10]. Muhammad et al. evaluated 38 patients with primary shoulder dislocation and found that patients with hypermobility (Beighton score >6) had a 60% chance of experiencing an additional instability event compared to 39% of patients without preexisting hypermobility [10].

Associated Lesions

Damage to the glenoid labrum, glenoid bone loss, and humeral head injuries (e.g., Hill-Sachs lesion) at the time of dislocation are also known risk factors for anterior shoulder instability. As the humeral head slides anteriorly during the dislocation event, the anterior glenoid labrum is sheared or the anterior rim of the glenoid rim is fractured, resulting in a loss of concavity of the glenoid surface, thereby affecting the stability of the glenohumeral relationship (Fig. 3.1) [7]. When the anterior glenoid labrum is sheared from its bony attachment, it is referred to as a Bankart lesion. This is the most common lesion found when evaluating for anterior shoulder instability and as such is referred to as the "essential lesion." A Perthes lesion, which is a variant of the Bankart lesion, results when the anteroinferior glenoid labrum is completely avulsed from the glenoid rim and the medial scapular neck periosteum is preserved (Table 3.1). Healing of the labrum in a displaced, nonanatomic position (i.e., medially on the scapular neck), is referred to as an anterior labroligamentous periosteal sleeve avulsion (ALPSA) lesion and contributes to increased rates of recurrence, along with bony Bankart lesions [11]. According to a study conducted by Baker et al., when evaluated arthroscopically, 28 of 45 patients with gross anterior shoulder instability were found to have sustained a bony Bankart lesion [12]. Although it is well known that glenoid bone loss contributes to shoulder instability, there has been much debate regarding treatment strategies when considering the size of the bony defect.

Injury to the glenohumeral ligaments has also been shown to play a significant role in recurrent

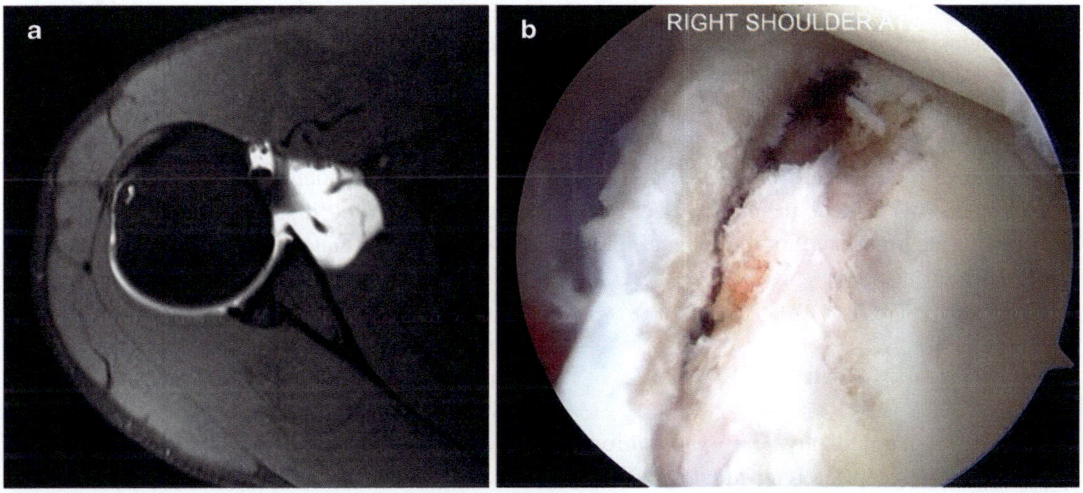

Fig. 3.1 Magnetic resonance arthrogram (MRA) showing a labral tear (**a**) along with an arthroscopic view of the right shoulder in the lateral decubitus position showing an anterior labral tear (**b**)

Table 3.1 Common intra-articular lesions associated with anterior shoulder instability [14]

Lesion	Description
Perthes	Bankart variant involving a complete avulsion of the anterior-inferior glenoid labrum complex with retention of the periosteal hinge
Bankart	Avulsion of the anterior-inferior glenoid labrum without retention of a periosteal hinge
Bony Bankart	Avulsion of the anterior-inferior glenoid labrum with an associated bony avulsion
ALPSA	Avulsion of the anterior-inferior glenoid labrum complex with preservation of the periosteal hinge. The loose fragment heals in an aberrant position at the medial glenoid neck
HAGL	Avulsion of the glenohumeral ligaments from the humeral insertion

anterior shoulder stability and development of glenohumeral arthritis if left untreated. Injury to these ligamentous structures commonly occur at the glenoid; however, they may also occur at the humeral insertion. When the damage occurs at the humeral insertion, it is termed a humeral avulsion of the glenohumeral ligament (HAGL) lesion and has an incidence of approximately 1–9%. When this is accompanied by a bony avulsion, it is referred to as a B-HAGL, pronounced "bagel" lesion [13].

Additionally, impaction fractures to the humeral head, also known as a Hill-Sachs lesion, plays a critical role in determining appropriate treatment and risk for recurrent instability. Hill-Sachs lesions result from impaction of the posterior aspect of the humeral head with the anterior surface of the glenoid during an acute dislocation event. The size of the bony defect is important. If this lesion extends medially and is large enough to engage with the glenoid (i.e., "on-track lesion), there is an increased risk of dislocation. A smaller humeral head defect that does not engage is referred to as an "off-track" lesion. According to Kaar et al., if the Hill-Sachs lesion is >5/8 of the humeral head radius, there is a statistically significant rate of recurrence if not addressed surgically due to the high likelihood of engaging with the glenoid surface [14].

Physical Examination

Performing a detailed physical examination is important to appropriately evaluate and diagnose anterior shoulder instability. The examination must be goal-directed and conducted in a precise and sequential manner beginning with a thorough inspection of the patient's topographical anatomy. This must be done with the shirt removed to evaluate for scars indicating previous history of trauma or surgical procedures. Atrophy of the shoulder girdle musculature, symmetry, and scapular positioning must also be evaluated, including the patient's resting posture. Once inspection is complete, the physician should perform an evaluation of the patient's arc of motion in all planes, including forward flexion, abduction, internal rotation, and external rotation. This should be done actively and passively to assess for generalized shoulder weakness, physical blocks to motion, and imbalance in the soft tissues surrounding the glenohumeral joint. It is important to note the degree of soft tissue mobility, as this may indicate underlying genetic factors, which could contribute to shoulder instability.

Bony landmarks must be palpated including the clavicle, coracoid, acromion, and acromioclavicular joint, as well as the insertion of the supraspinatus and infraspinatus tendons. A thorough neurological evaluation must then be performed comparing symmetry of muscular engagement, being mindful to evaluate each component of the rotator cuff as massive subscapularis tears that may manifest as clinical anterior shoulder instability [15].

Following the general physical exam, several specific provocative maneuvers should be performed. In the setting of anterior shoulder instability, the most accurate test is the apprehension-relocation test, which is performed by placing the patient in the supine position and the affected shoulder in 90° of abduction [16]. With the elbow at 90° of flexion, the shoulder is then externally rotated. This position places maximal tension on the inferior glenohumeral ligament (IGHL). If the IGHL is incompetent, the patient will feel a sense of apprehension, as if the shoulder is subluxed in the anterior direction. The physician may then place his/her hand on the anterior shoulder and apply gentle posterior pressure to relieve the patient's apprehension (i.e., relocation test) [16]. Without notice, the physician may release the hand to surprise the patient, as they experience a recurrence of their sense of anterior instability.

Additionally, anterior labral pathology may be assessed with the use of the load and shift maneuver. This is performed by placing both hands on the patient's upper arm directing pressure into the glenoid (Table 3.2). The shoulder is then "shifted" in the anterior and posterior position. Pain or sensation of instability with an anteriorly directed force indicates likely a tear of the anterior labrum.

Table 3.2 Grading system for anterior and posterior shoulder laxity. Increasing grade signifies worsening shoulder pathology

0	A humeral head that does not translate to the glenoid rim
1+	A humeral head that translates to but does not translate over the glenoid rim
2+	A humeral head that translates over the glenoid rim but spontaneously reduces
3+	A humeral head that translates over the glenoid rim and does not spontaneously reduce

Posterior Shoulder Instability

Case #3

A 28-year-old right-hand-dominant male with no past medical history is brought to the emergency department by his coworker because of right shoulder pain after he was observed having a seizure at work. He describes the pain as aching and worsens when he attempts to move the arm forward but denies any weakness in the arm. On physical examination, there is limited external rotation and forward flexion of the shoulder. There is a palpable mass on the posterior aspect of the shoulder and flattening of the anterior aspect of the shoulder. The patient mentions that this is the first time he has had a seizure.

Case #4

A 17-year-old left-hand-dominant male offensive lineman presents with a history of recurrent shoulder subluxation and weakness. On physical examination, he has a positive Jerk and Kim test. Posterior stress test produces pain and translation of the humeral head over the glenoid rim. The patient is concerned because the pain is negatively affecting his performance on the football field.

Background

Posterior shoulder instability is a relatively rare and challenging diagnosis to make, with a misdiagnosis rate of up to 79%. Delayed diagnosis may lead to unsatisfactory outcomes such as chronic pain, stiffness, osteoarthritis, functional disability, and chronic instability [17]. Several mechanisms may result in posterior shoulder dislocation including seizures, electric shock, and electroconvulsive therapy, all of which result in forced muscle contractions displacing the humeral head. The causes of recurrent posterior shoulder instability include acute traumatic injury, recurrent microtrauma, and ligamentous laxity [18]. Posterior shoulder instability ranges from recurrent posterior subluxation to a locked posterior shoulder dislocation [18]. Posterior shoulder instability is less common than anterior shoulder instability but is becoming increasingly recognized in athletes. Posterior instability often results from repetitive microtrauma occurring in a variety of loading conditions and arm positions (push-ups, bench press, etc.) [18].

Athletes that participate in volleyball, football, tennis, swimming, and weightlifting are among those at highest risk. A study of 336 college football players reported that 14% of offensive lineman, 8.1% of defensive lineman, and 4.5% of defensive backs experienced posterior shoulder instability [19]. Patients with posterior shoulder instability often complain of aching pain and weakness along the posterior joint line. Symptoms intensify with the arm in forward flexion, adduction, and internal rotation. Performing a good physical examination is necessary to distinguish joint laxity from a true posterior shoulder instability, which is defined as symptomatic translation of the shoulder joint. In the case of instability, patients have both a subjective feeling of discomfort and a feeling of joint laxity or shifting.

Associated Lesions

Posterior shoulder instability may be associated with bony or soft tissue injuries around the affected shoulder. Impaction of the anterior medial articular surface of the humeral head (i.e., reverse Hill-Sachs lesion) may occur in 86% of acute traumatic posterior shoulder dislocations. It is generally accepted that the reverse Hill-Sachs lesion is the most important factor responsible for

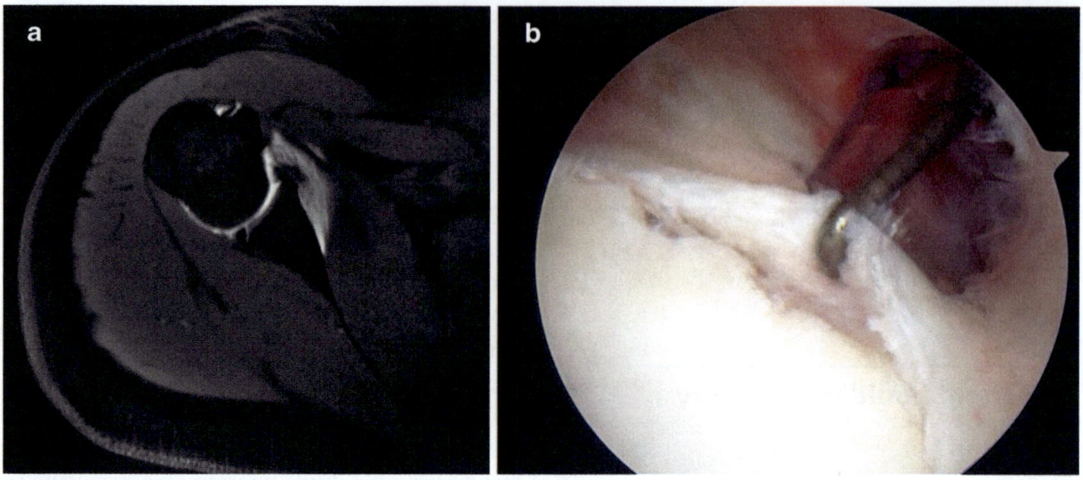

Fig. 3.2 Magnetic resonance imaging (MRI) (**a**) and arthroscopic view (**b**) of the left shoulder after an acute traumatic posterior subluxation event showing a large posterior labral tear

recurring instability [17]. Detachment of the posterior-inferior labrum and posterior capsular periosteum during posterior shoulder dislocation can also occur, which is termed a reverse Bankart lesion (Fig. 3.2). Recurrent instability is often associated with laxity or tearing of the posterior band of the inferior glenohumeral ligament.

History

It is important to obtain a detailed history when examining patients following a posterior shoulder dislocation. A history of epileptic seizures, recent electric shock, or trauma that resulted in the shoulder being held in an internally rotated position should be elicited [17]. The classic signs of posterior shoulder dislocation include a palpable mass on the posterior shoulder, coracoid prominence, and flattening of the anterior aspect of the shoulder. There may also be decreased or a complete lack of external rotation of the shoulder [17]. Patients do not always demonstrate the classic symptoms of posterior shoulder dislocation, and some patients may not be able to determine the direction of instability or weakness.

Patients with posterior shoulder instability typically complain of aching pain and weakness along the posterior joint line, biceps tendon, and/or superior aspect of the rotator cuff. These symptoms intensify when the arm is in 90° of forward flexion, adducted, and internally rotated [20]. The symptoms of recurrent posterior shoulder instability can also be nonspecific, which can make it difficult to diagnose. Symptoms may include pain with activity, patient reported weakness, crepitus, and episodes of intermittent subluxation. Loss of motion may be a complaint if a patient has a capsular contracture. Bradley et al. demonstrated that 90% of patients with recurrent posterior shoulder instability had clicking and crepitus with range of motion [18].

Physical Examination

The physical examination is an important component of the patient evaluation and begins with visual inspection of the skin. This should be done with the shirt off to see any obvious deformities, open wounds, asymmetry, or muscle atrophy. Patients with a posterior shoulder dislocation may have prominence of the coracoid process or axillary fullness by palpation. The patient is then assessed for tenderness to palpation over the posterior glenohumeral joint line, greater tuberosity, and biceps tendon. In patients with recurrent posterior shoulder instability, posterior joint line tenderness may be due to posterior rotator cuff tendinosis due to multiple episodes of instability.

Forward elevation, abduction in the scapular plane, external rotation with the arms at the side, and internal rotation with the hand behind the back to the highest vertebral level should be evaluated in both shoulders and recorded.

Shoulder range of motion should be measured in the sitting and supine position. While the patient is supine, the arm is abducted 90°, the scapula is stabilized, and glenohumeral external and internal rotations are measured. Total arc rotation is calculated by adding total external plus total internal rotation [18]. Patients who have glenohumeral internal rotation deficit (GIRD) may have a decrease in internal rotation compared to the contralateral extremity. Once inspection, palpation, and range of motion have been evaluated, specific provocative maneuvers for posterior shoulder instability should be conducted.

The jerk test is performed with the patient in a sitting position. The examiner stabilizes the scapula with one hand, and the patient's arm is abducted 90° and internally rotated 90°. An axial force is applied with the examiner's contralateral hand holding the patient's elbow and simultaneously applying a horizontal adduction force. A sharp pain with or without posterior clunk or click suggests a positive test result. Kim's test is performed with the patient in a sitting position with the arm in 90° of abduction. The examiner holds the elbow and the lateral aspect of the proximal arm, and an axial loading force is applied. While the arm is elevated 45° diagonally upward, a downward and backward force is applied to the proximal arm. A sudden onset of posterior shoulder pain indicates a positive result regardless of accompanying posterior clunk of the humeral head [21].

The posterior stress test is performed by stabilizing the medial border of the scapula with one hand, and with the other hand, the examiner applies a posteriorly directed force to the patient's shoulder while it is flexed at 90°, adducted, and internally rotated. The test is positive if posterior subluxation or pain is present [21]. The load and shift test is used to evaluate for subluxation of the humeral head and is reliable with a high specificity. The load and shift maneuver, which is performed with the arm held in 90° of abduction and neutral rotation, involves applying an axial load to the glenohumeral joint with an anterior directed force applied to test the anterior capsule, followed by a posterior directed force to test the posterior capsule. The amount of translation of the humeral head over the anterior or posterior glenoid rim is quantified as grade 0 to 3+ (Table 3.2) [18].

Table 3.3 Grading for a sulcus sign. A grade 2+ or greater is associated with multidirectional instability

1+	Acromiohumeral distance <1 cm
2+	Acromiohumeral distance between 1 and 2 cm
3+	Acromiohumeral distance >2 cm

The presence of a sulcus sign indicates excessive inferior glenohumeral ligament laxity and superior glenohumeral ligament laxity. While the patient is seated, downward traction is applied with the arm adducted and in neutral rotation. A positive sulcus sign suggests an inferior component of the instability, which is present in more than 75% of patients with posterior instability [22]. The test is repeated in 30° of external rotation. Laxity is quantified based on the acromiohumeral distance (Table 3.3). A sulcus sign that remains 2+ or greater in 30° of external rotation is considered pathognomonic for multidirectional instability [18].

Multidirectional Instability

Case # 5

A 24-year-old right-hand-dominant female volleyball player with a family history of Marfan syndrome presents with chronic right shoulder instability. She does not recall any inciting events and explains that she used to have a sense of shoulder instability and pain only when playing volleyball, but now it occurs more often. On physical examination, she has a Beighton score of 6, with a positive sulcus sign, and positive anterior and posterior load and shift tests. The patient has not had any improvement with rest.

Background

In 1980, Neer and Foster coined the term multidirectional instability (MDI), which is defined as anterior and posterior shoulder instability that is associated with involuntary inferior subluxation or dislocation [23]. MDI has also been described as pathologic shoulder instability in two or three directions and can be due to congenital laxity, which is often atraumatic and asymptomatic in nature, but can also present as instability in the setting of abnormal laxity [24]. In cases where there is instability or a traumatic event in a patient with underlying physiologic laxity, structural defects in the dynamic and static shoulder stabilizers may be present.

Laxity in the shoulder can be highly variable and is not the same as instability (Table 3.4). Many athletes use laxity to increase competitive performance and their periscapular muscles allow extreme ranges of motion without pathological instability [25]. Stability of the glenohumeral joint is provided by the dynamic and static shoulder stabilizers. Patients with MDI may have a shallow glenoid cavity or increased capsular redundancy [26, 27]. Capsular redundancy can be genetic, and it can also be associated with systemic diseases such as Marfan syndrome, Ehlers Danlos syndrome, and osteogenesis imperfecta [28–31]. It can also be acquired from repetitive microtrauma that stretches the capsuloligamentous restraints. A thorough history and physical exam is critical in making the diagnosis of MDI.

History

Patients may present with an insidious onset of activity-related shoulder pain or decreased athletic performance. It is important to determine which activities cause pain, as MDI is seen more often in overhead athletes who participate in sports such as swimming and volleyball. Physicians should inquire about any inciting traumatic events or daily repetitive motions that could be contributing. It should also be noted if the patient can voluntarily dislocate his/her shoulder, if there is a history of collagen disorders, and if the patient has any psychiatric conditions. Patients with concomitant psychiatric conditions have poorer outcomes with surgical intervention [33]. Clarifying whether the patient has subluxation or dislocation events may also be helpful, as well as the determining the primary direction of instability. Most patients do not have global instability, and it is necessary to determine whether it is true MDI or unidirectional instability with multidirectional laxity. Patients with a history of prior failed instability surgery should also be evaluated for MDI. It is also important to speak with the patient and discuss their overall treatment goals and expectations.

Table 3.4 Classification and description of dynamic shoulder instability [32]

Classification	Description
Unidirectional instability without hyperlaxity	Symptoms elicited in a single direction Traumatic capsulolabral lesions frequently present
Unidirectional with hyperlaxity	Symptoms elicited in single direction Patulous capsular tissue frequently present Presence of capsulolabral lesions less likely
Multidirectional instability without hyperlaxity	Symptoms elicited in two or more directions Anterior and posterior capsulolabral lesions frequently present
Multidirectional instability with hyperlaxity	Symptoms elicited in two or more directions Patulous capsular tissue frequently present Signs of generalized hyperlaxity frequently present Frequent recurrent subluxation

Table 3.5 Components of the Beighton score. A score >3 is indicative of hyperlaxity [34]

Characteristic	Score
Active elbow hyperextension beyond 10°	1 point per extremity
Passive thumb apposition to ipsilateral forearm	1 point per extremity
Passive dorsiflexion of little finger beyond 90°	1 point per extremity
Active knee hyperextension beyond 10°	1 point per extremity
Ability to place palms of hands on the floor with knees extended	1 point

Physical Examination

Visual inspection should always be performed with the patient's shirt off to evaluate for asymmetry, atrophy, scapular winging, or previous surgical scars. Scarring in skin folds, keloid formation, and hyper-elasticity may suggest a collagen disorder. Tenderness to palpation about the shoulder should be noted and range of motion should be evaluated. A thorough neurovascular exam should be performed. The cervical spine should also be examined on any patient with a complaint of shoulder pain.

In patients with suspected MDI, generalized ligamentous laxity should be evaluated by administering a Beighton examination (Table 3.5) [34]. Knee, elbow, thumb, and metacarpophalangeal hyperextension are given a point for each side, with another point if the patient can put their hands flat on the floor with their knees straight bending forward. Patients with a score greater than 3 are considered to have generalized ligamentous laxity [35].

The presence of a sulcus sign should also be noted when examining the patient. Inferior glenohumeral laxity can be examined with the hyperabduction test, described by Gagey and Gagey [35]. Patients with more than 105° of passive abduction under anesthesia are considered to have laxity of the inferior glenohumeral ligament.

Anterior and posterior instability should also be evaluated in patients with suspected MDI. Anterior instability can be assessed with the apprehension test and the anterior load and shift maneuver. To assess for posterior instability, the push-pull test can be performed, which is similar to the anterior load and shift test. The patient is positioned supine with the arm abducted to 90° in neutral rotation and 30° of horizontal adduction. A fulcrum is placed on the shoulder by grasping the patient's wrist with one hand (pull) and the humerus with the other and posteriorly loading the humerus (push) [36]. Evaluation of instability in all three directions is imperative when assessing for MDI.

It is critical to distinguish between instability and laxity when assessing patients for MDI. The examiner must have a thorough understanding of the different pathologies. A thorough history, physical exam, and determination of the direction of instability is important to determine the most appropriate treatment option for patients with MDI.

Conclusion

The shoulder is a complex joint with intricate anatomy and multiplanar mobility. Shoulder instability can occur from a traumatic event, repetitive microtrauma, and as a result of underlying pathology and hyperlaxity. It is imperative to be aware of the subtle differences in the presentation of patients with anterior, posterior, and multidirectional instability. A thorough understanding of the pathoanatomy can help facilitate early diagnosis and appropriate treatment.

References

1. Halder AM, Itoi E, An KN. Anatomy and biomechanics of the shoulder. Orthop Clin North Am. 2000;31(2) https://doi.org/10.1016/S0030-5898(05)70138-3.
2. Dumont GD, Russell RD, Robertson WJ. Anterior shoulder instability: a review of pathoanatomy, diagnosis and treatment. Curr Rev Musculoskelet Med. 2011;4(4) https://doi.org/10.1007/s12178-011-9092-9.
3. Hovelius L, Augustini BG, Fredin H, et al. Primary anterior dislocation of the shoulder in young

patients. A ten-year prospective study. J Bone Joint Surg Am. 1996;78(11):1677–84. https://doi.org/10.2106/00004623-199611000-00006.
4. Burkhead WZ, Rockwood CA. Treatment of instability of the shoulder with an exercise program. J Bone Joint Surg Am. 1992;74(6):890–6.
5. Dickens JF, Rue JP, Cameron KL, et al. Successful return to sport after arthroscopic shoulder stabilization versus nonoperative management in contact athletes with Anterior Shoulder Instability: a prospective multicenter study. Am J Sports Med. 2017;45(11):2540–6. https://doi.org/10.1177/0363546517712505.
6. Shanley E, Thigpen C, Brooks J, et al. Return to sport as an outcome measure for shoulder instability: surprising findings in nonoperative Management in a High School Athlete Population. Am J Sports Med. 2019;47(5):1062–7. https://doi.org/10.1177/0363546519829765.
7. Dickens JF, Slaven SE, Cameron KL, et al. Prospective evaluation of glenoid bone loss after first-time and recurrent anterior Glenohumeral instability events. Am J Sports Med. 2019;47(5):1082–9. https://doi.org/10.1177/0363546519831286.
8. Sachs RA, Lin D, Lou SM, et al. Can the need for future surgery for acute traumatic anterior shoulder dislocation be predicted? J Bone Joint Surg Am. 2007;89(8):1665–74. https://doi.org/10.2106/JBJS.F.00261.
9. Chahal J, Leiter J, McKee MD, et al. Generalized ligamentous laxity as a predisposing factor for primary traumatic anterior shoulder dislocation. J Shoulder Elb Surg. 2010;19(8) https://doi.org/10.1016/j.jse.2010.02.005.
10. Akhtar Muhammad A, Jenkins P, Ashton F, et al. Hypermobility- a risk factor for recurrent shoulder dislocations. Br J Sports Med. 2013;47(10) https://doi.org/10.1136/bjsports-2013-092558.11.
11. Neviaser TJ. The anterior labroligamentous periosteal sleeve avulsion lesion: a cause of anterior instability of the shoulder. Arthroscopy. 1993;9(1):17–21.
12. Baker CL, Uribe JW, Whitman C. Arthroscopic evaluation of acute initial anterior shoulder dislocations. Am J Sports Med. 1990;18(1) https://doi.org/10.1177/036354659001800104.
13. Bui-Mansfield LT, Taylor DC, Uhorchak JM, Tenuta JJ. Humeral avulsions of the glenohumeral ligament: imaging features and a review of the literature. Am J Roentgenol. 2002;179(3):649–55.
14. Kaar SG, Fening SD, Jones MH, et al. Effect of humeral head defect size on glenohumeral stability: a cadaveric study of simulated Hill-Sachs defects. Am J Sports Med. 2010;38(3):594–9. https://doi.org/10.1177/0363546509350295.
15. Antonio GE, Griffith JF, Yu AB, et al. First-time shoulder dislocation: high prevalence of labral injury and age-related differences revealed by MR arthrography. J Magn Reson Imaging. 2007;26(4) https://doi.org/10.1002/jmri.21092.
16. Hegedus EJ, Goode AP, Cook CE, et al. Which physical examination tests provide clinicians with the most value when examining the shoulder? Update of a systematic review with meta-analysis of individual tests. Br J Sports Med. 2012;46(14) https://doi.org/10.1136/bjsports-2012-091066.
17. Mi M, Zhang J-m, Jiang X-y, et al. Management of locked posterior shoulder dislocation with reverse Hill–Sachs lesions via anatomical reconstructions. Orthop Surg. 2021;13(7) https://doi.org/10.1111/os.13152.
18. Bradley J, Tjoumakaris FP. Posterior shoulder instability. In: DeLee, Drez and Miller's orthopaedic sports medicine, vol. 1; 2018.
19. Kaplan LD, Flanigan DC, Norwig J, Jost P, Bradley J. Prevalence and variance of shoulder injuries in elite collegiate football players. Am J Sports Med. 2005;33(8):1142–6.
20. Tannenbaum E, Sekiya JK. Evaluation and management of posterior shoulder instability. Sports Health. 2011;3(3):253–63. https://doi.org/10.1177/1941738111400562.
21. Kim SH, Park JS, Jeong WK, et al. The Kim test: a novel test for posteroinferior labral lesion of the shoulder – a comparison to the Jerk test. Am J Sports Med. 2005;33(8) https://doi.org/10.1177/0363546504272687.
22. Pollock RG, Bigliani LU. Recurrent posterior shoulder instability: diagnosis and treatment. Clin Orthop Relat Res. 1993;291:85–96.
23. Neer CS, Foster CR. Inferior capsular shift for involuntary inferior and multidirectional instability of the shoulder. A preliminary report. J Bone Joint Surg Am. 1980;62(6):897–908.
24. Werner A. Multidirectional shoulder instability. Nonoperative and operative treatment strategies. Der Orthopade. 2009;38(1):64–9. https://doi.org/10.1007/s00132-008-1357-7.
25. Halder AM, Kuhl SG, Zobitz ME, et al. Effects of the glenoid labrum and glenohumeral abduction on stability of the shoulder joint through concavity-compression : an in vitro study. J Bone Joint Surg Am. 2001;83(7):1062–9. https://doi.org/10.2106/00004623-200107000-00013.
26. Kim SH, Noh KC, Park JS, et al. Loss of chondrolabral containment of the glenohumeral joint in atraumatic posteroinferior multidirectional instability. J Bone Joint Surg Am. 2005;87(1):92–8. https://doi.org/10.2106/JBJS.C.01448.
27. von Eisenhart-Rothe R, Mayr HO, Hinterwimmer S, et al. Simultaneous 3D assessment of glenohumeral shape, humeral head centering, and scapular positioning in atraumatic shoulder instability: a magnetic resonance-based in vivo analysis. Am J Sports Med. 2010;38(2):375–82. https://doi.org/10.1177/0363546509347105.
28. Malfait F, Hakim AJ, de Paepe A, et al. The genetic basis of the joint hypermobility syndromes. Rheumatology (Oxford). 2006;45(5):502–7. https://doi.org/10.1093/rheumatology/kei268.
29. Maltz SB, Fantus RJ, Mellett MM, et al. Surgical complications of Ehlers-Danlos syn-

drome type IV: case report and review of the literature. J Trauma. 2001;51(2):387–90. https://doi.org/10.1097/00005373-200108000-00029.
30. Shafer BL, Mihata T, McGarry MH, et al. Effects of capsular plication and rotator interval closure in simulated multidirectional shoulder instability. J Bone Joint Surg Am. 2008;90(1):136–44. https://doi.org/10.2106/JBJS.F.00841.
31. Mallon WJ, Speer KP. Multidirectional instability: current concepts. J Shoulder Elbow Surg. 4(1 Pt 1):54–64. https://doi.org/10.1016/s1058-2746(10)80009-6.
32. Gerber C, Nyffeler RW. Classification of glenohumeral joint instability. Clin Orthop Relat Res. 2002;400:65–76. https://doi.org/10.1097/00003086-200207000-00009.
33. Carliste R, Tokish J. Multidirectional Instability of the Shoulder. In: DeLee, Drez, and Miller's Orthopaedic sports medicine, vol. 1 (Issue 5); 2019. p. 567–88.
34. Beighton P, Horan F. Orthopaedic aspects of the Ehlers-Danlos syndrome. J Bone Joint Surg Br. 1969;51(3):444–53.
35. Gagey OJ, Gagey N. The hyperabduction test: an assessment of the laxity of the inferior glenohumeral ligament. J Bone Joint Surg Br. 2001;83:69–74.
36. Tokish JM, Krishnan SG, Hawkins RJ. Clinical examination of the overhead athlete: the "differential-directed" approach. In: The shoulder and the overhead athlete. A holistic approach. Philadelphia: Lippincott Williams and Wilkins; 2004. p. 23–49.

Glenoid Bone Loss: How to Measure

4

Paolo Spinello and Giovanni Di Giacomo

Patient Presentation The patient, a 28-year-old professional rugby player, presented for evaluation the day following a self-reduced left shoulder dislocation, which occurred during a rugby match. This event marks the second instance of anterior shoulder dislocation, the first occurring roughly a year ago during a training session.

Chief Complaint The patient reports acute onset of left shoulder pain and instability following a fall during a game, consistent with his description of the initial injury.

History of Present Illness The patient had an anterior shoulder dislocation 1 year ago, which was managed with sedation, reduction, immobilization, and rehabilitation. He returned to professional rugby after receiving clearance but experienced a second dislocation after a fall in his second game back.

Past Medical History Notable for pollen allergy. Surgical history includes an appendectomy at age 16. No chronic conditions. The patient uses NSAIDs as needed.

P. Spinello · G. Di Giacomo (✉)
Department of Orthopaedic Surgery, Concordia Hospital, Rome, Italy

Social History The patient consumes alcohol socially and has no history of tobacco or illicit drug use. He lives in Rome with his girlfriend.

Clinical Examination

The left shoulder appeared swollen and bruised from the recent trauma. Tenderness was present over the anterior shoulder, especially over the glenohumeral joint and the bicipital groove. The patient showed discomfort, particularly during external rotation and abduction. Moderate pain and weakness were present during evaluation of the rotator cuff muscles for strength.

We observed a positive apprehension test, performed by externally rotating and abducting the arm to 90°.

Imaging

X-rays, including anteroposterior, lateral, and axillary views, were prescribed for an initial assessment to check for bony abnormalities. The detection of a "bony Bankart lesion" suggested glenoid bone loss, indicating the necessity for further imaging (Fig. 4.1).

CT scan: A 3D CT scan of the shoulder was then performed. Currently, 3D CT of the shoulder is considered the gold standard for the evaluation of the glenoid because it can provide accurate

© The Author(s), under exclusive license to Springer Nature Switzerland AG 2026
R. M. Frank, J. M. Tokish (eds.), *Management of Shoulder Instability*,
https://doi.org/10.1007/978-3-032-18089-6_4

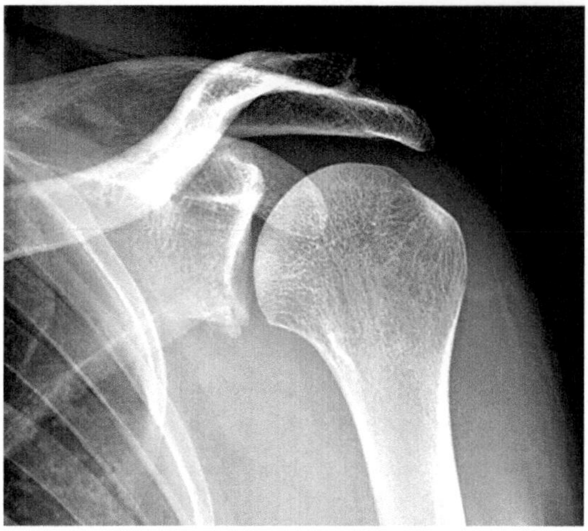

Fig. 4.1 Clinical case

information on its true anatomy [23]. A Glenoid bone loss was observed associated with a small bony Bankart fragment that likely underwent resorption over time since the first trauma [11]. Using the glenoid en face view of a 3D CT image, it is possible to quantify glenoid bone loss and an associated bony Bankart lesion as described in detail in the paragraph "How to measure glenoid bone loss with an associated bony Bankart lesion." The inferior part of the glenoid perimeter can be approximated to a true circle (Fig. 4.5) [9, 24]. Glenoid bone loss can then be calculated as a percentage, using the equation $\frac{b}{a}X100$, where (a) is the diameter of the fitted circle and (b) is the width of the defect. The bony Bankart width is then measured as (c). The ratio between the bony fragment and the glenoid width is calculated as a percentage using the formula $\frac{c}{a}X100$. In the case of a bony Bankart lesion, a mismatch between the glenoid bone loss and bony Bankart ratios is observed ($\frac{b}{a}X100 \uparrow \frac{c}{a}X100$). On the CT scan was also noted an Hill-Sachs lesion on the humerus. Given the critical role of both the glenoid cavity and the integrity of the humeral head in ensuring glenohumeral joint stability during mid-range movements, it's essential to accurately calculate the glenoid track and the Hill-Sachs interval. These measurements are pivotal in assessing the extent of shoulder injury and determining the most suitable surgical approach, whether to opt for arthroscopic bony Bankart repair or the Latarjet procedure. A detailed explanation of these considerations and the decision-making process will be provided later in the chapter. A Hill-Sachs lesion, which stays on the glenoid track (on-track lesion), cannot engage with the glenoid and cannot cause dislocation. On the other hand, a Hill-Sachs lesion, which is out of the glenoid track (off-track lesion), has a risk of engagement and dislocation. In this particular case, the Hill-Sachs interval exceeded the glenoid track so the lesion was considered off-track.

Clinical Decision

In this case, the glenoid bone loss was quantified at 24%. According to Itoi [3], Burkhart et al. [4], and Lo [5], glenoid bone loss exceeding 20–27% of the glenoid width can result in an inverted pear-shaped glenoid, which is considered critical and generally precludes arthroscopic intervention. Furthermore, the glenoid track was measured to be smaller than the Hill-Sachs interval, classifying the lesion as "off-track." Given the patient's high level of functional activity and the "off-track" nature of the lesion, a Latarjet procedure was deemed the most appropriate treatment option.

Outcome

The patient undergone surgery without complication. Four weeks of immobilization followed the procedure and a progressive rehabilitation was started.

The patient had a progressive return to his sport profession starting from 6 months post op. Now he is at 3 years follow-up with satisfactory stability, ROM, and strength.

Introduction

Glenoid bone loss (GBL) is one of the key factors to consider when planning surgical treatment for anteroinferior glenohumeral instability cases. After obtaining a detailed clinical history and a thorough physical examination, an orthopedic surgeon may suspect a labral lesion with associated GBL [1]. The next diagnostic step is to request imaging, either a radiograph, CT, or MRI scan, to quantify GBL. In patients with anteroinferior glenohumeral instability, GBL, in addition with humeral-sided Hill-Sachs lesions, are considered bipolar bone loss and should be assessed in the light of different types of injuries of the dynamic and static stabilizers of the shoulder (e.g., glenoid labrum, glenohumeral ligaments, and rotator cuff tears) [2]. The cause of GBL should also be assessed, considering whether the bone loss is due to the presence of an associated bony Bankart (fragment) or if it is the result of a flattening-type lesion. The extent of GBL is related to situations of different clinical relevance. GBL larger than 20% to 27% of the glenoid width can cause an inverted pear-shaped glenoid and, above that threshold, is considered critical, leading to the elimination of arthroscopy as a potential intervention [3–5]. GBL between 13% and 19% of the glenoid width is considered subcritical and has varying outcomes depending on the functional needs of patients [6–8]; worse functional scores have been observed after arthroscopic repair in high function demanding patients [7]. Therefore, imaging techniques not only provide a tool to identify and confirm the diagnosis of shoulder instability during clinical evaluation but also allow the quantification of the bone loss, an essential step for planning surgical treatment. Knowing how to measure GBL can help surgeons choose the most appropriate surgical treatments so as to obtain the best possible clinical outcomes, considering the functional needs of patients.

Classification of Glenoid Bone Loss and Its Relationship with Humeral Hill-Sachs Lesion

The cause of GBL should be assessed, considering if the bone loss is due to the presence of an associated bony Bankart (fragment) or if it is the result of a flattening-type lesion.

1. *Bony Bankart (Fragment-Type Bone Loss)*

   A bony Bankart is a triangle-shaped osseous Bankart lesion, defined as a displaced fracture of the anterior glenoid rim. The prevalence of an osseous Bankart lesion, confirmed by a preoperative 3D CT scan, is 16–50% [9, 10]. According to Griffith et al. [10], 16% of single-anterior dislocations presented with a bony fragment that is most likely caused by an avulsion mechanism, whereas 23% of bony Bankart lesions were observed in patients with recurrent anterior dislocations. The increase in frequency of the fragment type bone loss in these recurrent patients may be explained either by a newly created avulsion fracture in patients with a healed Bankart lesion or by a shear fracture in those with an unhealed Bankart lesion.
2. *Flattening-Type Bone Loss (the So-Called Erosion Type)*

   The pathogenesis of this type of bone loss is best described by a compression fracture mechanism rather than an erosion mechanism as it is caused by the collapse of trabecular bone of the articular surface of the glenoid [11–13]. As shown in the cadaveric study by Etoh et al., anterior flattening of the glenoid, or the so-called erosion-type bone loss, was observed only during stage two of their experiment, in an equilibrium position under muscle force. MicroCT revealed disruption of the subchondral trabeculae and articular cartilage at the anterior rim of the glenoid, confirming that a compression fracture had occurred. Anterior flattening is observed more in shoulders with recurrent dislocations compared to those with a single dislocation. Three possible mechanisms can explain this observation: (1) a new compression fracture, (2) the absorption of the bony fragment (i.e., conversion from the fragment type to the flattening type), or (3) a true erosion caused by repetitive dislocations. Thus, we propose calling this type of GBL "flattening-type," based on the morphology [12] since pathogenic mechanism is not yet clear.

How to Measure GBL

Radiography

Although shoulder X-ray images are not used in current clinical practice for quantitative assessment of GBL, they still are requested as the first imaging exam during the initial patient evaluation, allowing the orthopedic surgeon to identify suspect cases of anteroinferior glenohumeral instability.

Standard X-ray projections of the shoulder include the anterior-posterior view (AP), the "Y" view [14], and axial view of the shoulder. The AP view can provide useful information in cases of anteroinferior glenohumeral instability and can be acquired with the arm in external, neutral, or internal rotation. On a *true* AP view (or Grashey view), the anterior rim of the glenoid can be identified as a sclerotic line; the loss of this sclerotic line for more than 5 mm from the inferior glenoid edge is a sign of bony lesions of the anterior glenoid rim [15]. With the arm in internal rotation, a Hill-Sachs lesion can be observed on the proximal humerus in patients with a history of dislocation. The scapular "Y" and the axillary views have a high degree of accuracy and supplement the AP view, providing important information despite not having a role in GBL quantification [16]. The scapular "Y" view can show if the glenohumeral joint is dislocated with less painful positioning because abduction of the arm is not required, making it particularly useful in the trauma setting. The axillary view allows visualization of the glenoid rim, the glenoid version, and the possible presence of associated GBL; it can be far superior in recognizing Hill-Sachs's lesions compared to the "Y" view [17]. Other X-ray views of interest for studying the glenoid include the West Point and Bernageau views [16, 18, 19]. The West Point view can reveal obvious changes in glenoid length that are detectable but not decisively quantifiable [16]. Some authors showed that using the Bernageau view, it could be possible to assess the glenoid dimensions (e.g., the distance between the anterior and posterior glenoid rims), as the values they obtained were not significantly different to the measurements taken from 3D CT images [20, 21].

CT Scan

To obtain an accurate quantification of GBL, 2D and 3D computed tomography (CT) of the injured shoulder should be obtained. Different measurement techniques have been described in the literature, which are summarized below:

How to Measure GBL on 2D CT

Baudi et al. developed the Pico method [22], a technique that allows for the detection and measurement of GBL by processing 2D CT images using multiplanar reconstruction (MPR) and using the circle method to quantify changes in bone surface area. A CT scan of both shoulders is acquired. The images are processed through MPR on a dedicated CT workstation, maintaining working axes parallel to the glenoid surface. On the en face view of the healthy glenoid, a best-fitting circle is drawn on the inferior part of glenoid, considering the outer cortex of the inferior glenoid (from 3 to 9 o'clock) as reference points for the circumference of the circle. An identical circle is drawn on the affected glenoid. The area of the circle (*A*) and the area of the missing part of the circle (*D*) should be measured. The glenoid bone defect can be expressed as a percentage using the formula: *[(D) / (A)] *100* (Fig. 4.2).

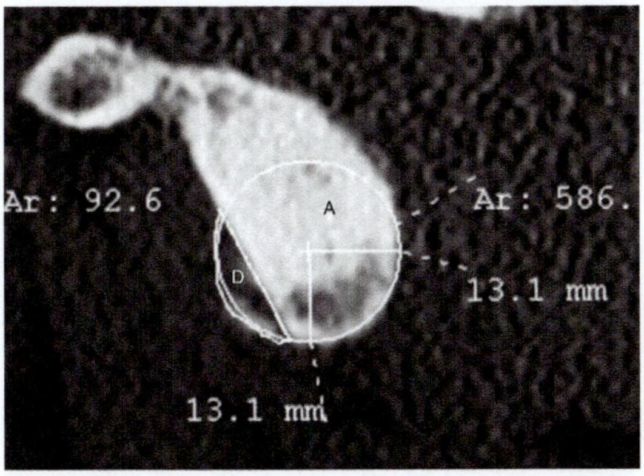

Fig. 4.2 The Pico method [22]. This technique allows providers to detect and measure GBL by processing 2D CT images using a best-fitting circle. The area of the circle (*A*) and the area of the missing part of the circle (*D*) should be measured. The glenoid bone defect can be expressed as a percentage using the formula: [(*D*) / (*A*)] *100

How to Measure GBL on 3D CT

Currently, 3D CT of the shoulder is considered the gold standard for the evaluation of the glenoid because it can provide accurate information on its true anatomy [23]. After acquiring the CT scans, 3D reconstruction and proximal humerus subtraction are made with the use of a dedicated image processing software so as to obtain an en face view of the glenoid. On this view, the uninjured glenoid appears pear-shaped [4], and the inferior part of the glenoid perimeter can be approximated as a true circle [9, 24, 25]. After obtaining this processed image, different techniques can be applied [26–28]:

- Barchilon et al. described how to assess the GBL directly using a femoral head gauge on the glenoid en face view [26]. The gauge is first used for identifying the best fitting circle. First, the radius (R) of the circle, a straight line from the center of the circle to its outside edge, is drawn. Then, a second line is drawn from the center of the circle to the anterior glenoid border where the bone defect is observed (d). The percentage of GBL is calculated by substituting these two values into a mathematical formula that calculates the area of GBL and the ratio between the area of the bone defect and the area of whole glenoid (Fig. 4.3):

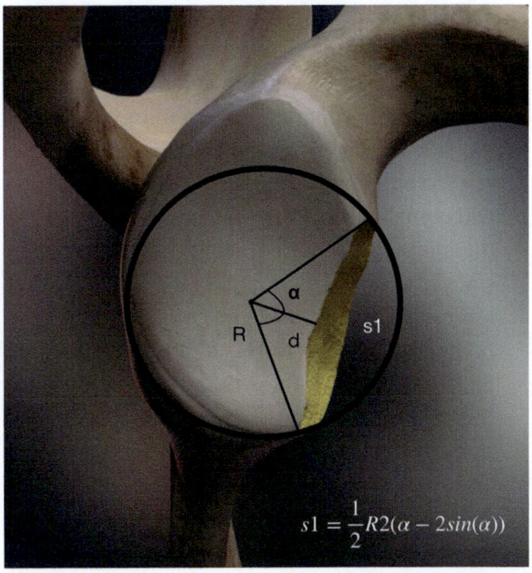

Fig. 4.3 How to assess the GBL using a femoral head gauge on the glenoid en face view [26]. The gauge is first used to identify the best fitting circle. The first line is the radius (*R*) of this circle, drawn from the center to the perimeter. A second line should be drawn from the center of the circle to the anterior glenoid border where the bone defect is observed (*d*). The percentage of GBL is calculated substituting these two values into a mathematical formula that calculates the area of GBL and the ratio between the area of the bone defect and the area of the whole glenoid

$$s1 = \frac{1}{2}R2\left(\alpha - 2\sin\alpha\right))$$

$$d = R\cos\left(\frac{\alpha}{2}\right)$$

$$0 \le \alpha \le \pi$$

- The ratio, q, between the affected area, s1, and the total area of the circle can be calculated:

$$q = \frac{s1}{\pi R^2} = \frac{1}{\pi}\left(\cos^{-1}\left(\frac{\mathrm{d}}{\mathrm{R}}\right) - \frac{d}{R}\sqrt{1-\left(\frac{d}{r}\right)^2}\right)$$

- GBL can be also assessed as the difference between pre- and post-injury glenoid width after obtaining an en face 3D CT reconstruction of the injured and healthy contralateral glenoid using a linear method [27]. Considering identical morphology between the sides, Chuang et al. described the following technique: on the healthy glenoid, identify and connect the highest and superior border of the glenoid (A1) with a line to the most inferior point of the glenoid (B1). This A1B1 line represents the normal glenoid height (H1). A perpendicular line to H1 is drawn the level of the maximum width of the glenoid (W1), and the points identified at the anterior (C1) and posterior (D1) glenoid margin are identified. The intersection of H1 and W1 is the center (O1) of the best fitting circle of the inferior healthy glenoid, and O1D1 is the radius (R1). Following the same steps, H2 (A2B2) is drawn on the injured glenoid. Assuming comparable morphology of the two shoulders, the radius (R2) of the best fitting circle of the injured glenoid can be calculated as R1/H1 = R2/H2, so R2 = (R1/H1)*H2. O2 is then identified by drawing a line with length R2 from the most inferior point of the injured glenoid (B2), and the rest of the circle, using R2 and O2, is drawn. A perpendicular line (W2) to H2, passing through O2, is drawn, and the points identified at the anterior (C2) and posterior (D2) glenoid margin are identified. The predicted preinjury width (W2') is calculated as W2' = (W1/H1)*H2. This formula is used for normalizing the preinjury width by accounting for any height difference between the injured and uninjured glenoid. A glenoid index is then quantified as W2/W2', and the obtained value expresses the residual percentage of uninjured glenoid (Fig. 4.4a–b).

- An area-based technique was proposed by Dumont [28], in which a best-fitting circle is drawn on the inferior part of the glenoid on an en face 3D CT view. The center of the circle is denoted (A). Where the circumference intersects the Bankart lesion, superior (B) and inferior (C) points are identified. The angle BAC (α) is determined using the angle tool on a dedicated image processing software (Fig. 4.5) and is then plotted in the following equation:

$$\text{Percentage Area of Glenoid Defect} = \left[(\alpha - \sin\alpha)/2\pi\right] \times 100$$

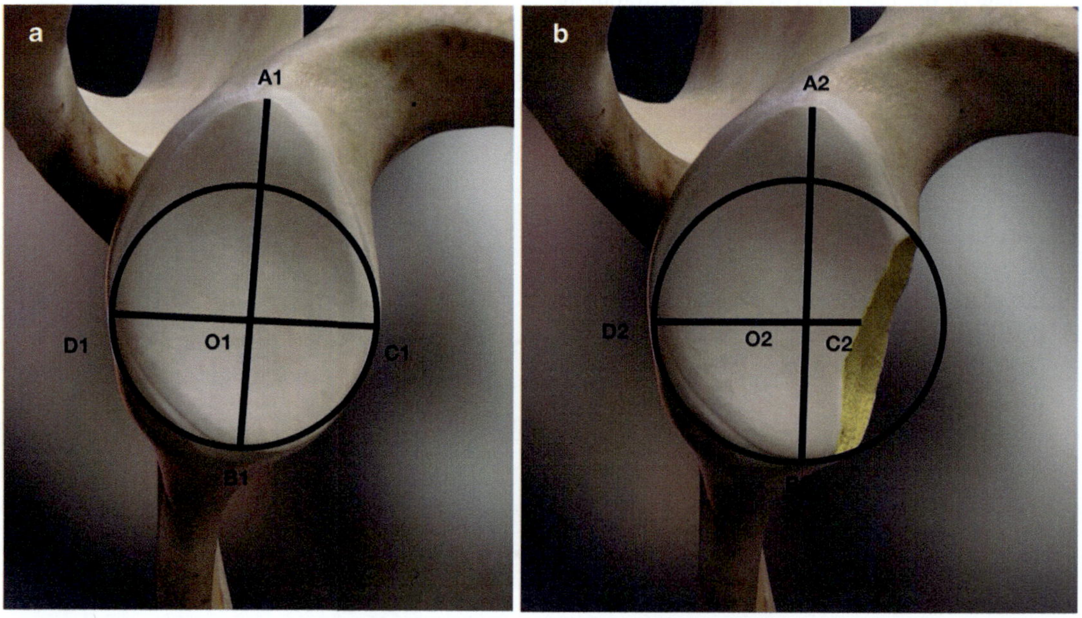

Fig. 4.4 GBL can be also assessed as a difference of pre- and post-injury glenoid width after obtaining an en face 3D CT reconstruction of the injured and healthy contralateral glenoid by the use of a linear method [27]. The details of this technique can be found in the text

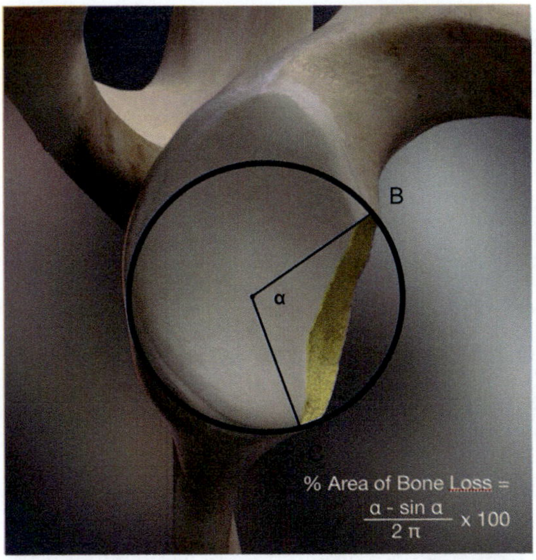

Fig. 4.5 An area-based technique [28] for assessing GBL after calculating the subtended angle identified at the level of the anterior bone loss

Three-dimensional CT reconstructions are considered the gold standard because they eliminate the effect of the gantry angle during image acquisition [29] and allow for a true en face view of the glenoid. The limits of this technique are the cost for the hospital and its availability in the different healthcare systems. On the other hand, 2D CT scans are more easily accessible, but the images require processing and alignment in the axial, sagittal, and coronal planes of the glenoid and the scapula using MPR so as to obtain accurate bone dimensions. Incorrect orientation in any one of the three planes affects the two other corresponding planes leading to improper alignment of the scans and inaccurate measurements of both the glenoid width and glenoid version [30].

Magnetic Resonance Imaging (MRI)

MRIs are routinely performed in the diagnostic evaluation of shoulder instability cases, providing essential information about associated soft tissue lesions. Some of the techniques described above [24, 28] can be applied on MRI scans as well. In a recent systematic review, it was observed that measurement techniques based on the best-fit circle are reliable and accurate for both CTs and MRIs; either can be used to quantify GBL. Like CTs, MRIs can be converted to 3D reconstructions and have additional benefits such as allowing for the evaluation of bone loss without the use of ionizing radiation or the additional cost of a CT exam [31].

Arthroscopy

Burkhart et al. described a technique for quantifying GBL during arthroscopy after observing that the glenoid bare spot is located in the central point of the circle that best fit the inferior part of the glenoid [32]. During an arthroscopic procedure, using an anterosuperior-viewing portal and a graduated probe, the distance from the bare spot to the posterior, anterior, and inferior glenoid rims can be measured. After calculating the full diameter of the inferior glenoid, the glenoid bone defect can be expressed as a percentage of the diameter of the intact anterior glenoid. However, this technique has limitations: studies based on CT imaging have showed that it is not reliable to consider the bare spot as the center of the best fit circle of the inferior part of the glenoid since it cannot always be identified [33, 34].

How to Measure GBL with an Associated Bony Bankart Lesion

Using the glenoid en face view of a 3D CT image, it is possible to quantify GBL and an associated bony Bankart lesion. The inferior part of the glenoid perimeter can be approximated to a true circle [9, 24] as previously described. GBL can then be calculated as a percentage, using the equation $\frac{b}{a}\text{X}100$, where (a) is the diameter of the fitted circle and (b) is the width of the defect. The bony Bankart width is then measured as (c). The ratio between the bony fragment and the glenoid width is calculated as a percentage using the formula $\frac{c}{a}\text{X}100$. In the case of a bony Bankart lesion, a mismatch between the GBL and bony

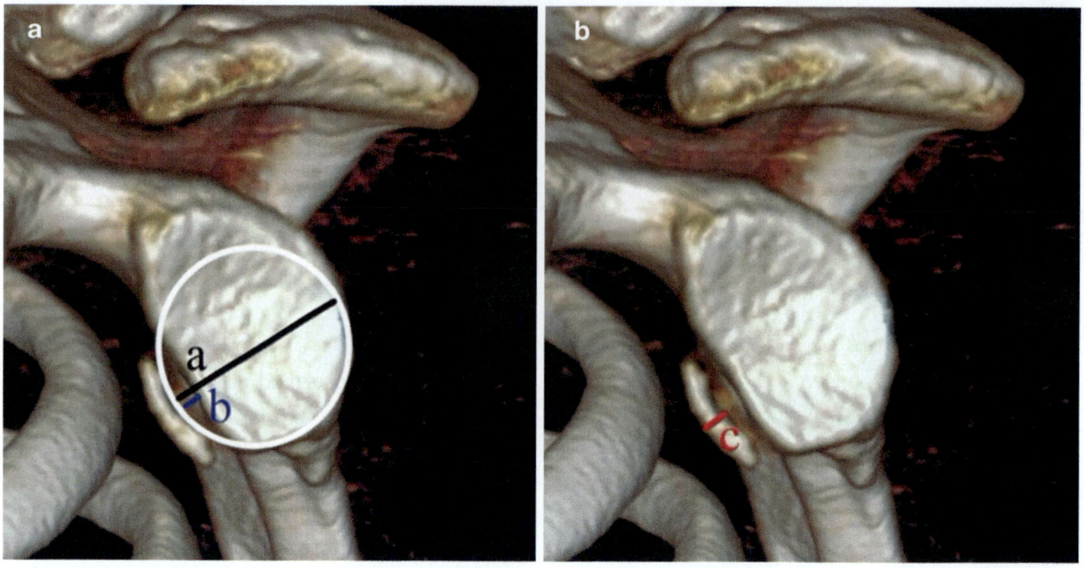

Fig. 4.6 Calculation of the preoperative glenoid defect size and bone fragment size. The glenoid defect size is calculated as a percentage of the normalized glenoid width ($\frac{b}{a}X100$), where (a) is the diameter of the best-fitting circle based on the contour of the inferior glenoid pole and (b) is the width of the defect. The same procedure is used to calculate the postoperative glenoid defect size. The bone fragment size is calculated as a percentage ($\frac{c}{a}X100$), where (c) is the width of the bone fragment

Bankart ratios is observed ($\frac{b}{a}X100 \uparrow \frac{c}{a}X100$). This occurs because bony Bankart lesions undergo extensive resorption within 1 year after their occurrence [11]. This phenomenon becomes more marked as the number of dislocations increases and the period after the primary trauma becomes lengthens. The expected (true) GBL should be then calculated as a percentage of the difference ($\frac{b-c}{a}$)X100 (Fig. 4.6).

Bipolar Bone Loss: Humeral Hill-Sachs Lesion, GBL, and Glenoid Track

In addition to the glenoid cavity, glenohumeral stability in mid-range motion is guaranteed by the integrity of the humeral head. Di Giacomo et al. [2] proposed the term "bipolar bone loss" to describe bone defects affecting both the glenoid and proximal humerus. The Hill-Sachs lesion is a compression fracture of the postero-lateral portion of the humeral head caused by collision of the glenoid and humerus during an anterior shoulder dislocation. Kawakami et al., in a 3D CT study of 100 patients with recurrent anterior dislocation of the shoulder, observed the position in which the Hill-Sachs humeral lesion perfectly fit the anterior rim of the glenoid. They hypothesized that Hill-Sachs lesions are not created at the time of dislocation but rather later in the midrange position [35]. This hypothesis was later confirmed by Etoh et al. in cadaveric study where no Hill-Sachs lesion were observed during stage one, the time of dislocation, but instead during stage two with the arm in equilibrium position under muscle force [13].

The paramount importance of the geometric interplay between the glenoid and humeral lesions is best explained by the glenoid track concept [37] and its relationship with the humeral on-track/off-track Hill-Sachs lesion [2, 36]:

The glenoid track (GT) is defined as the contact zone between the glenoid and the head of the humerus when the arm is moved along the poste-

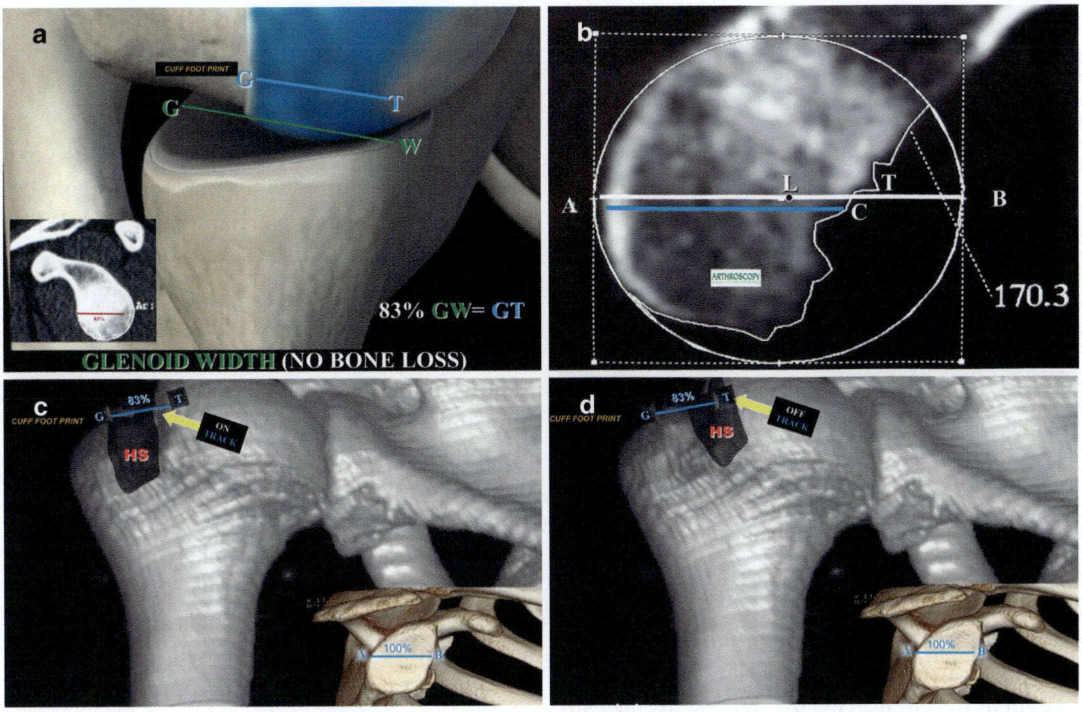

Fig. 4.7 The glenoid track (GT) is defined as the contact zone between the glenoid and the head of the humerus when the arm is moved along the posterior end-range of motion (**a**). The width of the GT is reduced in patients with a glenoid defect; GT is calculated with the following equation: GT = 0,83 × *AB* − *CB* where *AB* is the glenoid diameter and *CB* is the glenoid defect (**b**). A lesion is classified as on-track if the HSI falls within the GT (i.e., is smaller than the GT) (**c**), while it is considered off-track if it falls outside the GT (i.e., is larger than the GT) (**d**). An off-track lesion is at high risk for glenohumeral engagement

rior end-range of motion (Fig. 4.7a). This concept is crucial to assess the risk of a Hill-Sachs lesion engaging the glenoid rim with or without a glenoid defect. The width of the GT is reduced in patients with a glenoid defect; GT is calculated with the following equation: GT = 0.83 × AB − CB where AB is the glenoid diameter and CB is the glenoid defect (Fig. 4.7b).

In order to determine whether a Hill-Sachs lesion is on-track or off-track, a Hill-Sachs interval (HSI) must be assessed; on 3D CT image, the HSI is measured as the distance between the rotator cuff attachments and the medial aspect of the Hill-Sachs lesion. A lesion is classified as on-track if the HSI falls within the GT (i.e., the HSI is smaller than the GT) (Fig. 4.7c), while it is considered off-track if it falls outside the GT (i.e., the HSI is larger than the GT) (Fig. 4.7d). An off-track lesion is at high risk for glenohumeral engagement. A Hill-Sachs lesion can then be classified as a central or peripheral lesion [38]. A "peripheral-track" lesion is defined as a Hill-Sachs lesion with a medial margin very close to the periphery of the glenoid track. A "central-track" lesion is instead characterized by a Hill-Sachs occupancy that is less than 75% of the glenoid track width.

Magnetic Resonance Imaging (MRI) and On-/Off-Track Hill-Sachs Lesions

It is also possible to quantify bone loss in an on-track/off-track Hill-Sachs lesions using MRI.

GBL is assessed with the best-fit circle method: a best-fit circle is placed along the posterior and inferior margins of the glenoid. A hor-

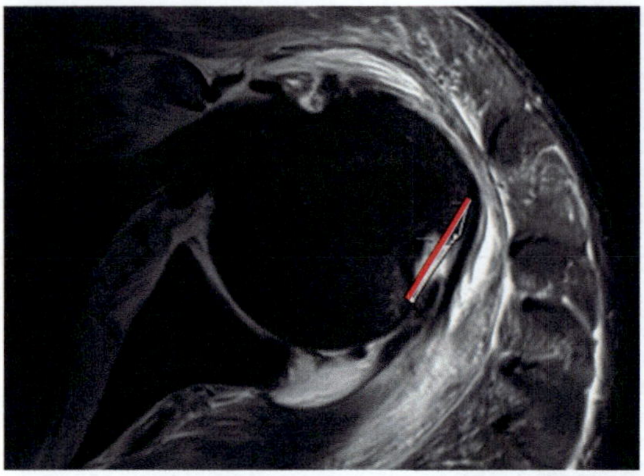

Fig. 4.8 T2-weighted magnetic resonance image using an axial view of the shoulder in the slice with the largest extension of the Hill-Sachs lesion. The Hill-Sachs interval is measured as the width of the Hill-Sachs lesion plus the width of the intact bone bridge between the rotator cuff and the Hill-Sachs lesion

izontal line, extending through the center of the circle, is drawn from the posterior to the anterior margin of the circle. This line represents the estimated diameter of the intact glenoid (*D*). A second horizontal line, also running through the middle of the circle, is drawn between the anterior margin of the circle and the anterior margin of the glenoid (*d*). This line represents the amount of anterior glenoid bone loss. According to the on-track/off-track concept, the glenoid track is calculated as $0.83 * D - d$ in which (*D*) represents the diameter of the intact glenoid in millimeters and (*d*) is the amount of glenoid bone loss in millimeters.

The HSI can be calculated as the width of the Hill-Sachs lesion in millimeters plus the width of the intact bone bridge in millimeters, located between the rotator cuff attachment and the lateral margin of the Hill-Sachs lesion. The HSI is assessed in all three MRI planes (axial, coronal, and sagittal). The measurement is made on the axial images at the point with the largest medial extent of the Hill-Sachs lesion. Lesions are considered off-track if the HSI exceeds the glenoid track and on-track if the HSI is smaller than the glenoid track (Fig. 4.8).

Glenoid Bone Loss and Hill-Sachs Lesion in the Surgical Decision-Making Process

Quantifying the critical amount of GBL that requires intervention with a bone grafting procedure remains a controversial topic [3–5]. While in prior literature, GBL greater than 20–25% of the native glenoid width was considered a critical threshold for excluding candidates for arthroscopic stabilization, recent studies have demonstrated that it is necessary to reduce this threshold to subcritical values as low as 13–19% to obtain satisfactory results [6–8]. Even at this lower cut-off, patients with higher functional demands were found to have worse functional scores post-arthroscopic Bankart reconstruction [7]. Accurate preoperative calculation of expected GBL and bony Bankart width, considering factors like time elapsed since primary trauma and the number of preoperative dislocations, is a useful tool in the surgical treatment algorithm for anterior glenohumeral instability [39, 40]. When uncertainty exists about a GBL defect that is *greater than* 13.5% (i.e., if it is a flattening type above 13.5% or an expected GBL associated with a bony Bankart lesion approaching the subcritical bone loss value), especially in a high function-demanding patient population, the Latarjet procedure could be the most robust choice in order to minimize risk of recurrence and maximize functional results. If the expected GBL or flattening type is lower than subcritical bone loss, an arthroscopic Bankart repair can be considered. Concerning the humeral-sided Hill-Sachs lesion, on-track Hill-Sachs lesions do not engage the glenoid rim, but further subclassification into peripheral-track and central-track lesions has been proposed [38]. Peripheral-track lesions, defined by a Hill-Sachs occupancy close to the medial border of the glenoid track, have been associated with inferior functional outcomes, particularly in high-demand or contact athletes. In such cases, restoration of the native glenoid track with a bony augmentation proce-

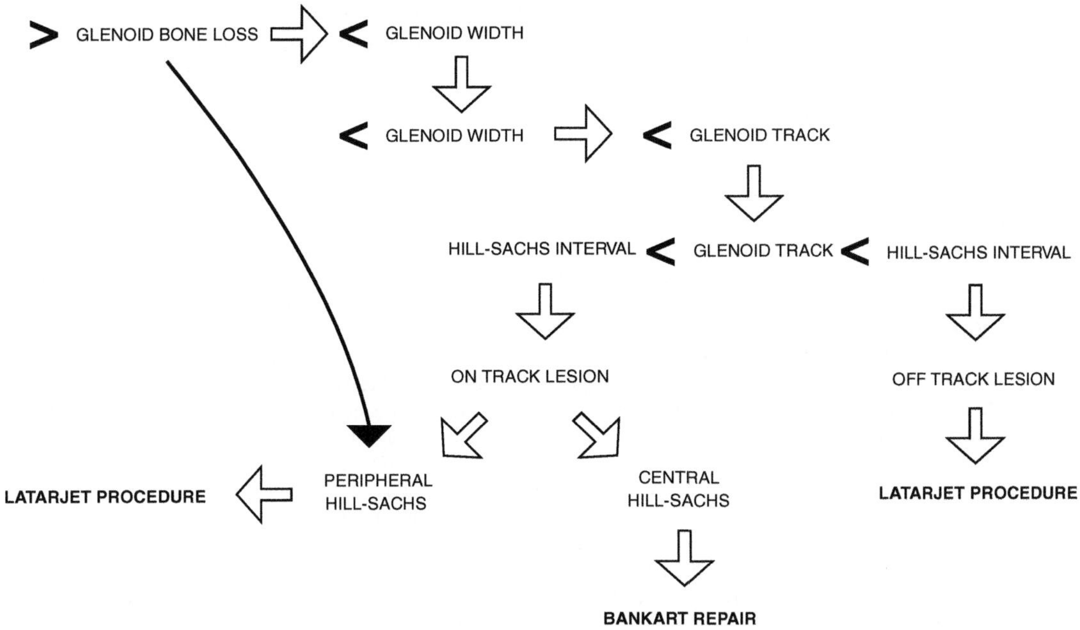

Fig. 4.9 The figure shows the surgical treatment algorithm based on the characteristics of the bipolar bone loss: glenoid width, glenoid track, and on−/off-track Hill-Sachs lesion

dure may be considered, whereas central-track lesions can generally be managed with standard Bankart repair (Fig. 4.9).

References

1. Provencher MT, Bhatia S, Ghodadra NS, et al. Recurrent shoulder instability: current concepts for evaluation and management of glenoid bone loss. J Bone Joint Surg Am. 2010;92(Suppl 2):133–51. https://doi.org/10.2106/JBJS.J.00906.
2. Di Giacomo G, Itoi E, Burkhart SS. Evolving concept of bipolar bone loss and the Hill-Sachs lesion: from "engaging/non-engaging" lesion to "on-track/off-track" lesion. Arthroscopy. 2014;30(1):90–8. https://doi.org/10.1016/j.arthro.2013.10.004.
3. Itoi E, Lee SB, Berglund LJ, Berge LL, An KN. The effect of a glenoid defect on anteroinferior stability of the shoulder after Bankart repair: a cadaveric study. J Bone Joint Surg Am. 2000;82(1):35–46. https://doi.org/10.2106/00004623-200001000-00005.
4. Burkhart SS, De Beer JF. Traumatic glenohumeral bone defects and their relationship to failure of arthroscopic Bankart repairs: significance of the inverted-pear glenoid and the humeral engaging Hill-Sachs lesion. Arthroscopy. 2000;16(7):677–94.
5. Lo IK, Parten PM, Burkhart SS. The inverted pear glenoid: an indicator of significant glenoid bone loss. Arthroscopy. 2004;20(2):169–74. https://doi.org/10.1016/j.arthro.2003.11.036.
6. Yamamoto N, Itoi E, Abe H, et al. Effect of an anterior glenoid defect on anterior shoulder stability: a cadaveric study. Am J Sports Med. 2009;37(5):949–54. https://doi.org/10.1177/0363546508330139.
7. Shaha JS, Cook JB, Song DJ, et al. Redefining "critical" bone loss in shoulder instability: functional outcomes worsen with "subcritical" bone loss. Am J Sports Med. 2015;43(7):1719–25. https://doi.org/10.1177/0363546515578250.
8. Shin SJ, Kim RG, Jeon YS, Kwon TH. Critical value of anterior glenoid bone loss that leads to recurrent Glenohumeral instability after arthroscopic Bankart repair. Am J Sports Med. 2017;45(9):1975–81. https://doi.org/10.1177/0363546517697963.
9. Sugaya H, Moriishi J, Dohi M, Kon Y, Tsuchiya A. Glenoid rim morphology in recurrent anterior glenohumeral instability. J Bone Joint Surg Am. 2003;85-a(5):878–84.
10. Griffith JF, Antonio GE, Yung PS, Wong EM, Yu AB, Ahuja AT, Chan KM. Prevalence, pattern, and spectrum of glenoid bone loss in anterior shoulder dislocation: CT analysis of 218 patients. AJR Am J Roentgenol. 2008 May;190(5):1247–54. https://doi.org/10.2214/AJR.07.3009.

11. Nakagawa S, Mizuno N, Hiramatsu K, Tachibana Y, Mae T. Absorption of the bone fragment in shoulders with bony Bankart lesions caused by recurrent anterior dislocations or subluxations: when does it occur? Am J Sports Med. 2013;41(6):1380–6.
12. Griffith JF, Antonio GE, Tong CW, Ming CK. Anterior shoulder dislocation: quantification of glenoid bone loss with CT. AJR Am J Roentgenol. 2003;180(5):1423–30.
13. Etoh T, Yamamoto N, Shinagawa K, Hatta T, Itoi E. Mechanism and patterns of bone loss in patients with anterior shoulder dislocation. J Shoulder Elb Surg. 2020;29(10):1974–80. https://doi.org/10.1016/j.jse.2020.03.022. Epub 2020 Jun 9. PMID: 32741565.
14. Rubin SA, Gray RL, Green WR. The scapular "Y": a diagnostic aid in shoulder trauma. Radiology. 1974 Mar;110(3):725–6. https://doi.org/10.1148/110.3.725.
15. Jankauskas L, Rüdiger HA, Pfirrmann CW, Jost B, Gerber C. Loss of the sclerotic line of the glenoid on anteroposterior radiographs of the shoulder: a diagnostic sign for an osseous defect of the anterior glenoid rim. J Shoulder Elb Surg. 2010 Jan;19(1):151–6. https://doi.org/10.1016/j.jse.2009.04.013.
16. Itoi E, Lee SB, Amrami KK, Wenger DE, An KN. Quantitative assessment of classic anteroinferior bony Bankart lesions by radiography and computed tomography. Am J Sports Med. 2003;31:112–8.
17. Silfverskiold JP, Straehley DJ, Jones WW. Roentgenographic evaluation of suspected shoulder dislocation: a prospective study comparing the axillary view and the scapular 'Y' view. Orthopedics. 1990 Jan;13(1):63–9. https://doi.org/10.3928/0147-7447-19900101-11.
18. Bernageau J, Patte D, Debeyre J, Ferrane J. Value of the glenoid profile in recurrent luxations of the shoulder. Rev Chir Orthop Reparatrice Appar Mot. 1976;62(2 suppl):142–7.
19. Edwards TB, Boulahia A, Walch G. Radiographic analysis of bone defects in chronic anterior shoulder instability. Arthroscopy. 2003;19(7):732–9.
20. Murachovsky J, Bueno RS, Nascimento LG, et al. Calculating anterior glenoid bone loss using the Bernageau profile view. Skeletal Radiol. 2012;41:1231–7. https://doi.org/10.1007/s00256-012-1439-9.
21. Pansard E, Klouche S, Billot N, et al. Reliability and validity assessment of a glenoid bone loss measurement using the Bernageau profile view in chronic anterior shoulder instability. J Shoulder Elbow Surg. 2013;22:1193–8. https://doi.org/10.1016/j.jse.2012.12.
22. Baudi P, Righi P, Bolognesi D, Rivetta S, Rossi Urtoler E, Guicciardi N, Carrara M. How to identify and calculate glenoid bone deficit. Chir Organi Mov. 2005;90:145–52.
23. Kwon YW, Powell KA, Yum JK, Brems JJ, Iannotti JP. Use of three-dimensional computed tomography for the analysis of the glenoid anatomy. J Shoulder Elb Surg. 2005;14:85–90.
24. Huysmans PE, Haen PS, Kidd M, Dhert WJ, Willems JW. The shape of the inferior part of the glenoid: a cadaveric study. J Shoulder Elb Surg. 2006;15:759–63.
25. Nofsinger C, Browning B, Burkhart SS, Pedowitz RA. Objective preoperative measurement of anterior glenoid bone loss: a pilot study of a computer-based method using unilateral 3-dimensional computed tomography. Arthroscopy. 2011;27:322–9.
26. Barchilon VS, Kotz E, Barchilon Ben-Av M, Glazer E, Nyska M. A simple method for quantitative evaluation of the missing area of the anterior glenoid in anterior instability of the glenohumeral joint. Skeletal Radiol. 2008;37:731–6.
27. Chuang TY, Adams CR, Burkhart SS. Use of preoperative three-dimensional computed tomography to quantify glenoid bone loss in shoulder instability. Arthroscopy. 2008;24:376–82.
28. Dumont GD, Russell RD, Browne MG, Robertson WJ. Area-based determination of bone loss using the glenoid arc angle. Arthroscopy. 2012 Jul;28(7):1030–5. https://doi.org/10.1016/j.arthro.2012.04.147.
29. Hsu JE, Ricchetti ET, Huffman GR, Iannotti JP, Glaser DL. Addressing glenoid bone deficiency and asymmetric posterior erosion in shoulder arthroplasty. J Shoulder Elb Surg. 2013;22(9):1298–308. https://doi.org/10.1016/j.jse.2013.04.014. Epub 2013 Jun 22. PMID: 23796384.
30. Gross DJ, Golijanin P, Dumont GD, Parada SA, Vopat BG, Reinert SE, Romeo AA, Provencher CD. The effect of sagittal rotation of the glenoid on axial glenoid width and glenoid version in computed tomography scan imaging. J Shoulder Elb Surg. 2016;25(1):61–8. https://doi.org/10.1016/j.jse.2015.06.017. Epub 2015 Sep 28. PMID: 26423023.
31. Walter WR, Samim M, LaPolla FWZ, Gyftopoulos S. Imaging quantification of glenoid bone loss in patients with Glenohumeral instability: a systematic review. AJR Am J Roentgenol. 2019:1–10. https://doi.org/10.2214/AJR.18.20504. Epub ahead of print. PMID: 30835517.
32. Burkhart SS, Debeer JF, Tehrany AM, Parten PM. Quantifying glenoid bone loss arthroscopically in shoulder instability. Arthroscopy. 2002;18:488–91.
33. Kralinger F, Aigner F, Longato S, Rieger M, Wambacher M. Is the bare spot a consistent landmark for shoulder arthroscopy? A study of 20 embalmed glenoids with 3-dimensional computed tomographic reconstruction. Arthroscopy. 2006;22:428–32.
34. Saintmard B, Lecouvet F, Rubini A, Dubuc JE. Is the bare spot a valid landmark for glenoid evaluation in arthroscopic Bankart surgery? Acta Orthop Belg. 2009 Dec;75(6):736–42.
35. Kawakami J, Yamamoto N, Hatta T, Shinagawa K, Itoi E. In which arm position is a hill-Sachs lesion created? Am J Sports Med. 2019;47(10):2464–8. https://doi.org/10.1177/0363546519858418. Epub 2019 Jun 27. PMID: 31246498.
36. Nakagawa S, Hirose T, Uchida R, Tanaka M, Mae T. Postoperative recurrence of instability after

arthroscopic Bankart repair for shoulders with primary instability compared with recurrent instability: influence of bipolar bone defect size. Am J Sports Med. 2020;48(1):48–55. https://doi.org/10.1177/0363546519880496.
37. Yamamoto N, Itoi E, Abe H, et al. Contact between the glenoid and the humeral head in abduction, external rotation, and horizontal extension: a new concept of glenoid track. J Shoulder Elb Surg. 2007;16:649–56.
38. Yamamoto N, Shinagawa K, Hatta T, Itoi E. Peripheral-track and central-Track Hill-Sachs lesions: a new concept of assessing an on-track lesion. Am J Sports Med. 2020;48(1):33–8. https://doi.org/10.1177/0363546519886319.
39. Spinello P, Golijanin P, Brindisino F, Moreno Rodriguez L, Di Giacomo G. Glenoid bone loss and patient history influence surgical decision-making for bony Bankart lesion: a mid-term followup retrospective study. J Shoulder Elbow Surg. 2025;34(7):1681–91. https://doi.org/10.1016/j.jse.2024.10.019. Epub 2024 Dec 22. PMID: 39716616.
40. Golijanin P, Spinello P, Brindisino F, de Gasperis N, Moreno Rodriguez L, Provencher MT, Di Giacomo G. Age, glenoid bone fragment, and glenoid bone loss increase recurrence risk after arthroscopic bony Bankart repair. Bone Joint J. 2026;108-B(2):202–8. https://doi.org/10.1302/0301-620X.108B2.BJJ-2024-1360.R3. PMID: 41619770)

Humeral Head Bone Loss: How to Measure for Treatment Decisions

5

Phob Ganokroj, Ryan J. Whalen, Anthony A. Romeo, and Matthew T. Provencher

Introduction

The glenohumeral (GH) joint consists of the humeral head, which is relatively large compared to the shallow glenoid fossa with which it articulates. This mismatch allows for greater mobility through the GH joint but sacrifices the stability of the joint. As a result, GH instability events in the general population are estimated to affect between 8 and 24 per 100,000 people, with the incidence rate significantly increasing with age, level of activity, military population, and contact athletes. Military personnel have been identified to be up to 20 times more likely to suffer from GH instability than the general US population. This population is engaged in a high amount of physical activity and is actively involved in contact/collision sports and training. These activities also lead to an increased likelihood of recurrent GH instability [1]. Literature has suggested that the rate of recurrent instability events following primary arthroscopic stabilization can be up to 25% [2]. Each recurrent instability event can further increase the possibility or extent of bony defects on the glenoid or the humeral head. The presence of HSL is estimated to increase by 14% in patients with primary dislocation compared to recurrent dislocations, and the incidence of HSL has been shown to be up to 100% in patients with recurrent shoulder dislocation [3, 4]. Patient identification is crucial in determining the treatment options in order to minimize the risk of further damage that comes with recurrent instability events.

Major risk factors for recurrent instability are bone loss in both glenoid and humeral bone loss, known as HSL. The amount of glenoid bone loss (GBL) is of clinical interest because it significantly correlates with an increased risk of recurrent dislocation [5]. Thus, the introduction of the on-track vs. off-track concept highlights the important contribution of both the HSL and GBL [6, 7]. A precise preoperative humeral bone loss measurement is essential to guide treatment decision-making and optimize the best outcomes after surgery. Various parameters such as size,

P. Ganokroj
The Steadman Philippon Research Institute, Vail, CO, USA

Faculty of Medicine Siriraj Hospital, Mahidol University, Bangkok, Thailand
e-mail: pganokroj@sprivail.org

R. J. Whalen
Center for Outcomes Based Orthopaedic Research, Steadman Philippon Research Institute, Vail, CO, USA
e-mail: rwhalen@sprivail.org

A. A. Romeo
DuPage Medical Group, Westmont, IL, USA

M. T. Provencher (✉)
Department of Orthopaedic Surgery and Sports Medicine, The Steadman Clinic and the Steadman Philippon Research Institute, Vail, CO, USA
e-mail: mprovencher@thesteadmanclinic.com

© The Author(s), under exclusive license to Springer Nature Switzerland AG 2026
R. M. Frank, J. M. Tokish (eds.), *Management of Shoulder Instability*,
https://doi.org/10.1007/978-3-032-18089-6_5

percentage of the humeral surface, depth, volume, location, or orientation are commonly reported in the literature using radiographs, CT scan, or magnetic resonance imaging (MRI) [8–14]. Recently, the 3D reconstruction image using an advanced 3D modeling software has been introduced to quantitatively and qualitatively describe the characteristics of the HSLs [15, 16]. A scoping review from Saliken et al. summarized the current studies on imaging and calculation of the humeral bone loss. They concluded that there is limited evidence to guide imaging of HSL measurement [8]. However, it is essential that physicians know all image modalities and limitations in determining humeral bone loss. This book chapter aims to review the image modalities' reliability in quantifying humeral head defects to properly care for patients with shoulder instability.

Illustrative Clinical Case

A 19-year-old right-hand-dominant female sustained a direct blow to the right shoulder from behind while playing rugby. She had pain and dislocation of the right shoulder. She was sent to the nearby hospital and underwent a closed reduction under general anesthesia in the operating room. The reduction was achieved, and she was instructed to put on the external rotation arm sling and treated conservatively. However, she has had persistent pain and a sensation of instability in the right shoulder. The preoperative radiographs, computed tomography (CT) scan, and three-dimensional (3D) reconstruction image are shown in Figs. 5.1 and 5.2. She was diagnosed with traumatic anterior shoulder instability with a large humeral head bone loss at the pos-

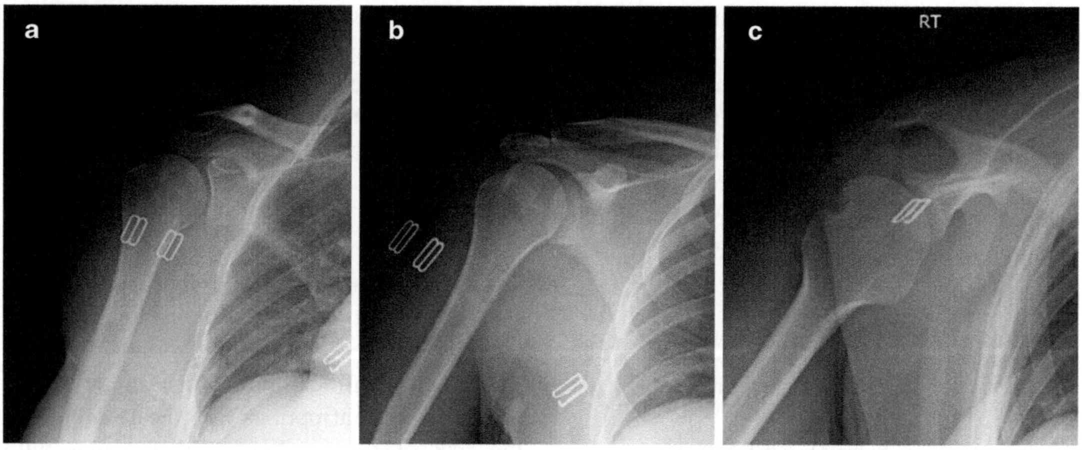

Fig. 5.1 The anteroposterior (AP) radiograph (**a**), AP radiograph with an arm in external rotation (**b**), and lateral axillary radiograph (**c**) of the right shoulder demonstrated a good reduction of the glenohumeral joint and a Hill-Sachs lesion (HSL) at the humeral head

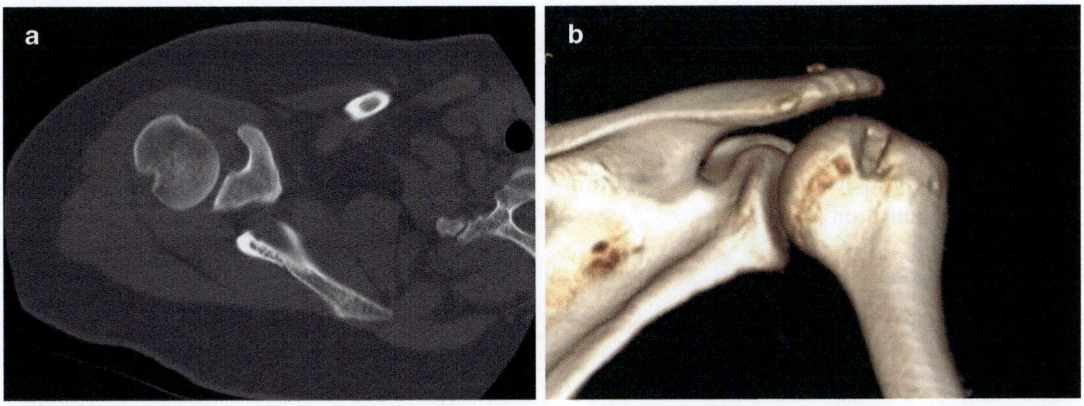

Fig. 5.2 The axial view CT scan (**a**) of the right shoulder showed a large HSL without significant glenoid bone loss. (**b**) the CT with the 3D reconstruction image demonstrated the large and medialized position of the HSL

terolateral aspect of the humeral head, known as a Hill-Sachs lesion (HSL).

Etiology

Hill-Sachs Lesions

Bony defects of the humeral head that are caused by anterior shoulder instability are termed the HSL. These lesions typically occur following an anteroinferior GH dislocation event where the shoulder is in approximately 74° abduction, 27° external rotation, and 3° horizontal flexion [4, 17]. This forces the humeral head out of the glenoid fossa anteriorly and causes the posterior superolateral aspect of the humeral head to forcefully come into contact with the anterior glenoid rim, causing a compression fracture of the humeral head [4, 18]. These lesions can also be accompanied by GBL, coined bipolar bone loss. Recurrent dislocation events increase the risk of developing or increasing the size of an HSL, which can cause chronic instability. HSLs can be classified as either "engaging," if the lesion comes in contact with the glenoid rim during abduction or external rotation, or "non-engaging" lesions [4, 6, 18].

Reverse Hill-Sachs Lesion

The reverse HSL is much less common and involves a bony defect to the anterior superomedial portion of the humeral head, caused by a posterior GH dislocation event [4, 19]. Posterior dislocations only comprise approximately 10% of all GH instability events [20]. Due to the location of the lesion, there is extensive anterior cartilage damage that exceeds the amount of posterior cartilage damage seen in traditional HSL patients [4, 19].

Diagnosis/Imaging

Physical Examination

A complete history and physical examination are imperative to guide the best treatment option for each patient. The mechanism of injury and number of instability events can provide key information to the possibility of an HSL, as well as the type or extent of the lesion. Traditional HSLs tend to have a distinct mechanism of injury that involves a traumatic anteroinferior GH dislocation, but reverse HSL tend to have vague complaints or, in rare cases, the patient experienced a traumatic posterior GH dislocation. Patients with an engaging lesion may report a sense of the humeral head "catching" during abduction or external rotation. The physical examination should include a bilateral comparison of apprehension, range of motion, strength, and sensation [4, 20].

Imaging

Imaging, along with the physical examination and history of the patient, can allow for a proper diagnosis of an HSL. Plain radiographs in the anteroposterior, lateral, and axillary views have been useful diagnostic tools, but radiography alone has been shown to miss up to 60% of bony lesions [21]. This has led to the use of other imaging modalities, such as ultrasound, CT scan, CT arthrography (CTA), 3D reconstruction CT, MRI, magnetic resonance arthrography (MRA), and 3D MRI or the emerging 3D modeling software [4, 15, 16].

Radiographs

X-rays are useful in the initial identification of bony defects in the shoulder, such as glenoid and humeral fractures. Patients typically undergo X-rays in the true anteroposterior (AP), axillary, west point, Grashey, and the Stryker notch views.

The standard AP radiograph radiographs done in the true AP view with the shoulder in internal rotation allow the beam to be directed on the postsuperolateral aspect of the humeral head to view the Hill-Sachs lesion. The axillary view is performed with the arm in abduction, with the beam directed toward the glenoid and the humeral head, and can identify bony lesions on the anterior aspect of the GH joint, such as bony Bankart defects that are often associated with Hill-Sachs lesions. The west point view has the patient lying prone with their arm in 90° of abduction and elbow flexed to 90° with the forearm hanging off the examination table, perpendicular to the ground. The beam is angled approximately 25° anterior and medially, which allows viewing of the inferior aspect of the glenoid rim and humeral head. For the Grashey view, the beam is directed 45° oblique to show any associated fractures, along with the Hill-Sachs lesion. The patient lies supine with their arm in approximately 120° of flexion and their palm on the top of their head for the Stryker notch view. The beam is directed 10° superiorly, which allows for visualization of the posterolateral aspect of the humeral head, where the HSL is found. Stryker notch view radiographs are generally considered the most reliable to detect and measure the HSL defect because the internal rotation makes the humerus's posterior aspect more visible [4].

Radiographs have displayed an 84% sensitivity and 83% specificity, with an accuracy of 83% and moderate intraobserver reliability [22, 23]. In terms of measuring HSL size, the sensitivity ranges from 8% to 81%; the specificity ranges from 91% to 100%; and the accuracy is 84%, with weak to minimal interobserver reliability [24, 25].

Ultrasound

The patient should be seated, with their arm flexed at the elbow, hanging at their side. In order to view the posterior aspect of the humerus, the placement of the transducer should be slightly under the scapular spine. The arm can then be externally rotated from a position of internal rotation. An HSL can be detected by a disruption that typically looks like a depression of the spherical humeral head [24]. The sensitivity of ultrasound has been measured to be between 74% and 96%, a specificity of 60 and 100%, and an accuracy of 91 and 97% in identifying an HSL. The interobserver reliability is relatively weak however. Regarding measuring the size of HSLs, ultrasound showed a sensitivity of 96%, specificity of 100%, and an accuracy of 97% [24, 26–28].

Computed Tomography (CT) Scans

Axial, coronal, and sagittal CT scans can detect and measure an HSL with the patient in a supine position and their arm in neutral rotation. Kodali et al. studied the accuracy of the CT measurement of the HSLs and found good (ICC of 0.88) inter-rater reliability for the depth measurement and moderate (ICC 0.72) inter-rater reliability for the width measurement. Individual observers were more accurate in depth rather than the width measurements [29]. Their study results suggest that the HSL depth can be reliably assessed using the standard CT scan (axial- or sagittal-planed).

The size of the HSL is measured on axial and coronal CT images where the largest size of the HSL is identified. A circle that includes the humeral articular surface is drawn on the axial CT image. The HSL width is defined as the distance between the medial and lateral end of the HSL located on the circle. The HSL depth is defined as the longest length between the base of the HSL and the corresponding arc. Each measurement will be divided by the humeral head diameter and recorded as a percentage (Fig. 5.3) [8, 14, 29].

The location of the lesion is essential to evaluate to determine if the HSL is "on-track" or "off-track." The glenoid track is the zone of contact between the posterosuperolateral portion of the humeral head and the glenoid. "Off-track" lesions extend over the medial border of the glenoid track (18.4 ± 2.5 mm medial from the footprint) and can lead to recurrent instability [7, 30]. A recent systemic review from Vopat et al. studies the image modalities to determine glenoid track in recurrent shoulder instability. Their group found evidence supporting the use of CT scan in accessing the glenoid track with high validity (sensitivity 92% and specificity 100%) and accuracy (96%) [31].

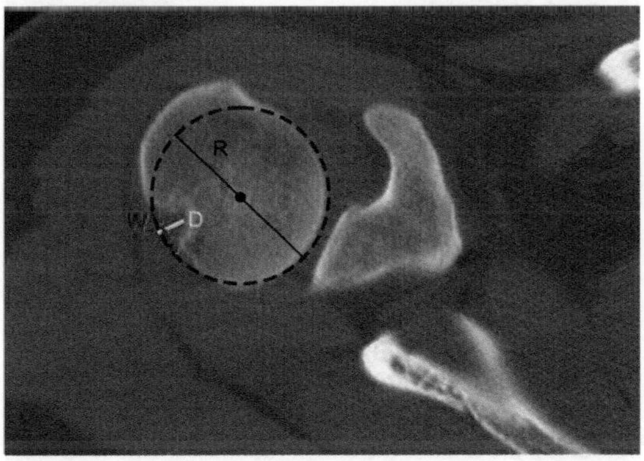

Fig. 5.3 The axial-image CT scan demonstrates how to measure the HSL width and depth. The HSL width (W) is defined as the distance between the medial and lateral end of the HSL, which is located on the circle. The HSL depth (D) is defined as the longest length between the base of the HSL and the corresponding arc. Each measurement will be divided by the humeral head diameter (2R) and recorded as a percentage

Computed Tomography Arthrogram (CTA)

Computed tomography arthrogram follows the same procedure as CT scans, but with the addition of a solution injected that contains an iodinated contrast. CTA median sensitivity was measured to be 94% (range, 50–100%), specificity ranged from 91% to 100%, and had a high median accuracy of 91% (range, 66 and 100%) [26, 32–36].

Three-Dimensional (3D) Reconstruction CT Scan

The 3D CT scans allow for a more accurate reconstruction of the bony anatomy of the shoulder and therefore is seen as the gold standard in imaging HSLs. The axial, coronal, and sagittal 2D CT scans are used to generate a 3D model using computer software [37]. The 3D CT scans have displayed interobserver and intraobserver reliabilities ranges that were almost perfect and moderate to almost perfect, respectively. In terms of HSL size, the sensitivity is 76.3%, the specificity is 100%, and the accuracy is 80.3%, with the interobserver and intraobserver reliabilities ranging from moderate to almost perfect and almost perfect, respectively [14, 38, 39].

Magnetic Resonance Imaging (MRI), MRA, and 3D MRI

MRI has been introduced to measure bone loss with the benefit of addressing the concomitant soft tissue pathologies and decreasing radiologic exposure. The range of sensitivity to HSL detection is 60–97%, specificity is 54%, and accuracy is 79–94%, with almost perfect interobserver reliability. Regarding HSL size, the interobserver reliability was weak to moderate, and the intraobserver reliability was almost perfect for length, moderate for the area, and minimal for depth [22, 35, 40–43]. Sgroi et al. compared the diagnostic precision and reliability of HSL measurement between CT scan and MRI. Their study showed the superiority of MRI in determining the Hill-Sachs interval (HSI); however, there was no difference in calculating the glenoid track or identifying off-track lesions [44]. Both CT and MRI are good imaging modalities to identify glenoid track and off-track lesions [31, 44].

MRA has a sensitivity ranging from 75% to 100%, specificity from 0 to 98%, and accuracy between 81% and 93%, with moderate interobserver reliability. In terms of the size of HSL, MRA displays strong intraobserver reliability [28, 36, 45–51].

The 3D MRIs use axial proton density (PD) fat-saturated (FS) turbo spin echo (TSE), coronal PD FS TSE, coronal T2 FS TSE, sagittal T2 TSE, sagittal T1 TSE, and axial T2 3D double-echo steady-state to recreate a three-dimensional osseous reconstruction. Literature has shown 3D MRI to be as accurate as the gold standard 3D CT, with the advantage of a lack of radiation exposure. But it is not practical to use in a clinical setting yet, due to the amount of time each reconstruction takes compared to a 3D CT scan [37].

The Emerging Technique Using an Advanced 3D Modeling Software

Recently, Golijanin et al. studied the characteristics of HSLs using the advanced 3D modeling software (MIMICS software, Materialise NV, Leuven, Belgium). All models were reconstructed from the patients' CT scan, and the volume, surface area (SA), width, and depth of identified HSLs were quantified along with their locations (medial, superior, and inferior extent) (Figs. 5.4 and 5.5) and HSL angles (Fig. 5.6). The result of their study showed that there was a direct association between the HSL location (medialization) and the HSL volume, position, and orientation. More medialized HSLs have a larger volume, greater width, more SA loss, higher lesion angles, and a more inferior position [15]. With this emerging technology, better quantified size, location, orientation, and impaction of the HSL can be addressed to study whether these parameters affect the risk of recurrent instability.

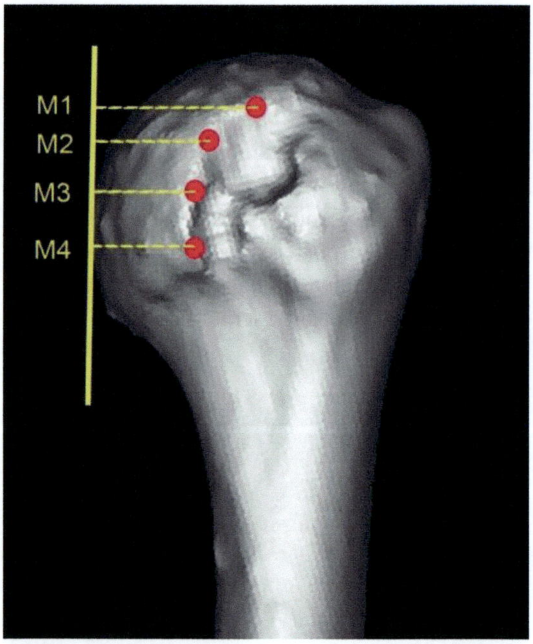

Fig. 5.4 The 3D image using the advanced 3D modeling software shows the measurement of the medialization of the HSL. Four points were measured at equidistant intervals along the total of the HSL. The most medialized HSL would be the smallest length of the medialization (M3)

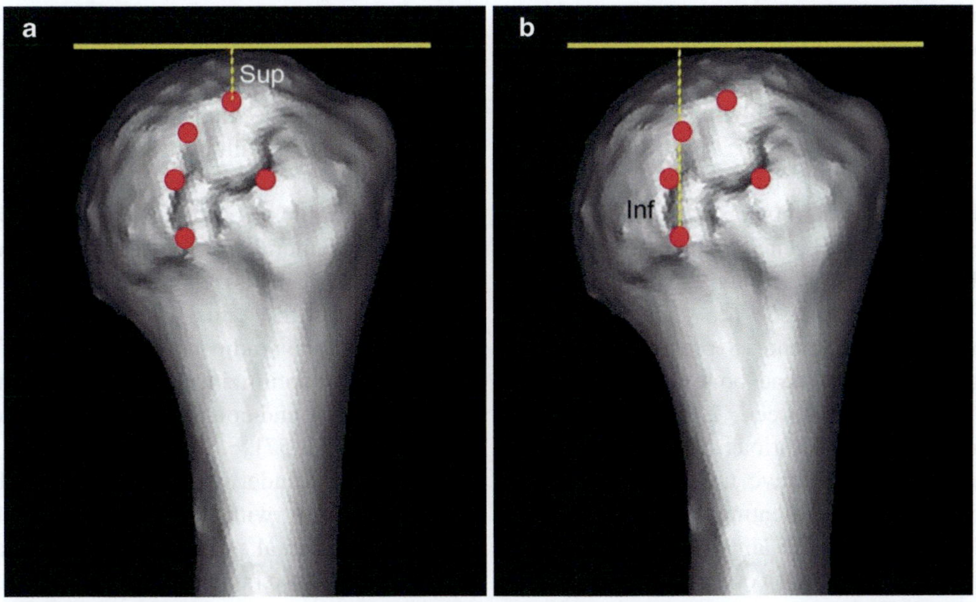

Fig. 5.5 The 3D image using the advanced 3D modeling software shows the measurement of the superior and inferior positions of the HSL. (**a**) The superior extent measurement is defined by the distance between a horizontal line that is orthogonal to the superior most portion of the humeral head and the most superior point of the HSL. (**b**) The inferior extension measures the distance from the previous horizontal line to the most inferior point of the HSL

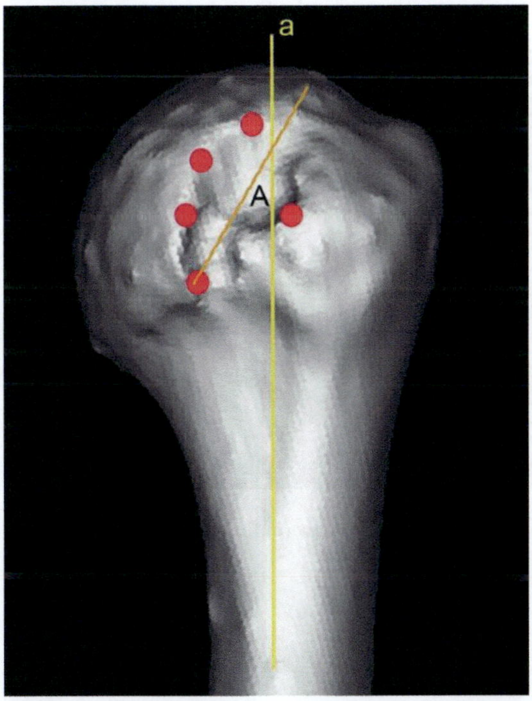

Fig. 5.6 The 3D image using the advanced 3D modeling software shows the measurement of the HS center angle (A). The HS center angled (HSLc) (A) is defined as the best fit line through the deepest aspect of the HSL and the humeral shaft diaphysis axis (a)

Surgical Management

Various HSL parameters such as size, location, and orientation increase the risk of recurrent instability in the current literature and need to be considered in treatment decision making [6, 12–14, 52]. It has been shown that patients with recurrent shoulder instability demonstrated deeper and larger HSLs [14, 52]. Kurokawa et al. reported two types of engaging or off-track lesions: (1) a large and wide type and (2) a narrow but medially located position. Medialization of the HSL is a risk factor for engagement even for a small HSL [12, 13]. Recently, Yamamoto et al. proposed a new concept, assessing on-track HSL lesions. They divided the lesion into the central-track lesion (<75% of HSL occupancy) and the peripheral-track lesion (≥75% of HSL occupancy). They found a lower functional outcome after arthroscopic Bankart repair in the peripheral-track group compared with the central-track group, $P = 0.03$ [53]. This study's result highlights the significance of HSL location (medialization) to treatment decision-making.

Orientation is another parameter that needs to be addressed preoperatively. Cho et al. demonstrated that the HS angle in an engaged lesion (25.6° ± 7.4°) was significantly higher than the nonengaged lesion (13.8° ± 6.2°), $P < 0.001$ [14].

Although there is no consensus as to how much bone loss is too much for the HSL defect, larger lesions have been associated with a higher number of instability events, as well as lesions that are "engaging" [2, 54]. Typically, nonoperative treatment is preferred in cases where the humeral head bone loss is less than 20%. However, between 20% and 40% of humeral bone loss, various patient factors will drive either nonoperative treatment or surgical options. Patients presenting with greater than 30–40% bone loss are almost always clinically significant and require an osteochondral allograft, a partial arthroplasty, or in severe cases, a hemiarthroplasty [2]. Many procedures have been proposed to treat HSLs, with the remplissage technique becoming more popular. Recently, bony augmentation has been shown to be successful in managing large HSLs. Osteoarticular humeral head allograft is a technically difficult procedure but allows for better restoration of the humeral head biomechanics [4, 18].

The fresh talus allograft has recently been proposed by Provencher et al. as an excellent alternative graft choice for anatomic reconstruction of the humeral head in recurrent shoulder instability [55]. This technique offers several advantages as the talus allograft has almost identical to the radius of curvature of the humeral head, optimizing restoration of humeral head sphericity and congruent arch of motion to the glenoid [56, 57].

This patient underwent the diagnostic shoulder arthroscopy with extensive debridement, open anterior labral repair with capsulorrhaphy, and open anatomic humeral reconstruction using a fresh talus allograft (sex-matched only). It is fixed with headless compression screws after a soak in platelet-rich plasma (PRP) from the patient. The postoperative radiographs are demonstrated in Fig. 5.7.

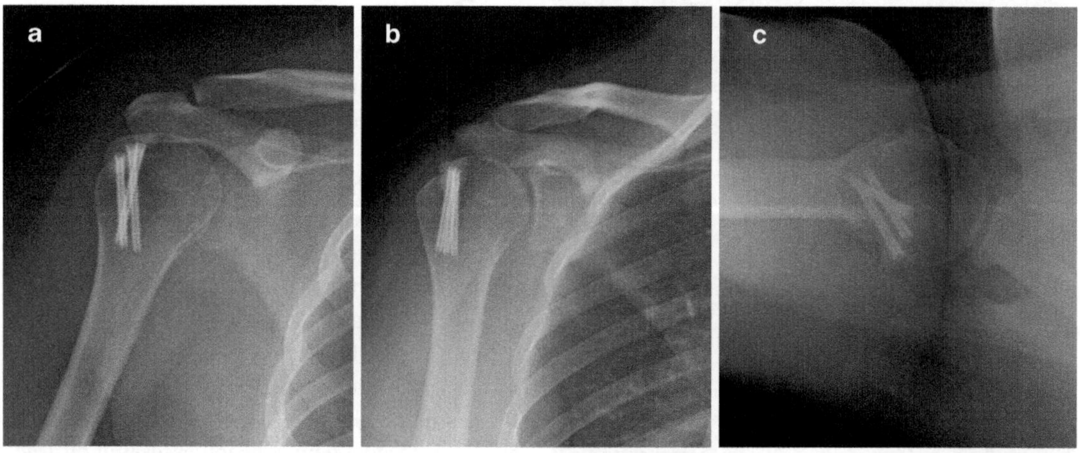

Fig. 5.7 Postoperative AP radiograph (**a**), Grashey view (**b**), and lateral axillary view (**c**) following anatomic humeral head reconstruction using a fresh talus allograft

Post-op After Open HSL Reconstruction

Postoperatively, the patient is instructed to place the shoulder in an abduction sling (neutral position) for the first 5 weeks and weaned off for 1 week after. Active-assist range of motion (ROM) is not allowed for the first 4 weeks, whereas passive flexion to 100° and 120° and external rotation (ER) to 30° and 60° are encouraged. Full passive ROM and active ROM are allowed at 5 weeks after surgery. Isometrics exercises are initiated at 3 weeks postoperatively, while the active ROM exercise (bench press series) and activities of daily living are allowed after 5 weeks postoperatively. Anterior capsule stretching is not allowed for the first 12 weeks. Between 4 and 6 months postoperatively, the patient is allowed to return to full, unrestricted activity.

References

1. Owens BD, Dawson L, Burks R, Cameron KL. Incidence of shoulder dislocation in the United States military: demographic considerations from a high-risk population. J Bone Joint Surg Am. 2009;91(4):791–6.
2. Kramer J, Gajudo G, Pandya NK. Risk of recurrent instability after arthroscopic stabilization for shoulder instability in adolescent patients. Orthop J Sports Med. 2019;7(9):2325967119868995.
3. Rutgers C, Verweij LPE, Priester-Vink S, van Deurzen DFP, Maas M, van den Bekerom MPJ. Recurrence in traumatic anterior shoulder dislocations increases the prevalence of Hill-Sachs and Bankart lesions: a systematic review and meta-analysis. Knee Surg Sports Traumatol Arthrosc. 2022;30(6):2130–40.
4. Provencher MT, Frank RM, Leclere LE, Metzger PD, Ryu JJ, Bernhardson A, et al. The Hill-Sachs lesion: diagnosis, classification, and management. J Am Acad Orthop Surg. 2012;20(4):242–52.
5. Burkhart SS, De Beer JF. Traumatic glenohumeral bone defects and their relationship to failure of arthroscopic Bankart repairs: significance of the inverted-pear glenoid and the humeral engaging Hill-Sachs lesion. Arthroscopy. 2000;16(7):677–94.
6. Di Giacomo G, Itoi E, Burkhart SS. Evolving concept of bipolar bone loss and the Hill-Sachs lesion: from "engaging/non-engaging" lesion to "on-track/off-track" lesion. Arthroscopy. 2014;30(1):90–8.
7. Yamamoto N, Itoi E, Abe H, Minagawa H, Seki N, Shimada Y, et al. Contact between the glenoid and the humeral head in abduction, external rotation, and horizontal extension: a new concept of glenoid track. J Shoulder Elb Surg. 2007;16(5):649–56.
8. Saliken DJ, Bornes TD, Bouliane MJ, Sheps DM, Beaupre LA. Imaging methods for quantifying glenoid and Hill-Sachs bone loss in traumatic instability of the shoulder: a scoping review. BMC Musculoskelet Disord. 2015;16:164.
9. Sommaire C, Penz C, Clavert P, Klouche S, Hardy P, Kempf JF. Recurrence after arthroscopic Bankart repair: is quantitative radiological analysis of bone loss of any predictive value? Orthop Traumatol Surg Res: OTSR. 2012;98(5):514–9.
10. Charousset C, Beauthier V, Bellaïche L, Guillin R, Brassart N, Thomazeau H. Can we improve radiological analysis of osseous lesions in chronic anterior shoulder instability? Orthop Traumatol Surg Res: OTSR. 2010;96(8 Suppl):S88–93.
11. França FO, Godinho A, Ribeiro E, Ranzzi A, Bittencourt BLL, Barreto BB. New quantitative method to measure the Hill-Sachs lesion: validation of Hardy's radiographic method for MRI/AMRI. Rev Bras Ortop. 2018;53(5):589–94.
12. Kurokawa D, Yamamoto N, Nagamoto H, Omori Y, Tanaka M, Sano H, et al. The prevalence of a large Hill-Sachs lesion that needs to be treated. J Shoulder Elb Surg. 2013;22(9):1285–9.
13. Gyftopoulos S, Yemin A, Beltran L, Babb J, Bencardino J. Engaging Hill-Sachs lesion: is there an association between this lesion and findings on MRI? AJR Am J Roentgenol. 2013;201(4):W633–8.
14. Cho SH, Cho NS, Rhee YG. Preoperative analysis of the Hill-Sachs lesion in anterior shoulder instability: how to predict engagement of the lesion. Am J Sports Med. 2011;39(11):2389–95.
15. Golijanin P, Peebles L, Arner JW, Douglass B, Peebles A, Rider D, et al. Advanced 3-dimensional characterization of hill-Sachs lesions in 100 anterior shoulder instability patients. Arthroscopy. 2021;37(11):3255–61.
16. Peebles LA, Golijanin P, Peebles AM, Douglass BW, Arner JW, Provencher MT. Glenoid bone loss directly Affects Hill-Sachs morphology: an advanced 3-dimensional analysis. Am J Sports Med. 2022;50(9):2469–75.
17. Kawakami J, Yamamoto N, Hatta T, Shinagawa K, Itoi E. In which arm position is a Hill-Sachs lesion created? Am J Sports Med. 2019;47(10):2464–8.
18. Fox JA, Sanchez A, Zajac TJ, Provencher MT. Understanding the Hill-Sachs lesion in its role in patients with recurrent anterior shoulder instability. Curr Rev Musculoskelet Med. 2017;10(4):469–79.
19. Brelin A, Dickens JF. Posterior shoulder instability. Sports Med Arthrosc Rev. 2017;25(3):136–43.
20. Owens BD, Duffey ML, Nelson BJ, DeBerardino TM, Taylor DC, Mountcastle SB. The incidence and characteristics of shoulder instability at the United States military academy. Am J Sports Med. 2007;35(7):1168–73.

21. Yiannakopoulos CK, Mataragas E, Antonogiannakis E. A comparison of the spectrum of intra-articular lesions in acute and chronic anterior shoulder instability. Arthroscopy. 2007;23(9):985–90.
22. Workman TL, Burkhard TK, Resnick D, Goff WB 2nd, Balsara ZN, Davis DJ, et al. Hill-Sachs lesion: comparison of detection with MR imaging, radiography, and arthroscopy. Radiology. 1992;185(3):847–52.
23. Charousset C, Beauthier V, Bellaiche L, Guillin R, Brassart N, Thomazeau H, et al. Can we improve radiological analysis of osseous lesions in chronic anterior shoulder instability? Orthop Traumatol Surg Res. 2010;96(8 Suppl):S88–93.
24. Cicak N, Bilic R, Delimar D. Hill-Sachs lesion in recurrent shoulder dislocation: sonographic detection. J Ultrasound Med. 1998;17(9):557–60.
25. Delage Royle A, Balg F, Bouliane MJ, Canet-Silvestri F, Garant-Saine L, Sheps DM, et al. Indication for computed tomography scan in shoulder instability: sensitivity and specificity of standard radiographs to predict bone defects after traumatic anterior Glenohumeral instability. Orthop J Sports Med. 2017;5(10):2325967117733660.
26. Farin PU, Kaukanen E, Jaroma H, Harju A, Vaatainen U. Hill-Sachs lesion: sonographic detection. Skeletal Radiol. 1996;25(6):559–62.
27. Pancione L, Gatti G, Mecozzi B. Diagnosis of Hill-Sachs lesion of the shoulder. Comparison between ultrasonography and arthro-CT. Acta Radiol. 1997;38(4 Pt 1):523–6.
28. Simao MN, Nogueira-Barbosa MH, Muglia VF, Barbieri CH. Anterior shoulder instability: correlation between magnetic resonance arthrography, ultrasound arthrography and intraoperative findings. Ultrasound Med Biol. 2012;38(4):551–60.
29. Kodali P, Jones MH, Polster J, Miniaci A, Fening SD. Accuracy of measurement of Hill-Sachs lesions with computed tomography. J Shoulder Elb Surg. 2011;20(8):1328–34.
30. Itoi E. 'On-track' and 'off-track' shoulder lesions. EFORT Open Rev. 2017;2(8):343–51.
31. Vopat ML, Hermanns CA, Midtgaard KS, Baker J, Coda RG, Cheema SG, et al. Imaging modalities for the glenoid track in recurrent shoulder instability: a systematic review. Orthop J Sports Med. 2021;9(6):23259671211006750.
32. Callaghan JJ, McNiesh LM, DeHaven JP, Savory CG, Polly DW Jr. A prospective comparison study of double contrast computed tomography (CT) arthrography and arthroscopy of the shoulder. Am J Sports Med. 1988;16(1):13–20.
33. Fanelli GP, D'Erme M, Francioso A, Flecca D, La Barbera L, Martinelli M, et al. 64-slice MDCT arthrography in shoulder instability: our experience. Radiol Med. 2007;112(4):572–80.
34. Fogerty S, King DG, Groves C, Scally A, Chandramohan M. Interobserver variation in reporting CT arthrograms of the shoulder. Eur J Radiol. 2011;80(3):811–3.
35. AH J Jr, Petersen SA, Neumann C, Steinbach L, Morgan F. A prospective comparison of computerized arthrotomography and magnetic resonance imaging of the glenohumeral joint. Am J Sports Med. 1992;20(6):695–700; discussion -1.
36. Oh JH, Kim JY, Choi JA, Kim WS. Effectiveness of multidetector computed tomography arthrography for the diagnosis of shoulder pathology: comparison with magnetic resonance imaging with arthroscopic correlation. J Shoulder Elb Surg. 2010;19(1):14–20.
37. Stillwater L, Koenig J, Maycher B, Davidson M. 3D-MR vs. 3D-CT of the shoulder in patients with glenohumeral instability. Skeletal Radiol. 2017;46(3):325–31.
38. Ho A, Kurdziel MD, Koueiter DM, Wiater JM. Three-dimensional computed tomography measurement accuracy of varying Hill-Sachs lesion size. J Shoulder Elb Surg. 2018;27(2):350–6.
39. Ozaki R, Nakagawa S, Mizuno N, Mae T, Yoneda M. Hill-sachs lesions in shoulders with traumatic anterior instability: evaluation using computed tomography with 3-dimensional reconstruction. Am J Sports Med. 2014;42(11):2597–605.
40. Denti M, Monteleone M, Trevisan C, De Romedis B, Barmettler F. Magnetic resonance imaging versus arthroscopy for the investigation of the osteochondral humeral defect in anterior shoulder instability. A double-blind prospective study. Knee Surg Sports Traumatol Arthrosc. 1995;3(3):184–6.
41. Hayes ML, Collins MS, Morgan JA, Wenger DE, Dahm DL. Efficacy of diagnostic magnetic resonance imaging for articular cartilage lesions of the glenohumeral joint in patients with instability. Skeletal Radiol. 2010;39(12):1199–204.
42. Kirkley A, Litchfield R, Thain L, Spouge A. Agreement between magnetic resonance imaging and arthroscopic evaluation of the shoulder joint in primary anterior dislocation of the shoulder. Clin J Sport Med. 2003;13(3):148–51.
43. Suder PA, Frich LH, Hougaard K, Lundorf E, Wulff JB. Magnetic resonance imaging evaluation of capsulolabral tears after traumatic primary anterior shoulder dislocation. A prospective comparison with arthroscopy of 25 cases. J Shoulder Elb Surg. 1995;4(6):419–28.
44. Sgroi M, Huzurudin H, Ludwig M, Dornacher D, Reichel H, Kappe T. With the exception of the Hill-Sachs interval, CT and MRI show no significant differences in the diagnostic value of the HSL measurement regardless of the measurement technique. Knee Surg Sports Traumatol Arthrosc. 2021;29(12):3981–8.
45. Chauvin NA, Jaimes C, Ho-Fung V, Wells L, Ganley T, Jaramillo D. Diagnostic performance of magnetic resonance arthrography of the shoulder in children. Pediatr Radiol. 2013;43(10):1309–15.
46. O'Brien J, Grebenyuk J, Leith J, Forster BB. Frequency of glenoid chondral lesions on MR arthrography in patients with anterior shoulder instability. Eur J Radiol. 2012;81(11):3461–5.

47. Probyn LJ, White LM, Salonen DC, Tomlinson G, Boynton EL. Recurrent symptoms after shoulder instability repair: direct MR arthrographic assessment–correlation with second-look surgical evaluation. Radiology. 2007;245(3):814–23.
48. Saqib R, Harris J, Funk L. Comparison of magnetic resonance arthrography with arthroscopy for imaging of shoulder injuries: retrospective study. Ann R Coll Surg Engl. 2017;99(4):271–4.
49. Tirman PF, Stauffer AE, Crues JV 3rd, Turner RM, Nottage WM, Schobert WE, et al. Saline magnetic resonance arthrography in the evaluation of glenohumeral instability. Arthroscopy. 1993;9(5):550–9.
50. van Grinsven S, Kesselring FO, van Wassenaer-van Hall HN, Lindeboom R, Lucas C, van Loon CJ. MR arthrography of traumatic anterior shoulder lesions showed modest reproducibility and accuracy when evaluated under clinical circumstances. Arch Orthop Trauma Surg. 2007;127(1):11–7.
51. Willemsen UF, Wiedemann E, Brunner U, Scheck R, Pfluger T, Kueffer G, et al. Prospective evaluation of MR arthrography performed with high-volume intraarticular saline enhancement in patients with recurrent anterior dislocations of the shoulder. AJR Am J Roentgenol. 1998;170(1):79–84.
52. Matsumura N, Oki S, Kitashiro M, Minemoto M, Ichikawa T, Matsumoto M, et al. Three-dimensional quantitative analysis of humeral head and glenoid bone defects with recurrent glenohumeral instability. J Shoulder Elb Surg. 2017;26(9):1662–9.
53. Yamamoto N, Shinagawa K, Hatta T, Itoi E. Peripheral-track and central-Track Hill-Sachs lesions: a new concept of assessing an on-track lesion. Am J Sports Med. 2020;48(1):33–8.
54. Valencia Mora M, Ruiz-Iban MA, Heredia JD, Ruiz Diaz R, Cuellar R. Management of humeral defects in anterior shoulder instability. Open Orthop J. 2017;11:1011–22.
55. Provencher MT, Sanchez G, Schantz K, Ferrari M, Sanchez A, Frangiamore S, et al. Anatomic humeral head reconstruction with fresh Osteochondral talus allograft for recurrent Glenohumeral instability with reverse hill-Sachs lesion. Arthrosc Tech. 2017;6(1):e255–e61.
56. Chan CM, LeVasseur MR, Lerner AL, Maloney MD, Voloshin I. Computer modeling analysis of the Talar dome as a graft for the humeral head. Arthroscopy. 2016;32(8):1671–5.
57. Griswold BG, Paré DW, Herzwurm ZP, Murphy CS, Morpeth BG, Provencher MT, et al. Utility of allograft talus as a source for grafting of concurrent humeral and glenoid defects associated with anterior Glenohumeral instability: an anthropometric analysis. Arthroscopy. 2021;37(3):845–51.

Part II

Anterior Shoulder Instability

The Bankart Repair in Lateral Decubitus: Indications, Technique, and Limits

6

Mark Getelman and Jonathan Erickson

Introduction

The glenohumeral joint is the most mobile major joint in the human body and affords excellent range of motion in all planes. Stability of the joint relies on a complex interplay between bony contact and the surrounding dynamic and static stabilizers. Limited bony congruency due to the relatively small size of the glenoid in comparison to the humeral head requires an intact capsulolabral complex for maintenance of glenohumeral joint stability. Imbalance caused by injury or excessive ligamentous laxity makes the shoulder joint the most frequently dislocated joint in the body with a reported incidence of 1.7%, with anterior instability being much more common than posterior [1]. Risk factors for shoulder instability include male sex, younger age, and higher activity levels [2]. Many factors are considered when determining the most appropriate management of shoulder instability, and controversy still exists with regard to first time dislocators. Primary shoulder stabilization may be considered for patients with high risk of recurrence or for elite athletes [3]. However, in many cases, surgical repair is only performed after a patient develops recurrent instability. Even with the many advances in arthroscopic management, enhanced imaging modalities, and better recognition of important pathology, selecting the appropriate patient for arthroscopic management is paramount to success. For patients with glenoid bone loss, there may be an unacceptable risk of recurrent instability, even with proper technique [4]. This chapter focuses on the arthroscopic Bankart repair for patients without glenoid bone loss performed in the lateral decubitus position and is just one technique available in the armamentarium of the shoulder specialist to appropriately manage the spectrum of shoulder instability.

Indications

A careful history and physical examination is the cornerstone to determining appropriate surgical indications. The diagnosis may be more obvious in the case of a frank dislocation requiring reduction on the athletic field or in the emergency department. However, some patients may have a much more subtle presentation with symptoms of pain, apprehension, activity avoidance, and minor subluxation events.

The physical exam is crucial in guiding treatment. Both shoulders are visualized for abnormal contour and atrophy, and the scapulothoracic contribution to motion is visualized. Range of motion is tested in both the upright and supine positions. Supine motion allows for scapular sta-

M. Getelman (✉) · J. Erickson
Southern California Orthopedic Institute,
Van Nuys, CA, USA
e-mail: mgetelman@scoi.com

© The Author(s), under exclusive license to Springer Nature Switzerland AG 2026
R. M. Frank, J. M. Tokish (eds.), *Management of Shoulder Instability*,
https://doi.org/10.1007/978-3-032-18089-6_6

bilization on the exam table for a more accurate assessment of the glenohumeral contribution to motion. Many physical exam maneuvers have been described, and we point out several key exam techniques of the shoulder when testing for anterior shoulder instability. For example, the apprehension/relocation test remains a crucial diagnostic tool that often recreates feelings of instability. Load and shift testing is also important and is always performed in the lateral position. This allows the patient to relax with the arm fully supported by the examiner, allowing it to be additionally performed under anesthesia just prior to surgical intervention.

Controversy still exists with regard to appropriate management of anterior shoulder instability. Much of the controversy exists around risk factors for instability recurrence and the appropriate surgical procedure, especially when considering young and active patients [5]. Many studies focus primarily on bone loss, but others have others shifted to patient specific risk factors such as age, gender, high risk sports, number of lifetime dislocations, and previous surgical interventions. It is also important to consider the glenoid track as on-track versus off-track lesions may be instrumental in guiding surgical planning. Given all the factors to consider, no definitive algorithm has been universally accepted.

Glenoid bone loss has been the most studied risk factor for recurrent dislocation and, along with glenoid track evaluation, is a good starting point when indicating an appropriate surgical procedure. In patients with minimal or no bone loss and on-track lesions, a Bankart repair is often the procedure of choice. The following is a preferred surgical technique for an arthroscopic Bankart repair with capsular plication in the lateral decubitus position.

Case Presentation

A 17-year-old male was injured making a tackle in a high school football game and sustained an anterior glenohumeral dislocation of his dominant right shoulder. He was reduced in the emergency department, and followed up 1 week later in orthopedic surgery, presenting in a sling. His pertinent examination findings included demonstration of positive apprehension in the abducted externally rotated position, with significant guarding. He had slightly decreased strength in external rotation. He did not display signs of hyperlaxity and was neurovascularly intact.

X-rays after reduction were normal, without evidence of a bony abnormality at the glenoid or a Hill-Sachs lesion on X-ray. The patient did get an MRI of the R shoulder. This showed a Bankart lesion on the axial and coronal imaging, without significant bone loss. There was edema in the posterosuperior humeral head, but with no significant Hill-Sachs depression.

Given the fact that this patient is a young male contact athlete with an anterior dislocation, he was deemed at a high risk for recurrence with nonoperative management. After a discussion with he and his parents, the patient and parents elected to go forward with surgical intervention. Given that this patient presented with a relatively isolated Bankart lesion without bone loss, it was felt that he would be an excellent candidate for an arthroscopic Bankart procedure.

Surgical Technique

The surgery is performed in the lateral decubitus position. The patient is placed laterally on a bean bag evacuation device with an axillary roll to protect the brachial plexus. The patient is allowed to roll back approximately 20 to 30 degrees to the keep the glenoid parallel to the floor. The knees and hips are flexed to stabilize the pelvis. The dependent lateral femoral cutaneous and peroneal nerves should be padded for protection. The bean bag is then evacuated.

A complete and thorough examination under anesthesia is performed, assessing forward elevation, abduction, and humeral rotation in adduction and in 90 degrees of abduction. A load and shift exam is then performed testing anterior, posterior, and inferior instability along with sulcus testing to assess the instability pattern. A shoulder positioner is used to place the arm in 70 degrees of abduction and 10 degrees of forward flexion.

The shoulder is draped in the standard fashion, and bony landmarks are drawn with a surgical marking pen. Correct portal placement is crucial for successful instability surgery. The standard posterior portal often lies 1 cm medial and 2 cm inferior to the posterior lateral acromial corner. However, in cases of shoulder instability, the incision is moved approximately 5 mm more superior and lateral to allow for a better trajectory when posterior labral work may be required. The anterior superior portal (ASP) is then established using an 18-gauge spinal needle in an outside-in fashion. This portal is typically made immediately adjacent to the anterior lateral corner of the acromion. The spinal needle pierces the rotator interval adjacent to the leading edge of the supraspinatus immediately behind the long head biceps. This high anterior portal is made close to, but without damaging the leading edge of the supraspinatus (Fig. 6.1). This helps avoid crowding within the rotator interval after the additional anterior mid glenoid working portal is created.

For all shoulder arthroscopy cases, a standard 15-point diagnostic exam is then completed documenting each point of pathology and confirming the surgical plan [6]. After the exam, the anterior mid glenoid (AMG) portal is then created. Prior to repair, the humeral head often sits subluxated anteriorly and inferiorly (Fig. 6.2). It is important to have the assistant apply a posteriorly directed force to center the humeral head on the glenoid prior to making this portal. Failure to reduce the head prior to making this portal may negatively impact trajectory for later anchor placement. The spinal needle is again used as a guide to verify trajectory. The needle is inserted in an outside-in fashion lateral to the coracoid and just superior to the subscapularis tendon. Ideally, the needle enters the joint just superior to the subscapularis and will easily reach the 5:30 position (Fig. 6.3). A working cannula of 7 mm or greater diameter is directed inferiorly and inserted into this portal.

For an isolated Bankart repair, the ASP is the primary viewing portal, and the AMG portal is the primary working portal. The arthroscope can be positioned posterior to the biceps while viewing from the ASP to avoid crowding the anterior working cannula. A 5-mm cannula is then placed in the posterior portal and is primarily used for shuttling sutures. On occasion, it is easier to make the inferior-most suture pass from the posterior side, and in those cases, an additional 7-mm cannula can be placed posteriorly to allow for better circumferential access.

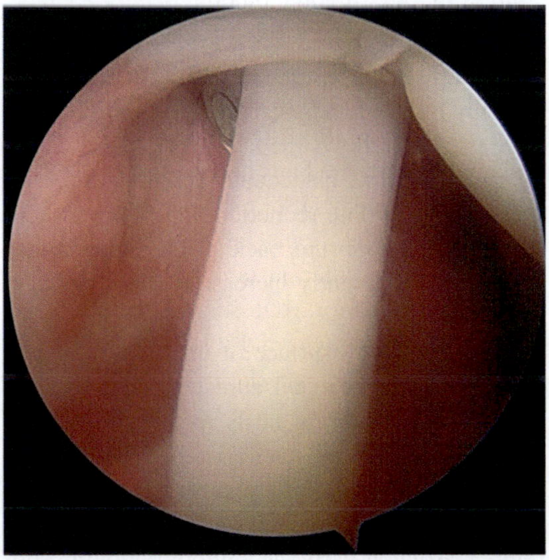

Fig. 6.1 The anterior superior portal (ASP) is established using outside-in technique

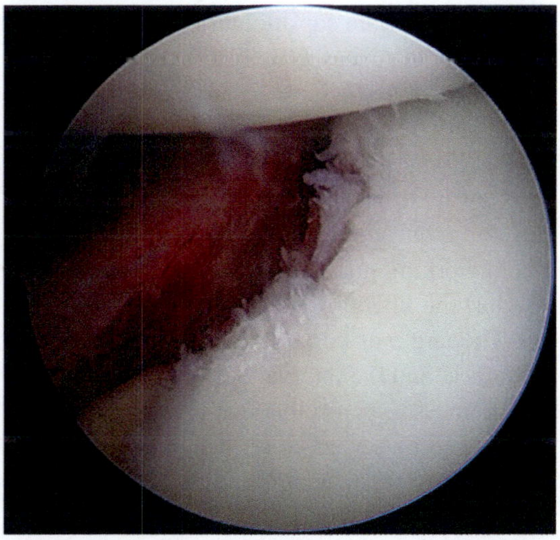

Fig. 6.2 Prior to Bankart repair, the humeral head will often sit subluxated anterior and inferior relative to the glenoid

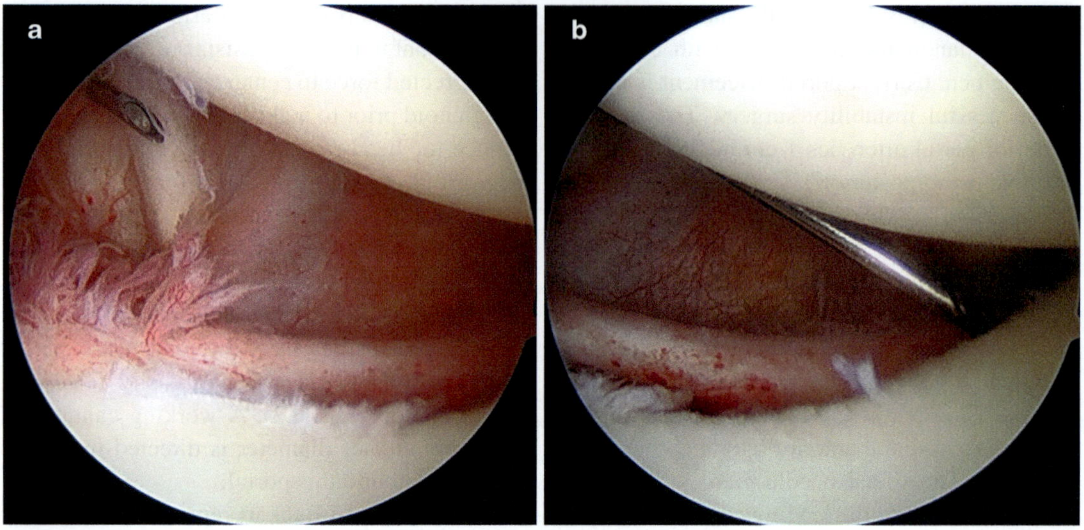

Fig. 6.3 (**a**) The anterior mid-glenoid (AMG) portal is established using the outside-in technique. (**b**) With the humeral head centered on the glenoid, a spinal needle is used to verify trajectory for later anchor placement

In most patients with chronic and recurrent anterior instability, the labrum and capsule have been torn from their anatomic position and heal medially on the glenoid neck. This disrupts the function of the labrum and often causes the humeral head to sit in an anterior and inferior subluxated position. The primary goal of a Bankart repair and capsular plication is to recenter the humeral head on the glenoid face and restore appropriate capsulolabral tension.

In order to successfully repair the labrum, the capsulolabral tissue must be advanced from inferior to superior and from medial to lateral. To do so, the tissue must first be appropriately mobilized away from the glenoid neck. A liberator elevator is introduced through the anterior midglenoid working portal. Working from superior to inferior, the liberator is used in a stepwise fashion. The angle of curve is faced toward the glenoid neck, and the interval between the bone and labrum must be carefully developed. Usually, the labrum can be separated with standard pressure, but on occasion, a small tap with the palm of the hand may be required to initially separate the labrum from the glenoid neck (Fig. 6.4). The sides of the liberator are also sharp, so care must be taken to avoid violating the labral border. After the plane is developed, the liberator elevator is exchanged for a blunted large Steinman pin on a chuck handle. This is used like a crow bar as a blunt dissection tool and a lever. By anchoring the distal end of the Steinmann pin along the medial glenoid neck, the adherent capsule can be levered away from the medial glenoid without risk of tool breakage or damage from the sharp edges of the liberator. Adhesions can then be released, and the labrum and capsule will become progressively more mobile. Adequate release is confirmed when the muscle fibers of the subscapularis are visualized (Fig. 6.5). Appropriate mobilization can also be seen with the pump pressure reduced and suction turned on. The negative pressure allows the labrum to "float" to the glenoid margin. Inadequate mobilization will prevent appropriate reduction and improper tensioning of the labrum back to the glenoid face and will subsequently increase the risk of instability recurrence.

Next, the bony surface of the glenoid is prepared using mechanical abrasion with a shaver and rasp. The labrum heals to a well-prepared bony surface and will not heal well to cartilage. A curette is then used to expose the peripheral medial glenoid rim (Fig. 6.6). Be careful to only remove articular cartilage without removing subchondral bone which may compromise later

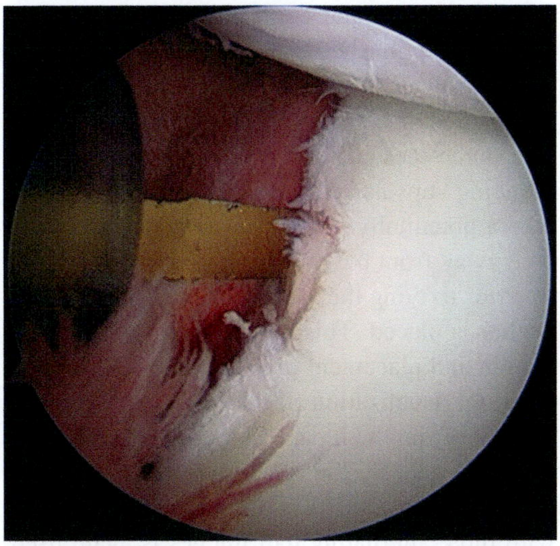

Fig. 6.4 The use of a liberator knife to separate the labrum from the glenoid neck

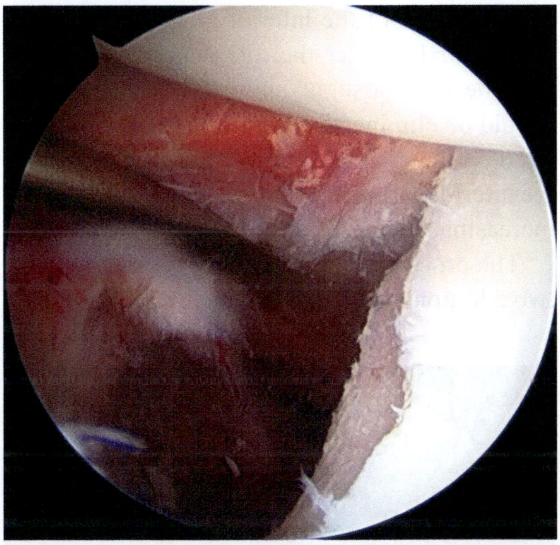

Fig. 6.5 The use of a Steinmann pin as a blunt dissection tool. Adequate release is confirmed with visualization of the subscapularis muscle fibers

anchor fixation. This step ensures the best opportunity for the labrum to heal to the glenoid face rather than adjacent to it.

The first anchor pilot hole is made at approximately the 5:30 position using a curved drill guide. Many suture anchor options are available, though preferred anchors are small, typically less than 3.5 mm, and are double loaded with #2 high tensile suture. Optimizing anchor

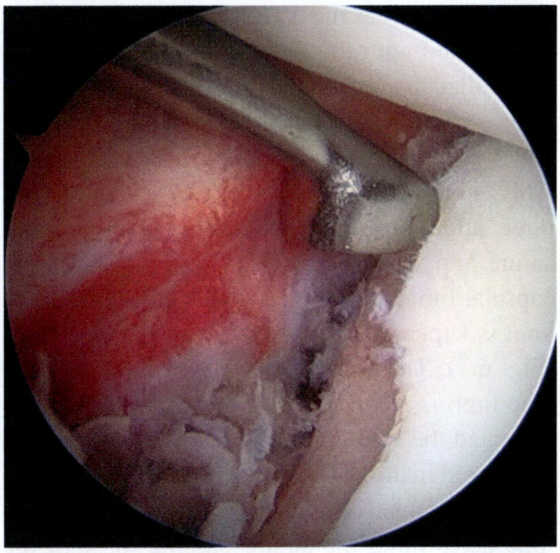

Fig. 6.6 Small curette removing 1 to 2 mm of the articular cartilage on the glenoid face

position is important, but an exact 6 o'clock anchor is not mandatory in all cases. The anchor is placed on the glenoid face near the edge to allow for appropriate lateral and superior advancement of the capsulolabral tissue. The more inferior 6 to 6:30 o'clock capsular tissue can be mobilized and advanced to the anchor at the 5:30 position. Using a double-loaded instead of a single-loaded suture anchor allows for added points of fixation at each drill hole. Double-loaded anchors also allow the capsule and labrum to be tensioned independently, creating the strongest repair construct.

After the double-loaded suture anchor is placed, the sutures can be stored outside the cannula, and a shuttling technique is used. It is critical to advance the capsulolabral tissue from inferior to superior, so it is often best to make the first capsular pass from the posterior portal. Retrieve the most inferior suture on the labral side through the anterior cannula. A 45-degree suture hook loaded with #1 PDS or other shuttling device is then used to penetrate the capsule 1 to 1.5 cm inferior to the anchor depending on the amount of inferior to superior shift required. The capsular tissue is penetrated, and the suture hook exits below the labrum inferior to the anchor. The shuttle is advanced and retrieved with a grasper out the AMG portal. The shuttle is then loaded with the previously retrieved suture and pulled back through the posterior cannula. The suture that is now in the posterior cannula, and the partner stitch can be retrieved through the AMG portal. A sliding-locking SMC knot with three alternating half hitches secures the first suture in place. The post is always placed on the capsular limb of the suture which ensures that the knot is kept well away from the glenoid surface (Fig. 6.7). The second suture is now addressed. One limb is retrieved back out the anterior cannula, and the suture to be passed is now retrieved and stored in the posterior cannula. A similar process is completed with the second suture, this time performing the suture passing through the AMG portal. There may be residual capsular redundancy after the first suture is tied. For the second pass, a plication technique is used to titrate the capsular volume. Therefore, the 45-degree suture hook is used in a pinch-tuck fashion to plicate and reduce the capsular volume. To complete the pinch-tuck method, the capsule is first independently pierced in a through and through fashion. The amount of capsule taken can be adjusted according to the amount of volume reduction desired. The suture hook is then passed beneath the labrum before the shuttling suture is advanced. This technique has been deemed the hospital corner repair and has been previously published [7]. The shuttling suture is then retrieved, loaded in the posterior cannula, and pulled back through the anterior cannula. The pinch-tuck method does an excellent job at reducing capsular redundancy without having to take a potentially dangerous deep bite and stays well away from the axillary nerve.

Prior to tying the second suture limb, the next anchor is placed. This allows for optimal visualization and placement of the next anchor without limiting visualization of the more proximal glenoid rim from the repair (Fig. 6.8). After the next anchor is placed, the remaining suture from the prior anchor is tied. A sliding-locking SMC knot with three alternating half hitches is again used. As the knot is tightened the labrum and inferior capsule will be advanced superiorly. This creates a robust repair, or bumper, and restores the appropriate tension of the inferior glenohumeral ligament (IGHL). After the first anchor sutures are tied, the anterior subluxation of the humeral head should be eliminated with the humeral head centered on the glenoid. If not, there is concern that the inferior capsular tension has not been restored, increasing the risk of recurrence.

The process is repeated, in general by placing two additional anchors with the goal of placing a

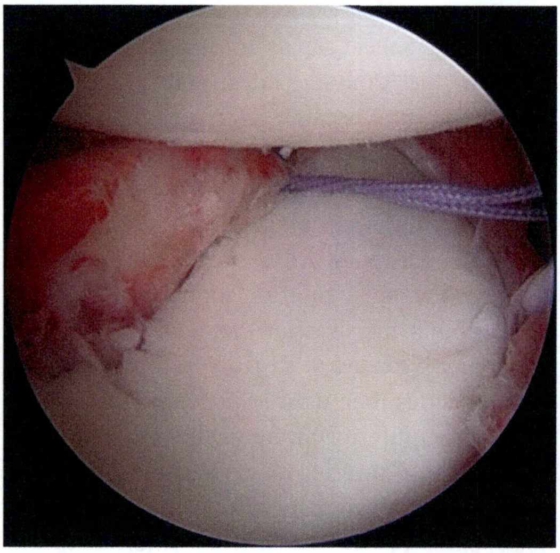

Fig. 6.7 First suture limb is tied down. The knot is well away from the glenoid face

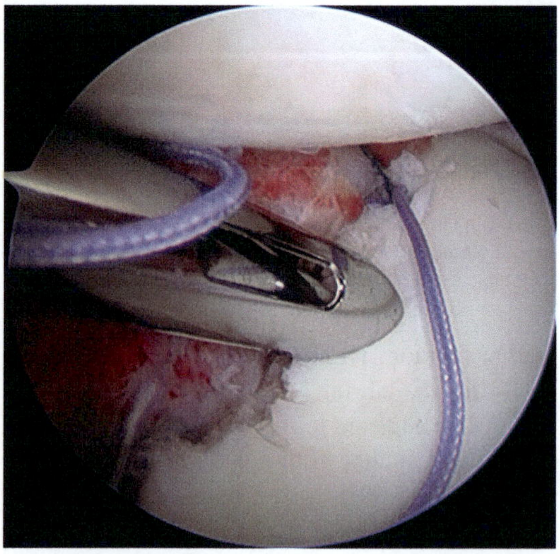

Fig. 6.8 Insert more proximal suture anchor before tying the second suture of inferior anchor to achieve ideal position with improved visualization

total of three anchors below the equator of the glenoid often in the 3, 4:30, and 5:30 to 6 o'clock positions.

After completion of the repair, the humeral head should be centered on the glenoid face with balanced tension of the anterior and posterior bands of the IGHL (Fig. 6.9). The completed hospital corner repair restores capsular tension, reduces excessive volume, and advances the disrupted labrum from inferior and medial to its anatomic position that is more superior and lateral on the glenoid face. The first stitch of each respective anchor secures the labrum, and the second stitch addresses capsular redundancy and provides additional labral fixation. The completed Bankart repair anatomically reduces the labrum, provides multiple points of fixation, reduces capsular redundancy, and appropriately restores its chock-block function (Fig. 6.10).

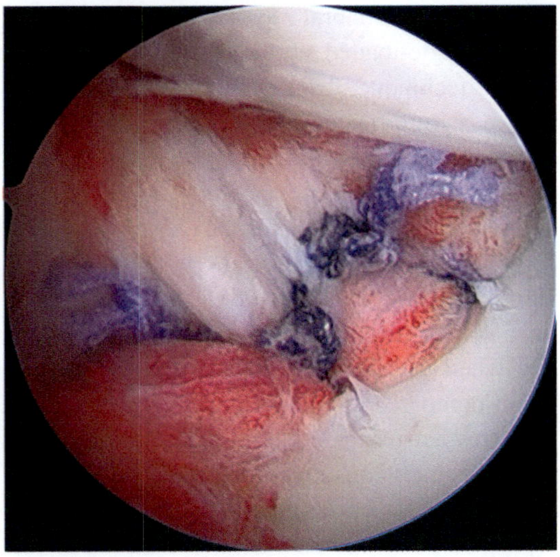

Fig. 6.10 Completed Bankart repair

Discussion/Limitations

Management of shoulder instability is complex. Appropriate patient selection and surgical indications are crucial to a successful outcome. This chapter provides only a basic template for patient selection but a detailed description of the Bankart repair itself. To have successful outcomes surgeons must also identify and treat concomitant pathology with additional techniques as discussed in subsequent chapters, including remplissage as needed. The principles remain the same when adding a remplissage, but the order of incorporation changes. It is recommended that the Bankart lesion be mobilized and the glenoid prepared first. The remplissage preparation, anchor insertion, and suture passing are then completed but not tied or tensioned. Tensioning the remplissage sutures ahead of the Bankart repair may limit visualization and could compromise the Bankart advancement. The Bankart repair is then completed, and the remplissage sutures are subsequently tied blind or visualized via a subacromial approach as the final step of the repair.

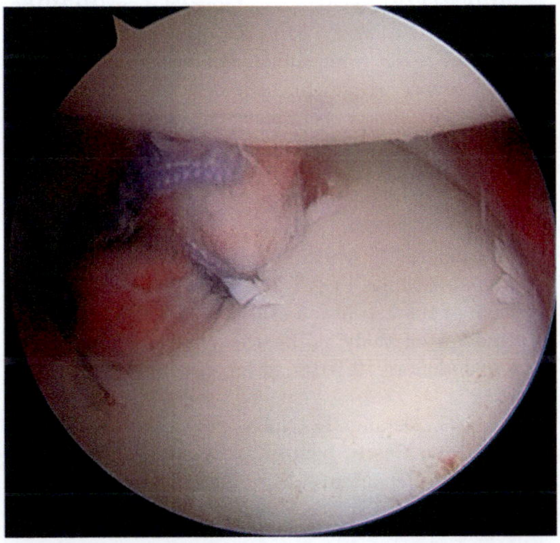

Fig. 6.9 The humeral head should be centered on the glenoid face after completion of the repair

The arthroscopic Bankart repair is a commonly utilized procedure when treating anterior shoulder instability. Although open and arthroscopic techniques have been described, there continues to be trend toward arthroscopic techniques for appropriately selected patients. Clinical outcomes and recurrence rates have been shown to be similar using both techniques [8]. However, arthroscopic repair has been associated with reduced surgical time, better cosmesis, faster recovery, and improved ability to identify and treat additional intra-articular pathology [9].

Arthroscopic labral repair may be performed with a single-loaded suture anchor or a knotless anchor technique. Our technique uses double-loaded suture anchors and arthroscopic knot tying. This allows preferential repair of the labrum to its anatomic position with the first suture limb and plication of the capsule and reinforcement of the labral repair with the second suture limb. Cadaveric biomechanical studies have shown that forces are higher at the repair site when capsular plication is added to labral repair compared to a labral repair alone [10]. We theorize that using a double-loaded anchor creates a stronger construct more resistant to failure by better distributing the stresses across the repair. Stability has been shown to increase with the number of anchors used, but this may also increase the risk of a postage stamp fracture, particularly in young, active male patients [11].

Depending on surgeon preference, shoulder instability can be managed in beach chair or lateral decubitus positions. Our preference is the lateral position as it affords the best visualization and access to the inferior glenoid and capsule. Recent evidence has shown that surgeons utilizing the lateral position placed anchors in the 6 o'clock position more frequently than their beach chair counterparts [12]. In addition, systematic reviews have shown the risk of recurrent instability to be lower in the lateral position when compared to beach chair [13].

Limitations of our technique include a more technically demanding procedure that requires more advanced suture management, advanced suture hook maneuvering (pinch-tuck), arthroscopic knot tying, and requisite increased surgical time. Also, for those not accustomed to the lateral position, setup, orientation, visualization, and manipulation require a learning curve.

The surgeon has many options for treating shoulder instability. This chapter demonstrates the Bankart repair in the lateral decubitus position and is just one technique in the armamentarium of the shoulder specialist to appropriately manage the spectrum of shoulder instability.

References

1. Hovelius L. Incidence of shoulder dislocation in Sweden. Clin Orthop Relat Res. 1982;166:127–31.
2. Gibbs DB, Lynch TS, Nuber ED, Nuber GW. Common shoulder injuries in American football athletes. Curr Sports Med Rep. 2015;14(5):413–9. https://doi.org/10.1249/JSR.0000000000000190. PMID: 26359844.
3. Dickens JF, Rue JP, Cameron KL, Tokish JM, Peck KY, Allred CD, Svoboda SJ, Sullivan R, Kilcoyne KG, Owens BD. Successful return to sport after arthroscopic shoulder stabilization versus nonoperative management in contact athletes with anterior shoulder instability: a prospective multicenter study. Am J Sports Med. 2017;45(11):2540–6. https://doi.org/10.1177/0363546517712505. Epub 2017 Jun 28. PMID: 28657778.
4. Torrance E, Clarke CJ, Monga P, Funk L, Walton MJ. Recurrence after arthroscopic labral repair for traumatic anterior instability in adolescent rugby and contact athletes. Am J Sports Med. 2018;46(12):2969–74. https://doi.org/10.1177/0363546518794673. Epub 2018 Sep 10. PMID: 30198752.
5. Bottoni CR, Wilckens JH, DeBerardino TM, D'Alleyrand JC, Rooney RC, Harpstrite JK, Arciero RA. A prospective, randomized evaluation of arthroscopic stabilization versus nonoperative treatment in patients with acute, traumatic, first-time shoulder dislocations. Am J Sports Med. 2002;30(4):576–80. https://doi.org/10.1177/03635465020300041801. PMID: 12130413.
6. Snyder SJ, Fasulo GJ. Shoulder arthroscopy: surgical technique. Surg Technol Int. 1993;2:447–53. PMID: 25951601.
7. Wang DW, Getelman MH. "Hospital-corner repair" for shoulder instability. Arthroscopy. 2010;26(12):1706–9. https://doi.org/10.1016/j.arthro.2010.08.009. PMID: 21112479.
8. Bottoni CR, Smith EL, Berkowitz MJ, Towle RB, Moore JH. Arthroscopic versus open shoulder stabilization for recurrent anterior instability: a prospective randomized clinical trial. Am J Sports Med. 2006;34(11):1730–7. https://doi.org/10.1177/0363546506288239. Epub 2006 May 30. PMID: 16735589.
9. Fabbriciani C, Milano G, Demontis A, Fadda S, Ziranu F, Mulas PD. Arthroscopic versus open treatment of Bankart lesion of the shoulder: a prospective randomized study. Arthroscopy. 2004;20(5):456–62. https://doi.org/10.1016/j.arthro.2004.03.001. PMID: 15122134.
10. Penna J, Deramo D, Nelson CO, Sileo MJ, Levin SM, Tompkins B, Ianuzzi A. Determination of anterior labral repair stress during passive arm motion in

a cadaveric model. Arthroscopy. 2008;24(8):930–5. https://doi.org/10.1016/j.arthro.2008.03.010. Epub 2008 May 15. PMID: 18657742.

11. Woolnough T, Shah A, Sheean AJ, Lesniak BP, Wong I, de Sa D. "Postage stamp" fractures: a systematic review of patient and suture anchor profiles causing anterior glenoid rim fractures after Bankart repair. Arthroscopy. 2019;35(8):2501–2508.e2. https://doi.org/10.1016/j.arthro.2019.02.047. PMID: 31395192.
12. Baron JE, Duchman KR, Hettrich CM, Glass NA, Ortiz SF, MOON Shoulder Group, Baumgarten KM, Bishop JY, Bollier MJ, Bravman JT, Brophy RH, Carpenter JE, Cox CL, Feeley BT, Frank RM, Grant JA, Jones GL, Kuhn JE, Lansdown DA, Benjamin Ma C, Marx RG, McCarty EC, Miller BS, Neviaser AS, Seidl AJ, Smith MV, Wright RW, Zhang AL, Wolf BR. Beach chair versus lateral decubitus position: differences in suture anchor position and number during arthroscopic anterior shoulder stabilization. Am J Sports Med. 2021;49(8):2020–6. https://doi.org/10.1177/03635465211013709. Epub 2021 May 21. PMID: 34019439.
13. Frank RM, Saccomanno MF, McDonald LS, Moric M, Romeo AA, Provencher MT. Outcomes of arthroscopic anterior shoulder instability in the beach chair versus lateral decubitus position: a systematic review and meta-regression analysis. Arthroscopy. 2014;30(10):1349–65. https://doi.org/10.1016/j.arthro.2014.05.008. Epub 2014 Jul 4. PMID: 25000864.

7 The Bankart Repair in Beach Chair: Indications, Technique, and Limits

Stephen D. Daniels, Alex Lencioni, and Adam Seidl

Introduction

The humeral head, as it articulates with the glenoid, has a large range of motion that is stabilized by both static and dynamic stabilizers. The glenohumeral joint is a diarthrodial, multiaxial joint involving the humeral head and the glenoid as the main articulation in the shoulder gridle. The glenoid has a shallow cavity relying on static and dynamic stabilizing structures to prevent instability [1]. As a primary static stabilizer, the labrum is a fibro-osseous complex surrounding the outer rim of the glenoid, deepening the fossa by ~50%, contributing significantly to the stability to the glenohumeral joint [2]. The disruption of this soft tissue structure can result in instability of the shoulder. Anterior shoulder instability is the most common type of shoulder instability and can be the consequence of both traumatic and atraumatic etiologies. This condition typically occurs as a consequence of anterior shoulder dislocation, often associated with injury to the anteroinferior labrum resulting in the classically described Bankart lesion [3].

Treatment strategies for this condition include both nonoperative and surgical management. Nonsurgical management consists of a brief period of immobilization followed by early rehabilitation and return to sport determined by clinical symptoms. However, patients with Bankart lesions that experience recurrent symptomatic instability typically require surgical stabilization. Surgical strategies include both open and arthroscopic procedures. With comparable long-term outcomes of both open and arthroscopic techniques, arthroscopic stabilization is highly effective and the preferred method for both orthopedic surgeons and patients due to the minimally invasive nature of the procedure [4].

Positioning of the patient during arthroscopic Bankart repair is a topic for debate. There are two mainstay positions in which this procedure may be performed, lateral decubitus and beach chair, each of which has advantages and disadvantages [5]. For the purpose of this chapter, we will focus on detailing arthroscopic Bankart repair in the beach chair position, discuss pros and cons, outcomes, and complications associated with this technique.

S. D. Daniels · A. Lencioni · A. Seidl (✉)
Department of Orthopedic Surgery, University of Colorado, Aurora, CO, USA
e-mail: stephen.d.daniels@cuanschutz.edu; alex.lencioni@cuanschutz.edu; adam.seidl@cuanschutz.edu

© The Author(s), under exclusive license to Springer Nature Switzerland AG 2026

R. M. Frank, J. M. Tokish (eds.), *Management of Shoulder Instability*,
https://doi.org/10.1007/978-3-032-18089-6_7

Patient History and Preoperative Assessment

A thorough evaluation of a patient with shoulder instability, after an initial or recurrent event, is essential to the physician's ability to properly manage this injury. An appropriate workup of the patient should be completed. This includes a detailed event and medical history, mechanism of injury, prior instability events, treatments, activity level, occupation, and a detailed physical exam performed. Gross deformities such as a sulcus sign and atrophy should be noted utilizing the contralateral shoulder for reference. Active and passive range of motion, rotator cuff strength, and neurologic deficits should be assessed in all patients as a method of good practice. Generalized ligamentous laxity may be evaluated utilizing Beighton's criteria [6]. Specific maneuvers assessing anterior glenohumeral instability should be performed. Among these include anterior apprehension and relocation signs, along with load and shift testing [2]. A detailed and precise physical exam is a critical component to isolating pathology, indicating appropriate intervention, and should be further correlated with radiographs and advanced imaging.

Appropriate imaging of the patient with shoulder instability includes plain radiographs (anterior-posterior, axillary, scapular Y, and Grashey views) which should be carefully scrutinized for signs of glenoid or humeral bone loss. Concern for bone loss can further be evaluated with a CT scan and an MRI will detail soft tissue injury. Patients most appropriate for an isolated arthroscopic Bankart repair are those with an anteroinferior labral tear without significant glenoid bone loss. Preoperative assessment tools such as the Instability Severity Index Score (ISIS) proposed by Balg and Boileau, can be helpful to predict patients at risk for recurrent instability following isolated soft tissue procedures and identify patients that may require some form of anterior bone block to supplement associated glenoid bone loss [7]. Once the patient has been appropriately worked up and indicated, arthroscopic Bankart repair may be pursued.

Operating Room Setup and Beach Chair Positioning

An operating room table that breaks at the patients waist, allowing the torso and chest to be upright is utilized. The patient is initially placed supine on the operating table. General endotracheal (ET) anesthesia, which is preferred for this positioning, is induced by the anesthesia staff, and then the endotracheal tube is placed and secured exiting the contralateral side of the mouth away from the operative side. The patient's head is then centered in a well-padded head positioner to maintain a neutral position of the neck throughout the entire procedure. Bony prominences such as the heels are padded to prevent pressure sores. The contralateral arm is placed onto a well-padded holder with the wrist in neutral to prevent ulnar nerve irritation. A padded face mask is placed to assist in maintaining safe head positioning throughout the entirety of the case while allowing access to the ET tube. A pillow or pad is placed under the patient's knees. The surgical bed is then lowered and placed in slight Trendelenburg position; the feet are lowered slightly with a bend at the knees. The table is then adjusted to position the patient 60–90° to the horizontal [5, 8, 9]. As the patient is brought from supine into this upright position, communication with the anesthesia team is essential as monitoring for hypotension is critical in this moment to assess for risk of cerebral ischemia (a reported potential complication that will be discussed later in the chapter). Once the patient is properly positioned, the head and neck are checked again and confirmed in neutral/physiologic alignment. An exam under anesthesia should be performed. Range of motion and a load and shift on both the operative and nonoperative side are documented. The operative side is then draped to expose as much of the shoulder girdle as possible, and prepped in a standard sterile fashion. The operative arm is wrapped in a sterile stockinette, wrapped in a self-adhesive wrap, and can remain free on a padded mayo stand or be placed into a self-adjustable mechanical arm positioner to assist in arm positioning throughout the procedure (Fig. 7.1).

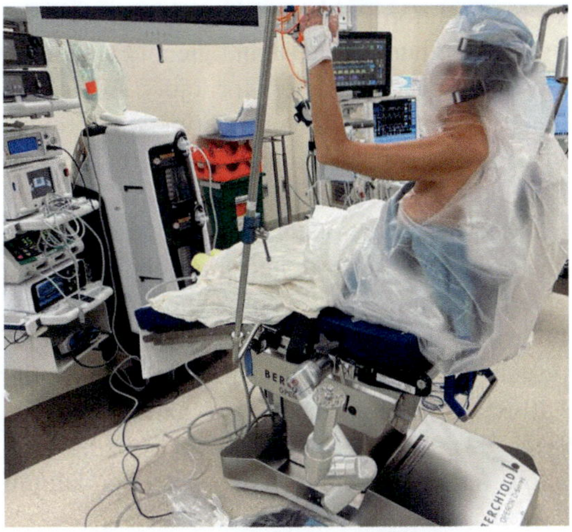

Fig. 7.1 The beach chair position places the patient at 60–90° relative to the floor. The contralateral arm is placed on an arm holder, a pillow under the knees, and a well-padded head positioner. Non-sterile drapes should be placed to expose as much of the shoulder girdle possible to prevent draping out for the procedure

Once the patient has been positioned and instrumentations set up, attention should then be turned to surgical landmarks. The external bony anatomy of the shoulder girdle should be palpated and drawn out with a surgical marking pen to identify the clavicle, acromion, acromial clavicular joint, and coracoid. The authors anticipate the initial posterior portal to be placed generally 1–2 cm inferior and 1–2 cm medial to the posterior lateral aspect of the acromion (Fig. 7.2). This portal can vary slightly based on patient specific anatomy and is more accurately identified by placing the thumb in the sulcus between the glenoid and humeral head, index finger at Neviaser's portal, and small finger over the coracoid. A shucking maneuver with the fingers held in this position will help identify the appropriate trajectory into the GH joint. The anterior portals are established through the rotator interval under direct visualization from the posterior portal by

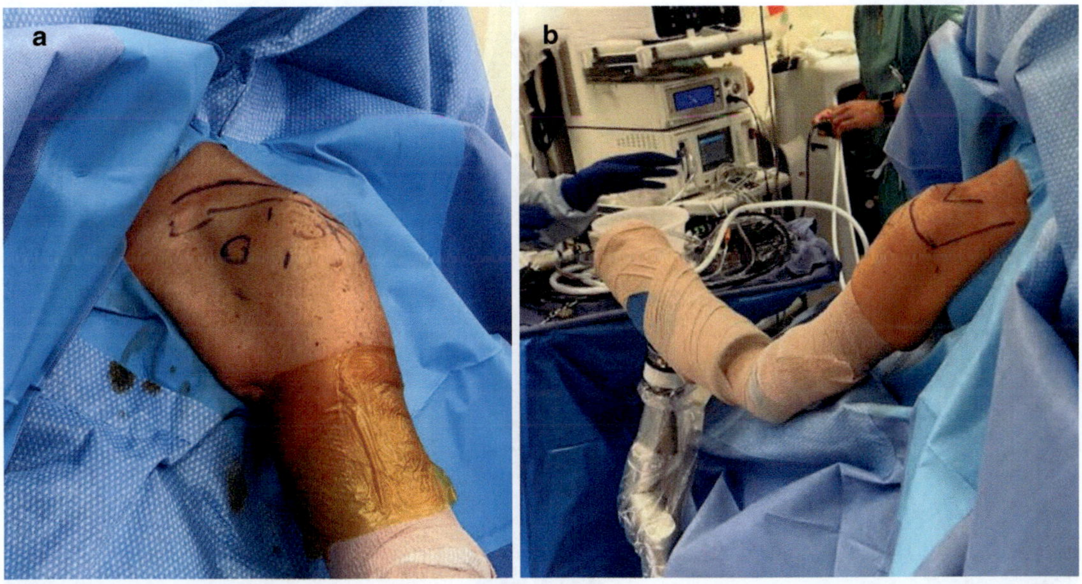

Fig. 7.2 Anatomy of the shoulder should be identified and marked before the procedure. The coracoid, clavicle, and acromion are marked out to aid with portal placement. The initial entry portal is placed approximately 1–2 cm inferior and medial referenced off of the posterolateral border of the acromion (B). This point is also identified by palpating for the sulcus between the glenohumeral articulation. The anterior portals are marked above but are appropriately made under direct visualization from the posterior portal. A high rotator interval portal, as well as an anteroinferior portal targeting the upper border of the subscapularis is also created under direct visualization

placing a spinal needle into the joint. Accessory working portals are created in a similar fashion [10, 11].

Diagnostic Arthroscopy

A standard diagnostic arthroscopy is performed through the posterior portal to assess the superior labrum and biceps anchor. Rotating the scope inferiorly exposes the middle glenohumeral ligament, subscapularis tendon, and the anterior superior labrum. Here it is essential to carefully evaluate for anatomic variants in these structures such as a Buford complex. The articular cartilage of both the humeral head and glenoid should be closely inspected to assess for injury. Advancing the camera to view anteroinferior will provide visualization of the Bankart lesion, as demonstrated in Fig. 7.3b. The articular side of the superior and posterior rotator cuff can be inspected, and positioning the arm into slight abduction and external rotation can help achieve this view. Following the articular margin of the rotator cuff posteriorly allows for visualization of potential Hill-Sachs lesion and the axillary recess (Fig. 7.3). Turning the scope back medial will allow for visualization of the posterior labrum

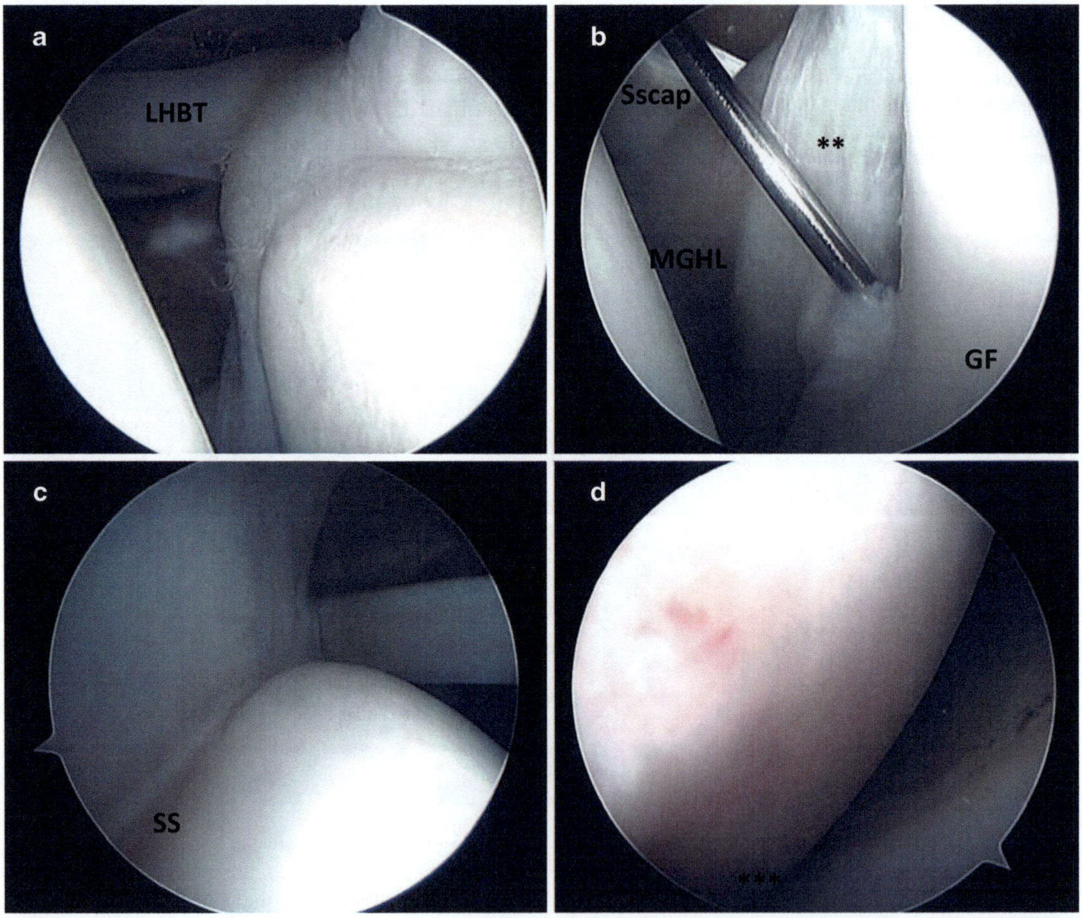

Fig. 7.3 A diagnostic scope from primarily the posterior portal is performed to begin the case. The insertion of the long head biceps tendon (LHBT) at the superior labrum is assessed for instability and lesions (**a**). The glenoid face (GF) and anterior labrum is then evaluated for Bankart lesions such as the one demonstrated in (**b**) (**). The subscapularis (Sscap) and middle glenohumeral ligament (MGHL) may also be evaluated. The insertion of the supraspinatus (SS) and superior rotator cuff is identified at its footprint on the humeral head (HH) (**c**). Finally, the posterior humeral head is then visualized to identify Hill-Sach's lesions (***) (**d**)

and completion of the diagnostic arthroscopy. This upright anatomy is an advantage of beach chair positioning, creating ease of a familiar working orientation.

Bankart Repair

The authors preferred method for arthroscopic Bankart repair is with 1.6 mm all-suture, suture anchors. The first cannula is placed through the rotator interval just above the subscapularis. This should be placed lateral enough to achieve a good angle for drilling and suture anchor placement. Anticipating this trajectory with a spinal needle upon establishing this anterior portal can assist with proper placement. Once the cannula is inserted, a shaver is introduced, and debridement of any frayed tissue is performed. Mobilization of the labrum and capsule is performed with a liberator or a radiofrequency ablation device at the zone of injury to release scarred labral tissue from the glenoid rim. Once this is initiated, the authors preferred technique involves moving the arthroscope anteriorly through a high-rotator interval portal, allowing visualization down the anterior neck of the glenoid. Further mobilization of the capsulolabral complex is performed. Complete mobilization of the lesion is essential to allow for adequate repair. Adequate mobilization is classically achieved when subscapularis muscle fibers are visualized through the released anteroinferior labrum. The neck of the glenoid is then debrided with a shaver, and a rasp is utilized to stimulate a healing surface. At this point, the author prefers to establish an accessory posterior portal and insert a cannula to assist in anchor placement and suture passing. The first suture anchor as close to the 5:30/6 O'clock glenoid position is then placed, either from the posterior or anterior cannula, depending on the extension of the tear. A suture shuttling device is used to capture a small portion of the capsule with the labrum, bringing tissue from inferior to superior. Sutures can be passed in a simple fashion (one limb through the tissue), or in a horizontal mattress configuration (both limbs through the tissue with space between the limbs). The horizontal mattress technique is helpful in preventing the suture knot stack from encroaching on the face of the glenoid. This suture is then tied, establishing an anteroinferior bumper, as well as an inferior to superior capsular shift. Additional anchors are placed and passed in similar fashion, moving from inferior to superior on the anterior glenoid, with the goal of placing four or more anchors throughout the repair to prevent additional risks of failure [12] (Fig. 7.4).

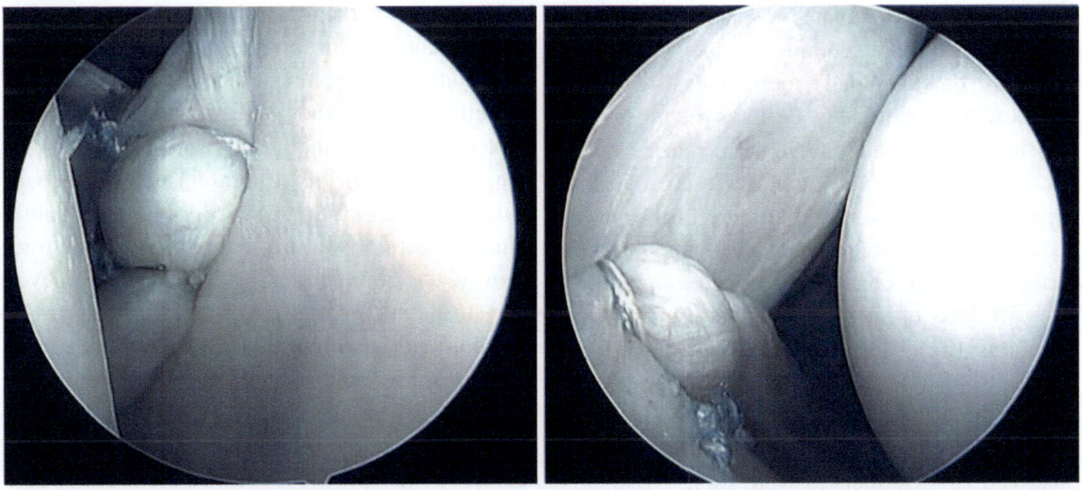

Fig. 7.4 The authors prefer to utilize suture anchors for Bankart repairs. A minimum of four anchors should be inserted along the anteroinferior labrum to secure the labrum to the glenoid

Outcomes Following Arthroscopic Bankart Repair in Beach Chair Positioning

The literature on arthroscopic Bankart repair supports excellent outcomes when performed on the appropriately indicated patient. This includes high rates of return to sport and low rates of recurrent instability [13]. In general, this portends to patients diagnosed with Bankart lesions in the absence of significant glenoid bone loss. Historically, glenoid bone loss approaching 20–25% was accepted as a critical cutoff, at which point the bone loss should be addressed. However, recent data suggest glenoid bone loss as low as 13.5% has led to unacceptable outcomes with isolated soft tissue procedures [14]. Previous studies have demonstrated independent risk factors for recurrent instability after arthroscopic Bankart repair to be young age (<19 years), contact/collision athletes, history of closed reduction prior to surgical intervention, and revision arthroscopic Bankart repair [7, 15, 16].

Despite encouraging results, some studies cite recurrent instability rates up to 30%, necessitating research focused on factors related to failure. The influence of patient position in beach chair or lateral decubitus for the repair is often cited. [17–21]. To date, there is no conclusive data demonstrating clear superiority of one technique over the other as it relates to patient outcomes. One of the more comprehensive systematic reviews to date included a meta-analysis comparing these two techniques. Perhaps the most critical findings was an overall recurrence rate of instability after suture anchor fixation of 12%, regardless of position. The authors further noted a 12.6% recurrence rate in those repairs performed in beach chair positioning, compared to an 8.3% rate of recurrent instability in lateral decubitus [22]. A second study evaluated the influence of positioning on total number of anchors used, frequency of 6 o'clock anchor placement, and surgeon-reported tear lengt, demonstrated sutures anchors were more frequently placed at the 6 o'clock position in lateral decubitus. Further, surgeons more frequently achieved placement of at least 4 anchors when repairing from a lateral position [23]. Interestingly, a cadaveric study demonstrated the most accurate view for analyzing glenoid anchor placement was done with a 30-degree scope in the posterior portal of beach chair position [24].

Importantly, while we are starting to see potential differences in outcomes of lateral vs beach chair positioning, this data should be interpreted with caution. Studies commonly do not directly compare positioning modalities, and there are many other important factors that affect the outcomes of arthroscopic Bankart repair. Overall, excellent outcomes can be achieved in either position if performed with good technique on the appropriately indicated patient.

Advantages of Beach Chair Shoulder Arthroscopy

Placing the patient in the upright position permits a shoulder examination under anesthesia with greater ease. The scapula can be properly stabilized when in this orientation, and the glenohumeral joint manipulated through its maximum range of motion in all planes. For the arthroscopic procedure, the extremity may be manually manipulated and placed on a padded table such as a mayo stand for the duration of the procedure. Alternatively, surgeons commonly utilize a mechanical arm holder for positioning and to maintain the shoulder in a desired amount of rotation. Rotation affects visualization of structures within the glenohumeral joint and is also a factor that should be taken into consideration when repairing structures such as the capsule and labrum that are susceptible to the subtle alterations in position of repair. Finally, distraction of the glenohumeral joint can be achieved and sustained, creating a workable space between the humeral head and glenoid face. This can be aided by used of a sterile towel bump placed between the humerus and the rib cage. The use of a mechanical arm holder has the advantage of precise positioning. This can be particularly useful when performing a tension-free capsular repair.

Anatomic/Upright Orientation

Visualization of the glenohumeral joint in an upright position can be less disorienting to trainees and those less familiar with shoulder arthroscopy. Cadaveric studies have demonstrated the most consistent and reproducible view of the shoulder is performed from the posterior portal utilizing a 30-degree scope with the patient in beach chair positioning [24].

The placement of anchors below 4 o'clock on the glenoid face can be performed in this upright position, and access improved through establishment of an accessory 5 o'clock anteroinferior portal. Importantly, creating this portal in beach chair positioning has been demonstrated to pose less risk to the musculocutaneous nerve when compared to lateral decubitus positioning [25]. Lastly, the upright positioning of beach chair portends an easy transition to an open procedure if needed.

Complications of Beach Chair Positioning

Cerebral Hypotension

It is essential surgeons operating in the beach chair position understand all nuances of this technique which includes the potential physiologic strain of cerebral ischemia that may occur while patients are elevated into the beach chair position. The potential for cerebral desaturation events (CDE) have been identified as a potential complication, specifically when raising the patient from a supine to upright position. CDEs have historically been defined as a decrease in regional blood oxygen by 20% of baseline values. Several prior investigations have demonstrated CDEs in up to 80% of patients subject to beach chair positioning, on occassion associated with increased postoperative nausea and vomiting [26]. However, despite these early postoperative symptoms, no increased incidence of longer term neurological deficits have been reported. Notably, many of the studies assessing postoperative effects have not been adequately powered to detect differences in psychometric testing. Despite the unlikelihood of long-term effects, it is important for the orthopedic surgeon to be aware of this physiologic process as there are several strategies that can be employed to manage intraoperative hypotension.

Effective communication and teamwork with anesthesia colleagues and nursing staff should be a priority throughout the case. Anesthesiologists closely regulate ventilation rate and hemodynamic status (goal to maintain systolic BP >90 mm Hg, and decrease in mean arterial pressures no more than 20%) to decrease cerebral hypotension. The use of sequential compression device (SCD) on the lower extremities has been demonstrated to assist in the maintenance of Mean Arterial Pressure (MAP) and reduce incidence of hypotension from 64% to 28% [27]. Lastly, the risk of neurological injury is related to duration of the desaturation event. Accordingly, it is always important for the operating physician to be mindful of the patient's time on the table, working efficiently and safely to complete the operation at hand.

Peripheral Nerve Injury

Neuropraxia after arthroscopic shoulder surgery is well documented. Nerve injury is typically caused through excessive traction or as a consequence of portal placement. Fortunately, by nature of arm position, beach chair is less subject to traction-based injuries than lateral decubitus. Despite this advantage, there have been cases reported in the literature.

Iatrogenic injury to the axillary nerve is the most often reported nerve complication in beach chair positioning. While some studies cite incidence of up to 21% specific to thermal injury during procedures such as capsulorrhaphy, the incidence of axillary nerve injury specific to arthroscopic Bankart repair is much lower. A large cohort study reported a 0.05% incidence of axillary nerve injury associated with isolated arthroscopic Bankart repair in beach chair—a transient neuropraxia that spontaneously resolved. Notably, rates of axillary nerve injury in isolated Bankart repair were significantly lower than incidence of nerve injury in capsular and humeral avulsion of glenohumeral ligament (HAGL) repair [28]. Although injury to the axillary nerve is uncommon, with an average reported distance of 2.5 mm from the inferior glenohumeral ligament, this is certainly an anatomical consideration the operating surgeon should be mindful of [29].

A small case series examined four patients presenting with anterior interosseous nerve (AIN) palsy after arthroscopic shoulder surgery, three of which were performed in beach chair. Although neurological testing demonstrated this to be a mixed palsy, AIN deficits were the most clinically prevalent. Although the exact etiology remained unclear, it was hypothesized the palsy could be a manifestation of potentially tight intraoperative forearm dressings, regional anesthesia, fluid extravasation causing median nerve compression, the use of shoulder sling, or likely a combination of these factors. Two patients in this cohort recovered spontaneously, while the other two required surgical decompression [30].

Although more commonly noted as a complication related to lateral decubitus positioning, based on its anatomical location, the musculocutaneous nerve can be at risk if utilizing anteroinferior/trans subscapular portals for inferior glenoid anchor placement. A cadaveric study demonstrated injury to the musculocutaneous in 0.08% of cadavers when simulating drilling the glenoid from an anteroinferior portal [25].

Additional nerve complications related to beach chair position include cutaneous facial neuropraxia from inadequate padding around the head. Changes in neck positioning are theorized to have resulted in hypoglossal nerve injury. Finally, the cervical spinal cord is at risk for injury with improper management of the patient's head and neck that could result in excessive neck flexion or extension. Although not reported as a complication related to arthroscopic shoulder surgery, this has been demonstrated in the spine and neurosurgery literature [5].

Chapter Summary

Overall, arthroscopic Bankart repair performed in the beach chair position has been well established to be a reliable technique producing excellent patient outcomes with minimal complications. Ultimately, patient position is at the discretion and comfort of the performing surgeon. The purpose of this chapter was to serve as a guide to beach chair for arthroscopic Bankart repair and provide insight into some of the advantages, pearls, and pitfalls of the technique as summarized in Table 7.1.

Table 7.1 This table summarizes some of the advantages, complications, and potential solutions to consider for beach chair positioning

Advantages	Complications/pitfalls	Solution
Anatomic/upright orientation	Cerebral hypotension and theoretical neurologic complications	Proper communication with anesthesia team related to hemodynamic monitoring Maximize efficiency to limit patient time on the table
Ease of extremity manipulation	Upper extremity peripheral nerve injury	Mindful of anatomy when placing portals, performing capsular repair Gentle arm manipulation to reduce traction injury Loose intraoperative upper extremity dressings
Readily converted to open procedure (rare)	Facial neuropraxia/ cervical spinal cord injury	Ensure the head is appropriately padded Gentle, mindful manipulation of the neck when positioning
Low rates of nerve injury/ limited traction placed on nerves and soft tissues	Need for assistant without mechanical arm	

References

1. Chang L-R, Anand P, Varacallo M. Anatomy, shoulder and upper limb, Glenohumeral joint. StatPearls; 2021.
2. Bakhsh W, Nicandri G. Anatomy and physical examination of the shoulder. Sports Med Arthrosc Rev. 2018;26:e10–22.
3. Provencher MT, Midtgaard KS, Owens BD, Tokish JM. Diagnosis and management of traumatic anterior shoulder instability. J Am Acad Orthop Surg. 2021;29:e51–61.
4. Bottoni CR, Johnson JD, Zhou L, Raybin SG, Shaha JS, Cruz CA, Lindell KK, Thoma DC. Arthroscopic versus open anterior shoulder stabilization: a prospective randomized clinical trial with 15-year follow-up with an assessment of the glenoid being "on-track" and "off-track" as a predictor of failure. Am J Sports Med. 2021;49:1999–2005.
5. Li X, Eichinger JK, Hartshorn T, Zhou H, Matzkin EG, Warner JP. A comparison of the lateral decubitus and beach-chair positions for shoulder surgery: advantages and complications. J Am Acad Orthop Surg. 2015;23:18–28.
6. Engelbert RH, Rombaut L. Clinimetrics: assessment of generalised joint hypermobility: the Beighton score. J Physiother. 2022; https://doi.org/10.1016/J.JPHYS.2022.02.004.
7. Balg F, Boileau P. The instability severity index score. A simple pre-operative score to select patients for arthroscopic or open shoulder stabilisation. J Bone Joint Surg Br. 2007;89:1470–7.
8. Mannava S, Jinnah AH, Plate JF, Stone A v, Tuohy CJ, Freehill MT. Basic shoulder arthroscopy: beach chair patient positioning. Arthrosc Tech. 2016;5:e731.
9. Higgins JD, Frank RM, Hamamoto JT, Provencher MT, Romeo AA, Verma NN. Shoulder arthroscopy in the beach chair position. Arthrosc Tech. 2017;6:e1153–8.
10. Paxton ES, Backus J, Keener J, Brophy RH. Shoulder arthroscopy: basic principles of positioning, anesthesia, and portal anatomy. J Am Acad Orthop Surg. 2013;21:332–42.
11. Farmer KW, Wright TW. Shoulder arthroscopy: the basics. J Hand Surg Am. 2015;40:817–21.
12. Boileau P, Villalba M, Héry JY, Balg F, Ahrens P, Neyton L. Risk factors for recurrence of shoulder instability after arthroscopic Bankart repair. J Bone Joint Surg Am. 2006;88:1755–63.
13. Blonna D, Bellato E, Caranzano F, Assom M, Rossi R, Castoldi F. Arthroscopic Bankart repair versus open Bristow-Latarjet for shoulder instability: a matched-pair multicenter study focused on return to sport. Am J Sports Med. 2016;44:3198–205.
14. Shaha JS, Cook JB, Song DJ, Rowles DJ, Bottoni CR, Shaha SH, Tokish JM. Redefining "critical" bone loss in shoulder instability: functional outcomes worsen with "subcritical" bone loss. Am J Sports Med. 2015;43:1719–25.
15. Mahure SA, Mollon B, Capogna BM, Zuckerman JD, Kwon YW, Rokito AS. Risk factors for recurrent instability or revision surgery following arthroscopic Bankart repair. Bone Joint J. 2018;100-B:324–30.
16. Imhoff AB, Ansah P, Tischer T, Reiter C, Bartl C, Hench M, Spang JT, Vogt S. Arthroscopic repair of anterior-inferior glenohumeral instability using a portal at the 5:30-o'clock position: analysis of the effects of age, fixation method, and concomitant shoulder injury on surgical outcomes. Am J Sports Med. 2010;38:1795–803.
17. Randelli P, Ragone V, Carminati S, Cabitza P. Risk factors for recurrence after Bankart repair a systematic review. Knee Surg Sports Traumatol Arthrosc. 2012;20:2129–38.
18. Owens BD, Deberardino TM, Nelson BJ, Thurman J, Cameron KL, Taylor DC, Uhorchak JM, Arciero RA. Long-term follow-up of acute arthroscopic Bankart repair for initial anterior shoulder dislocations in young athletes. Am J Sports Med. 2009;37:669–73.
19. van der Linde JA, van Kampen DA, Terwee CB, Dijksman LM, Kleinjan G, Willems WJ. Long-term results after arthroscopic shoulder stabilization using suture anchors: an 8- to 10-year follow-up. Am J Sports Med. 2011;39:2396–403.
20. Lenters TR, Franta AK, Wolf FM, Leopold SS, Matsen FA. Arthroscopic compared with open repairs for recurrent anterior shoulder instability. A systematic review and meta-analysis of the literature. J Bone Joint Surg Am. 2007;89:244–54.
21. Harris JD, Gupta AK, Mall NA, Abrams GD, McCormick FM, Cole BJ, Bach BR, Romeo AA, Verma NN. Long-term outcomes after Bankart shoulder stabilization. Arthroscopy. 2013;29:920–33.
22. Frank RM, Saccomanno MF, McDonald LS, Moric M, Romeo AA, Provencher MT. Outcomes of arthroscopic anterior shoulder instability in the beach chair versus lateral decubitus position: a systematic review and meta-regression analysis. Arthroscopy. 2014;30:1349–65.
23. Baron JE, Duchman KR, Hettrich CM, et al. Beach chair versus lateral decubitus position: differences in suture anchor position and number during arthroscopic anterior shoulder stabilization. Am J Sports Med. 2021;49:2020–6.
24. Jong BY, MacDonald PB, Regan WD, Leiter JR, Sayre EC, Sasyniuk TM, Goel DP. Perceived vs. true glenoid anchor placement: a cadaveric comparison of the beach chair and lateral position. JSES Int. 2020;5:66–71.
25. Gelber PE, Reina F, Caceres E, Monllau JC. A comparison of risk between the lateral decubitus and the beach-chair position when establishing an anteroinferior shoulder portal: a cadaveric study. Arthroscopy. 2007;23:522–8.
26. Aguirre JA, Etzensperger F, Brada M, Guzzella S, Saporito A, Blumenthal S, Bühler P, Borgeat A. The beach chair position for shoulder surgery in intravenous general anesthesia and controlled hypoten-

sion: impact on cerebral oxygenation, cerebral blood flow and neurobehavioral outcome. J Clin Anesth. 2019;53:40–8.
27. Murphy GS, Greenberg SB, Szokol JW. Safety of beach chair position shoulder surgery: a review of the current literature. Anesth Analg. 2019;129:101–18.
28. Hamada H, Sugaya H, Takahashi N, Matsuki K, Tokai M, Ueda Y, Hoshika S, Kuniyoshi K. Incidence of axillary nerve injury after arthroscopic shoulder stabilization. Arthroscopy. 2020;36:1555–64.
29. Price MR, Tillett ED, Acland RD, Nettleton GS. Determining the relationship of the axillary nerve to the shoulder joint capsule from an arthroscopic perspective. J Bone Joint Surg Am. 2004;86:2135–42.
30. Pope D, Wottowa C. Mixed neuropathy presenting clinically as an anterior interosseous nerve palsy following shoulder arthroscopy: a report of four cases. J Shoulder Elb Surg. 2016;25:1699–703.

The HAGL Lesion: Recognition and Arthroscopic Surgical Technique

8

Jasan Dannaway, Sumit Raniga, and Desmond Bokor

Introduction

Avulsion of the glenohumeral ligaments is associated with traumatic shoulder instability. Recurrent post-traumatic instability is often caused by lesions of the glenoid labrum but can also be attributed to capsular or glenohumeral ligament injury, albeit less frequently. In 1942, Nicola noted avulsion of the capsular ligaments in four out of five patients that were operatively explored after acute dislocations [1]. However, further research into capsular lesions was not pursued at that time as focus turned toward Bankart lesions which were becoming established as the "essential lesion" responsible for glenohumeral instability [2]. In 1988, Bach et al. once again noted this pathology in their report of two cases of "lateral capsular avulsion" which were managed successfully with surgery [3].

The current term for this lesion, humeral avulsion of the glenohumeral ligaments (HAGL), was first presented by Wolf et al. in 1995 [4]. They presented a series of 64 patients with the diagnosis of anterior shoulder instability, whom they evaluated arthroscopically. Six shoulders (9.3%) were found to have HAGL lesions. They emphasized the importance of recognizing this lesion in the absence of a concurrent Bankart lesion and concluded that repair can restore anterior stability. In 1999, Bokor et al. presented a series of 547 shoulders undergoing operations for instability [5]. In 41 (7.5%) shoulders, the cause of instability was deemed to be a HAGL lesion. Of the primary cases, 33 (94.3%) dislocations were caused by violent injury, and 4 (11.4%) had a Bankart lesion. In patients whose first dislocation was a violent injury, who did not have a Bankart lesion, and had no suggestion of multidirectional laxity, the incidence of HAGL was 39%. In 2019, Patzkowski et al. reported HAGL lesions in 25% (9/36) of a cohort of female college athletes, most of whom were injured in collision or contact sporting environments [6].

A small number of HAGLs are associated with injury to the posterior capsular components. Reports of posterior capsule failure at the humeral insertion have been documented in the orthopedic literature since 1995 and in the radiological literature since 1998, but there has been no official standardization of the injury definition [7, 8]. Most commonly, these injuries have been classified as posterior HAGL. However, in 2010, Bokor et al. proposed three distinct entities within the HAGL spectrum: the HAGL (or anterior humeral avulsion of the glenohumeral ligament), the posterior HAGL (avulsion of the inferior glenohumeral ligament's posterior band), and the reverse HAGL (posterior capsule avulsion with or without involvement of the posterior band of the infe-

J. Dannaway · S. Raniga · D. Bokor (✉)
Faculty of Medicine, Health and Human Sciences, Macquarie University, Sydney, NSW, Australia
e-mail: jasan.dannaway@mqhealth.org.au; sumit.raniga@mqhealth.org.au

© The Author(s), under exclusive license to Springer Nature Switzerland AG 2026
R. M. Frank, J. M. Tokish (eds.), *Management of Shoulder Instability*,
https://doi.org/10.1007/978-3-032-18089-6_8

rior glenohumeral ligaments) [9]. They hypothesized that they are present in separate patient groups with varying clinical presentations and injury mechanisms.

A HAGL lesion is an established cause of shoulder instability, and a high index of suspicion is required, especially in cases where associated lesions, such as Bankart lesions, are not present.

Illustrative Clinical Case: Management of Traumatic Shoulder Instability in a 22-Year-Old Basketball Player

This case describes a 22-year-old male accountant who presented with ongoing right shoulder apprehension and occasional pain following a basketball injury 3 months prior. The injury occurred when he landed in a hyper-flexed position while attempting to rebound, causing a sensation of shoulder dislocation, though it relocated spontaneously. There were no associated neurovascular symptoms at the time of injury. He rested for 1 week, and his pain improved rapidly without the need for immobilization or analgesia. However, despite returning to work, the patient continued to experience apprehension particularly during overhead movements and occasional pain. He initiated physiotherapy several weeks after the injury, but the symptoms persisted, prompting him to seek specialist advice as he was eager to return to basketball.

On examination, the patient exhibited a positive anterior apprehension test and Gagey sign, consistent with anterior shoulder instability. His past medical history was unremarkable, and there were no signs of generalized ligamentous laxity. The specialist recommended an MRI to further evaluate the extent of the injury. Imaging revealed a small Hill-Sachs lesion, a Bankart lesion, and a humeral avulsion of the glenohumeral ligament (HAGL) lesion (Fig. 8.7).

A diagnosis of anterior shoulder instability secondary to a first-time traumatic dislocation was made. Initial treatment involved a course of physiotherapy focusing on proprioception and scapular stabilization exercises. However, after 2 months of physiotherapy, the patient's instability symptoms persisted, with even simple activities like reaching for a bus handrail exacerbating his pain. Given the failure of conservative management, the decision was made to proceed with surgical intervention.

The patient underwent arthroscopic labral repair and HAGL repair using suture anchors (Fig. 8.7). The surgery addressed both the Bankart and HAGL lesions successfully. Unfortunately, in the immediate postoperative period, the patient developed pain and dysesthesia over the axillary nerve distribution, which disrupted his rehabilitation process. A period of observation yielded no resolution of the neurological symptoms. A repeat MRI showed a satisfactory shoulder repair and no evidence of nerve-related injury.

Due to the persistent axillary nerve symptoms, referral was made for a second opinion and continued management. An open surgical exploration was performed. Intraoperatively, it was found that one of the inferior capsular sutures had inadvertently been passed through the axillary nerve. A neurolysis was performed, and the suture was removed (Fig. 8.7). Postoperatively, the patient experienced immediate improvement in his axillary nerve function. Over the following 3 months, the nerve-related symptoms completely resolved, allowing him to resume routine rehabilitation.

At 9 months post-surgery, the patient reported full resolution of his shoulder instability symptoms and was able to return to recreational basketball without any further complications.

Anatomy

The glenohumeral joint is extremely mobile and hence prone to instability. Its stability is maintained by a combination of dynamic and static stabilizers. The deltoid, rotator cuff, and biceps long head are all dynamic stabilizers. Static stabilizers include the articulation between the humeral head and the glenoid cavity, the glenoid labrum, the joint capsule, and the glenohumeral ligaments. The glenoid labrum connects the glenohumeral ligaments and works to enlarge the glenoid cavity. The coracohumeral ligament, superior glenohumeral ligament, middle glenohumeral ligament, and inferior glenohumeral ligament (IGHL) make up the capsuloligamentous complex.

The IGHL complex is made up of three components: the anterior band (AIGHL), the posterior band (PIGHL), and the axillary pouch. On the anterior and posterior portions of the glenoid, the pouch and bands form a hammock-like structure [10–13]. The AIGHL begins between two and four on the anterior aspect of the glenoid when projected clockwise [3, 11, 14]. The PIGHL originates between seven and nine on the glenoid's posterior aspect [10]. Both bands are positioned on the labrum's inferior third. They originate predominantly from the labrum, with a similar connection to that of a tendon inserted directly. Early investigations of the anatomy of the IGHL's attachment to the humeral neck showed two unique attachment types. The capsule is linked either directly to the juxta chondral edge or in a "V" configuration to the humeral neck, with an equal distribution [15]. Pouliart and Gagey's further dissection revealed that the genuine functional capsular insertion was the "V" attachment of the humeral neck and that the juxta chondral attachment was a capsular recess filled with tissue they termed "frenula capsulae" [13]. The humeral attachment of the AIGHL and PIGHL both span 12 mm from the 4:05 to 5:10 and 7:40 to 8:50, respectively, on a humeral head clock face [16]. In a cadaveric biomechanical investigation, Southgate et al. verified that the capsule should be attached about 10 mm below the chondral neck onto the medial humeral neck to restore "normal" glenohumeral joint laxity after simulated HAGL lesions and repair [17]. Between the AIGHL and PIGHL, the axillary pouch extends from the inferior two-thirds of the anterior glenoid to the inferior one-third of the humeral head [14, 15]. The IGHL's function is determined by the arm's position. The anterior band of the IGHL covers the midportion of the anterior glenohumeral joint when the arm is in 90° of abduction both in neutral and external rotation, restricting anterior and inferior humeral translation [10, 15, 18, 19]. The posterior band of the IGHL covers the midportion of the posterior glenohumeral joint, while the arm is in flexion and internal rotation, providing posterior stability [10, 14, 15, 19].

Mechanism and Pathophysiology

Anterior HAGL Lesions

The glenohumeral ligaments act as key capsular stabilizers, preventing the shoulder from dislocating. Ninety-five percent of the time, the shoulder dislocates anteriorly [20]. Turkel et al. demonstrated the contribution of the glenohumeral ligaments to stability depending on the abduction angle (0, 45°, or 90°) in external rotation [18]. Biomechanical studies have indicated that when stress/load increases, the IGHL will experience strain/deformation and ultimately fail at the glenoid (40%), inside the capsule (35%), or at the humeral connection (25%) [21].

Nicola originally characterized the process by which an anterior HAGL might be created as hyperabduction combined with external rotation moving the humeral head into the glenohumeral pouch [1]. As hyperabduction increases, the head displaces out of the joint and may tear the capsule at the humeral connection. When an axial stress is also applied, the head may tear the inferior labrum from the glenoid, resulting in the "floating anterior band." Similarly, Gagey et al. demonstrated that hyperabduction of the humerus with an axial load results in HAGL (Fig. 8.1) but can also cause the same range of concomitant injuries as previously documented, including labral and rotator cuff tears [22]. A more recent investigation indicated that significant capsule and labral tearing is necessary before dislocation occurs by simulating instability with successive separation of the humeral sided capsule [23]. This does not necessarily correspond with surgical findings [24].

A number of associated lesions can be present with anterior HAGL. In Bokor's series of 514 shoulders, 400 patients had a Bankart lesion. One hundred thirty shoulders did not

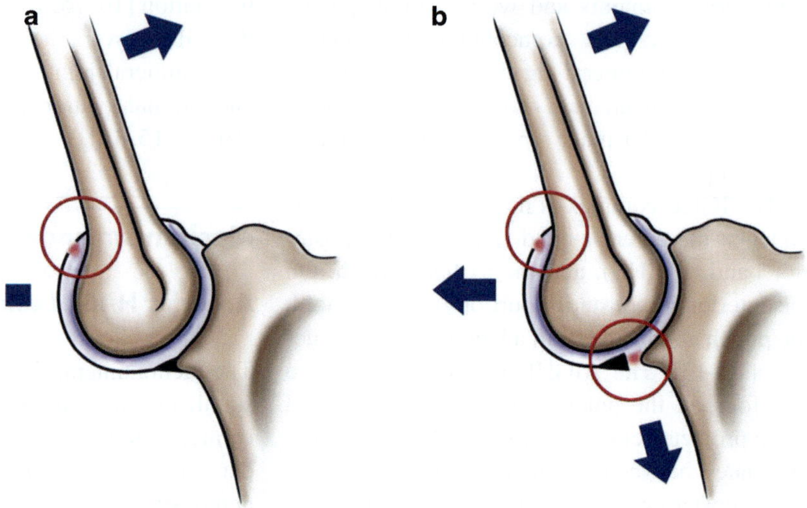

Fig. 8.1 Frontal view demonstrating mechanism of anterior HAGL with hyperabduction. (**a**) Increased external rotation levers humeral head anteriorly with capsular tearing. (**b**) Axial load pushes humeral head onto anteroinferior glenoid rim causing capsular tearing with concurrent Bankart lesion

have a Bankart lesion [5]. Of those patients, 35 had HAGL, suggesting a 26.9% chance of encountering HAGL in a patient with anterior instability but no Bankart lesion. In the HAGL groups, both primary and revision, 15 patients had rotator cuff tears: 8 had scarring of the inferior portion of the subscapularis; 6 had a partial avulsion of the subscapularis, usually involving the lowermost fibers, or other rotator cuff tears; and 1 had a partial tear of both the subscapularis and supraspinatus. Cuff injuries were more common in the older individuals in their study. Rotator cuff pathology with anterior instability in the older patient is a known association. In 1993, Neviaser published their series of 37 patients, mostly over 40 years old, which described subscapularis ruptures in patients subsequent to anterior dislocation [25].

Posterior HAGL Lesions

The mechanism behind posterior HAGL is less understood. Forced cross-body adduction, with or without a component of posteriorly directed translation of the proximal humerus, was the mechanism most often described in the largest series [9]. The authors hypothesized that a reverse HAGL (posterior capsule avulsion) is more likely to occur when the arm is forwards flexed, adducted, and rotates somewhat externally (Fig. 8.2). In this posture, the posterior band of the inferior glenohumeral ligament provides just minor support, with the whole stress imposed on the thinner posterior capsule. When the arm is forced into adduction across the chest, the cantilever action on the humeral head results in tensile pressures on the posterior capsule that exceed its failure limit. They hypothesized that this resulted in an avulsion injury to the posterior capsule with failure at the humeral insertion. They suggested that posterior capsule overload, rather than poste-

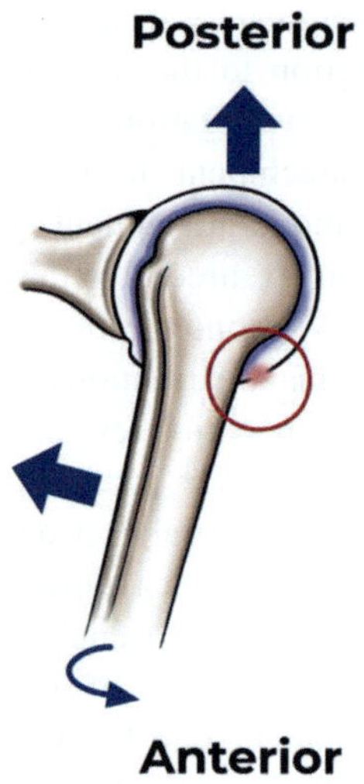

Fig. 8.2 Axial view demonstrating mechanism of posterior HAGL. The arm is forward flexed, adducted with slight external rotation

riorly directed translation of the humeral head via the posterior shoulder structures, accounted for the very uncommon (26%) occurrence of a reverse Bankart lesion in their group.

Associated injuries with posterior HAGL are common. In a cohort of 19 patients described by Bokor in 2010, labral pathology was the most prevalent concomitant diagnosis with fraying of the labrum observed in 11 of the patients [9]. The posterior labrum was detached in five of the individuals (posterior Bankart lesion), a SLAP lesion was found in six cases, and in two individuals, the posterior capsular damage spread into the inferior glenohumeral ligament's posterior band. Chondral lesions were found in four individuals, two of which had both glenoid and humeral deficiencies, the third had an isolated humeral defect, and the fourth had an isolated glenoid defect. Four of the patients had rotator cuff injuries, and two of them had full-thickness tears of the infraspinatus and supraspinatus. A further two individuals suffered partial thickness rotator cuff injuries.

Classification

Classification of HAGL lesions are descriptive which may increase awareness and improve communication, but how they are used to determine management is unclear. Bui-Mansfield et al. created the West Point categorization system to organize the IGHL complex's several concurrent injuries [19]. The authors defined six distinct subtypes of HAGL lesion based on their anterior or posterior location, the presence or absence of bony avulsion, and the presence or absence of associated labral pathology: anterior HAGL, anterior bony HAGL (with associated bony avulsion), floating anterior IGHL (HAGL lesion with concurrent anteroinferior labrum detachment), posterior HAGL, and posterior bony HAGL (HAGL lesion with concurrent detachment of the posterior inferior labrum). Anterior HAGL accounts for 93% of reported instances, while posterior HAGL accounts for only 7% of reported cases [19].

While anterior HAGL is more widely documented, posterior HAGL has a more ambiguous classification. The injury has been described as a "lateral capsular disruption of the posterior aspect of the shoulder"; a "humeral detachment along the posterior humeral head, called a reverse humeral glenohumeral ligament avulsion or rHAGL lesion"; and a "posterior humeral avulsion of the posterior portion of the inferior glenohumeral ligament" [7, 26–28]. The radiology literature mentions pathology of the inferior glenohumeral ligament's posterior band [29, 30]. In 2010, Bokor et al. characterized a reverse humeral avulsion of the glenohumeral ligament as an avulsion of the glenohumeral joint's posterior capsule above the level of the inferior glenohumeral ligament's posterior band that may or may not extend into the IGHL's posterior band [9]. This is different from IGHL disruptions that only affect the posterior band and not the posterior capsule or that may be a result of an anterior capsular avulsion. They highlighted this difference to distinguish this damage from an injury to the IGHL complex caused by anterior, anteroinferior, or multidirectional instability, which has a different proposed mechanism of injury. Because it is a considerably less frequent entity, references to it in the literature continue to remain somewhat unclear.

Recently, a modification of the classification has been proposed to include axillary pouch humeral avulsion of the glenohumeral ligament (APHAGL) (Fig. 8.3) [31]. This lesion was described in 2011 in four volleyball players without a known trauma or dislocation event [32]. It was hypothesized that repetitive volleyball-related overhead activity may lead to avulsion of the central pouch of the IGHL. In 2019, Patzkowski et al. found APHAGL in 8 of the 9 HAGL lesions in their cohort of 36 female college athletes playing volleyball, although this observation may be a separate entity to HAGL [6].

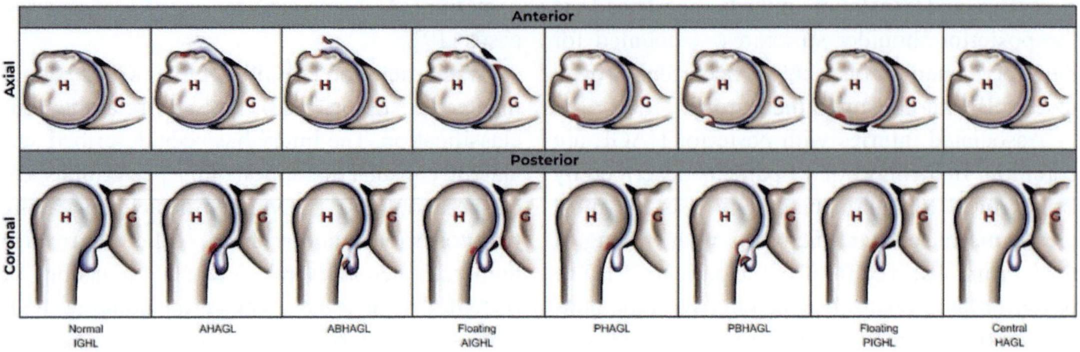

Fig. 8.3 Modified West Point classification. H humerus, G glenoid, IGHL inferior glenohumeral ligament, AHAGL anterior HAGL, ABHAGL anterior HAGL with a bony avulsion, AIGHL anterior band of the inferior glenohumeral ligament, PHAGL posterior HAGL, PBHAGL posterior HAGL with a bony avulsion, and PIGHL posterior band of the inferior glenohumeral ligament

Diagnosis

Clinical

While traumatic shoulder injury caused by a HAGL lesion frequently manifests as recurrent subluxation or dislocation, the specific damage is not always obvious. A thorough history is garnered, including the arm's position at the moment of injury, the direction of instability, and any history of recurrent instability. Patients often arrive with vague symptoms, such as weakness, discomfort, or impaired function, rather than obvious instability. Those with anterior HAGL may have greater anterior shoulder discomfort than patients with normal shoulder instability [33]. Posterior joint line pain was noted in all patients with posterior HAGL in the largest reported series [9]. The history may be contradictory, and a strong index of suspicion is required for HAGL lesions, especially in patients who have previously had unsuccessful stabilization surgery.

Range of motion should be measured both actively and passively, as well as deltoid and rotator cuff strength and subscapularis function. Generalized ligamentous laxity should be assessed using tools such as the modified Beighton scale. Apprehension, relocation, load-and-shift, posterior stress, and posterior jerk tests are all provocative maneuvers used to determine stability. For comparison, the contralateral shoulder should be evaluated. Multidirectional instability should be assessed including the sulcus sign in neutral and exterior rotation to assess the rotator interval. According to Gagey, injury to the IGHL might result in higher shoulder hyperabduction relative to the opposing side [34]. Positive posterior load shift, posterior glide, or posterior jerk signs along with history is likely to lead to a diagnosis of posterior HAGL [9]. Prior interventions, surgical records, and photos should also be examined.

Imaging

Standard radiographs include a true anterior to posterior (AP) view of the scapula in neutral and internal rotation in addition to scapular Y and axillary views. These can be utilized to assess for concentric glenohumeral alignment, a humeral head impaction fracture (Hill-Sachs lesion), a glenoid rim fracture, and glenoid hypoplasia. On the AP view, scalloping of the medial portion of the humeral neck may be indicative of a HAGL lesion [35]. Bony HAGL, an avulsion fracture of the medial cortex of the humeral anatomic neck, may be present as a fleck of bone inferior to the humeral anatomic neck [36]. The Garth view of the glenohumeral joint (45° oblique radiograph of the shoulder in the anterior plane) may be used to see the bone fragments [10]. The axillary view is used to assess glenoid anatomy including version. Abnormalities may be a consequence of chronic instability causing glenoid erosion or underlying glenoid hypoplasia. The West Point view will provide additional information about the anterior glenoid rim, and the Stryker notch view will help to characterize Hill-Sachs lesions.

MRI/MRA is the preferred imaging modality for assessing a suspected HAGL lesion. Coronal oblique or sagittal oblique T2-weighted fat-suppressed magnetic resonance images are optimal for evaluating the IGHL complex [37]. Due to the fluid distension of the axillary pouch, the normal IGHL anatomy appears as a U-shaped structure. In the presence of a HAGL lesion, the normally U-shaped axillary pouch may appear J-shaped due to the extravasation of contrast or joint fluid over the ruptured capsule and ligament (Fig. 8.4) [35]. The presence of glenohumeral joint effusion or the injection of intra-articular contrast dye aids in the detection of a HAGL lesion. However, the accuracy of MRI remains debatable, with many case reports of false-positive imaging of suspected HAGL lesions [38]. Liavaag et al. studied the optimal time for plain MRI or MR arthrography (MRA) [37]. They discovered that more than two thirds of the HAGL lesions seen on the first MRI (mean 7 days post injury) had healed by the time of the following MR arthrogram (mean 30 days post injury). They suggested that the clinical significance of pathological abnormalities inside the capsular ligaments seen on the first MRI be interpreted cautiously and that a follow-up MR arthrogram be performed 2 months later before deciding on surgical intervention. Chronic HAGL lesions can be more difficult to identify. Imaging (MR arthrogram in 11 and MRI in one of 12 cases) has been shown to successfully identify 83% (10 of 12 cases) of lesions that were later confirmed by arthroscopy [39]. A CT arthrogram may be used if an MRI/MRA is contraindicated (Fig. 8.4).

Arthroscopy

Arthroscopy of the glenohumeral joint with examination of the whole capsule, labrum, rotator cuff, and chondral surfaces is the gold standard of diagnostic study. The two distinctive findings during arthroscopy are visualization of subscapularis fibers via the avulsed capsule and the rupture of the IGHL's inferior wave-like attachment to the humerus as seen from the posterior portal (Fig. 8.5) [4, 5]. A 70° arthroscope allows for a more comprehensive view of the axillary pouch [40].

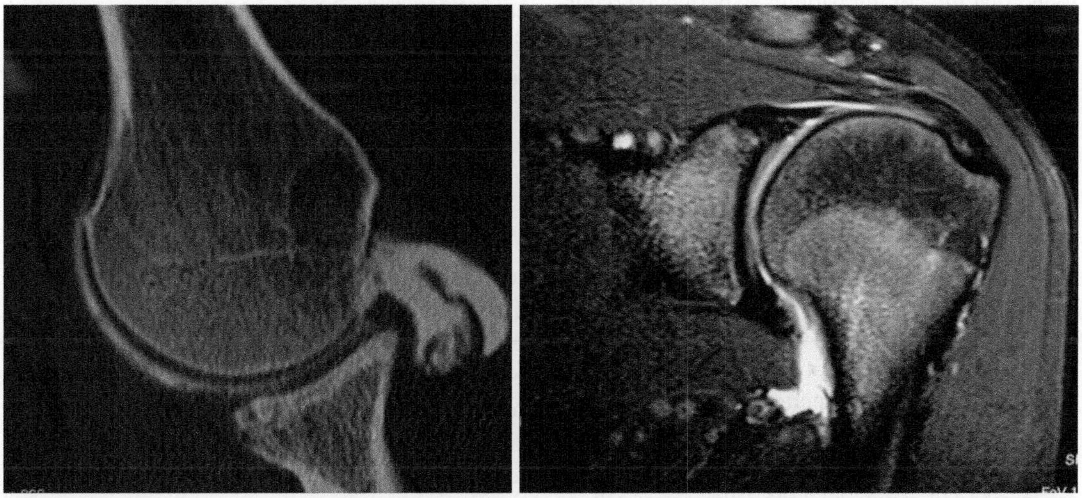

Fig. 8.4 (Left) CT arthrogram demonstrating posterior HAGL. (Right) MRI demonstrating HAGL

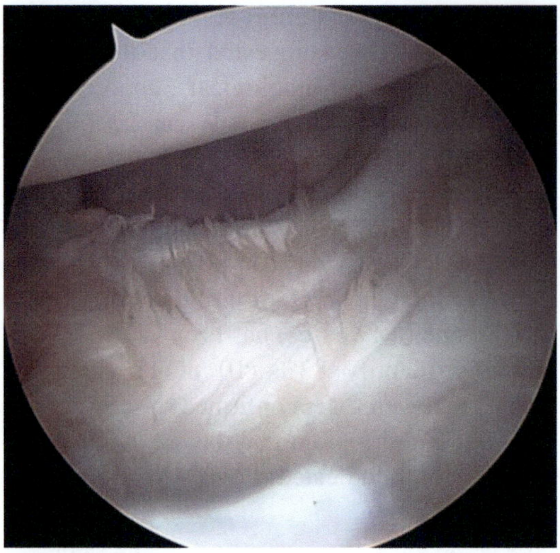

Fig. 8.5 Arthroscopic image demonstrating HAGL

Management

Nonoperative

Nonsurgical management of HAGL lesions is indicated but needs to be assessed with regard to concurrent injuries. It involves initial sling immobilization followed by physiotherapy and activity moderation. Small studies have demonstrated the successful nonoperative management of HAGL lesions [41–43]. However, a systematic review found that nine of ten patients experienced recurrent instability, necessitating surgical management [44]. The history and probability of conservative therapy failing resulting in additional instability in patients with a HAGL lesion have not been studied in comparison to the general instability group.

Surgery

Surgical intervention is indicated when instability, pain, or loss of function remains. Surgery may also be recommended preferentially for young athletes and manual laborers. If surgery is recommended, it may be done arthroscopically or open. The presence of associated injuries needs to be taken into account and may affect technique and order of management.

Open

HAGL open surgical repair includes a deltopectoral approach with a subscapularis tenotomy. Scarring in the inferior portion of the subscapularis may indicate the presence of a HAGL lesion. The lesion may be detected after blunt dissociation of the subscapularis from the capsule. Typically, the lesion is located in the inferior pouch of the shoulder, just below the level of the subscapularis [5]. This relates to a point on the humeral neck between about 6 and 8 o'clock in the right shoulder [45]. The capsule often has a thicker rolling edge, and care must be taken to dissect this free while identifying and protecting the axillary nerve, which is frequently located very near the capsular border. Anchors or transosseous sutures via bone tunnels should be used to secure the capsule to the medial humeral neck around 10 mm below the chondral margin.

Techniques that spare the subscapularis are referred to as mini open surgery. Arciero and Mazzocca presented an approach that included making an L-shaped incision in the lower portion of the subscapularis tendon [45]. The vertical limb of the incision extends 1.5 cm medial to the lesser tuberosity, from the inferior half of the subscapularis insertion to just above the anterior humeral circumflex vessels. The incision's transverse limb is made immediately superior to the circumflex vessels. This procedure saves the subscapularis tendon's inferior half. In eight patients treated with this technique, they observed no recurrence of instability, but the duration of follow-up was not specified. The benefit of this technique is that the upper section of the subscapularis is not incised. Bhatia et al. presented a technique that avoids any incision of the subscapularis [46]. The anterior humeral circumflex vessels define the subscapularis inferior boundary. The superior border of the pectoralis major tendon is retracted inferiorly, and a curved hemostat is slipped under the inferior border of the subscapularis to gently separate it from the anterior capsule. The subscapularis is then superiorly retracted. According to the authors, this approach may be utilized to get enough exposure in around two-thirds of patients. In the remaining patients, the subscapularis requires an L-shaped incision as previously described. No clinical results were reported. Bhatia and Das Gupta developed a combined medial subscapularis splitting method to repair the Bankart lesion and fix the coracoid transfer, known as the Latarjet procedure. Further, a "lateral subscapularis window" was described as retracting the subscapularis fibers superiorly and anchoring the HAGL lesion below [47].

In order to access the PHAGL, a posterior incision is performed, and the deltoid is bluntly extended in line with its fibers. To get access to the posterior glenohumeral capsule, the space between the infraspinatus and teres minor is dissected. Suture anchors are used to prepare the bone and restore the avulsed capsule. Only case studies have described successful open repair of posterior HAGL [7, 48, 49].

Arthroscopic

The beach chair or lateral position can be utilized although conversion to an open technique is easier from the beach chair position. To begin, the conventional posterior portal is created, and a comprehensive diagnostic examination is undertaken to rule out any concurrent injuries, including a careful assessment of the anterior capsulolabral tissue. The anterior portal is placed dependent on additional lesions and planned procedures. The IGHL complex is examined via the axillary recess from the posterior portal using a 30° arthroscope. The IGHL complex is avulsed from its attachment on the humeral neck in a HAGL lesion, exposing the subscapularis muscle fibers. The capsule will not be in the typical U form; rather, it will be narrow and attenuated. Internal and external rotation might aid in seeing the whole humeral neck in its entirety. Anterior lesions are best examined with a 70° arthroscope with the arm in internal rotation via the anterosuperior portal.

Once identified, attention needs to be paid to the exact location of the HAGL in order to determine the position of additional portals. Typically, a three-port method is required. A conventional posterior portal, an anterior portal above the subscapularis, and at least one axillary portal, anterior or posterior, depending on the location of the HAGL and other associated lesions, are required. When coexisting pathology is present, typically one should begin with the HAGL repair due to its greater technical difficulty. Labral repair or capsulorrhaphy can tighten the capsule, hence making HAGL repair more difficult [35, 50].

Anterior HAGL Lesions

The anteroinferior portal is the most often utilized portal for HAGL lesions that are anteriorly situated (between 4 and 5 o'clock). It is inserted via an outside-in technique, through the subscapularis muscle at the 5 o'clock position [51]. To protect the musculocutaneous nerve, the shoulder should not be abducted. The portal is roughly 1 cm inferior to the upper border of the subscapularis tendon and as lateral as possible (Fig. 8.6). Inserting the suture anchor at this location has been identified as one of the most challenging steps of the procedure and was even dubbed the "killer angle" by Huberty and Burkhart due to its obliquity [50]. Prior to creating the portal, a spinal needle should be utilized to verify the portal's appropriate location and access to the humeral neck. Once the portal is established, the arm can then be abducted and externally rotated as necessary to reach the humeral insertion point. A burr can be used to roughen the humeral neck, and suture anchors can be inserted. Sutures are retrieved via the rotator interval portal. Sutures are then passed through the IGHL, avoiding deep bites of tissue and the 6 o'clock position due to the axillary nerve's close proximity. Because the nerve is typically 4.9 mm from the lesion's free border, although this distance is often underestimated on MRI, axillary nerve injury after repair can occur; special care must be taken to prevent iatrogenic injury (Fig. 8.7) [6, 52]. Capsular tissue is attached to the humeral neck using horizontal mattress sutures. Following suture passage, the surgeon should visually ensure that the glenohumeral ligaments have been reduced to the proximal humerus, at which point the sutures are routinely knotted.

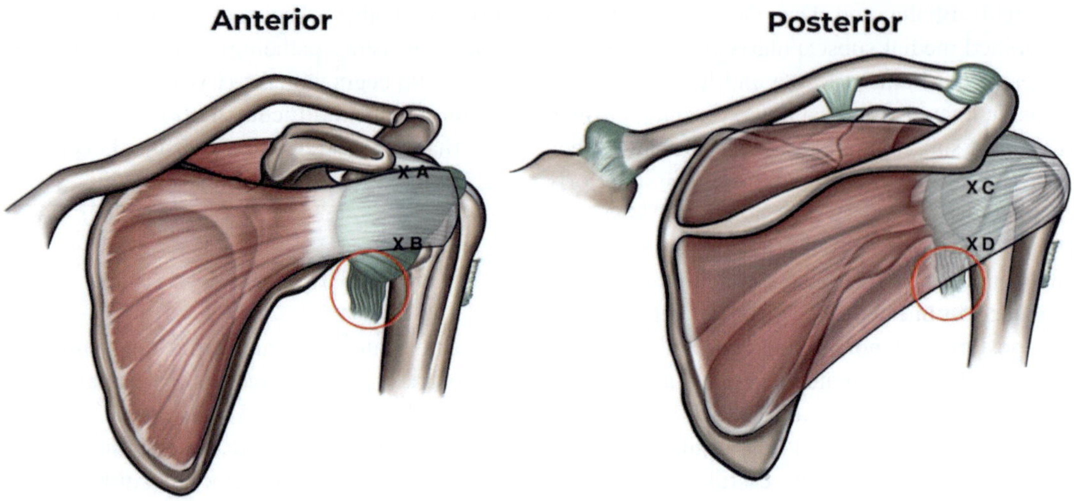

Fig. 8.6 Anterior and posterior view to demonstrate arthroscopic portal placement for management of HAGL lesions. Red circle demonstrates area of HAGL lesion. (**a**) Anterior portal. (**b**) Five o'clock portal. (**c**) Posterior portal. (**d**) Posteroinferior (7 o'clock) portal

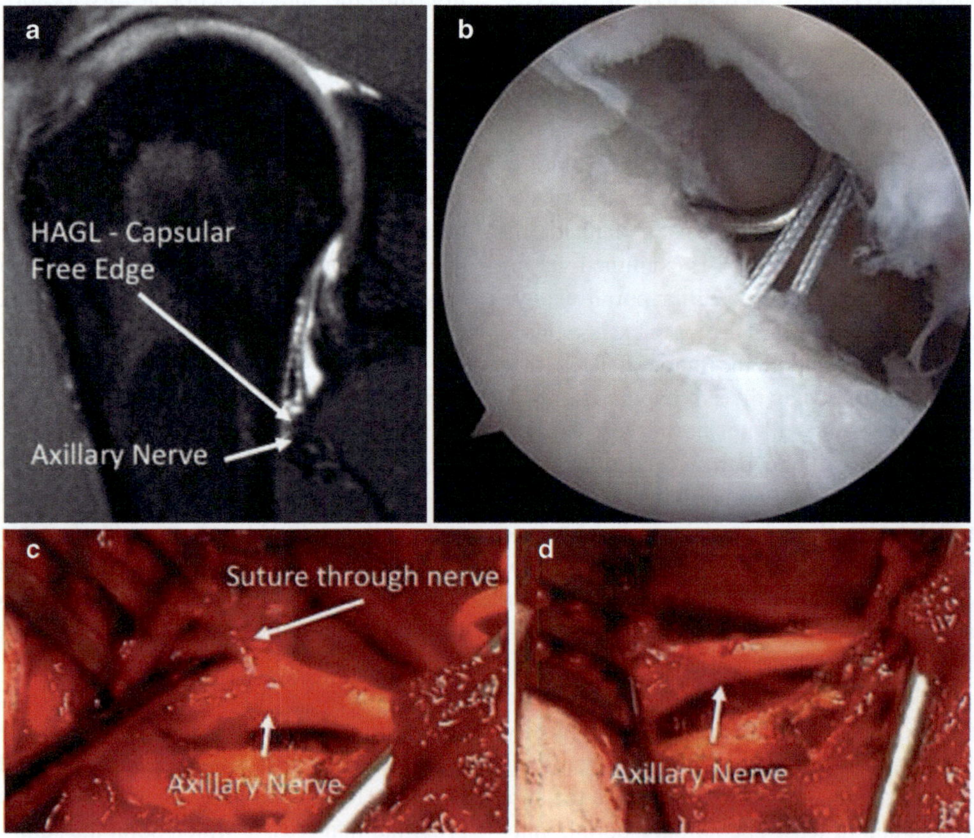

Fig. 8.7 (**a**) MRI demonstrating HAGL lesion and proximity of axillary nerve. (**b**) Arthroscopic image demonstrating suture position of HAGL lesion repair. (**c**) Clinical image of suture through axillary nerve and (**d**) subsequent release of nerve

Posterior HAGL Lesions

To treat posterior HAGL lesions, two alternative ports have been described: the axillary pouch and the 7 o'clock portal. The axillary pouch portal (also known as the Bhatia portal) is created using an outside-in approach, with the insertion location marked with a needle [53]. It is positioned about 2 to 3 cm inferior to the lower margin of the posterolateral acromial angle, approximately 1 to 2 cm lateral to the typical posterior viewing portal. In the axial plane, the portal will eventually be inclined 30° medially and somewhat inferiorly in the sagittal plane. If positioned properly, it will be proximal to the IGHL's posterior band, providing access to the whole IGHL complex, including the anterior portion. The insertion of the complete IGHL into the humerus is best seen via this portal when a 70-degree arthroscope is used.

The 7 o'clock posteroinferior portal can also be utilized and is performed via an outside-in technique, as described by Davidson and Rivenburgh [54]. The portal is placed about 2 to 3 cm posterior to the posterior viewing portal. While this portal is often needed for reverse Bankart lesions, it is not necessary for a HAGL repair, which may be accomplished via a standard posterior portal (Fig. 8.8). Once again, an arthroscopic burr is used to prepare the humeral neck. Suture anchors are inserted into the posterior humeral neck, and a horizontal mattress suture is formed to connect the IGHL's posterior band to the humeral head. Tensioning should be done with caution to avoid over tightening the posterior capsule [27].

Outcomes

Likely due to the limited prevalence and detection of HAGL lesions, their outcomes are often discussed in case reports or limited series. The majority of published HAGL repair series consist of less than ten patients with a short length of follow-up. Although the authors report a high rate of success in stabilizing the joint, they do not provide an in depth discussion on the number of patients who return to sport, especially in high collision settings.

In 2016, Longo et al. performed a systematic review and included 42 HAGL lesions of which 25 were managed operatively [44]. Another review in 2017 by Bozzo et al. included 18 HAGL repair studies with a total of 118 patients, but the way in which outcomes were reported varied and was inconsistent [55]. Only 2 of the 79 patients who had surgical management were unable to

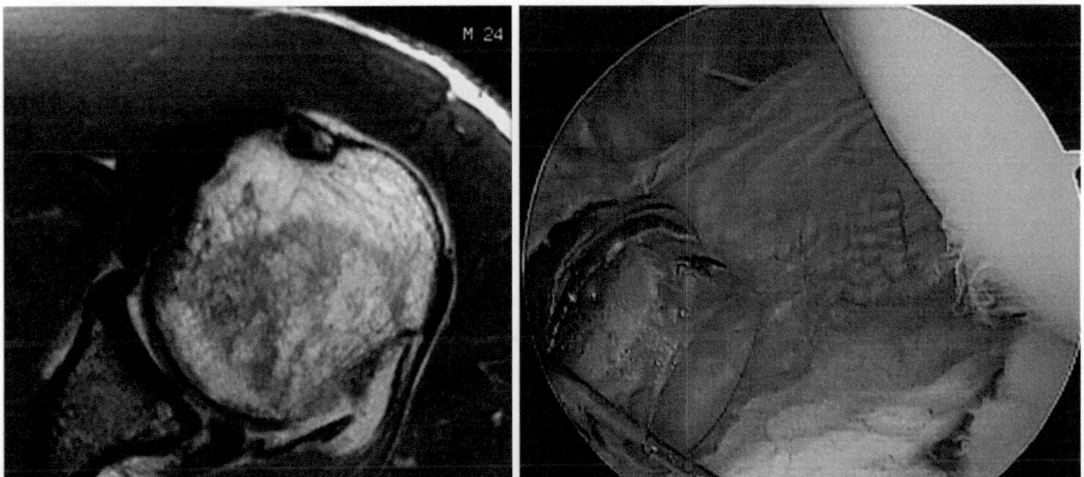

Fig. 8.8 MRI and arthroscopic image demonstrating floating posterior HAGL

return to their prior levels of sport. In 34 patients, there was no reported discomfort or clinical instability (using the apprehension test). Sixteen patients completed the Rowe score for shoulder instability, which averaged 94% postoperatively. Thirty patients completed the Western Ontario Shoulder Instability Index, with an average preoperative score of 54% and a postoperative score of 13%. Fifteen patients were evaluated using both the UCLA (University of California, Los Angeles) Shoulder Rating Scale and the Constant Shoulder Score and demonstrated average pre- and postoperative UCLA scores of 17 and 34 and Constant scores of 60 and 83, respectively. Notably, one of the two patients treated nonoperatively had ongoing symptomatic instability. A few case reports have been published describing patients who received HAGL repairs and were unable to resume athletic activities due to limited range of motion. Castagna et al. reported decreased internal rotation thought to be the result of excessive tightening in the posterior capsule [27]. Schmiddem et al. published a small case series in which five of nine patients were unable to return to sports up to 59 months after the surgery due to reduced external rotation, which might be attributed to the fact that 89% of patients had concurrent shoulder lesions [56]. In an retrospective review of the senior author's (D.B.) own series of open HAGL repairs [57], 10/47 (21%) patients experienced further instability episodes (dislocation or subluxation) postoperatively. These were observed over long-term follow-up (16–247 months). Furthermore, all except one recurrent dislocation and three subluxations occurred with a new violent/collision event. This may suggest that open HAGL repair delivers a stable joint; however, the resilience of the repair may be challenged by high risk exposures, similar to other anatomical repairs.

Arthroscopy and open procedures seem to provide comparable outcomes (Table 8.1) [55]. However, open procedures enable visualization and may therefore improve protection of nerves [52].

Table 8.1 Summary of outcomes reported by current literature

Author	Number of cases	Duration of follow-up (months)	Recurrence of instability	Arthroscopic vs open
Wolf et al. (1995)	6	40	Nil	Arthro 4, open 2
Oberlander et al. (1996)	3	28 (24–36)	Nil	Open 2, 1 non op
Field et al. (1997)	5	26	Nil	Open
Warner et al. (1997)	1	26	Nil	Open
Schippinger et al. (2001)	1	12	Nil	Arthro
Gehrmann et al. (2003)	1	13	Nil	Open
Chabra et al. (2004)	1	9	Nil	Arthro
Kon et al. (2005)	3	16	Nil	Arthro
Huberty et al. (2006)	6	32	Nil	Arthro
Rhee et al. (2007)	6	39	Nil	Open 5, arthro 1
Castanga et al. (2007)	9	34 (28–39)	Nil	Arthro
Rothberg et al. (2009)	2	12	Nil	Arthro
Shah et al. (2010)	1	36	Nil	Open
Taljanovic et al. (2011)	4	24	Nil	Arthro
Bahtia et al. (2013)	7	20	Nil	Mini open (with Latarjet)
Smith et al. (2014)	1	2	Nil	Arthro
Chang et al. (2014)	4	4	Nil	3 arthro, 1 non op
Provencher et al. (2014)	23	68	Nil	14 open, 9 arthro
Schmiddem et al. (2019)	18	59 (16–104)	1	Arthro
Patzkowski et al. (2019)	9	59 (25–110)	1	Arthro
Dannaway et al. (2024)	47	105 (16–247)	10	Open

Conclusion

Humeral avulsion of the glenohumeral ligament is a rare but a significant cause of recurrent anterior and posterior shoulder instability. Anterior HAGL is caused by hyperabduction and axial force, and posterior HAGL by forced cross-body adduction. Arthroscopic surgical repair can be technically challenging, but it does seem to offer satisfactory results in small studies; further follow-up and detailed outcomes are required.

References

1. Nicola T. Anterior dislocation of the shoulder: the role of the articular capsule. J Bone Joint Surg Am. 1942;25:614–6.
2. Rowe CR, Patel D, Southmayd WW. The Bankart procedure: a long-term end-result study. J Bone Joint Surg Am. 1978;60(1):1–16.
3. Bach BR, Warren RF, Fronek J. Disruption of the lateral capsule of the shoulder. A cause of recurrent dislocation. J Bone Joint Surg Br. 1988;70-B(2):274–6.
4. Wolf EM, Cheng JC, Dickson K. Humeral avulsion of glenohumeral ligaments as a cause of anterior shoulder instability. Arthroscopy. 1995;11(5):600–7.
5. Bokor DJ, Conboy VB, Olson C. Anterior instability of the glenohumeral joint with humeral avulsion of the glenohumeral ligament. A review of 41 cases. J Bone Joint Surg Br. 1999;81(1):93–6.
6. Patzkowski JC, Jonathan DF, Cameron KL, Bokshan SL, Garcia E'SJ, Owens BD. Pathoanatomy of shoulder instability in collegiate female athletes. Am J Sports Med. 2019;47(8):1909–14.
7. Laurencin CT, Paletta GA, Potter HG, Wickiewicz TL. Disruption of the posterior-lateral shoulder capsule. J Shoulder Elb Surg. 1995;4(5):391–4.
8. Hottya GA, Tirman PF, Bost FW, Montgomery WH, Wolf EM, Genant HK. Tear of the posterior shoulder stabilizers after posterior dislocation: MR imaging and MR arthrographic findings with arthroscopic correlation. AJR Am J Roentgenol. 1998;171(3):763–8.
9. Bokor DJ, Brett F. Posterior shoulder instability secondary to reverse humeral avulsion of the glenohumeral ligament. J Shoulder Elb Surg. 2010;19(6):853–8.
10. Bui-Mansfield LT, Taylor DC, Uhorchak JM, Tenuta JJ. Humeral avulsions of the glenohumeral ligament: imaging features and a review of the literature. AJR Am J Roentgenol. 2002;179(3):649–55.
11. Cooper DE, Arnoczky SP, O'Brien SJ, Warren RF, DiCarlo EF, Allen AA. Anatomy, histology, and vascularity of the glenoid labrum. An anatomical study. J Bone Joint Surg Am. 1992;74(1):46–52.
12. Ticker JB, Bigliani LU, Soslowsky LJ, Pawluk RJ, Flatow EL, Van Mow C. Inferior glenohumeral ligament: geometric and strain-rate dependent properties. J Shoulder Elb Surg. 1996;5(4):269–79.
13. Pouliart N, Gagey O. Reconciling arthroscopic and anatomic morphology of the humeral insertion of the inferior glenohumeral ligament. Arthroscopy. 2005;21(8):979–84.
14. Burkart A, Debski RE. Anatomy and function of the glenohumeral ligaments in anterior shoulder instability. Clin Orthop. 2002;400(400):32–9.
15. O'Brien SJ, Neves MC, Arnoczky SP, Rozbruck SR, DiCarlo EF, Warren RF, et al. The anatomy and histology of the inferior glenohumeral ligament complex of the shoulder. Am J Sports Med. 1990;18(5):449–56.
16. Dekker TJ, Zachary AS, Peebles LA, Storaci HW, Chahla J, Millett PJ, Provencher MT. Quantitative and qualitative analyses of the glenohumeral ligaments: an anatomic study. Am J Sports Med. 2020;48(8):1837–45.
17. Southgate DF, Bokor DJ, Longo UG, Wallace AL, Bull AM. The effect of humeral avulsion of the glenohumeral ligaments and humeral repair site on joint laxity: a biomechanical study. Arthroscopy. 2013;29(6):990–7.
18. Turkel SJ, Panio MW, Marshall JL, Girgis FG. Stabilizing mechanisms preventing anterior dislocation of the glenohumeral joint. J Bone Joint Surg Am. 1981;63(8):1208–17.
19. Bui-Mansfield LT, Banks KP, Taylor DC. Humeral avulsion of the glenohumeral ligaments the HAGL lesion. Am J Sports Med. 2007;35(11):1960–6.
20. Chandnani VP, Gagliardi J, Murnane TG, Bradley YC, DeBerardino TA, Spaeth J, Hansen MF. Glenohumeral ligaments and shoulder capsular mechanism: evaluation with MR arthrography. Radiology. 1995;196(1):27–32.
21. Bigliani LU, Pollock RG, Soslowsky LJ, Flatow EL, Pawluk RJ, Mow VC. Tensile properties of the inferior glenohumeral ligament. J Orthop Res. 1992;10(2):187–97.
22. Gagey O, Gagey N, Boisrenoult P, Hue E, Mazas F. Experimental study of dislocations of the scapulohumeral joint. Rev Chir Orthop Reparatrice Appar Mot. 1993;79(1):13–21.
23. Pouliart N, Olivier G. Simulated humeral avulsion of the glenohumeral ligaments: a new instability model. J Shoulder Elb Surg. 2006;15(6):728–35.
24. Bokor D, Arama Y. Biomechanics and management of HAGL lesions in anterior instability. Asian J Arthrosc. 2017;2(1):36–9.
25. Neviaser RJ, Neviaser TJ, Neviaser JS. Anterior dislocation of the shoulder and rotator cuff rupture. Clin Orthop. 1993;291:103–6.
26. Abrams JS. Arthroscopic repair of posterior instability and reverse humeral glenohumeral ligament avulsion lesions. Orthop Clin North Am. 2003;34(4):475–83.
27. Castagna A, Snyder SJ, Conti M, Borroni M, Massazza G, Garofalo R. Posterior humeral avulsion

of the glenohumeral ligament: a clinical review of 9 cases. Arthroscopy. 2007;23(8):809–15.
28. Safran OD, Michael J, Hatem SF, Iannotti JP. Posterior humeral avulsion of the glenohumeral ligament as a cause of posterior shoulder instability. A case report. J Bone Joint Surg Am. 2004;86(12):2732–6.
29. Chung CB, Steven S, Dwek JR, Resnick D. Humeral avulsion of the posterior band of the inferior glenohumeral ligament: MR arthrography and clinical correlation in 17 patients. AJR Am J Roentgenol. 2004;183(2):355–9.
30. Harish S, Arpit N, Moro J, Pugh D, Rebello R, O'Neill J. Imaging findings in posterior instability of the shoulder. Skeletal Radiol. 2008;37(8):693–707.
31. Krueger VS, Shigley C, Bokshan SL, Owens BD. Humeral avulsion of the glenohumeral ligament: diagnosis and management. JBJS Rev. 2022;10(2)
32. Taljanovic MS, N Jon K, Hunter TB, Cohen RP, Rogers LF. Humeral avulsion of the inferior glenohumeral ligament in college female volleyball players caused by repetitive microtrauma. Am J Sports Med. 2011;39(5):1067–76.
33. George M, Khazzam M, Kuhn J. Humeral avulsion of glenohumeral ligaments. J Am Acad Orthop Surg JAAOS. 2011;19(3):127–33.
34. Gagey OJ, Gagey N. The hyperabduction test. J Bone Joint Surg Br. 2001;83(1):69–74.
35. Parameswaran AD, Provencher MT, Bach BR, Verma NN, Romeo AA. Humeral avulsion of the glenohumeral ligament: injury pattern and arthroscopic repair techniques. Orthopedics. 2008;31(8):773–9.
36. Oberlander MA, Morgan BE, Visotsky JL. The BHAGL lesion: a new variant of anterior shoulder instability. Arthroscopy. 1996;12(5):627–33.
37. Liavaag S, Stiris MG, Svenningsen S, Enger M, Pripp AH, Brox JI. Capsular lesions with glenohumeral ligament injuries in patients with primary shoulder dislocation: magnetic resonance imaging and magnetic resonance arthrography evaluation. Scand J Med Sci Sports. 2011;21(6):e291–7.
38. Melvin JS, MacKenzie JD, Nacke E, Sennett BJ, Wells L. MRI of HAGL lesions: four arthroscopically confirmed cases of false-positive diagnosis. AJR Am J Roentgenol. 2008;191(3):730–4.
39. Maldjian C, Khanna V, Bradley J, Adam R. Evaluation of contrast extravasation as a diagnostic criterion in the evaluation of arthroscopically proven HAGL/pHAGL lesions. Radiol Res Pract. 2014;2014:283575.
40. Richards DP, Burkhart SS. Arthroscopic humeral avulsion of the glenohumeral ligaments (HAGL) repair. Arthroscopy. 2004;20(6):134–41.
41. Yiannakopoulos CK, Elias M, Antonogiannakis E. A comparison of the spectrum of intra-articular lesions in acute and chronic anterior shoulder instability. Arthrosc J Arthrosc Relat Surg. 2007;23(9):985–90.
42. Murphy DT, K George, Gopez AG, Kavanagh EC. Humeral avulsion of the glenohumeral ligament. AJR Am J Roentgenol. 2009;193(1):W74–5; author reply W76.
43. Ernat JJ, Bottoni CR, Rowles DJ. Successful nonoperative management of HAGL (Humeral Avulsion of Glenohumeral Ligament) lesion with concurrent axillary nerve injury in an active-duty US navy SEAL. Am J Orthop Belle Mead NJ. 2016;45(5):E236–9.
44. Longo UG, Rizzello G, Ciuffreda M, Locher J, Berton A, Salvatore G, et al. Humeral avulsion of the glenohumeral ligaments: a systematic review. Arthroscopy. 2016;32(9):1868–76.
45. Arciero RA, Mazzocca AD. Mini-open repair technique of HAGL (Humeral Avulsion of the Glenohumeral Ligament) lesion. Arthroscopy. 2005;21(9):1152.
46. Bhatia DN, DeBeer JF, van Rooyen KS. The "subscapularis-sparing" approach: a new mini-open technique to repair a humeral avulsion of the glenohumeral ligament lesion. Arthroscopy. 2009;25(6):686–90.
47. Bhatia DN, DasGupta B. Surgical treatment of significant glenoid bone defects and associated humeral avulsions of glenohumeral ligament (HAGL) lesions in anterior shoulder instability. Knee Surg Sports Traumatol Arthrosc. 2013;21(7):1603–9.
48. Hasan SS, Fleckenstein CM, Albright J. Open treatment of posterior humeral avulsion of the glenohumeral ligaments: a case report and review of the literature. J Shoulder Elb Surg. 2007;16(4):e3–5.
49. Weinberg J, McFarland EG. Posterior capsular avulsion in a college football player. Am J Sports Med. 1999;27(2):235–7.
50. Huberty DP, Burkhart SS. Arthroscopic repair of anterior humeral avulsion of the glenohumeral ligaments. Tech Shoulder Elb Surg. 2006;7(4):186–90.
51. Navasartian DJ, Robert H, DeBerardino T, Burkhart S. Arthroscopic repair of humeral avulsion of the glenohumeral ligaments based on location. Arthrosc Tech. 2019;8(8):e841–5.
52. LeBrun DG, Sneag DB, Feinberg JH, McCarthy MM, Gulotta LV, Lee SK, et al. Surgical treatment of iatrogenic nerve injury following arthroscopic capsulolabral repair. J Hand Surg. 2021;46(12):1121.e1–1121.e11.
53. Bhatia DN, de Beer JF. The axillary pouch portal: a new posterior portal for visualization and instrumentation in the inferior glenohumeral recess. Arthroscopy. 2007;23(11):1241.e1–5.
54. Davidson PA, Rivenburgh DW. The 7-o'clock posteroinferior portal for shoulder arthroscopy. Am J Sports Med. 2002;30(5):693–6.
55. Bozzo A, Oitment C, Thornley P, Yan J, Habib A, Hoppe DJ, et al. Humeral avulsion of the glenohumeral ligament: indications for surgical treatment and outcomes—A systematic review. Orthop J Sports Med. 2017;5(8):2325967117723329.
56. Schmiddem U, Watson A, Perriman DM, Liodakis E, Page RS. Arthroscopic repair of HAGL lesions yields good clinical results, but may not allow return to former level of sport. Knee Surg Sports Traumatol Arthrosc. 2019;27(10):3246–53.
57. Dannaway J, Raniga S, Bokor D. Long-term outcomes after open repair of humeral avulsion of the glenohumeral ligament. Orthop J Sports Med. 2024;12(6):23259671241247544. https://doi.org/10.1177/23259671241247544. PMID: 38831871; PMCID: PMC11144362.

The HAGL Lesion: When to Go Open and How to Do It

9

James C. Messina, Antonio Cusano, and Robert A. Arciero

Introduction

Traumatic anterior shoulder instability can cause significant patient morbidity, preventing return to work or sport [1]. The cause is a complex problem that may involve either osseous, chondral, labral, and/or capsuloligamentous structures or a combination of that [2, 3]. A majority of these patients sustain a Bankart lesion (detachment of the anteroinferior labrum), but a less common injury termed a humeral avulsion of the glenohumeral ligament (HAGL) can also occur [4, 5]. First described by Nikola [6] in 1942 and coined by Wolf [7] in 1995, this avulsion of the glenohumeral ligament from the humerus as opposed to the glenoid rim (Bankart lesion) was largely ignored in the literature for many years until Bach [8] identified two similar cases, involving lateral capsular bony avulsions from the humerus. The difficulty in identification stems largely from the intimate relationship and difficult dissection of the subscapularis from the capsule [7, 9]. It is now reported that the prevalence of arthroscopically confirmed HAGL lesions ranges from 7.5% to 9.3%of cases of primary shoulder instability, but this prevalence may be higher in certain subgroups [2, 3, 7, 10, 11]. Other shoulder lesions are often associated with HAGL lesions, such as tears of the rotator cuff, Bankart lesions, Hill-Sachs lesions, and labral tears [2, 3, 7, 10, 11]. Recently, it has been determined that HAGL lesions are an infrequent, yet important contributor to recurrent instability after shoulder injury. Diagnosing HAGL lesions can be particularly challenging and can be addressed via anterior or posterior approaches. Although many anterior or posterior HAGL lesions can be repaired arthroscopically, an extensive anterior/inferior HAGL lesion may be best managed more completely and safely via an open approach. The purpose of this chapter is to describe our indications and preferred technique to surgically address an anterior inferior HAGL lesion through an open approach.

Case Presentation

A 21-year-old recreational athlete (football, wrestling) presented to clinic for evaluation of shoulder pain and instability. His first dislocation event occurred approximately 2 weeks prior to presentation. On evaluation, he described feelings of pain about the shoulder and apprehension. Physical examination was notable for pain-free forward flexion and abduction to 170° and 160°, respectively, with a fully intact rotator cuff on strength testing. The patient had a mild sulcus sign upon inferior stress of the extremity, equivo-

J. C. Messina (✉) · A. Cusano · R. A. Arciero
Department of Orthopaedic Surgery, University of Connecticut, Farmington, CT, USA
e-mail: jmessina@uchc.edu; acusano@uchc.edu; arciero@uchc.edu

© The Author(s), under exclusive license to Springer Nature Switzerland AG 2026
R. M. Frank, J. M. Tokish (eds.), *Management of Shoulder Instability*, https://doi.org/10.1007/978-3-032-18089-6_9

cal apprehension relocation, and a 1+ shift on anterior. Negative posterior load testing is done while in the supine position. Radiographs did not reveal any obvious glenohumeral joint subluxation or acute fracture/dislocation.

MRI showed torn anterior inferior glenohumeral ligament avulsion (Fig. 9.4). Given that he was at an elevated risk for recurrent instability and was involved in a contact sport with overhead activity, he was surgically indicated for an open HAGL repair.

Anatomy and Pathophysiology

The inferior glenohumeral ligament (IGHL) is the primary anterior stabilizer of the shoulder when the arm is at 90° of abduction and external rotation. It is composed of an anterior band, which originates between the 2 and 4 o'clock positions (right shoulder); a posterior band, emanating at the 7 to 9 o'clock positions; and an interposed axillary pouch. The IGHL complex has been described to attach to the humerus just below the articular margin of the humeral head in either a collar-like or a V-shaped attachment, where the entire IGHL labral complex inserts just below the anatomical neck of the humerus. Six forms of the HAGL lesion have been described based on anterior or posterior involvement, the presence or absence of bony avulsions or concomitant labral lesions. They are anterior and posterior HAGL, anterior and posterior bony HAGL (BHAGL), and a floating anterior or posterior IGHL (HAGL lesion with concurrent detachment of inferior labrum). Anterior HAGLs represent 93% of reported cases, whereas reverse or PHAGLs represent only 7% of cases. Not all anterior lesions are equivalent however. There are some that are almost purely anterior (Fig. 9.1) and others that are more extensive involving the entire inferior glenohumeral ligament (Fig. 9.2).

Trauma, especially athletic trauma, plays a significant role in recurrent anterior instability. Disruption typically occurs in the setting of an anterior dislocation of the shoulder when the IGHL is stressed, typically in a position of abduction and external rotation [12]. Biomechanical studies by Nicola and Mcmahon have shown a correlation between avulsion location site and arm positioning at the time of injury, namely, that there is an increased likelihood of a HAGL lesion with the arm in 105° of hyperabduction and external rotation, whereas a Bankart lesion occurs after more hyperabduction and compression [6, 12, 14]. Rarely, however, is the exact positioning of the arm identified at time of injury to help elucidate these subtleties. In the senior author's experience, HAGL lesions are more commonly seen in wrestler's and higher-

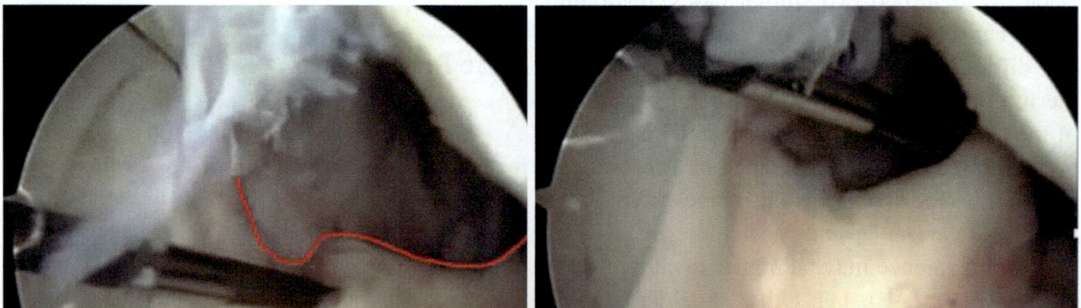

Fig. 9.1 Arthroscopic view of shoulder from posterior portal demonstrating isolated anterior HAGL lesion. Red line demonstrating extent of HAGL on left. Right demonstrating easy mobilization and repair on right

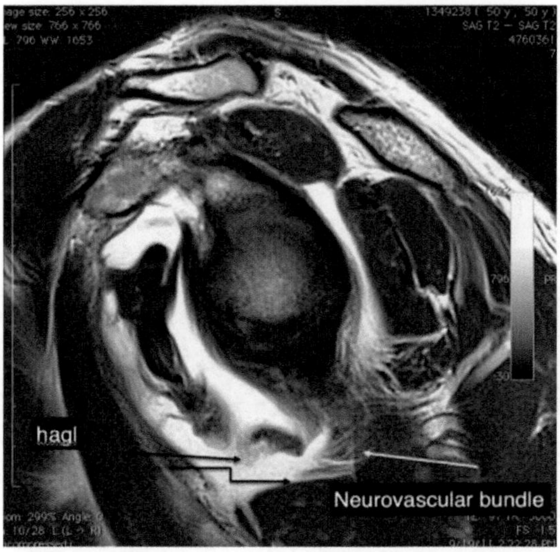

Fig. 9.2 Sagittal magnetic resonance imaging demonstrating proximity of humeral avulsion of the glenohumeral ligament lesion (upper black arrow), to the neurovascular bundle (lower black arrow and yellow arrow)

energy trauma such as a fall on an outstretched arm in skiing and snowboarding. Injury to the IGHL most commonly occurs at the level of the glenoid insertion and may or may not be associated with concomitant injuries to the capsule or labrum [2, 11, 15]. More seldomly seen, however, are disruptions at the humeral insertion or midsubstance [10, 15, 16].

Preop Planning

Proper diagnosis and management of HAGL lesions requires a high index of clinical suspicion, as there is much clinical overlap between patients with HAGL lesions to those of traumatic anteroinferior shoulder instability. Failure to diagnose is associated with 90% recurrent instability rates [11]. HAGL lesions should be highly suspected in patients with recurrent anterior instability without a distinct Bankart lesion. All physical examination findings should be compared with the uninjured, contralateral shoulder.

Standard radiographs including anteroposterior, scapular-Y, and axillary views should be obtained to assess for any bony lesions, such as glenoid fracture or Hill-Sachs lesions or in rare cases, a bony avulsion of the humeral neck. Currently magnetic resonance imaging (MRI) with intra-articular contrast, in particular T2 fat-suppressed sequencing, is the best modality for identifying an HAGL lesion and should be obtained when a HAGL lesion is suspected. [9, 17] On a coronal view, a HAGL lesion will result in contrast extravasation from the joint capsule inferiorly into the soft tissues of the arm, and the appearance of a J-shaped axillary pouch in lieu of the conventional U-shaped one [9]. Additionally, the extent of the humeral avulsion more inferiorly and toward the posterior portion of the IGHL can sometimes be appreciated in the sagittal view (Fig. 9.2). Nonetheless, while all these imaging modalities are helpful, the "gold standard" for diagnosis of a HAGL lesion is arthroscopic evaluation.

The appearance of HAGL in the acute setting is rather distinctive. Preoperative imaging and MRI should lead to a high index of suspicion for HAGL, but visualization of the fibers of the subscapularis through the avulsed inferior capsule is a key arthroscopic sign in addition to the reflection of the inferior capsule onto the humeral neck described as the "wave" sign (Fig. 9.1) [2, 7]. This is well delineated in the acute setting. In the chronic setting, HAGL lesions may be difficult to visualize secondary to scarring of the IGHL back to its attachment on the humerus and from attenuation and scarring into the anterior subscapularis. In these cases the separation between the two is more difficult, and more time and dissection using arthroscopic elevators and other arthroscopic tools may be necessary to delineate and define the HAGL lesion.

Surgical Technique and Postoperative Rehab

Surgical management of HAGL lesions includes open, mini open, and arthroscopic approaches [17, 18]. Arthroscopic techniques are probably advantageous in that they can be used to identify and treat radiologically missed HAGL lesions with concomitant pathology [14, 15]. Further, recent anatomic studies and advances in

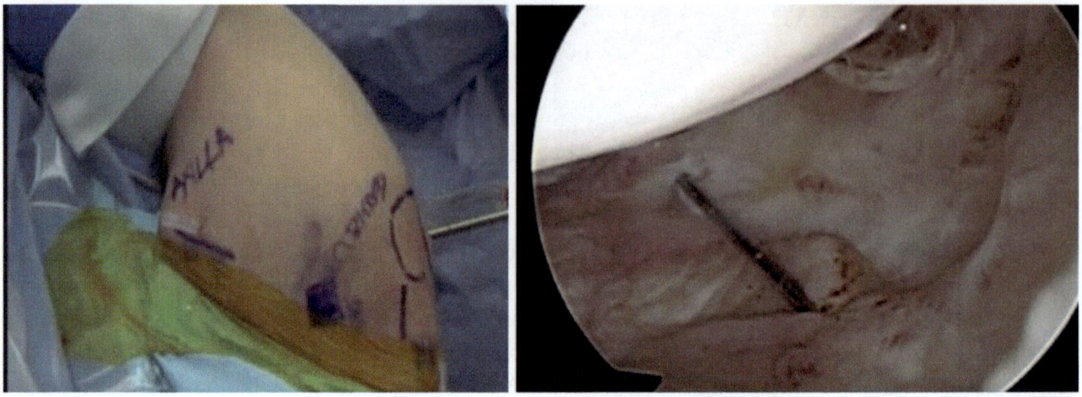

Fig. 9.3 Arthroscopic view from the posterior portal of the left shoulder showing ideal portal placement (right) and correlating surface anatomy location (left)

arthroscopic techniques now theoretically permit safe arthroscopic access to anterior and posterior aspects of the inferior glenohumeral recess (IGHR) [19–21]. However, this comes with the caveat that arthroscopic approaches can be technically challenging instrumenting the inferior portion of the pouch or IGHL. The proximity of the axillary nerve makes direct access to the inferior portion of the IGHL risky (Figs. 9.2 and 9.3). This makes placement of several anchors and the ability to firmly reattach the humeral ligament avulsion technically difficult. For this reason and because of the unique location where the humeral avulsion most typically occurs, the authors describe a limited open approach that essentially spares the important superior 2/3 of the subscapularis tendon. [18]

Arthroscopic Versus Open

The main indication for operative management of a HAGL lesion is instability, followed by pain. Two systematic reviews have demonstrated that a majority of patients (58–75%) underwent arthroscopic surgical management of their HAGL lesions, though there has been no reported difference in outcome shown between open and arthroscopic management [3, 11]. The majority of surgical patients demonstrated resolution of their instability and pain. All operative patients demonstrated lower rates of recurrence and better outcomes than those that underwent nonoperative management. Main advantages argued for open versus arthroscopic stem from increased visualization and safety accessing the inferior portion of the avulsed ligament in order to perform an accurate and anatomical repair of it [18, 22]. The open nature of the approach also lends itself to increased visualization of potential neurovascular structures that are potentially in danger of iatrogenic injury (i.e., axillary, musculocutaneous nerve, anterior circumflex humeral artery, and vein) (Fig. 9.2). However, this exposure may also inherently put these structures at greater risk as well. An open approach may also increase risk of postoperative swelling and inflammation that may lead to arthrofibrosis and stiffness. These risks are theoretical, nonetheless, and currently literature does not support a difference in outcomes. Currently decision of approach, open vs arthroscopic, mainly relies on location (anterior/posterior), extent of avulsion (isolated vs circumferential), surgeon comfort, and additional pathology being addressed. Below we detail the author's preference of when to go open.

When to Go Open

The open subscapularis-sparing approach is useful when addressing HAGL lesions that not only involve the anterior band (Fig. 9.1) but also extend inferiorly and including the inferior pouch, a complete avulsion of the inferior glenohumeral ligament (Fig. 9.2). Posterior lesions or isolated posterior are challenging to access via this approach and may be best suited for arthroscopic techniques [23]. Further, 19% of patients also suffer from some form of rotator cuff tear or scarring, while 13% of patients have concurrent glenoid bone loss [3]. Depending on the amount of bone loss or other pathologies, an open technique may also be preferred. Arthroscopic repair should be avoided in these patients or those with circumferential capsuloligamentous lesion, as this will lead to rapid extravasation of arthroscopy fluid with soft tissue swelling and inadequate joint distension [24]. As mentioned above, these large lesions put the neurovascular structures at greater risk and necessitate portal placement in dangerous zones (Fig. 9.3).

The presence of significant osseous defects of the glenoid, where adequate access to perform either a modified Latarjet or bone graft procedure, and a simultaneous HAGL repair can also be treated with an open approach.

Surgical Technique

Preop Planning

Preoperative evaluation starts with a thorough history and physical examination followed by diagnostic imaging including shoulder radiographs to assess for osseous abnormality and bone loss. The authors' preferred special views for all shoulder dislocations include the Stryker notch view to assess for the Hill-Sachs lesion and the West Point view to assess for anterior glenoid fracture [25]. In some instances of HAGL lesions, a bony avulsion off of the humerus may be seen radiographically [26].

The authors' preferred modality for all shoulder dislocations is magnetic resonance imaging (MRI) which allows confirmation of the size and extent of the HAGL lesion, as well as any concomitant pathology (labral, chondral, loose bodies). The injury at the humeral neck, where the aIGHL tears, is best seen on a T2-weighted oblique coronal image17 (Fig. 9.4). The extent of the HAGL anterior to posterior and the proximity of the axillary nerve can be visualized on the sagittal image (Fig. 9.3). In contrast, the Bankart lesion, which may occur in association with a HAGL, is best seen on axial images at the level of the mid to inferior glenoid [15]. Although not typically ordered by the senior author, as these patients typically already have a large joint effusion that causes distension and proves helpful in visualization of the defect, an arthrogram image demonstrating contrast extravasation and has been shown to be a positive predictor of HAGL in 83% of cases as a means of diagnosis [14, 16]. Both images in the setting of a HAGL may demonstrate attenuated inferior capsular pouch that forms a J shape rather than its normal U shape due to extension of intra-articular contrast or effusion down the glenoid neck (Fig. 9.5) [27].

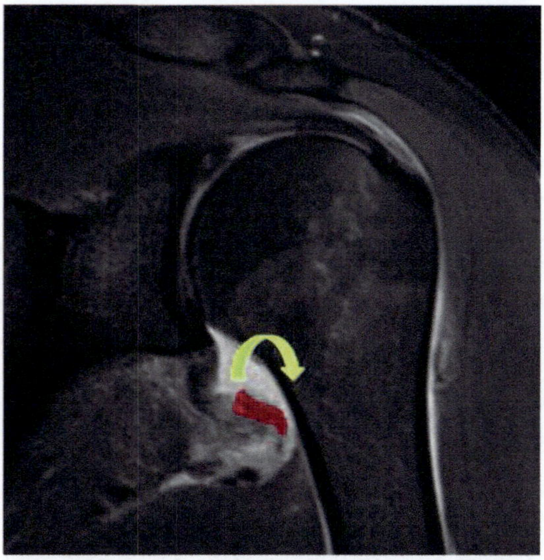

Fig. 9.4 Coronal T2-weighted magnetic resonance imaging sequence of left shoulder showing avulsion of the inferior glenohumeral ligament (red outline) from its native attachment site on the medial humeral neck (yellow arrow)

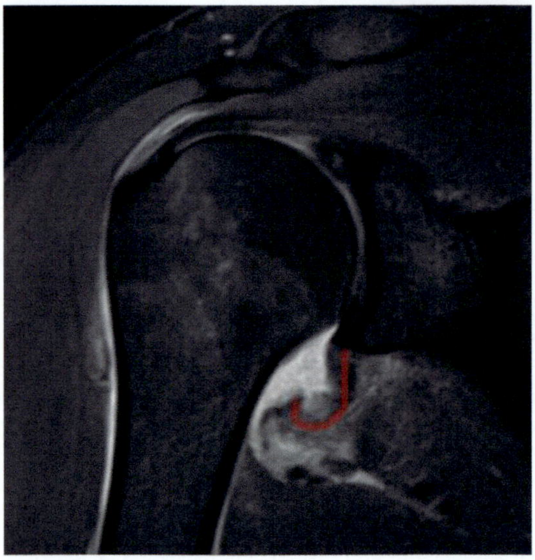

Fig. 9.5 Illustrating J sign of the torn anterior inferior glenohumeral ligament from its humeral attachment (red outline)

Patient Positioning/Diagnostic Scope

Under general anesthesia, the patient is positioned in a beach chair position with the back tilted 20–30°. This results in a more reclined position than the classic beach chair. A padded Mayo stand is used to support the arm. A diagnostic glenohumeral arthroscopy is performed in a standard fashion using a 4-mm arthroscope with a 30-degree-angle lens, through a standard posterior portal established 2 cm inferior and 1–2 cm medial to posterolateral acromial corner.

The IGHL and the inferior ligament complex should be evaluated through the standard posterior portal and switched over to the anterior portal to inspect the entirety of the recess. Arthroscopic confirmation of the HAGL lesion is followed by determination of the approach for repair (Fig. 9.3).

In this case an 18-gauge spinal needle can be seen close to the axilla from an outside view. However, arthroscopically the needle is observed to enter into the anterior most part of the HAGL. The majority of the lesion extends far inferior and posterior and would essentially require instrumenting through the axilla. Therefore, decision was made to change to an open approach.

Addressing the HAGL

An anterior skin incision measuring approximately 3–4 cm is then made, extending from the axillary fold toward the coracoid process (Fig. 9.6). A standard deltopectoral interval is opened, retracting the cephalic vein laterally. The clavipectoral fascia is then incised and extended to the tip of the coracoid, being careful to avoid any abnormal pathway of the musculocutaneous nerve. The conjoined tendon is then retracted medially, and the deltoid musculature is retracted laterally with a Kolbel retractor.

This provides exposure of the subscapularis tendon and inferior circumflex vessels (Fig. 9.7). A key portion of the procedure involves an L-shaped incision made in the lower third of the subscapularis tendon (Fig. 9.7). The vertical limb of the incision is started at the inferior half of the subscapularis insertion 1.5 cm medial to the lesser tuberosity. This vertical incision is extended, stopping just proximal to the circumflex vessels. The subscapularis tendon and muscle fibers are then gently extended medially a distance of approximately 1.5 to 2 cm, creating the horizontal portion of the L (Fig. 9.7). Before making the horizontal portion of this incision in the subscapularis tendon, a finger should be placed to palpate for the axillary nerve and ensure that it is medial and inferior.

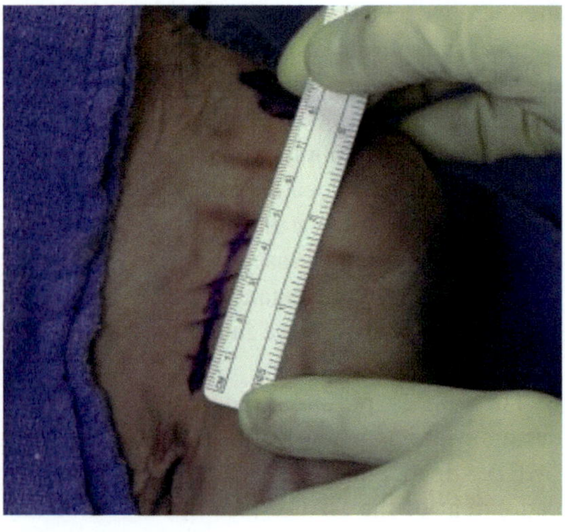

Fig. 9.6 The skin incision is made in line with the axillary fold and extends 3–4 cm toward the coracoid process

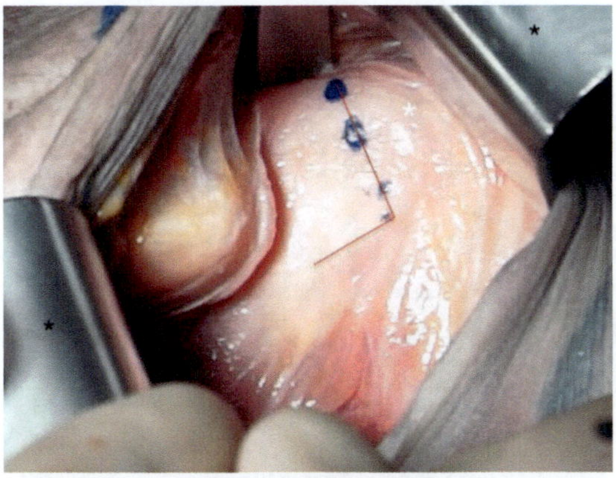

Fig. 9.7 Kolbel retractor in place (black asterisks) with exposed subscapularis tendon and planned L-shaped split (red line). This leaves the remaining subscapularis tendon intact (white asterisk)

One can now use a blunt Cobb or Metzenbaum scissors to spread the fibers of the subscapularis just proximal to the circumflex vessels. By gently spreading medially through the fibers and by retracting on the inferior corner of the subscapularis tendon superiorly, the HAGL lesion should be immediately encountered (Fig. 9.9). In the senior author's experience, this lesion is typically located in the anterior-inferior aspect of the glenohumeral joint. On a left shoulder, this would correspond to a position from approximately 8 to 6 o'clock on the humeral neck. One can now place a tag suture into the leading edge of the avulsed inferior glenohumeral ligament and, with retraction, inspect the joint using any of a number of humeral head retractors.

A tagging suture using a high strength No. 2 braided suture is placed in the leading edge of the avulsed inferior glenohumeral ligament (Fig. 9.8). Traction is placed on the tag suture to allow for inspection of the joint using a humeral head retractor if needed. Depending on the timing of the surgery since the initial injury, it is not uncommon to see scarring of the inferior muscular portion of the subscapularis and capsule near the insertion of the HAGL lesion on the humerus. It is therefore important to remove this tissue to expose the footprint of the avulsed capsuloligamentous complex to support a healthy surface for healing. The medial humeral neck is roughened to create a bleeding bony surface. This can be done using a rongeur to remove soft tissue and then a rasp to roughen the cortical bone. Alternatively, a 3-mm high-speed bur (Stryker, Kalamazoo, MI) can be used to gently decorticate the cortical bone to a healthy bleeding bone bed.

After this, the senior author, on average, uses two doubled-loaded suture anchors placed on the neck of the humerus, and the avulsed inferior glenohumeral ligament is repaired in a horizontal mattress fashion (Fig. 9.9). The inferior half of the subscapularis tendon insertion is repaired anatomically with side-to-side sutures [10]. The open wound is irrigated with copious amounts of sterile fluid, and closure is performed sequentially in layers.

The deltopectoral interval is reapproximated with 0 Vicryl suture in a simple running fashion. The subcutaneous tissue closed with a 2–0 Vicryl suture in a simple interrupted fashion, and the skin is closed with a nonabsorbable monofilament suture in a running subcuticular fashion, which is to be removed 2 weeks postoperatively. Steri-Strips are placed over the incision and remain in place until they fall off (typically 10 to 14 days). Sterile dressings are applied with a clear adherent dressing that should remain in place until the 1-week follow-up visit.

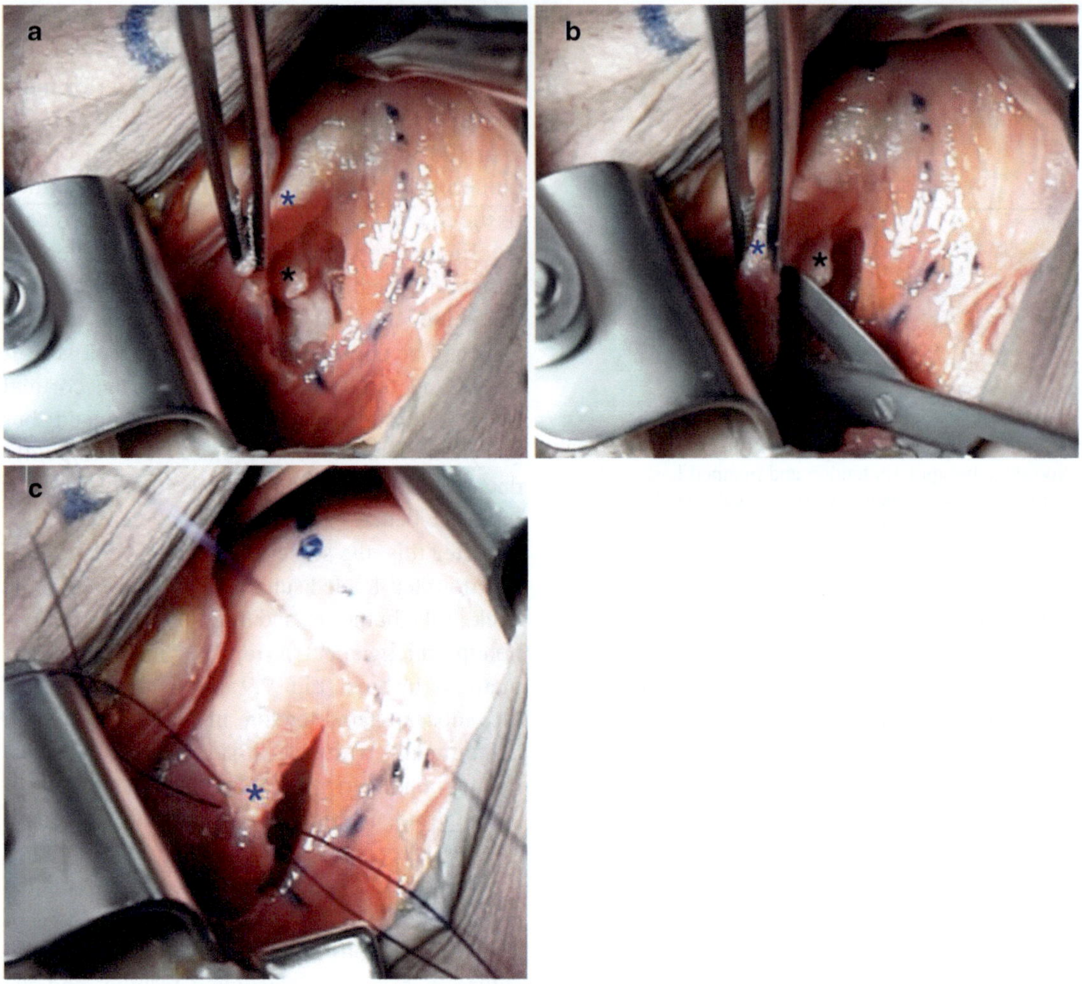

Fig. 9.8 (**a**) Humeral avulsion of the glenohumeral ligament (HAGL) lesion exposed (black asterisk) beneath inferior aspect of subscapularis tendon (blue asterisk). (**b**) Interval between Humeral avulsion of the glenohumeral ligament (HAGL) and inferior aspect of subscapularis tendon (blue asterisk) developed using curved mayo scissors. (**c**) Tag sutures placed in the inferior aspect of the subscapularis tendon for later retraction (blue asterisk)

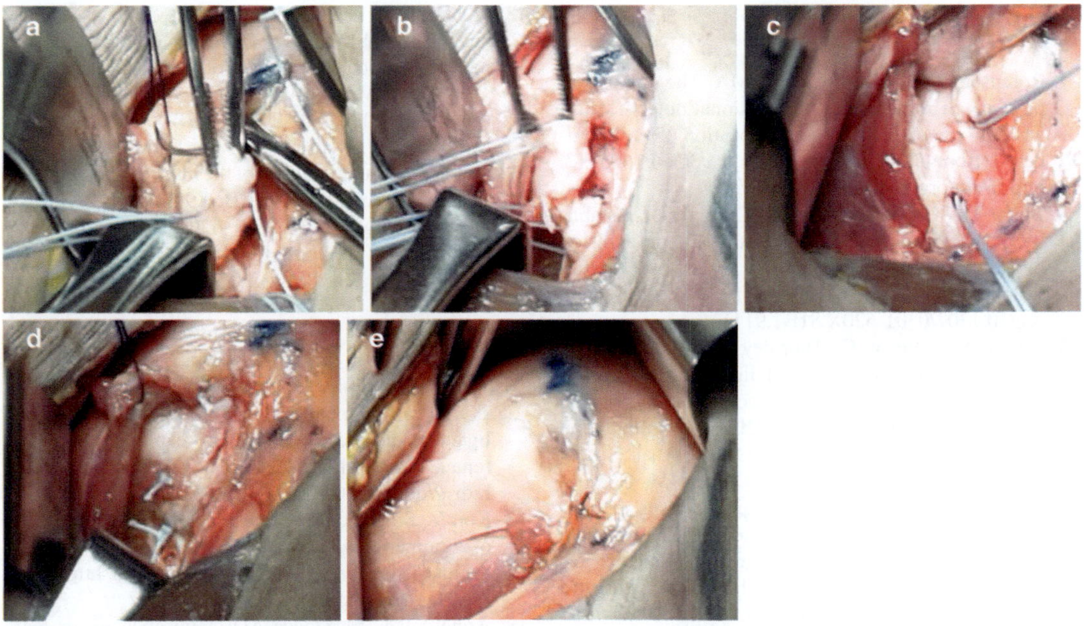

Fig 9.9 (**a**, **b**) Two double-loaded suture anchors are placed in the humerus with sutures passed in horizontal mattress fashion through the HAGL. (**c**, **d**) Sutures are tied sequentially from distal to proximal completing the humeral avulsion of the glenohumeral ligament repair. (**e**) The inferior aspect of subscapularis tendon is repaired back with side-to-side sutures

Postoperative Management

The arm is placed into a shoulder immobilizer, maintaining the arm in neutral or slight internal rotation for approximately 4 weeks. The patient is permitted to perform Codman exercises and supine well-arm-assisted forward elevation for the first 3–4 weeks. From 4 to 6 weeks postoperatively, range of motion exercises are used that specifically increase external rotation. Isometric exercises involving all components of the rotator cuff can be initiated within 2 to 3 weeks after surgery. Progressive resistance training using bands, cords, or weights is permitted 6 weeks after surgery. After 4 months, the patient is allowed to return to all activities, including contact sports.

Conclusion

Anterior HAGL lesions, though less common than other shoulder, pathology require a high index of suspicion for making a diagnosis. Proper diagnosis starts with a thorough physical examination and advanced imaging studies. With regard to treatment, some studies argue that conservative management may be sufficient for some HAGL lesions [16, 28]; however, others have suggested that operative management is associated with decreased recurrence and pain. Both open and arthroscopic repair have shown excellent outcomes in terms of restoring shoulder stability and improving shoulder pain. The proper surgical approach is largely dependent on surgeon preference, as well as the presence of concomitant shoulder pathology and location. In the surgeons' experience, we believe isolated small HAGLs are more than amenable for arthroscopic repair. Larger lesions that involve the entire pouch and band put significant risk to neurovascular structures, and the author elects for an open approach and elevation of the lower 1/3 of the subscapularis, which we believe allows for improved visualization of the lesion and a reliable way to completely restore the native anatomy for an anterior HAGL lesion.

References

1. Robinson CM, Seah M, Akhtar MA. The epidemiology, risk of recurrence, and functional outcome after an acute traumatic posterior dislocation of the shoulder. J Bone Joint Surg Am. 2011;93(17):1605–13. https://doi.org/10.2106/JBJS.J.00973.
2. Bokor DJ, Conboy VB, Olson C. Anterior instability of the glenohumeral joint with humeral avulsion of the glenohumeral ligament. A review of 41 cases. J Bone Joint Surg Br. 1999;81(1):93–6. https://doi.org/10.1302/0301-620X.81B1.9111.
3. Bozzo A, Oitment C, Thornley P, et al. Humeral avulsion of the glenohumeral ligament: indications for surgical treatment and outcomes—a systematic review. Orthop J Sports Med. 2017;5(8) https://doi.org/10.1177/2325967117723329.
4. Longo UG, van der Linde JA, Loppini M, Coco V, Poolman RW, Denaro V. Surgical versus nonoperative treatment in patients up to 18 years old with traumatic shoulder instability: a systematic review and quantitative synthesis of the literature. Arthrosc J Arthrosc Relat Surg. 2016;32(5):944–52. https://doi.org/10.1016/j.arthro.2015.10.020.
5. Warner JJP, Beim GM. Combined Bankart and HAGL lesion associated with anterior shoulder instability. Arthroscopy. 1997;13(6):749–52. https://doi.org/10.1016/S0749-8063(97)90012-8.
6. Nicola T. Anterior dislocation of the shoulder: the rôle of the articular capsule. JBJS. 1942;24(3). https://journals.lww.com/jbjsjournal/Fulltext/1942/24030/ANTERIOR_DISLOCATION_OF_THE_SHOULDER__The_R_le_of.10.aspx.
7. Wolf EM, Cheng JC, Dickson K. Humeral avulsion of glenohumeral ligaments as a cause of anterior shoulder instability. Arthroscopy. 1995;11(5):600–7. https://doi.org/10.1016/0749-8063(95)90139-6.
8. Bach B, Warren R, Fronek J. Disruption of the lateral capsule of the shoulder. A cause of recurrent dislocation. J Bone Joint Surg Br. 1988;70-B(2):274–6. https://doi.org/10.1302/0301-620X.70B2.3346302.
9. Bui-Mansfield LT, Banks KP, Taylor DC. Humeral avulsion of the glenohumeral ligaments. Am J Sports Med. 2007;35(11):1960–6. https://doi.org/10.1177/0363546507301081.
10. Southgate DFL, Bokor DJ, Longo UG, Wallace AL, Bull AMJ. The effect of humeral avulsion of the glenohumeral ligaments and humeral repair site on joint laxity: a biomechanical study. Arthroscopy. 2013;29(6):990–7. https://doi.org/10.1016/j.arthro.2013.02.021.
11. Longo UG, Rizzello G, Ciuffreda M, et al. Humeral avulsion of the glenohumeral ligaments: a systematic review. Arthroscopy. 2016;32(9):1868–76. https://doi.org/10.1016/j.arthro.2016.03.009.
12. O'Connell PW, Nuber GW, Mileski RA, Lautenschlager E. The contribution of the glenohumeral ligaments to anterior stability of the shoulder joint. Am J Sports Med. 1990;18(6):579–84. https://doi.org/10.1177/036354659001800604.
13. O'Brien SJ, Neves MC, Arnoczky SP, et al. The anatomy and histology of the inferior glenohumeral ligament complex of the shoulder. Am J Sports Med. 1990;18(5):449–56. https://doi.org/10.1177/036354659001800501.
14. McMahon PJ, Dettling J, Sandusky MD, Tibone JE, Lee TQ. The anterior band of the inferior glenohumeral ligament. J Bone Joint Surg Br. 1999;81-B(3):406–13. https://doi.org/10.1302/0301-620X.81B3.0810406.
15. Bigliani LU, Pollock RG, Soslowsky LJ, Flatow EL, Pawluk RJ, Mow VC. Tensile properties of the inferior glenohumeral ligament. J Orthop Res. 1992;10(2):187–97. https://doi.org/10.1002/jor.1100100205.
16. Park KJ, Tamboli M, Nguyen LY, McGarry MH, Lee TQ. A large humeral avulsion of the glenohumeral ligaments decreases stability that can be restored with repair. Clin Orthop Relat Res. 2014;472(8):2372–9. https://doi.org/10.1007/s11999-014-3476-2.
17. Kon Y, Shiozaki H, Sugaya H. Arthroscopic repair of a humeral avulsion of the glenohumeral ligament lesion. Arthroscopy. 2005;21(5):632.e1–6. https://doi.org/10.1016/J.ARTHRO.2005.02.004.
18. Arciero RA, Mazzocca AD. Mini-open repair technique of HAGL (humeral avulsion of the glenohumeral ligament) lesion. Arthroscopy. 2005;21(9):1152.e1–4. https://doi.org/10.1016/j.arthro.2005.06.009.
19. Page RS, Bhatia DN. Arthroscopic repair of humeral avulsion of glenohumeral ligament lesion. Tech Hand Up Extrem Surg. 2009;13(2):98–103. https://doi.org/10.1097/BTH.0b013e3181976ecf.
20. Bhatia DN, de Beer JF. The axillary pouch portal: a new posterior portal for visualization and instrumentation in the inferior glenohumeral recess. Arthroscopy. 2007;23(11):1241.e1–5. https://doi.org/10.1016/J.ARTHRO.2006.12.016.
21. Bhatia DN, de Beer JF, duToit DF. An anatomic study of inferior glenohumeral recess portals: comparative anatomy at risk. Arthroscopy. 2008;24(5):506–13. https://doi.org/10.1016/j.arthro.2007.11.018.
22. Godin JA, Sanchez G, Kennedy NI, Ferrari MB, Provencher MT. Open repair of an anterior humeral avulsion of the glenohumeral ligament. Arthrosc Tech. 2017;6(4):e1367–71. https://doi.org/10.1016/J.EATS.2017.05.019.
23. Pokabla C, Hobgood ER, Field LD. Identification and management of "floating" posterior inferior glenohumeral ligament lesions. J Shoulder Elb Surg. 2010;19(2):314–7. https://doi.org/10.1016/J.JSE.2009.08.002.
24. Bhatia DN, de Beer JF, van Rooyen KS, du Toit DF. The reverse terrible triad of the shoulder: circumferential glenohumeral musculoligamentous disruption and neurologic injury associated with posterior shoulder dislocation. J Shoulder Elb Surg. 2007;16(3):e13–7. https://doi.org/10.1016/J.JSE.2006.07.013.
25. Engebretsen L, Craig EV. Radiologic features of shoulder instability. Clin Orthop Relat Res. 1993;291:29–44. http://www.ncbi.nlm.nih.gov/pubmed/8504609.

26. Bui-Mansfield LT, Taylor DC, Uhorchak JM, Tenuta JJ. Humeral avulsions of the glenohumeral ligament: imaging features and a review of the literature. Am J Roentgenol. 2002;179(3):649–55. https://doi.org/10.2214/ajr.179.3.1790649.
27. Maldjian C, Khanna V, Bradley J, Adam R. Evaluation of contrast extravasation as a diagnostic criterion in the evaluation of arthroscopically proven HAGL/pHAGL lesions. Radiol Res Pract. 2014;2014:1–9. https://doi.org/10.1155/2014/283575.
28. Murphy DT, Koulouris GC, Gopez AG, Kavanagh EC. Humeral avulsion of the glenohumeral ligament. Am J Roentgenol. 2009;193(1) https://doi.org/10.2214/AJR.08.2228.

The HAGL Lesion: Recognition and Surgical Technique

10

Clayton W. Nuelle, Conor Smith, and Matthew Smith

Introduction

Anterior shoulder instability represents the most common type of shoulder instability and is typically the result of a traumatic event such as during sports or work-related activities [1]. There are a number of injury pathologies that may contribute to anterior instability, including, but not limited to, glenoid labral tears, glenoid bone loss, anterior labral periosteal sleeve avulsion (ALPSA), and glenoid labrum anterior disruption (GLAD). A less common, but often significant injury is capsular ligament de-attachment from the humerus, otherwise known as a humeral avulsion of the glenohumeral ligament (HAGL). This chapter summarizes the anatomy of the capsular ligamentous structures, the incidence of the HAGL lesion, its associated injuries, diagnosis and evaluation, and treatment options.

The incidence of shoulder dislocation in the USA is 23.9 per 100,000, with the majority (48%) occurring between the ages of 20 and 28 [1]. Football has been reported to have the highest incidence of shoulder dislocation and subluxation events, and it is suggested that contact during competition is the most common mode of injury. HAGL lesions represent a small subset of the sequelae from traumatic dislocations, and thus a high index of suspicion during examination, imaging, and diagnosis must remain regarding this injury.

C. W. Nuelle (✉) · C. Smith · M. Smith
Mizzou Joint Preservation Center, Department of Orthopaedic Surgery, University of Missouri, Columbia, MO, USA
e-mail: nuellec@umsystem.edu; smithmj@health.missouri.edu

Anatomy

The shoulder joint normally has a large arc of motion and therefore requires a complex balance of both static and dynamic stabilizers to maintain glenohumeral stability. This, in addition to its high degree of baseline motion, makes the shoulder one of the most commonly dislocated joints. Stabilizers of the shoulder are separated into two distinct groups: static and dynamic, with the interplay between these structures giving the shoulder its functional stability. Static stabilizers are classified broadly as structures whose primary purpose is to limit translation in a particular direction while in a specific position. They can be further subdivided into bone, ligament, and labrum. Dynamic stabilization of the shoulder is accomplished through musculotendinous structures, including the rotator cuff, latissimus, biceps, deltoid, and pectoralis major.

Bony anatomy is crucial in affording the shoulder joint its range of motion, given the relatively shallow bony glenoid and the congruent humeral head [2]. Additional depth to the glenohumeral joint is afforded by the glenoid labrum,

© The Author(s), under exclusive license to Springer Nature Switzerland AG 2026
R. M. Frank, J. M. Tokish (eds.), *Management of Shoulder Instability*,
https://doi.org/10.1007/978-3-032-18089-6_10

which has been described to deepen the glenoid cavity by as much as 50%. The function of the glenoid labrum as an attachment site for multiple static stabilizers of the shoulder cannot be overemphasized. The attachment of these surrounding structures creates a suction effect and allows for "concavity compression" in conjunction with the dynamic stabilizers [3–5]. Structures attaching to the glenoid labrum include the biceps tendon, joint capsule, and the glenohumeral ligaments. Given this anatomy and its role in joint congruity, the glenoid labrum is the most commonly injured structure after a shoulder instability episode, occurring in anywhere between 73% and 100% of patients. In some cases, however, the labrum may remain intact, resulting in injury to other shoulder stabilizers, such as the glenohumeral ligaments [6–9].

The glenohumeral ligaments (GHLs) represent four distinct thickenings of the glenohumeral capsule which afford stability in various positions of the shoulder. Anteriorly, the superior (SGHL), middle (MGHL), and anterior band of the inferior glenohumeral ligament (anterior band IGHL) resist anterior translation. Posteriorly, the posterior band of the IGHL is present and, together with the anterior band of the IGHL, represent the most important stabilizers of the shoulder.

When conceptualized as structures that limit translation of the humeral head on the glenoid surface, these four structures assist in stabilizing the shoulder in several described planes of motion, typically involving abduction of the shoulder and rotation (either internal or external). At 0 degree of abduction, the SGHL prevents inferior displacement of the humerus and anterior translation of the humeral head. When the arm is raised to 45 degrees of abduction, the middle glenohumeral ligament becomes taut and prevents anterior translation of the humeral head. At 90 degrees of abduction, the IGHL (both anterior and posterior bands) becomes taut. External rotation increases tension across the anterior band, while internal rotation increases tension across the posterior bands.

The IGHL complex is a "hammock-like" structure that prevents inferior subluxation of the humeral head. The capsular segment between two distinct bands of the IGHL is coined the axillary pouch, and forms the "netting" of the hammock. In general, the IGHL inserts onto the glenoid labrum anteriorly in the three o'clock position, while the posterior band inserts at the 8 o'clock position.

On the humeral side, the attachment of the IGHL to the humerus has two main descriptors: either collar shaped or V shaped. In a cadaveric study with 200 shoulders, as well as 100 living subjects undergoing shoulder arthroscopy, Pouilart and Gagey found a V-shaped insertion, whereby the tip of the V is covered by the latissimus dorsi tendon (Fig. 10.1).

It has also been described as a collar-like insertion when viewed during arthroscopy [10–15]. The insertion has been described by several authors as inserting inferior to the lesser tuberosity along the articular margin anteriorly, and inferior to the greater tuberosity posteriorly. Blood supply to the capsuloligamentous structures is derived from several sources and robust anastomoses. The suprascapular and circumflex scapular arteries supply some of the capsule, but the predominant blood supply is the anterior and posterior circumflex humeral vessels, which ascend along the humeral insertion before spreading medially [10, 14]. As described by Andary and Petersen, both bands of the IGHL are less vascular compared to the rest of the capsule, receiving contributions from branches of the intracapsular vessels which run parallel to the bands as they spread medially [16].

When Bankart first published his findings in regard to anterior shoulder instability, he described a scenario in which the humeral head "shears off the fibrous or fibrocartilaginous glenoid ligament from its attachment to bone." This has been aptly described as the Bankart lesion. Since the original description, we have expanded our knowledge of anterior shoulder instability include a wide variety and combination of injuries to the labrum and capsule labral complex particularly, the HAGL lesion.

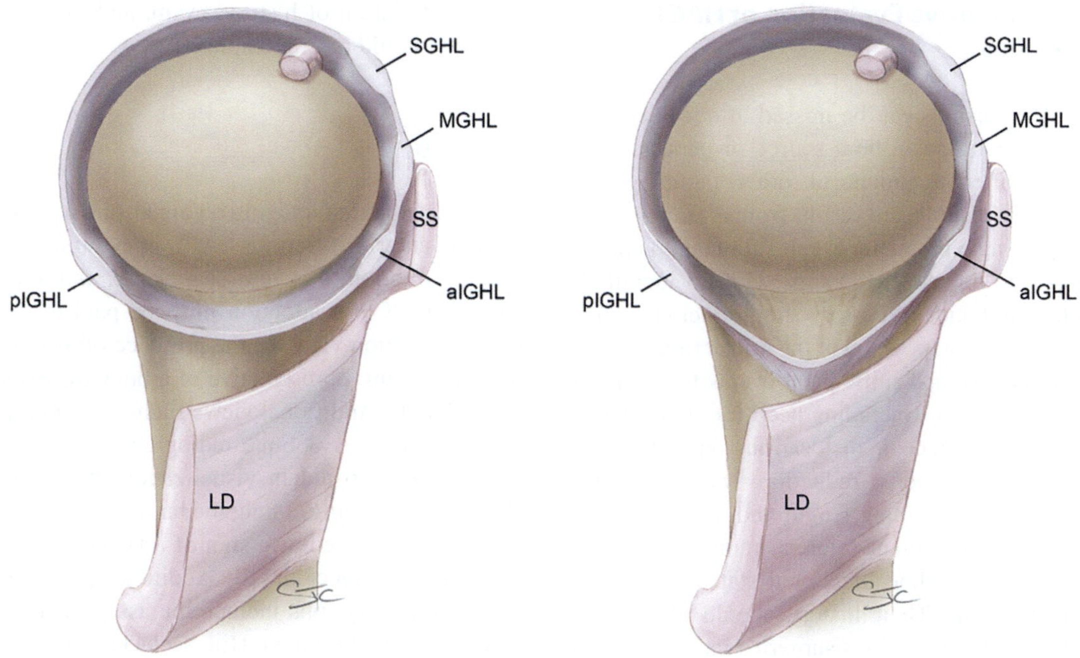

Fig. 10.1 Illustration in the sagittal plane demonstrating the anatomic variations of the inferior glenohumeral ligament (IGHL) complex, with a "collar" configuration shown on the left and a "V-shaped" configuration on the right with the latissimus dorsi (LD) tendon overlying the tip of the "V." SGHL superior glenohumeral ligament, MGHL middle glenohumeral ligament, SS subscapularis tendon. (© Copyright 2022 by the Curators of the University of Missouri, a public corporation)

Pathology

The HAGL lesion was initially described by Nicola in 1942 in which "hyperabduction tears the capsule from the neck of the humerus" [17]. Bach published case reports of two patients with this injury in the setting of recurrent anterior instability, but minimal Bankart type injury [18]. Wolf et al. were the first to coin the term "humeral avulsion of the glenohumeral ligament" in their 1995 article in a series of 64 patients with anterior instability in which they found HAGL lesions to be present in 9.3% of their patients [19]. HAGL lesions can be difficult to identify on physical exam and preoperative imaging, however, and therefore may be underdiagnosed in practice.

Classification of HAGL lesions was first described by Bui-Mansfield et al. and is referred to as the West Point classification system, which also incorporates associated injuries [20]. Six distinct HAGL variations were described relating to involvement of either anterior or posterior IGHL, presence or absence of bony involvement, and the presence of associated glenoid-sided pathology (Table 10.1). By far, the anterior HAGL lesion is the most common, representing up to 93% of all HAGL lesions [20].

Table 10.1 Proposed HAGL classification by Bui-Mansfield et al. including breakdown by location and including the presence of glenoid-sided pathology

Humeral avulsion of the glenohumeral ligament (HAGL) by type			
		N	%
Anterior subtype			
	Anterior HAGL	39	55
93%	Anterior BHAGL	12	17
	Floating AIGHL	15	21
Posterior subtype			
	Posterior HAGL	2	3
7%	Posterior BHAGL	0	0
	Floating PIGHL	3	34

Preoperative Evaluation of HAGL Lesions

HAGL lesions can be missed after initial injury episodes and can be a source of persistent pain even after treatment of other pathologies. A HAGL lesion can result from various factors including a traumatic event, subluxation episode, or even an unclear history with no identifiable inciting incident. History should include activity participation; position of the arm at time of injury (if known); and subsequent events following the injury episode, including need for medical assistance to reduce a dislocation, on field versus emergency room reduction, pain following reduction (including length and nature of symptoms), concomitant injuries, return to play, and return to baseline functional status after a traumatic event. Their history should also include details about previous surgeries including symptom resolution, rehabilitation protocols used, and return to previous levels of activity. When presenting to clinic, the symptoms of HAGL lesions may involve instability but can also include more vague descriptions such as pain, weakness, and distrust of their shoulder.

Physical examination includes assessment of a patient's active and passive range of motion, surrounding structures including the AC joint, strength of the rotator cuff musculature, deltoid function, and neurologic status. Provocative instability-specific tests may be used to further narrow the scope of pathology, particularly when compared to the uninjured contralateral side. The most common tests include anterior apprehension, relocation, posterior stress, jerk test, load and shift, and Mayo labral sheer testing. Multidirectional instability predisposition must also be assessed using Beighton's score and examination for a sulcus sign. No singular physical exam maneuver has been identified to be specific for an isolated HAGL lesion, but rather the full constellation of history, exam, and imaging findings should be contemplated.

Imaging

X-rays are the first imaging obtained, and usually include anterior-posterior (AP) in neutral and internal rotation, Grashey, scapular Y, and axillary views. Close attention must be paid to the internal rotation view for the presence of a small bony fragment representative of a bony avulsion of the IGHL. Additional views such as the Garth view (15 degrees oblique radiograph in the AP plane) may also aid in visualization of a bony HAGL. "Scalloping" along the humeral neck has also been described as a sign of a HAGL lesion by Parameswaran et al. [20]. Additional points of focus for radiographs include the assessment of glenohumeral alignment, Hill-Sachs lesions, glenoid hypoplasia or excessive retroversion, and bone loss of the glenoid due to either fracture or attrition. When there is a bony HAGL (BHAGL) lesion present, X-rays may only detect the injury 20% of the time [19].

MRI remains the modality of choice for thorough characterization of IGHL lesions and are often obtained in the setting of anterior instability to aid in both diagnosis and surgical planning. Stoller et al. first described a HAGL lesion on MRI sequences and suspected that a HAGL may only be appreciated in the setting of a large effusion or MR arthrography utilizing contrast dye [21]. These lesions are usually appreciated on T2-weighted fat-suppressed sequences, including coronal, sagittal, and axial cuts. In patients without a HAGL lesion, the axillary pouch has a characteristic U-shaped structure. In HAGL affected shoulders, the axillary pouch takes on a J shaped appearance due to the humeral attachment "falling" down and away, allowing contrast or effusion to "leak" into the surrounding tissues (Fig. 10.2).

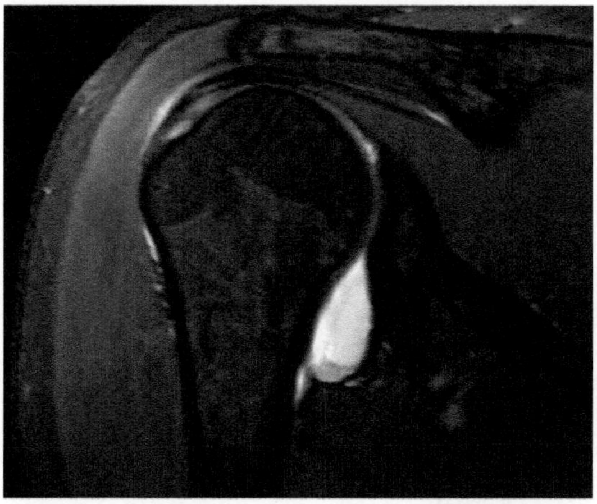

Fig. 10.2 A coronal T2-weighted magnetic resonance image demonstrating contrast dye inferior to the humeral head due to a humeral avulsion of the glenohumeral ligament (HAGL) lesion

Management of HAGL Lesions

Nonoperative

Nonoperative management of a HAGL lesion may be employed in small or partial tears. In cases where there is concomitant pathology (such as a labral tear), care should be taken to fully evaluate the joint capsule after surgical repair of the concurrent pathology. Missed HAGL lesions have been shown to be a potential generator of continued pain even after labral repair.

Surgical repair is indicated for complete HAGL lesions in patients who present with pain or shoulder instability. Repair of a HAGL lesion may be performed either arthroscopically or via an open approach based on the size and location of the lesion and the surgeon's comfort level and preference for repair.

Operative

Open or mini-open techniques have been described for anterior HAGL (aHAGL) lesions, most notably by Provencher et al. Their approach includes a standard deltopectoral incision and a subsequent L shape incision in the inferior aspect of the subscapularis. The vertical incision is made 0.5 cm medial to the medial edge of the bicipital groove at the midpoint of the tendon in the cranial-caudal orientation to but not through the anterior circumflex vessels. The transverse portion of the L-incision extends medially 2 cm. The subscapularis muscle is then carefully peeled off the capsule, protecting the axillary nerve. The lesion is then repaired in 30 to 40 degrees of external rotation. Humeral preparation for repair is performed utilizing a rasp or burr, and horizontal sutures secured with suture anchors were performed [8].

Arthroscopic techniques for both aHAGL and posterior HAGL (pHAGL) lesions have been described with favorable outcomes. Bhatia first published the arthroscopic technique for both aHAGL and pHAGL lesions [7]. For pHAGL lesions, Smith et al. describe their technique in the lateral decubitus position and incorporate a knotless suture anchor for final fixation of the pHAGL lesion [9].

Example Surgical Technique

An arthroscopic repair may be performed in the beach chair or lateral decubitus position but is typically performed in the lateral position to allowed easier access to the axillary pouch and inferior aspect of the humeral head and neck. Multiple portals are utilized, beginning with a standard anterior and posterior portal. Accessory portals are also beneficial, including either a 5 o'clock inferior portal for a aHAGL or a 7 o'clock inferior portal for a pHAGL. These portals may be made via a percutaneous insertion. Diagnostic arthroscopy is performed with a standard 30-degree arthroscope, followed by a 70-degree arthroscope to visualize the humeral neck and the entirety of the HAGL lesion (Fig. 10.3).

After appropriate visualization, the preparation of the humerus may be performed. A combination of curettes, shavers, and burrs are utilized to debride down to bare, bleeding bone to create an appropriate healing insertion point (Fig. 10.4). Next, a drill guide may be brought in from the accessory inferior portal and placed at the inferior aspect of the humeral head. The bony bed is drilled, and a suture anchor is placed (Fig. 10.5). A suture passing device is then utilized to pass a nitinol wire through the healthy glenohumeral

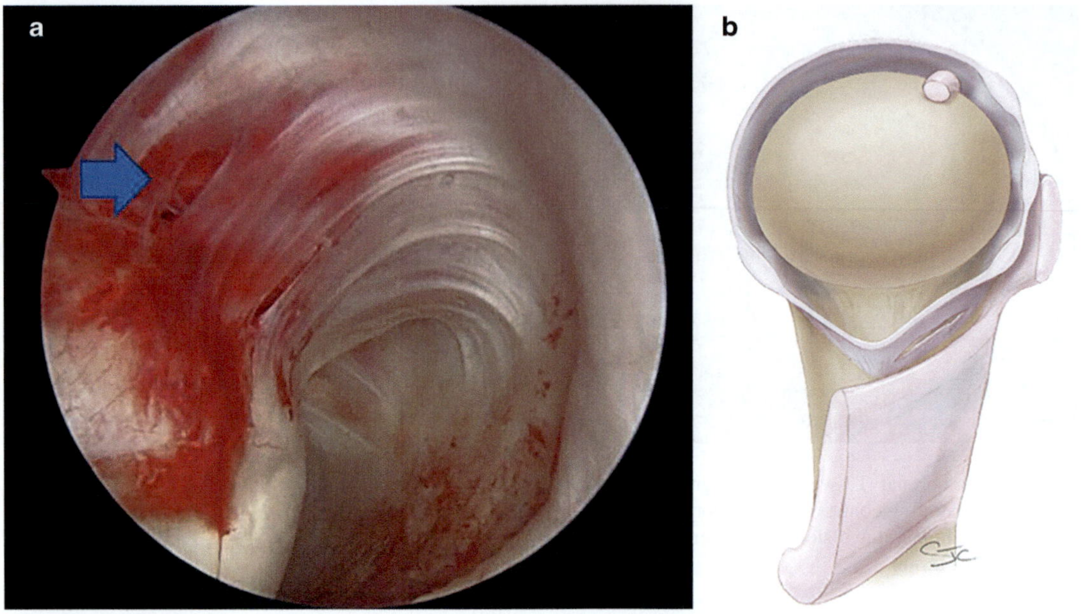

Fig. 10.3 (**a**) Intraoperative image of a right shoulder in the lateral decubitus position viewing from a standard posterolateral portal demonstrating a humeral avulsion of the glenohumeral ligament (HAGL) tear (blue arrow). (**b**) Illustration of a HAGL tear viewed in the sagittal plane. (© Copyright 2022 by the Curators of the University of Missouri, a public corporation)

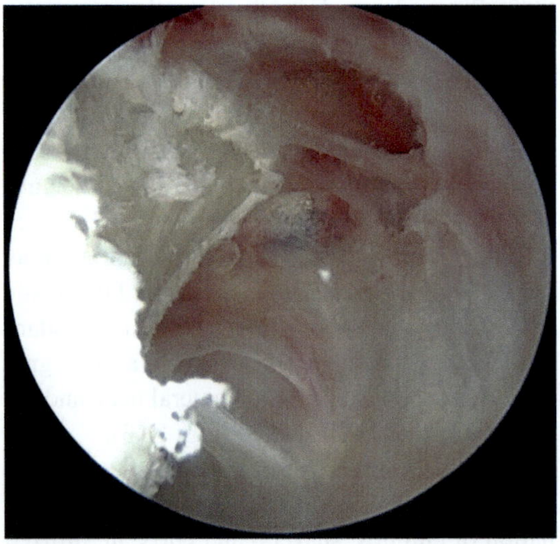

Fig. 10.4 Intraoperative image of a right shoulder in the lateral decubitus position viewing from a standard posterolateral portal demonstrating bony preparation of the humerus prior to repair of a humeral avulsion of the glenohumeral ligament (HAGL) tear

ligament tissue which can later be utilized to pull the sutures through the tissue and across the HAGL lesion (Fig. 10.6). If utilizing a standard anchor, the sutures are tied over the top of the lesion to secure it to bone. Alternatively, knotless suture anchors can be utilized, with repair and pull sutures incorporated to reduce the glenohumeral ligament to the humerus. The completed repair demonstrates closure of the defect and appropriate apposition of the glenohumeral ligament to the humerus (Fig. 10.7).

Outcomes

Reported outcomes following surgical repair of HAGL lesions are largely favorable but are limited by small sample sizes. A systematic review of the literature by Bozzo et al. included only 79 patients with HAGL repairs, with both open and

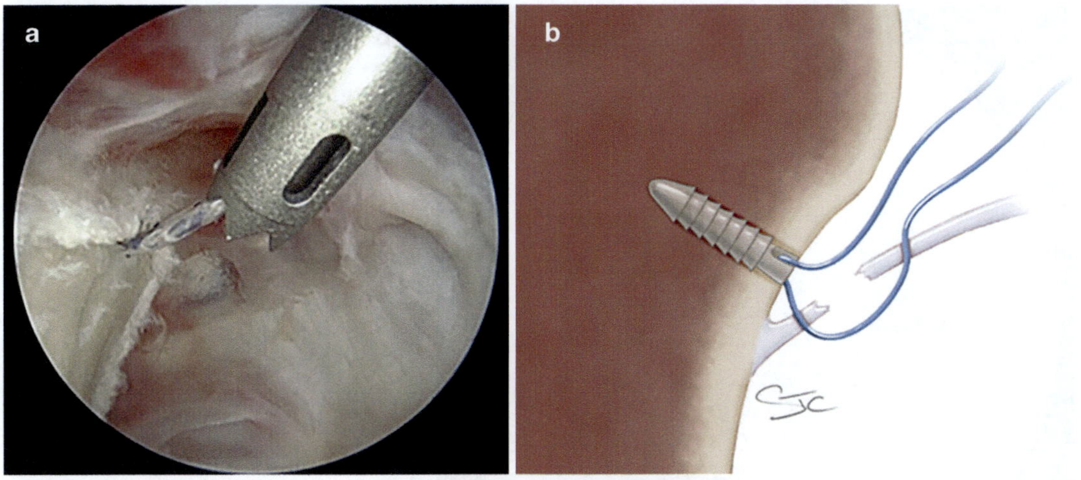

Fig. 10.5 (**a**) Intraoperative image of a right shoulder in the lateral decubitus position viewing from a standard posterolateral portal demonstrating suture anchor placement into the inferior aspect of the humeral head during repair of a humeral avulsion of the glenohumeral ligament (HAGL) tear. (**b**) Illustration of suture anchor placement in the humerus with sutures passed through the glenohumeral ligament tissue. (© Copyright 2022 by the Curators of the University of Missouri, a public corporation)

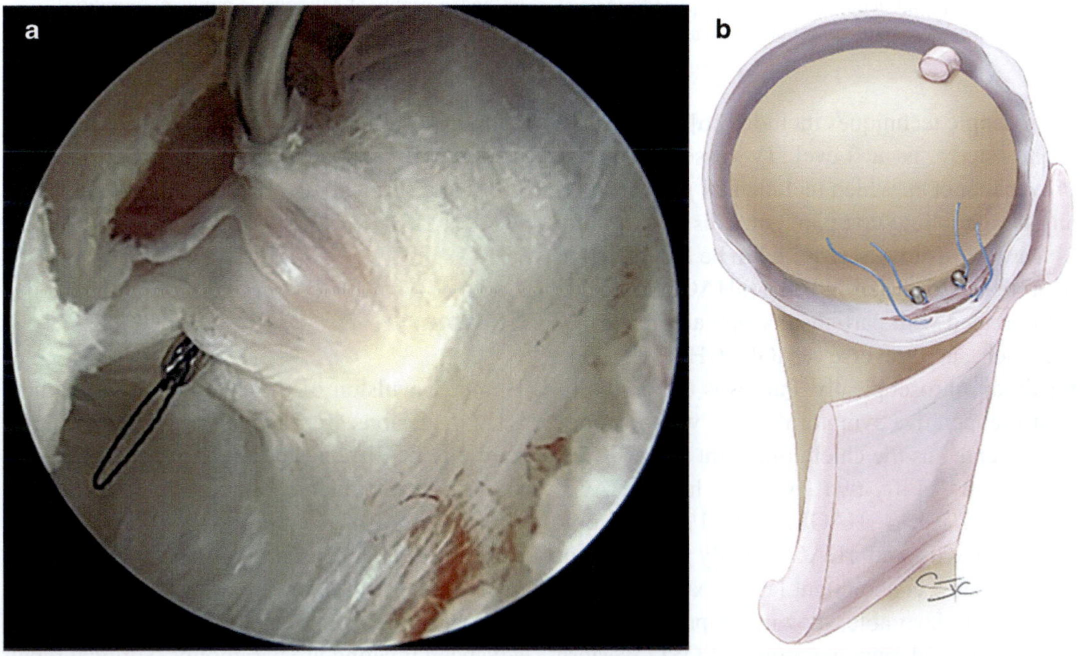

Fig. 10.6 (**a**) Intraoperative image of a right shoulder in the lateral decubitus position viewing from a standard posterolateral portal demonstrating nitinol wire passage through the avulsed glenohumeral ligament during repair of a humeral avulsion of the glenohumeral ligament (HAGL) tear. (**b**) Illustration in the sagittal plane demonstrating suture passage across a humeral avulsion of the glenohumeral ligament (HAGL) tear. (© Copyright 2022 by the Curators of the University of Missouri, a public corporation)

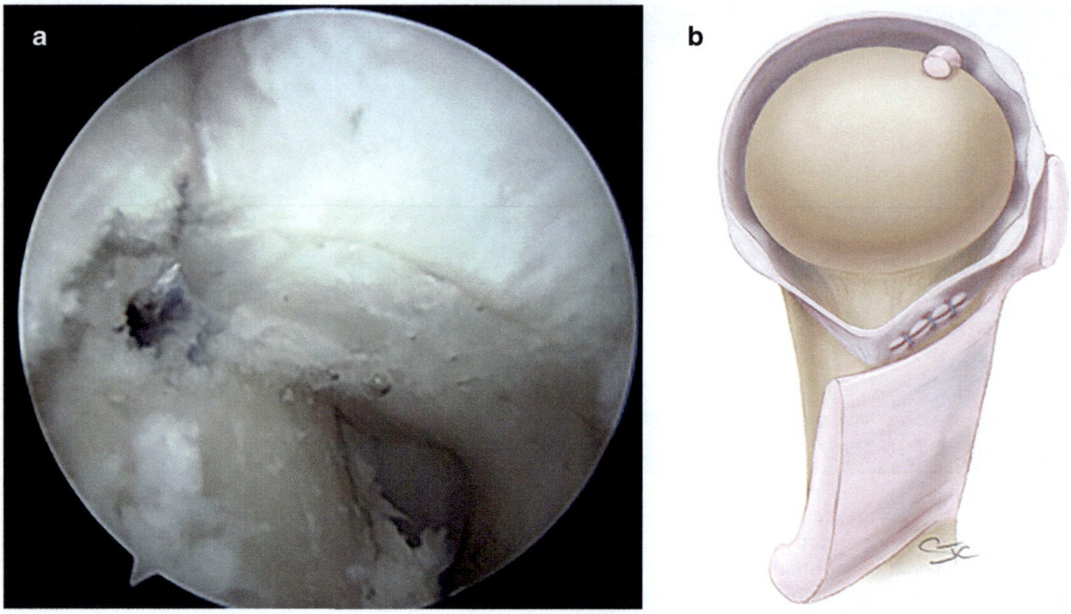

Fig. 10.7 (**a**) Intraoperative image of a right shoulder in the lateral decubitus position viewing from a standard posterolateral portal demonstrating a completed repair of a humeral avulsion of the glenohumeral ligament (HAGL) tear. (**b**) Illustration in the sagittal plane depicting a completed HAGL repair. (© Copyright 2022 by the Curators of the University of Missouri, a public corporation)

arthroscopic techniques included [6]. The largest single study is a Level IV case series by Provencher et al. which included 27 patients with an average follow-up of 36.2 months (a minimum 2-year follow-up was required to be included). In their study, anterior HAGL (aHAGL) patients were treated with partial subscapularis tenotomy approach, and reverse HAGL (rHAGL) were repaired arthroscopically. Pain was the predominant preoperative symptom (85%) with instability presented as the chief complaint in only 15% of patients. Fifty-two percent had aHAGL lesions, 37% had rHAGL, and 11% had combined aHAGL and rHAGL. Only 37% of all patients had a concomitant labral tear. Their outcomes were favorable, showing improvements in patient reported outcome scores, WOSI (Western Ontario Shoulder Instability Index) and SANE (single assessment numeric evaluation), from 54% to 88% for WOSI and 50–91% for SANE [8]. Similar case series by other authors describing outcomes of all arthroscopic techniques by Schmidden et al., Flury et al., and Bhatia et al. also report positive patient reported outcomes following surgical intervention for HAGL lesions [11, 13, 15].

Summary

Humeral avulsion of the glenohumeral ligament (HAGL) lesions are relatively infrequent injuries that may be difficult to diagnose but can lead to significant shoulder dysfunction and instability when present. These injuries should therefore be carefully evaluated after an acute traumatic event or in patients with persistent symptoms. A thorough history, exam, and careful evaluation of advanced imaging are paramount. Surgical repair is indicated for full-thickness tears in patients with pain or persistent shoulder instability. Both arthroscopic and open repair techniques have been described and have been shown to have excellent overall clinical outcomes.

References

1. Yamamoto N, Itoi E, Abe H, et al. Contact between the glenoid and the humeral head in abduction, external rotation, and horizontal extension: a new concept of glenoid track. J Shoulder Elb Surg. 2007;16(5):649–56. https://doi.org/10.1016/j.jse.2006.12.012.
2. Imagawa K, Zuo J, Hatta T, et al. The articular cartilage thickness of the glenoid in the Japanese population: a histological analysis. Osteoarthritis Cartilage. 2012;20:S223–4. https://doi.org/10.1016/j.joca.2012.02.363.
3. Bankart A. The pathology and treatment of recurrent dislocation of the shoulder. Br J Surg. 1938;26:23–9.
4. Cain PR, Mutschler TA, Fu FH, Lee SK. Anterior stability of the glenohumeral joint. A dynamic model. Am J Sports Med. 1987;15(2):144–8. https://doi.org/10.1177/036354658701500209.
5. Lippitt SB, Vanderhooft JE, Harris SL, Sidles JA, Harryman DT, Matsen FA. Glenohumeral stability from concavity-compression: a quantitative analysis. J Shoulder Elb Surg. 1993;2(1):27–35. https://doi.org/10.1016/S1058-2746(09)80134-1.
6. Cole BJ, Romeo AA. Arthroscopic shoulder stabilization with suture anchors: technique, technology, and pitfalls. Clin Orthop. 2001;390:17–30. https://doi.org/10.1097/00003086-200109000-00005.
7. Gates ME, Kou JX, Demetropoulos CK, Jurist KA, Guettler JH. Effects of zone-specific superior labral detachment on biceps anchor stability. Am J Sports Med. 2009;37(12):2445–50. https://doi.org/10.1177/0363546509343468.
8. Hill AM, Hoerning EJ, Brook K, et al. Collagenous microstructure of the glenoid labrum and biceps anchor. J Anat. 2008;212(6):853–62. https://doi.org/10.1111/j.1469 7580.2008.00904.x.
9. Ockert B, Braunstein V, Sprecher CM, Shinohara Y, Milz S. Fibrocartilage in various regions of the human glenoid labrum. An immunohistochemical study on human cadavers. Knee Surg Sports Traumatol Arthrosc. 2012;20(6):1036–41. https://doi.org/10.1007/s00167-011-1686-7.
10. Dekker TJ, Aman ZS, Peebles LA, et al. Quantitative and qualitative analyses of the glenohumeral ligaments: an anatomic study. Am J Sports Med. 2020;48(8):1837–45. https://doi.org/10.1177/0363546520917665.
11. Massimini DF, Boyer PJ, Papannagari R, Gill TJ, Warner JP, Li G. In-vivo glenohumeral translation and ligament elongation during abduction and abduction with internal and external rotation. J Orthop Surg. 2012;7:29. https://doi.org/10.1186/1749-799X-7-29.
12. Mihata T, Lee Y, McGarry MH, Abe M, Lee TQ. Excessive humeral external rotation results in increased shoulder laxity. Am J Sports Med. 2004;32(5):1278–85. https://doi.org/10.1177/0363546503262188.
13. O'Brien SJ, Neves MC, Arnoczky SP, et al. The anatomy and histology of the inferior glenohumeral ligament complex of the shoulder. Am J Sports Med. 1990;18(5):449–56. https://doi.org/10.1177/036354659001800501.
14. Passanante GJ, Skalski MR, Patel DB, et al. Inferior glenohumeral ligament (IGHL) complex: anatomy, injuries, imaging features, and treatment options. Emerg Radiol. 2017;24(1):65–71. https://doi.org/10.1007/s10140-016-1431-0.
15. Pouliart N, Gagey O. Reconciling arthroscopic and anatomic morphology of the humeral insertion of the inferior glenohumeral ligament. Arthroscopy. 2005;21(8):979–84. https://doi.org/10.1016/j.arthro.2005.04.111.
16. Andary JL, Petersen SA. The vascular anatomy of the glenohumeral capsule and ligaments: an anatomic study. J Bone Joint Surg Am. 2002;84(12):2258–65. https://doi.org/10.2106/00004623-200212000-00020.
17. Nicola T. Anterior dislocation of the shoulder: the rôle of the articular capsule. JBJS. 1942;24(3):614–6.
18. Bach BR, Warren RF, Fronek J. Disruption of the lateral capsule of the shoulder. A cause of recurrent dislocation. J Bone Joint Surg Br. 1988;70(2):274–6. https://doi.org/10.1302/0301-620X.70B2.3346302.
19. Wolf EM, Cheng JC, Dickson K. Humeral avulsion of glenohumeral ligaments as a cause of anterior shoulder instability. Arthroscopy. 1995;11(5):600–7. https://doi.org/10.1016/0749-8063(95)90139-6.
20. Bui-Mansfield LT, Banks KP, Taylor DC. Humeral avulsion of the glenohumeral ligaments: the HAGL lesion. Am J Sports Med. 2007;35(11):1960–6. https://doi.org/10.1177/0363546507301081.
21. Stoller DW. MR arthrography of the glenohumeral joint. Radiol Clin North Am. 1997;35(1):97–116.

References

The ASA Procedure: Partial Subscapularis Tenodesis with Bankart Repair

11

Marco Maiotti and Carlo Massoni

Introduction

The treatment of chronic anterior shoulder instability remains challenging for orthopedic surgeons since the cause of instability is multifactorial. Soft tissue dysfunction and damage, like the elongation of the coracohumeral ligament, capsular deficiency, and laxity of the upper third of the subscapularis, play an essential role in compromising shoulder stability especially in younger patients practicing contact sports [3]. Furthermore, glenoid and humeral bone loss has been well demonstrated to be an important risk factor for recurrence in patients with chronic shoulder instability [4, 5].

For almost three decades, arthroscopic Bankart repair (ABR) has been the most popular surgical option to treat recurrent anterior dislocation of the shoulder joint. However, some studies have reported that its failure rate may be higher than 20% in the presence of risk factors including bony defects, shoulder hyperlaxity, and anterior capsular deficiency [3–6].

Therefore, the Latarjet procedure in a patient with an ISIS score greater than three may be recommended due to its relatively low recurrence rate of 0–5% [7]. Nevertheless, Latarjet procedure is a non-anatomical procedure with high intra- and postoperative complications [8, 9]. In addition, the use coracoid bone plug with the conjoined tendon or other kinds of bone transfer procedures in active, young patients with shoulder hyperlaxity without glenoid bone loss (GBL) remains controversial [10, 11].

Recently, the remplissage procedure has been widely suggested to address humeral bone defects (e.g., engaging Hill-Sachs lesions) and has become very popular in the USA [12, 13]. This procedure, consisting of a tenodesis of the infraspinatus in the posterior humeral bone defect, seems to be an effective augmentation to ABR and acts pulling back the humeral head from behind but can be less effective in the presence of anterior capsular deficiency, with failure rates ranging from 4% to 15% [13]. More recently, arthroscopic subscapularis augmentation (ASA) combined with Bankart repair, consisting of a tenodesis of the upper third of the subscapularis, has been proposed by Maiotti [14] to treat patients with poor anterior glenohumeral ligaments. The ASA has a triple effect: it restores coracohumeral tension, addresses the stretched part of the subscapularis tendon, and augments capsule-labral insufficiency without causing external rotation restriction [3, 14–18].

M. Maiotti (✉) · C. Massoni
Shoulder and Knee Unit Mediterranea Hospital, Naples, Italy

Shoulder Unit Villa Stuart Hospital, Rome, Italy

© The Author(s), under exclusive license to Springer Nature Switzerland AG 2026
R. M. Frank, J. M. Tokish (eds.), *Management of Shoulder Instability*,
https://doi.org/10.1007/978-3-032-18089-6_11

Illustrative Clinical Case

We present a case of a 22-year-old, right-hand-dominant, patient who practices judo (contact sport) competitively. He reports a primary dislocation at 17 years old followed by other two dislocations and one subluxation. Clinical examinations highlighted a positive sulcus sign and positive Coudane Walch test [1]. The patient's history and examination pointed to two clinical features: coracohumeral ligament laxity and a redundant anterior inferior capsule with widening of the rotator interval. A glenoid bone defect of 10% was measured with the Pico area method (Fig. 11.1) [2]. A Hill-Sachs lesion was additionally seen on arthro-MRI (Fig. 11.2). According to ISIS criteria, the patient was scored as eight.

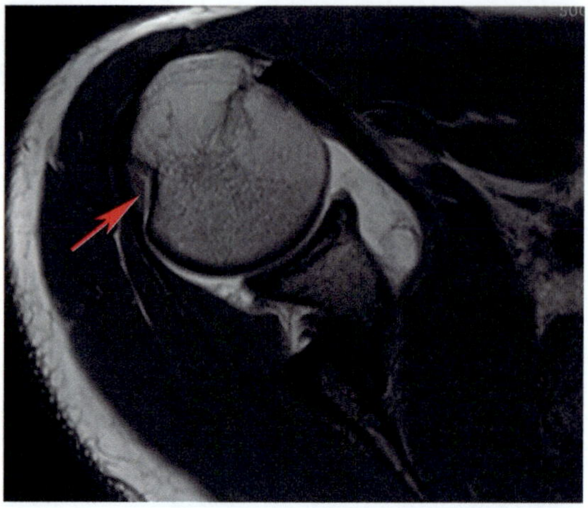

Fig. 11.2 Hill-Sachs lesion (red arrow) arthro-MRI

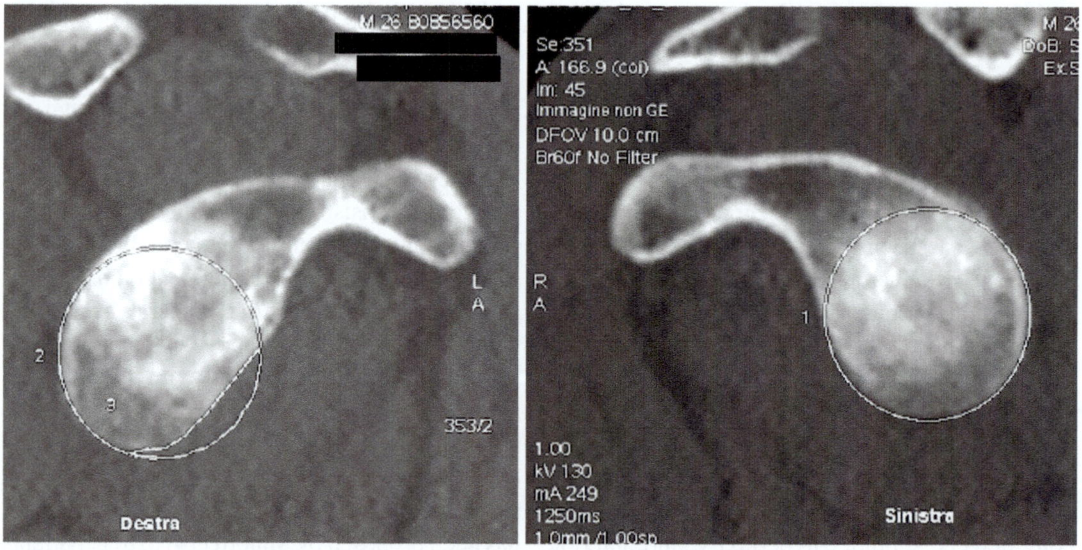

Fig. 11.1 Glenoid bone loss of 10% (right Shoulder) using the Pico area method

Surgical Management

Right Shoulder

The procedure is performed with the patient under an interscalene block or blended anesthesia in the lateral decubitus position. Standard posterior-anterior and anterosuperior portals are used.

The anterior and posterior glenohumeral joint structures are inspected, from posterior or anterior portals to assess for any anteroinferior labral insufficiency or redundancy and Hill-Sachs lesions. An anterior glenoid defect, the anterior displacement of the humeral head concerning the glenoid cavity (Fig. 11.3a), and rotator interval widening (Fig. 11.3b) are clearly noted. The labrum repair (Bankart) is performed using one or two FiberTak Anchors (Arthrex, Naples, FL, USA). A subscapularis fixation bone hole should be made slightly posterior to the anterior margin of the glenoid surface to ensure good bone stock for the anchor fixation (Fig. 11.3c) at the 2 o'clock position to allow for proper tissue tension.

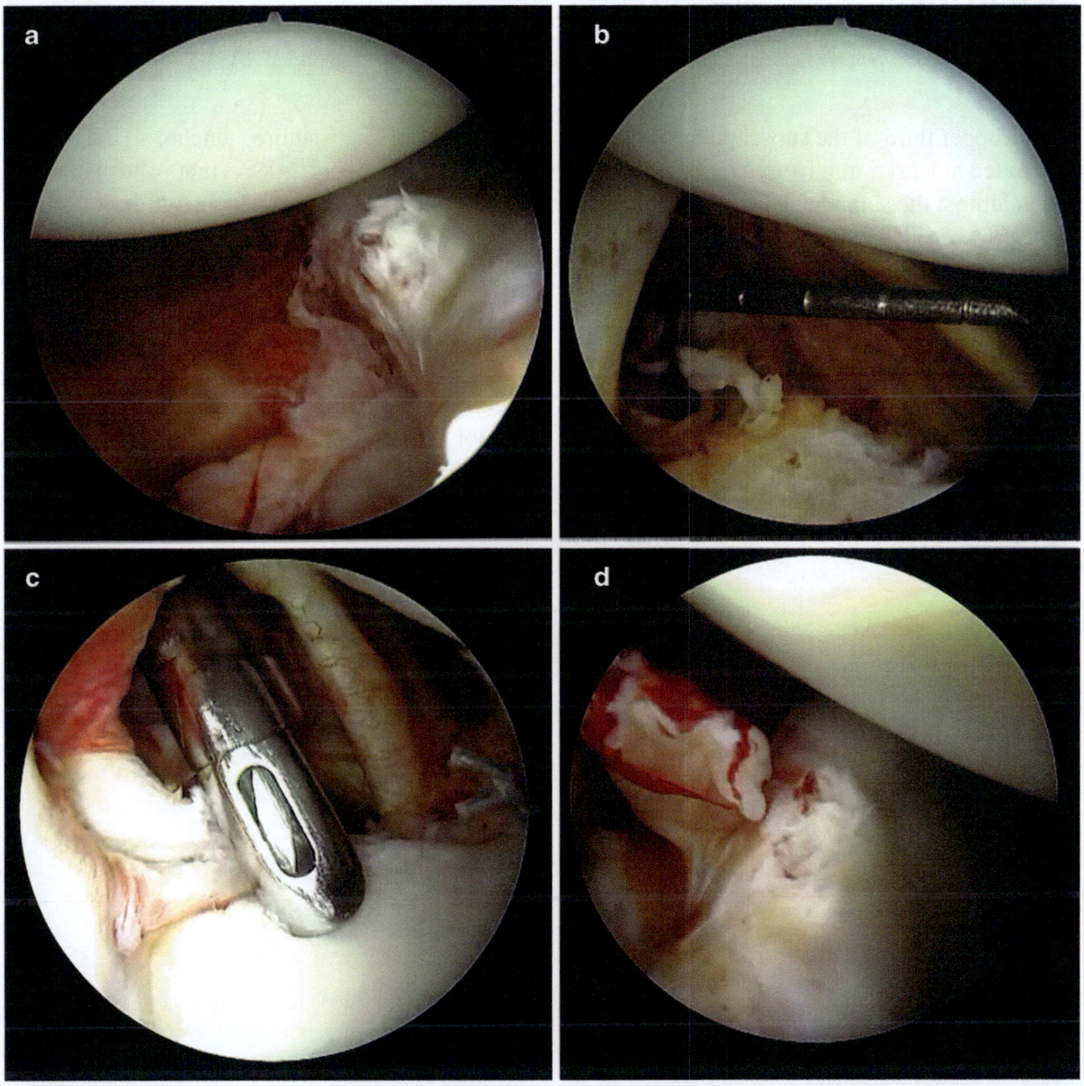

Fig. 11.3 An arthroscopic view of the humeral head that shows the anterior capsular deficiency and humeral head displacement (**a**). Viewing from antero-superior portal; the widening of the rotator interval (**b**). Viewing from posterior portal. Glenoid bone hole, at 2-o'clock position for subscapularis tenodesis (**c**). Tendon penetration at least 5 mm from its upper border (**d**)

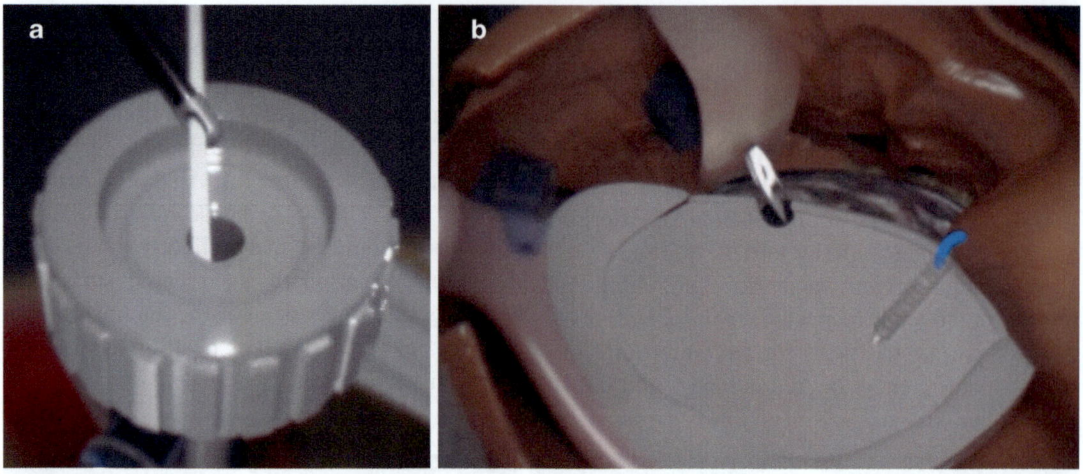

Fig. 11.4 The Push-lock is made to slide along the tape (**a**). The anchor is then impacted (**b**)

The upper third of the subscapularis tendon is penetrated at least 5 mm from its superior border and at almost the same level of the articular glenoid surface with a penetrator punch loaded with multistrand tape (FiberTape; Arthrex, Naples, FL, USA) (Fig. 11.3d). The tape is then retrieved from the upper cannula and passed again through the lower cannula so that the free ends of the tape remain accessible through the same lower cannula. A loop is created by passing the two ends of tape through the loop in the middle of the suture. At this point, both free ends of the tape are passed through the eyelet's anchor (2.9-mm knotless PEEK suture anchor (Push-lock) (Arthrex, Naples, FL, USA) that is pushed along the tape toward the bone hole. While impacting the anchor (Fig. 11.4), care is taken to keep the patient's arm in neutral rotation to avoid excessive tensioning on the tenodesis. The repair, including the complete closure of the anterior capsule, centering of the humeral head in the glenoid cavity (Fig. 11.5a), and closure of the rotator interval (Fig. 11.5b), are assessed by arthroscopic examination from the posterior and anterosuperior portals.

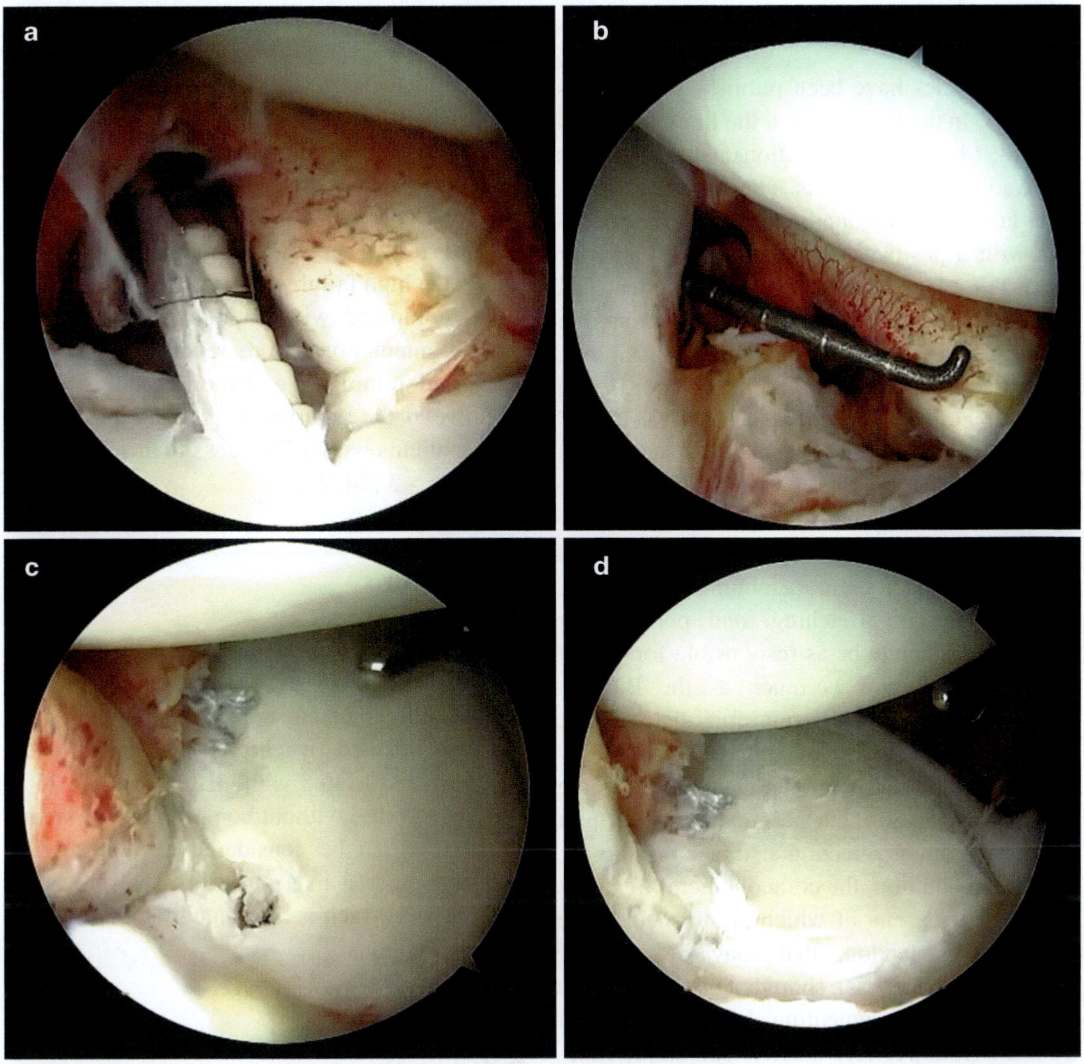

Fig. 11.5 Closure of the anterior capsule and recentering of the humeral head. (**a**) The Push-lock anchor is impacted toward the glenoid housing. (**b**) Viewing from the posterior portal. The probe is used to assess the subscapularis tendon fixation and closure of the rotator interval. (**c**) Viewing from anterosuperior portal of Bankar repair and subscapularis augmentation. (**d**) Another view from anterosuperior portal with Bankart repair and subscapularis augmentation

Postoperative Considerations

After surgical repair, the shoulder is immobilized in a sling with the arm in adduction for 4 weeks. At the end of the fourth week, the sling is removed, and pendulum exercises and active-assisted range of motion are instituted.

The rehabilitation program consists of four phases. The first phase is conducted at the fifth week in which patients perform exercises to increase their range of motion. The second phase occurs between the sixth and eighth weeks and focuses on recovering full range of motion. The third phase begins at the eighth or ninth week, and strength and proprioceptive abilities are recovered. The fourth phase occurs at the tenth week and includes the recovery of athletic gestures. Return to sports is allowed at 4 months.

Additional Considerations

Several articles have been published about this technique in the last 10 years, the first of those in 2013 [3, 14–18]. The indications include patients involved in contact sports, coracohumeral ligament laxity, and a redundant antero-inferior capsule with a positive sulcus sign (Neer) anterior laxity with a positive Coudane-Walch test [1], GBL less than 15% .The contraindications are GBL greater than 15%, voluntary instability, multidirectional instability (MDI), preexisting glenohumeral osteoarthritis, and "overhead" sports activities, assuming that a loss of external rotation might interfere with the sport-specific gesture of throwing athletes.

Several studies [19, 20] have demonstrated that elongation of the coracohumeral ligament, anterior capsular stretching, and poor-quality capsular tissue may be as responsible for glenohumeral dislocation as much as the Bankart lesion. Furthermore, after multiple dislocations, the humeral head comes out anteriorly and inferiorly and the rotator interval widening allows the shoulder dislocation. Furthermore the upper part of the subscapularis tendon also becomes lax [3, 21–23]. In addition, the coracohumeral ligament has two bands, one of which is attached to the subscapularis tendon, that may be torn or stretched with anterior shoulder instability. The ASA technique, augmenting the Bankart lesion from the front, restores anterior soft tissue function and recenters the humeral head, pushing it posteriorly [3, 14]. Moreover, when the subscapularis tenodesis with ASA is performed, a triple effect is produced: the stretched portion of the subscapularis is addressed, capsular insufficiency is amended, and physiological coracohumeral ligament tension is restored so that it will work without causing external rotation restriction [3].

A multicentric study [3] was conducted on 397 patients with evidence of shoulder hyperlaxity (positive sulcus sign in ER1 position and Coudane-Walch test greater than 85°). The patients were involved in contact sports, and their GBL was less than 15%. The minimum follow-up was 24 months with a maximum follow-up of 109. The mean final WOSI score was 321 to 335; the mean Rowe score rose from 68.5 to 92.5 ($p = 0.037$), and the ASES score increased from 71.5 to 97.4 ($p = 0.041$). Seven patients (1.6%) had atraumatic redislocation, and nine (2.2%) had post-traumatic redislocation. No intra- or early postoperative complications related to the ASA procedure were found. In another study, Ren [18] reported a drastic reduction in the high failure rate of the simple Bankart repair compared with patients with subscapularis augmentation. More recently in a study, ASA and remplissage demonstrated to be as effective as the Latarjet in restoring joint stability in patients with a GBL less than 15% and an ISI score > 3 [24, 25].

Conclusions

The Bankart repair plus ASA procedure has been demonstrated to be safe and effective in restoring joint stability in patients practicing contact sports who are affected by chronic anterior shoulder instability associated with GBL (less than 15%) and hyperlaxity, without compromising external rotation. It can be considered a valid surgical option compared to a more invasive procedure like Latarjet which is associated with a high rate of complications.

References

1. Ropars M, Fournier A, Campillo B, Bonan I, Delamarche P. Clinical assessment of external rotation for the diagnosis of anterior shoulder hyperlaxity. Orthop Traum Surg Res. 2010;96:S84–7. https://doi.org/10.1016/j.otsr.2010.09.002.
2. Baudi P, Campochiaro G, Rebuzzi M, Matino G, Catani F. Assessment of bone defects in anterior shoulder instability. Joints. 2013;1(1):40–8. eCollection 2013.
3. Maiotti M, Russo R, Zanini A, et al. Bankart repair with subscapularis augmentation in athletes with shoulder hyperlaxity. Arthroscopy. 2021;37(7):2055–62. https://doi.org/10.1016/j.arthro.2021.01.062.
4. Randelli P, Ragone V, Carminati S, Cabiza P. Risk factors for recurrence after Bankart repair. A systematic review. Knee Surg Sports Traumatol Arthrosc. 2012;20(11):2129–38. https://doi.org/10.1007/s00167-012-2140-1.

5. Boileau P, Vilialba M, Héry JV, Balq F, Ahrens P, Neyton L. Risk factors for recurrence of shoulder instability after arthroscopic Bankart repair. J Bone Joint Surg Am. 2006;88:1755–63. https://doi.org/10.2106/JBJS.E.00817.
6. Shah AS, Karadsheh MS, Sekiya JK. Failure of operative treatment for glenohumeral instability: etiology and management. Arthroscopy. 2011;27(5):681–94. https://doi.org/10.1016/j.arthro.2010.11.057. PMID: 21663724.
7. Lafosse L, Lejeune E, Bouchard A, Kakuda C, Gobezie R, Kochhar T. The arthroscopic Latarjet procedure for the treatment of anterior shoulder instability. Arthroscopy. 2007;23:1242.e1–5.
8. Griesser MJ, Harris JD, McCoy BW, et al. Complications and re-operations after Bristow-Latarjet shoulder stabilization: a systematic review. J Shoulder Elb Surg. 2013;22:286–92.
9. Randelli P, Fossati C, Stoppani C, Evola FR, De Girolamo L. Open Latarjet versus arthroscopic Latarjet: clinical results and cost analysis. Knee Surg Sports Traumatol Arthrosc. 2016;24:526–32.
10. Taverna E, D'Ambrosi R, Perfetti C, Garavaglia G. Arthroscopic bone graft procedure for anterior inferior glenohumeral instability. Arthros Tech. 2014;3(6):351 e653–60. https://doi.org/10.1016/j.eats.2014.08.002.
11. Pauzemberg L, Dyrna F, Obopilwe E, Heuberer PR, Arciero RA, Anderl W, Mazzocca AD. Biomechanical evaluation of glenoid reconstruction with an implant-free J-bone graft for anterior glenoid bone loss. Am J Sports Med. 2017;45(12):2849–57. https://doi.org/10.1177/0363546517716927.
12. Shu Yang J, Mehran N, Mazzocca AD, Pearl ML, Chen VW, Arciero RA. Remplissage versus modified Latarjet for off-track hill-sachs lesions with subcritical glenoid bone loss. Am J Sports Med. 2018;46(8):1885–91. https://doi.org/10.1177/0363546518767850. Epub 2018 Apr 19.
13. Hurley ET, Toale JP, Davey MS, Colasanti CA, Pauzenberger L, Strauss EJ, Mullett H. Remplissage for anterior shoulder instability with Hill-Sachs lesions: a systematic review and meta-analysis. J Shoulder Elbow Surg. 2020;29(12):2487–94. https://doi.org/10.1016/j.jse.2020.06.021.Epub.
14. Maiotti M, Massoni C. Arthroscopic augmentation with subscapularis tendon in anterior shoulder instability with capsulolabral deficiency arthroscopy techniques. Arthrosc Tech. 2013;2(3):e303–10.
15. Maiotti M, Massoni C, Russo R, Schroter S, Zanini A, Bianchedi D. Arthroscopic subscapularis augmentation of Bankart repair in chronic anterior shoulder instability with bone loss less than 25% and capsular deficiency: clinical multicenter study. Arthroscopy. 2017;33(5):902–9. https://doi.org/10.1016/j.arthro.2016.09.008. Epub 2016 Nov 19. PMID: 27876488.
16. Russo R, Della Rotonda G, Cautiero F, et al. Arthroscopic Bankart repair associated with subscapularis augmentation (ASA) versus open Latarjet to treat recurrent anterior shoulder instability with moderate glenoid bone loss: clinical comparison of two series. Musculoskelet Surg. 2017;101(1):75–83. https://doi.org/10.1007/s12306-016-0446-8.
17. Maiotti M, Russo R, Zanini A, Schröter S, Massoni C, Bianchedi D. Arthroscopic Bankart repair and subscapularis augmentation: an alternative technique treating anterior shoulder instability with bone loss. J Shoulder Elbow Surg. 2016;25(6):898–906. https://doi.org/10.1016/j.jse.2015.09.025. Epub 2015 Nov 21. PMID: 26613984.
18. Ren S, Zhang X, Zhou R, You T, Jiang X, Zhang W. Arthroscopic subscapularis augmentation combined with capsulolabral reconstruction is safe and reliable. Knee Surg Sports Traumatol Arthrosc. 2019;27(12):3997–4004. https://doi.org/10.1007/s00167-019-05648-3. Epub 2019 Aug 3. PMID: 31377825.
19. Bernhard J, Koch PP, Gerber C. Anatomy and functional aspects of the rotator interval. J Shoulder Elbow Surg. 2000;9(4):336–41. https://doi.org/10.1067/mse.2000.106746.
20. Turkel SJ, Panio MW, Marshall JL, Girgis FG. Stabilizing mechanisms preventing anterior dislocation of the glenohumeral joint. J Bone Joint Surg Am. 1981;63(8):1208–17. PMID: 7287791.
21. Klapper RC, Jobe FW, Matsuura P. The subscapularis muscle and its glenohumeral ligament-like bands. A histomorphologic study. Am J Sports Med. 1992;20(3):307–10. https://doi.org/10.1177/036354659202000312. PMID: 1379007.
22. Symeonides PP. The significance of the subscapularis muscle in the pathogenesis of recurrent anterior dislocation of the shoulder. J Bone Joint Surg Br. 1972;54(3):476–83. PMID: 5053891.
23. Tuoheti Y, Itoi E, Minagawa H, Wakabayashi I, Kobayashi M, Okada K, Shimada Y. Quantitative assessment of thinning of the subscapularis tendon in recurrent anterior dislocation of the shoulder by use of magnetic resonance imaging. J Shoulder Elbow Surg. 2005;14(1):11–5. https://doi.org/10.1016/j.jse.2004.04.009. PMID: 15723008.
24. Maiotti M, De Vita A, De Benedetto M, Cerciello S, Massoni C, Di Giunta A, Raffelini F, Lo Cascio R, Pirani P, Castricini R. Clinical outcomes and recurrence rate of 4 procedures for recurrent anterior shoulder instability: ASA, remplissage, open, and arthroscopic Latarjet: a multicenter study. J Shoulder Elb Surg. 2023;32:931–8. https://doi.org/10.1016/j.jse.2022.10.030.
25. Dekker TJ, Peebles LA, Bernhardson AS, Golijanin P, Di Giacomo G, Hackett TR, et al. Limited predictive value of the instability severity index score: evaluation of 217 consecutive cases of recurrent anterior shoulder instability. Arthoscopy. 2021;37(5):1381–91. https://doi.org/10.1016/j.arthro.2020.12.185. Epub 2020 Dec 17.

The Bony Bankart: Strategies to Incorporate the Bone

12

Rony-Orijit Dey Hazra, Maria E. Dey Hazra, Jared A. Hanson, Michael J. Foster, and Peter J. Millett

Introduction

The bony and soft tissue anatomy of the glenohumeral joint allows for a wide range of motion and functional capabilities of the upper extremity. The benefits of which are countered by the inherent instability of the shoulder joint with roughly 1.7% of the general population experiencing an anterior shoulder dislocation in their lifetime [1]. Anterior shoulder instability (ASI) is most common in young, active males [2], with even higher rates being reported in subgroups such as contact athletes and military personnel [3–5]. Episodes of traumatic shoulder dislocations result in disruption of the anteroinferior glenoid labrum, termed a Bankart lesion [6], in nearly all patients with varying rates of concomitant glenoid bone loss (GBL) [7, 8]. When the detachment of the glenoid labrum is associated with an avulsion fracture of the anterior glenoid rim and the fracture fragment is present, the resulting lesion is termed a bony Bankart lesion (BBL).

BBLs have been reported to occur in 7.9–50% of patients who experience a traumatic shoulder dislocation [9–14]. The presence of the fracture fragment in BBLs differs from other forms of GBL such as erosion or compression fractures because fracture fixation may be possible, ultimately preserving native glenoid bone stock. However, the identification of osseous fragments on initial evaluation is integral to patient management. Nakagawe et al. [15] reported that, in patients without surgical fixation of the fragment, resorption of the fragment occurs to some extent in 100% of shoulders evaluated with postoperative computed tomography (CT) and increases over time. In a patient cohort of 92 shoulders, mean resorption was 52% at <1 year, 65% between 1 and 2 years, and 70% at >2 years after trauma [15]. Further, resorption rates have been shown to be higher in smaller fracture fragments when compared to larger fragments [15, 16].

Several classification systems have been proposed to both define and guide treatment of glenoid fractures. Initially, Bigliani et al. [9] described three distinct types of glenoid fractures based on their characteristics. However, subsequent classifications or groupings of BBL's have

R.-O. D. Hazra · M. E. Dey Hazra
Steadman Philippon Research Institute, Vail, CO, USA
e-mail: Rony@Deyhazra.de; Maria@Deyhazra.de

J. A. Hanson
Steadman Philippon Research Institute, Vail, CO, USA

University of Colorado School of Medicine, Aurora, CO, USA
e-mail: jared.hanson@cuanschutz.edu

M. J. Foster · P. J. Millett (✉)
Steadman Philippon Research Institute, Vail, CO, USA

The Steadman Clinic, Vail, CO, USA
e-mail: mfoster@thesteadmanclinic.com; drmillett@thesteadmanclinic.com

© The Author(s), under exclusive license to Springer Nature Switzerland AG 2026

R. M. Frank, J. M. Tokish (eds.), *Management of Shoulder Instability*,
https://doi.org/10.1007/978-3-032-18089-6_12

focused on size-based definitions expressed as a percentage of the native glenoid [13, 17, 18]. These sized-based definitions of BBL's provide valuable insight into rates of bone union and recurrent instability. Park et al. [16] demonstrated that following arthroscopic bony Bankart repair, complete union occurred in 50% of fragments <5% of the glenoid diameter, 56% of fragments 5–10% of the glenoid diameter, and 87% of fragments >10% of the glenoid diameter. In their cohort, patients who united also experienced lower rates of recurrent ASI [16]. As a result of the importance of GBL and its relationship with recurrent shoulder instability [7, 9, 19–21], the integration of this knowledge with other patient-specific factors such as activity level, sex, and chronicity is important to provide appropriate treatment to patients [22].

Imaging

Multiple imaging modalities should be combined to detect all factors that contribute to and modify glenohumeral instability. The initial imaging usually consists of plain radiographs in three planes (anteroposterior, axillary, and scapular "Y" views). Additional radiographs like the West Point axillary lateral view, which illustrates anteroinferior glenoid rim fractures and/or BBLs from prior glenohumeral dislocations [23], or the Bernageau view, which can be performed in cases of recurrent instability to assess the anterior glenoid rim may be performed. However, radiographs sensitivity, specificity, and reliability for accurately detecting BBLs is inferior to CT.

GBL lesions should be distinguished between fragment-type and erosion-type lesions (Fig. 12.1). If a Hill-Sachs lesion (HSL) is present in conjunction with a bony lesion to the glenoid, the lesion is termed a "bipolar lesion." Another important concept to the diagnosis and management of ASI describes the glenoid track, which is the contact area between the humeral head as it articulates with the posterior articular margin of the glenoid with arm movement. An HSL can either be on-track

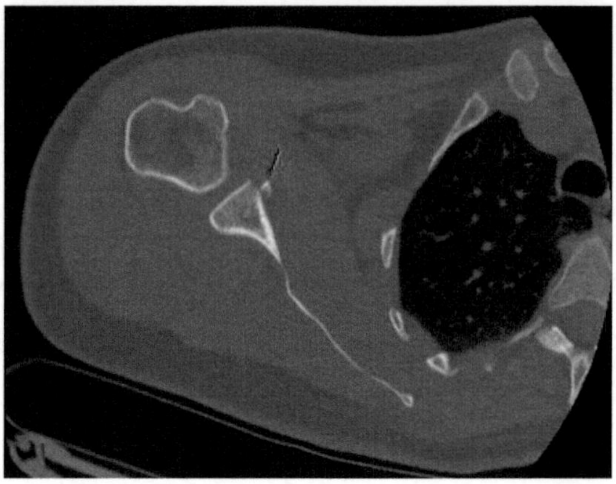

Fig. 12.1 Bony Bankart fracture of a 58-year-old female. The bony fragment (red arrow) comprises 15% of the glenoid face

(non-engaging) or off-track (with risk of engagement) [24, 25]. Intraoperative manual assessment for HSL engagement has been shown to be inferior to three-dimensional (3D) CT scan in establishing the presence of off-track defects putting patients at higher risk for recurrent dislocation [26]. Therefore, high-resolution 3D CT and reconstruction allows for the assessment of GBL (when removing the humeral head in 3D CT reconstruction utilizing the best fit circle method) [27], bony fragment, and glenoid retroversion. Additionally, soft tissue imaging should be obtained utilizing MRI, with or without contrast media, to detect labral injuries [27]. While CT classically provides a superior evaluation of osseous structures, some studies have shown that improved MRI capabilities have rendered MRIs to be comparable to CT for bone loss evaluation [28–31]. The joint congruency should always be assessed and subluxation or dislocation of the glenohumeral joint in the setting of BBLs lesions are indications for surgery.

Social and Economic Importance

No cost-effectiveness study has been performed regarding operative versus nonoperative management of acute BBLs, but early surgical intervention is recommended when certain risk factors are present (young age, male sex, and contact sport participation) [32, 33]. Postoperative admission to the hospital was the largest cost driver for arthroscopic Bankart repair and the Latarjet procedure. High-volume surgery centers had lower costs when compared with low-volume surgery centers [34]. Regional anesthesia increased costs in the arthroscopic Bankart group [34].

Treatment Options

Different strategies to incorporate the bone fragment have been reported. These range from soft tissue repair, doubl-row repair such as the bony Bankart bridge technique, and open versus arthroscopically assisted fixation with screws. When determining whether a fracture fragment is amenable to bone incorporation and/or fixation, it is important to consider factors such as acuity/chronicity, size of the fragment, amount of preoperative fragment resorption, fracture fragmentation or comminution, and whether the clinical scenario truly represents an avulsed bone fragment versus attritional bone loss [22].

Once it has been determined, the BBL is amenable to incorporation/fixation, the authors of this chapter advocate a fragment-size orientated approach. Various authors, including Bigliani et al. [9] and Sugaya et al. [13], have proposed size-oriented classification systems. Kim et al. [17] illustrated a classification system with fragment size <12.5% of the glenoid width classified as small, 12.5–25% of the glenoid width classified as medium, and > 25% classified as large. In cases with medium to large amounts of bone loss, and a large amount of bone fragment resorption is encountered, as in chronic cases, or no fragment is present, a bone block procedure, such as the Latarjet, should be utilized [22].

Soft Tissue Repair with Simple Incorporation of Bone Fragment

Technically the soft tissue repair is comparable to an arthroscopic Bankart repair. The senior author's surgical preferred technique contains one posterior portal and two anterior portals using a 5.0-mm anterosuperior cannula and an 8.25-mm anteroinferior cannula [35]. First, diagnostic arthroscopy is performed to confirm the diagnosis as well as assess concomitant injuries.

Next, the Bankart lesion and bony fragment are prepared for repair. The labral lesion and fracture are mobilized until the capsulolabral fragment can be freely elevated onto the glenoid rim without tension or tethering. If the fragment is small, it can be simply incoporated with the soft tissue repair. After the anteroinferior capsulolabral-fragment complex is mobilized, a 25°-angulated shuttling device is placed through the anteroinferior cannula and penetrates the capsule from inferior and lateral to the glenoid to create a capsulolabral sleeve and reattach it to the glenoid rim. The first anchor is typically placed at the 5:30 o'clock position. If a knot-tying technique is used, the shuttling device can shuttle a limb of suture from the anchor through the tissue, and knots can be tied securing the advanced and imbricated capsulolabral tissue in place. Knotless anchor options, which are now preferred by the senior author, are also available and can be utilized with either suture first or anchor placement first depending on the anchor that is selected. However, the principle of tissue imbrication, advancement, and repair remains the same. A minimum of three, but preferably four or five, anchors are used progressing counterclockwise up the glenoid rim to complete the stabilization [36]. The aforementioned article by Kim et al. reported low recurrence rates of 6.3% with significant improvements of the clinicals scores in a 2-year follow-up [17]. Likewise, Plath et al. illustrated in 82-month follow-up on

45 patients, a recurrence rate of 6.6% with ROWE score at follow-up of 85.9 points [37]. Given the high recurrence rate after nonoperative treatment, the authors of this article advocate an arthroscopic soft tissue repair for small bony Bankart fractures [37].

Double Row Repair/Bony Bankart Bridge

The bony Bankart bridge was originally described by the senior author to treat moderate sized bone fragments (Table 12.1). It compressed the fragment on the glenoid rim anatomically, preventing tilting of the fragment which can happen with single-row repairs and obviating the risk of further comminution which can occur when the fragment is penetrated [38]. Like other arthroscopic stabilization techniques, the bony Bankart bridge technique can be performed with the patient positioned in the beach chair or lateral position. After an examination under anesthesia is performed to confirm the level of instability, a standard posterior portal is established. A diagnostic arthroscopy is then completed, and concomitant pathologies are identified [38].

Next, it is the senior author's preference to create a high anterosuperior portal with a 5.0-mm cannula in the rotator interval [38]. A subsequent accessory anteroinferior portal is established, entering the joint low in the rotator interval just above the subscapularis tendon, with an 8.25 mm-cannula [38]. A 70° arthroscope is then utilized to visualize the bony Bankart fragment, the neck of the glenoid, and the medial aspect of the fracture.

Table 12.1 Pearls for successful arthroscopic bony Bankart bridge repair

Pearls
Visualize utilizing a 70° arthroscope from posterior viewing portal
Use an elevator for sufficient elevation of the fragment and optimized medial anchor positioning
Osteotomize in chronic settings
Use a spinal needle to place the medial anchor percutaneous in addition to suture anchor guide
After the medial anchor is placed, the drill guide can be used to shuttle the sutures anterior

Using a combination of instruments placed through the anterior portals, the bony fragment and the associated capsulolabral tissues are mobilized [38]. In almost all cases, the labrum and inferior glenohumeral ligament (IGHL) are attached to the bony fragment, and thus care must be taken to mobilize the complex as one continuous sleeve, preserving the soft tissue attachments [38]. Occasionally, in the more chronic setting, the fracture fragment may need to be osteotomized for adequate mobilization.

Once the fracture and associated tissues are appropriately mobilized (Fig. 12.2), the glenoid rim and fractured surface are prepared using a shaver and/or burr to create bleeding surfaces to enhance bone and labral healing. Next, attention is turned to medial anchor placement, which can be achieved one of two ways. One method of medial anchor placement is to insert the drill guide through the fracture site and to place the anchor medial to the fracture on the glenoid neck. If one anchor is being placed, it is placed in the midpoint of the fracture in the sagittal plane [38]. With this approach, the medial row sutures are then passed through the capsule, medial to the bony piece, via a shuttling device [38]. An alternative technique for medial anchor placement, and the one that is now preferred by

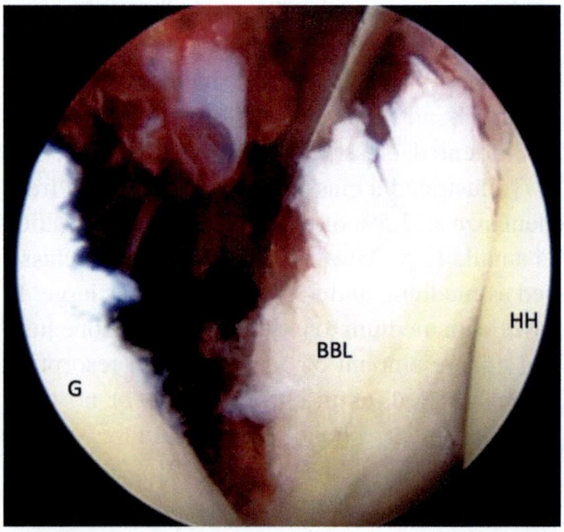

Fig. 12.2 Arthroscopic view of the fracture fragment previously demonstrated on CT after careful mobilization. The fragment comprises 15% of the glenoid. G glenoid, BBL bony Bankart lesion, HH humeral head

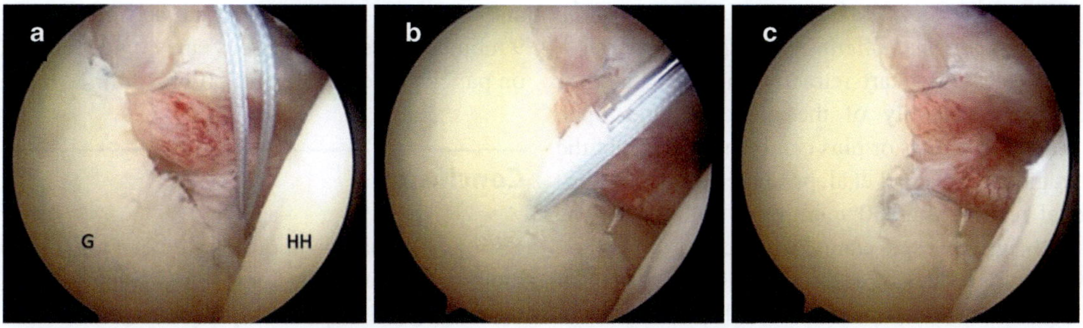

Fig. 12.3 Following careful mobilization and lavage of the fragment, the medial anchors are placed at fracture site and the drill guide can then be used to shuttle the sutures anteriorly (**a**). A second suture anchor is placed inferior to the fracture fragment, and a third another suture anchor is placed superior to the fracture fragment. The medial suture is then passed and secured in a standard arthroscopic repair fashion (**b**). At the end of the procedure, the medial anchor sutures are then retrieved and secured on the glenoid face at the cartilage-fracture margin in a knotless fashion (**c**)

the senior author, is to percutaneously place the anchor through the capsule medial to the fracture on the glenoid neck. Once the anchor is drilled and placed, the drill guide is then used to shuttle the sutures anterior and lateral to the bony fragment while remaining posterior to the subscapularis. The drill guide and sutures can then be "popped" through the capsule lateral to the bone fragment. This allows the sutures to be passed without the use of a shuttling device. The sutures are then parked outside a cannula (Fig. 12.3a). With either technique, multiple medial row anchors can be placed based on the size of the fracture fragment [38].

Next, a suture anchor is placed inferior to the fracture fragment, and the medial suture is passed through the inferior labrum and IGHL complex in a standard arthroscopic repair fashion, securing the labrum inferiorly to the bone fragment. The suture is then secured, shifting the inferior labrum and IGHL superiorly and medially [38]. Following this, another suture anchor is placed superior to the fracture fragment. The suture is then passed and secured in a standard arthroscopic repair fashion [38]. This secures the superior aspect of the bone fragment. Lastly, the medial anchor sutures, which were placed first, are then retrieved and secured on the glenoid face (Fig. 12.3b) at the cartilage-fracture margin in a knotless fashion with a push-in, screw in, or shuttled type anchor (Fig. 12.3b) [38]. The bridging double-row fixation can be achieved with knotless tensionable anchors, allowing fracture compression without tilting of the fragment (Fig. 12.3c) [38, 39].

Biomechanically, double-row arthroscopic bony Bankart repair techniques have been demonstrated to yield better fracture reduction, increased stability, and less displacement compared to single-row fixation [40, 41]. Clinically, Godin et al. reported on 13 patients with a mean follow-up of 6.7 years after treatment of BBLs with the bony Bankart bridge technique [42]. In this cohort, they demonstrated a mean postoperative ASES score of 93.1 (PMID 30485124). While 23% of patients reported subjective recurrent instability, none required further shoulder surgery [42].

Open Reduction and Internal Fixation

Large glenoid fragments are characterized by a size exceeding 20–25% of the native glenoid [17, 19, 21, 22]. Historically, an arthroscopic surgical treatment was reported to lead to high recurrence rates; therefore, an open approach and fixation was adopted as a valid alternative [43–45]. The open approach begins with a slightly medial deltopectoral approach in standardized fashion. After carefully protection of the cephalic vein, a subscapularis split is performed to expose the glenoid. *Pearl: a "Fukuda-like" retractor can be used to keep the humeral head out of the surgical field.* Next, Bankart retractors are facilitated to increase visibility of the glenoid. After open reduction screws or pins can be utilized to fix the fragment. Scheibel et al. presented excellent clinical results after 30 months of follow-up. The study group used cannulated screws and illustrated high rates of bony consolidation (9 out of 10) with no cases of recurrent shoulder dislocation [46]. Maier et al. performed open reduction and fixation with bioabsorbable pins [47]. After 6-year follow-up on 15 patients, the authors reported a constant score of 86.1 points, ROWE score of 95 points, and a simple shoulder test if 10.8 points [47]. Further, Bonnevialle et al. illustrated similar functional outcomes in open and arthroscopic repair [48]. However, concerns remain regarding the functionality and strength of the subscapularis muscle in open approaches [49]. While Caubère et al. reported deficits in internal/external rotation and endurance compared to the contralateral side 1 year after open an subscapularis split (Latarjet procedure), Hiemstra et al. [50] showed no differences between open and arthroscopic approach with both having strength deficiencies after 1 year.

Postoperative Rehabilitation

In general, the postoperative protocol is similar to the postoperative protocol for the more commonly performed arthroscopic Bankart repair. A short-term postoperative sling is utilized to provide comfort, and surgical site protection is recommended. Further, immediate postoperative range of motion exercises consisting of passive and active assisted motion is recommended. However, patient-specific factors such as bone quality, fracture fixation stability, and acuity should be considered. These fracture morphologies may require a more restrained postoperative protocol with a limitation of the external rotation for 5–6 weeks in 30° [10, 22, 38, 42, 51]. In general, preoperative strength can be achieved from 6 to 8 weeks postoperatively. Noncontact sport can be permitted after 3–4 months with contact and overhead sports permitted between 5 and 9 months. These time frames can vary depending on patient-specific strength [10, 37, 52].

Conclusion

Various surgical techniques have been utilized in the past to treat anterior "bony" Bankart fractures. Surgical treatment options range from soft tissue repair, "bony" augmentation after removal of the fragment, or open repair with screws. Small fragments under 12.5% of the native glenoid can be treated with an isolated soft-tissue repair, while fragments over 12.5% need fracture reduction and fixation. A key factor for a good clinical outcome is bony union of the BBL and the glenoid [15, 17, 18]. The authors of this article believe the above illustrated bony Bankart double-row bridge provides the best means of reduction and fixation. In particular, the two-point fixation results in less tilting of the fracture and increased contact pressure on the fracture site which enhances bony healing. Although biomechanical cadaveric studies have shown "suture crossing" on chondral tissue to theoretically increase contact pressures, excellent short- and mid-term results did not reveal it to be clinical [10, 42]. However, the senior author of the technical description recommends an acute reduction and fixation, with small all-suture anchors [10, 22, 38, 41, 51].

References

1. Hovelius L. Incidence of shoulder dislocation in Sweden. Clin Orthop Relat Res. 1982;166:127–31.
2. Leroux T, Wasserstein D, Veillette C, et al. Epidemiology of primary anterior shoulder dislocation requiring closed reduction in Ontario, Canada. Am J Sports Med. 2014;42(2):442–50. https://doi.org/10.1177/0363546513510391.
3. Mannava S, Frangiamore SJ, Murphy CP, et al. Prevalence of shoulder labral injury in collegiate football players at the National Football League Scouting Combine. Orthop J Sports Med. 2018;6(7):2325967118783982. https://doi.org/10.1177/2325967118783982.
4. Owens BD, Agel J, Mountcastle SB, Cameron KL, Nelson BJ. Incidence of glenohu-

meral instability in collegiate athletics. Am J Sports Med. 2009;37(9):1750–4. https://doi.org/10.1177/0363546509334591.
5. Owens BD, Dawson L, Burks R, Cameron KL. Incidence of shoulder dislocation in the United States military: demographic considerations from a high-risk population. J Bone Joint Surg Am. 2009;91(4):791–6. https://doi.org/10.2106/JBJS.H.00514.
6. Bankart AS. Recurrent or habitual dislocation of the shoulder-joint. Br Med J. 1923;2(3285):1132–3. https://doi.org/10.1136/bmj.2.3285.1132.
7. Dickens JF, Slaven SE, Cameron KL, et al. Prospective evaluation of glenoid bone loss after first-time and recurrent anterior glenohumeral instability events. Am J Sports Med. 2019;47(5):1082–9. https://doi.org/10.1177/0363546519831286.
8. Singson RD, Feldman F, Bigliani L. CT arthrographic patterns in recurrent glenohumeral instability. AJR Am J Roentgenol. 1987;149(4):749–53. https://doi.org/10.2214/ajr.149.4.749.
9. Bigliani LU, Newton PM, Steinmann SP, Connor PM, McLlveen SJ. Glenoid rim lesions associated with recurrent anterior dislocation of the shoulder. Am J Sports Med. 1998;26(1):41–5. https://doi.org/10.1177/03635465980260012301.
10. Millett PJ, Horan MP, Martetschlager F. The "bony Bankart bridge" technique for restoration of anterior shoulder stability. Am J Sports Med. 2013;41(3):608–14. https://doi.org/10.1177/0363546512472880.
11. Porcellini G, Paladini P, Campi F, Paganelli M. Long-term outcome of acute versus chronic bony Bankart lesions managed arthroscopically. Am J Sports Med. 2007;35(12):2067–72. https://doi.org/10.1177/0363546507305011.
12. Saito H, Itoi E, Sugaya H, Minagawa H, Yamamoto N, Tuoheti Y. Location of the glenoid defect in shoulders with recurrent anterior dislocation. Am J Sports Med. 2005;33(6):889–93. https://doi.org/10.1177/0363546504271521.
13. Sugaya H, Moriishi J, Dohi M, Kon Y, Tsuchiya A. Glenoid rim morphology in recurrent anterior glenohumeral instability. J Bone Joint Surg Am. 2003;85(5):878–84. https://doi.org/10.2106/00004623-200305000-00016.
14. Sugaya H, Moriishi J, Kanisawa I, Tsuchiya A. Arthroscopic osseous Bankart repair for chronic recurrent traumatic anterior glenohumeral instability. Surgical technique. J Bone Joint Surg Am. 2006;88(Suppl 1 Pt 2):159–69. https://doi.org/10.2106/JBJS.F.00319.
15. Nakagawa S, Mizuno N, Hiramatsu K, Tachibana Y, Mae T. Absorption of the bone fragment in shoulders with bony Bankart lesions caused by recurrent anterior dislocations or subluxations: when does it occur? Am J Sports Med. 2013;41(6):1380–6. https://doi.org/10.1177/0363546513483087.
16. Park I, Lee JH, Hyun HS, Oh MJ, Shin SJ. Effects of bone incorporation after arthroscopic stabilization surgery for bony Bankart lesion based on preoperative glenoid defect size. Am J Sports Med. 2018;46(9):2177–84. https://doi.org/10.1177/0363546518773317.
17. Kim YK, Cho SH, Son WS, Moon SH. Arthroscopic repair of small and medium-sized bony Bankart lesions. Am J Sports Med. 2014;42(1):86–94. https://doi.org/10.1177/0363546513509062.
18. Nakagawa S, Ozaki R, Take Y, Mae T, Hayashida K. Bone fragment union and remodeling after arthroscopic bony bankart repair for traumatic anterior shoulder instability with a glenoid defect: influence on postoperative recurrence of instability. Am J Sports Med. 2015;43(6):1438–47. https://doi.org/10.1177/0363546515571555.
19. Itoi E, Lee SB, Berglund LJ, Berge LL, An KN. The effect of a glenoid defect on anteroinferior stability of the shoulder after Bankart repair: a cadaveric study. J Bone Joint Surg Am. 2000;82(1):35–46. https://doi.org/10.2106/00004623-200001000-00005.
20. Provencher MT, Bhatia S, Ghodadra NS, et al. Recurrent shoulder instability: current concepts for evaluation and management of glenoid bone loss. J Bone Joint Surg Am. 2010;92(Suppl 2):133–51. https://doi.org/10.2106/JBJS.J.00906.
21. Yamamoto N, Itoi E, Abe H, et al. Effect of an anterior glenoid defect on anterior shoulder stability: a cadaveric study. Am J Sports Med. 2009;37(5):949–54. https://doi.org/10.1177/0363546508330139.
22. Nolte PC, Elrick BP, Bernholt DL, Lacheta L, Millett PJ. The bony Bankart: clinical and technical considerations. Sports Med Arthrosc Rev. 2020;28(4):146–52. https://doi.org/10.1097/JSA.0000000000000286.
23. Walter WR, Samim M, LaPolla FWZ, Gyftopoulos S. Imaging quantification of glenoid bone loss in patients with Glenohumeral instability: a systematic review. AJR Am J Roentgenol. 2019;5:1–10. https://doi.org/10.2214/AJR.18.20504.
24. Itoi E. 'On-track' and 'off-track' shoulder lesions. EFORT Open Rev. 2017;2(8):343–51. https://doi.org/10.1302/2058-5241.2.170007.
25. Mook WR, Petri M, Greenspoon JA, Horan MP, Dornan GJ, Millett PJ. Clinical and anatomic predictors of outcomes after the Latarjet procedure for the treatment of anterior glenohumeral instability with combined glenoid and humeral bone defects. Am J Sports Med. 2016;44(6):1407–16. https://doi.org/10.1177/0363546516634089.
26. Lee YJ, Kim C, Kim SJ, Yoon TH, Cho JY, Chun YM. Does an "off-track" Hill-Sachs lesion that is misclassified as "non-engaging" affect outcomes from Bankart repair alone compared with Bankart repair combined with Remplissage? Arthroscopy. 2021;37(2):450–6. https://doi.org/10.1016/j.arthro.2020.09.037.
27. Skupinski J, Piechota MZ, Wawrzynek W, Maczuch J, Babinska A. The bony Bankart lesion: how to measure the glenoid bone loss. Pol J Radiol. 2017;82:58–63. https://doi.org/10.12659/PJR.898566.
28. Gyftopoulos S, Beltran LS, Yemin A, et al. Use of 3D MR reconstructions in the evaluation of glenoid bone loss: a clinical study. Skeletal Radiol.

2014;43(2):213–8. https://doi.org/10.1007/s00256-013-1774-5.
29. Stecco A, Guenzi E, Cascone T, et al. MRI can assess glenoid bone loss after shoulder luxation: inter- and intra-individual comparison with CT. Radiol Med. 2013;118(8):1335–43. https://doi.org/10.1007/s11547-013-0927-x.
30. Bishop JY, Jones GL, Rerko MA, Donaldson C, Group MS. 3-D CT is the most reliable imaging modality when quantifying glenoid bone loss. Clin Orthop Relat Res. 2013;471(4):1251–6. https://doi.org/10.1007/s11999-012-2607-x.
31. Moroder P, Resch H, Schnaitmann S, Hoffelner T, Tauber M. The importance of CT for the pre-operative surgical planning in recurrent anterior shoulder instability. Arch Orthop Trauma Surg. 2013;133(2):219–26. https://doi.org/10.1007/s00402-012-1656-7.
32. Provencher CMT, Midtgaard KS. Editorial commentary: evidence to support surgical intervention for first-time shoulder instability: stabilize them early! Arthroscopy. 2020;36(9):2533–6. https://doi.org/10.1016/j.arthro.2020.07.034.
33. Hurley ET, Manjunath AK, Bloom DA, et al. Arthroscopic Bankart repair versus conservative management for first-time traumatic anterior shoulder instability: a systematic review and meta-analysis. Arthroscopy. 2020;36(9):2526–32. https://doi.org/10.1016/j.arthro.2020.04.046.
34. Li LT, Bokshan SL, Levins JG, Owens BD. Cost drivers associated with anterior shoulder stabilization surgery. Orthop J Sports Med. 2020;8(6):2325967120926465. https://doi.org/10.1177/2325967120926465.
35. Lacheta L, Dekker TJ, Anderson N, Goldenberg B, Millett PJ. Arthroscopic knotless, tensionable all-suture anchor Bankart repair. Arthrosc Tech. 2019;8(6):e647–53. https://doi.org/10.1016/j.eats.2019.02.010.
36. Sugaya H, Kon Y, Tsuchiya A. Arthroscopic repair of glenoid fractures using suture anchors. Arthroscopy. 2005;21(5):635. https://doi.org/10.1016/j.arthro.2005.02.006.
37. Plath JE, Feucht MJ, Bangoj R, et al. Arthroscopic suture anchor fixation of bony Bankart lesions: clinical outcome, magnetic resonance imaging results, and return to sports. Arthroscopy. 2015;31(8):1472–81. https://doi.org/10.1016/j.arthro.2015.03.005.
38. Millett PJ, Braun S. The "bony Bankart bridge" procedure: a new arthroscopic technique for reduction and internal fixation of a bony Bankart lesion. Arthroscopy. 2009;25(1):102–5. https://doi.org/10.1016/j.arthro.2008.07.005.
39. Liles J, Fletcher A, Johnston T, Riboh J. Arthroscopic double-row bony Bankart bridge repair using a tensionable knotless system. Arthrosc Tech. 2021;10(4):e957–62. https://doi.org/10.1016/j.eats.2020.11.009.
40. Greenstein AS, Chen RE, Knapp E, et al. A biomechanical, cadaveric evaluation of single- versus double-row repair techniques on stability of bony Bankart lesions. Am J Sports Med. 2021;49(3):773–9. https://doi.org/10.1177/0363546520985184.
41. Spiegl UJ, Smith SD, Todd JN, Coatney GA, Wijdicks CA, Millett PJ. Biomechanical comparison of arthroscopic single- and double-row repair techniques for acute bony Bankart lesions. Am J Sports Med. 2014;42(8):1939–46. https://doi.org/10.1177/0363546514532782.
42. Godin JA, Altintas B, Horan MP, et al. Midterm results of the bony Bankart bridge technique for the treatment of bony Bankart lesions. Am J Sports Med. 2019;47(1):158–64. https://doi.org/10.1177/0363546518808495.
43. Boileau P, Villalba M, Hery JY, Balg F, Ahrens P, Neyton L. Risk factors for recurrence of shoulder instability after arthroscopic Bankart repair. J Bone Joint Surg Am. 2006;88(8):1755–63. https://doi.org/10.2106/JBJS.E.00817.
44. Burkhart SS, De Beer JF. Traumatic glenohumeral bone defects and their relationship to failure of arthroscopic Bankart repairs: significance of the inverted-pear glenoid and the humeral engaging Hill-Sachs lesion. Arthroscopy. 2000;16(7):677–94. https://doi.org/10.1053/jars.2000.17715.
45. Lo IK, Parten PM, Burkhart SS. The inverted pear glenoid: an indicator of significant glenoid bone loss. Arthroscopy. 2004;20(2):169–74. https://doi.org/10.1016/j.arthro.2003.11.036.
46. Scheibel M, Magosch P, Lichtenberg S, Habermeyer P. Open reconstruction of anterior glenoid rim fractures. Knee Surg Sports Traumatol Arthrosc. 2004;12(6):568–73. https://doi.org/10.1007/s00167-004-0495-7.
47. Maier D, Izadpanah K, Ogon P, et al. Open fixation of acute anterior glenoid rim fractures with bioresorbable pins: analysis of clinical and radiological outcome. Arch Orthop Trauma Surg. 2015;135(7):953–61. https://doi.org/10.1007/s00402-015-2242-6.
48. Bonnevialle N, Clavert P, Arboucalot M, et al. Contribution of arthroscopy in the treatment of anterior glenoid rim fractures: a comparison with open surgery. J Shoulder Elb Surg. 2019;28(1):42–7. https://doi.org/10.1016/j.jse.2018.07.008.
49. Caubere A, Lami D, Boileau P, Parratte S, Ollivier M, Argenson JN. Is the subscapularis normal after the open Latarjet procedure? An isokinetic and magnetic resonance imaging evaluation. J Shoulder Elb Surg. 2017;26(10):1775–81. https://doi.org/10.1016/j.jse.2017.03.034.
50. Hiemstra LA, Sasyniuk TM, Mohtadi NG, Fick GH. Shoulder strength after open versus arthroscopic stabilization. Am J Sports Med. 2008;36(5):861–7. https://doi.org/10.1177/0363546508314429.
51. Spiegl UJ, Braun S, Euler SA, Warth RJ, Millett PJ. Bony Bankart lesions. Unfallchirurg. 2014;117(12):1125–38; quiz 1138-40. Die ossare Bankart-Lasion. https://doi.org/10.1007/s00113-014-2703-3.
52. Porcellini G, Campi F, Paladini P. Arthroscopic approach to acute bony Bankart lesion. Arthroscopy. 2002;18(7):764–9. https://doi.org/10.1053/jars.2002.35266.

The Remplissage: Indications and Surgical Technique

13

Nicholas A. Ott, Robert L. Parisien, Joshua Chiang, Ann Marie Kelly, and John D. A. Kelly IV

Introduction

Anterior shoulder instability remains a difficult clinical problem to reconcile. With every shoulder dislocation, there is inherent risk of bone loss to both the glenoid and the humeral head [1, 2]. With accruing bone loss, more constraining procedures become necessary to prevent dislocation. As Burkhart and De Beer have illustrated, untreated bone loss results in woefully inadequate results with soft tissue procedures alone [1].

The concept of the glenoid track introduced by Yammamoto et al. helps us to recognize the synergistic effects of bone loss on both the glenoid and humeral side in potentiating recurrence [3]. A key element of the glenoid track concept is that glenoid bone loss narrows the "track" and increases the likelihood that a Hill-Sachs lesion will engage. Similarly, the more medial a Hill-Sachs lesion extends, the more likely it is to engage the anterior rim of the glenoid [3].

The Hill-Sachs lesion is simply an impression defect located on the posterolateral humeral head which occurs either at time of dislocation or upon reduction. The size and depth of the Hill-Sachs lesion has been shown to correlate with recurrence rates. Some data suggests that a lesion greater than 19% of humeral head diameter may indicate a "critical" amount of affected humeral head with increased risk of potentiating recurrence [4].

In summary, lesions that are larger, deeper, and more medial will have an increased tendency to "engage" during the abducted external rotation position and therefore will need to be addressed surgically (Fig. 13.1).

Possible treatment options for the Hill-Sachs lesion include disimpaction [5, 6], metallic prosthetic implant [7], extension of the "glenoid track" with coracoid transfer [8, 9], or osteochondral allograft [10, 11]. All these options confer appreciable morbidity. Both the Latarjet and, to a lesser extent, the Bristow procedure violate the origins of the coracoacromial ligament, the short head of the biceps, coracobrachialis, and pectoralis minor. Furthermore, although coracoid

N. A. Ott
Andrews Research and Education Foundation, Andrews Institute, Gulf Breeze, FL, USA

R. L. Parisien
Orthopaedic Surgery and Sports Medicine, Mount Sinai Health System, New York, NY, USA
e-mail: robert.parisien@mountsinai.org

J. Chiang
Perelman School of Medicine, University of Pennsylvania, Philadelphia, PA, USA
e-mail: joshua.chiang@pennmedicine.upenn.edu

A. M. Kelly
Orthopaedic Surgery, Dartmouth-Hitchcock Medical Center, Lebanon, NH, USA

J. D. A. Kelly IV (✉)
Orthopaedic Surgery, Sports Medicine, University of Pennsylvania, Philadelphia, PA, USA
e-mail: john.kelly@pennmedicine.upenn.edu

© The Author(s), under exclusive license to Springer Nature Switzerland AG 2026
R. M. Frank, J. M. Tokish (eds.), *Management of Shoulder Instability*,
https://doi.org/10.1007/978-3-032-18089-6_13

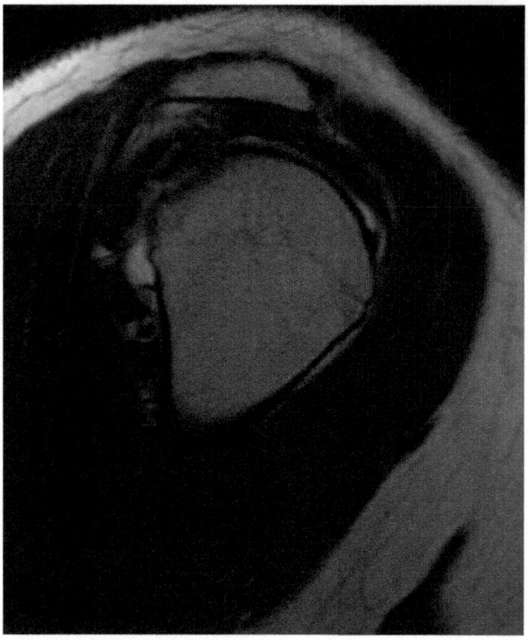

Fig. 13.1 Hill-Sachs lesion

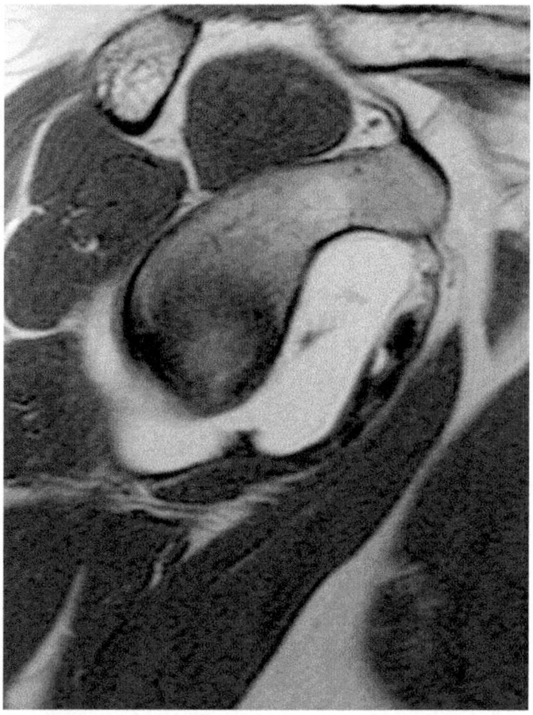

Fig. 13.2 Sagittal view of glenoid

transfer does indeed enlarge the glenoid track, coracoid width may prove to be insufficient to prevent engagement [12].

Mechanically, remplissage has been shown to shift the glenoid track medially, in addition to providing a biologic "fill" of the Hill-Sachs lesion. This twofold benefit likely explains the significant benefit afforded by this minimally invasive procedure.

In addition, current paradigms in management of the unstable shoulder regard glenoid bone loss of greater than 13.4% to require some form of boney augmentation [13]. We submit that a properly executed remplissage with the possible addition of glenoid bone grafting obviates the need for coracoid transfer in most cases.

Case

A 31-year-old right-hand-dominant male presented with a 6-year history of recurrent instability in the right shoulder. On examination, he demonstrated both apprehension and a positive relocation test. His MRI demonstrated a Hill-Sachs lesion (Fig. 13.1) as well as approximately 20% glenoid bone loss (Fig. 13.2). He failed to gain any appreciable relief from physical therapy and consented to undergo surgical intervention.

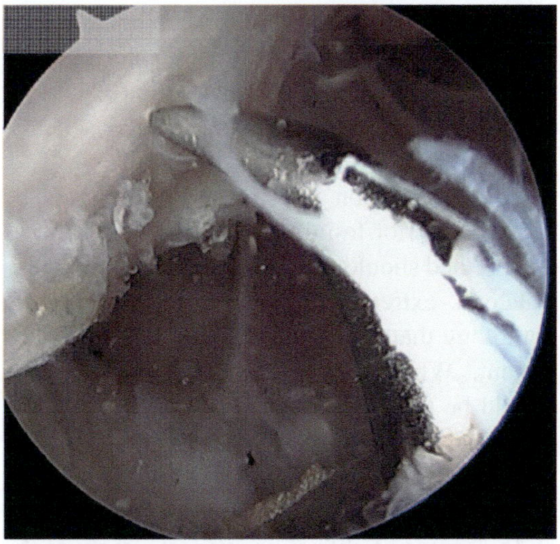

Fig. 13.3 Arthroscopic view of Hill Sachs lesion

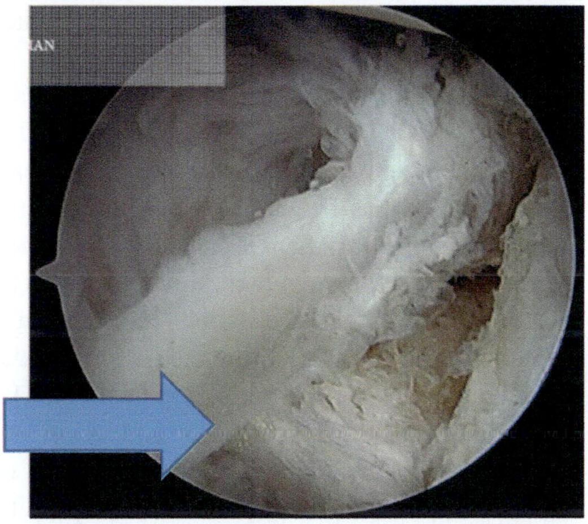

Fig. 13.4 Bankart with cancellous graft place between glenoid and labrum

In the lateral decubitus position, he was found to have an approximately 1.5-cm Hill-Sachs lesion (Fig. 13.3) in addition to a Bankart lesion

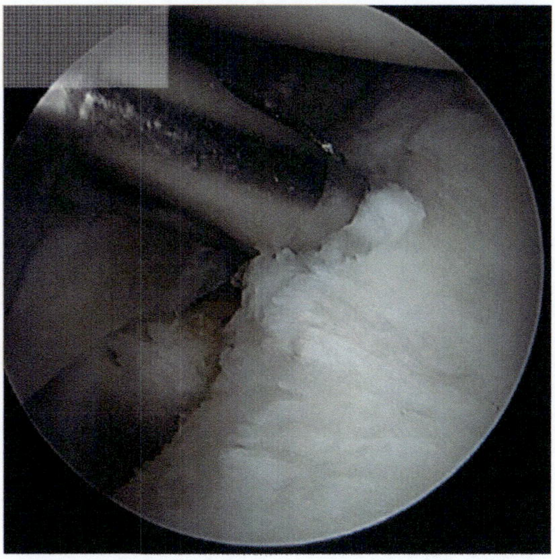

Fig. 13.5 Anchors fixed over bone grafted bankart

with moderate glenoid bone loss. He underwent remplissage in addition to cancellous bone grafting to the glenoid (Figs. 13.4 and 13.5). The anterior graft was enveloped by the labral repair, which consisted of horizontal mattress sutures.

After 5 weeks of wearing a sling and physical therapy, he returned to work at approximately 4 months postoperatively and has not experienced any recurrence of symptoms.

Indications

The senior author believes that essentially all Hill-Sachs lesions should be considered for remplissage since the procedure has minimal morbidity and, in his experience and that of others, there has been no appreciable loss of motion [14, 15].

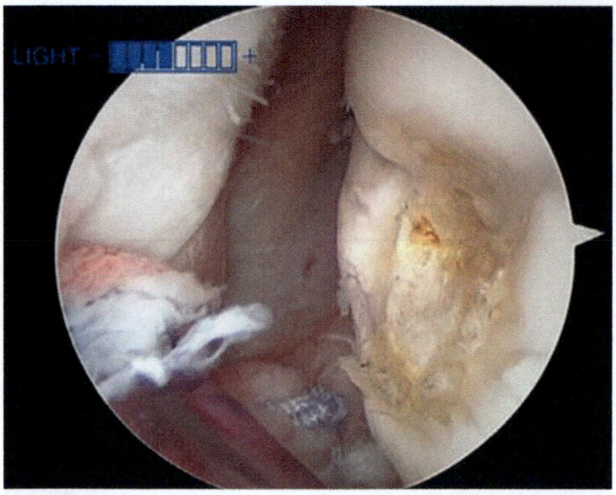

Fig. 13.6 Smaller, more medial Hill-Sachs lesion

Exceptions to remplissage include excessively large lesions—greater than 35–40% of humeral head circumference—where osteochondral allograft would be a more favorable option [10].

In addition, smaller and very medial lesions (Fig. 13.6), while more likely to engage, may sacrifice normal articular cartilage if remplissage is executed.

Physical examination plays an important role since pain and or apprehension in lower degrees of abduction indicates more profound bone loss. As Bushnell and his colleagues have articulated, discomfort in the abducted external rotation position in 45 degrees of abduction has a strong correlation with glenoid bone loss greater than 25% and/or Hill-Sachs lesion greater than 2 cm in length [16]. Although this boney apprehension test has been disputed by James et al., we still find it useful in predicting the magnitude of effect of bone loss on stability [17].

Technique

The literature is replete with several techniques for remplissage performance, and many investigators favor knotless [18–20] and "pulley" constructs [21]. However, the senior author has used standard shoulder anchors, a standard suture retriever, and "blind tying" (not viewing the subacromial space during knot tying) with excellent results. This technique is simple, reproducible, and has endured the test of time. While knotless and pulley constructs may confer greater mechanical strength, we are concerned that excessive compression of the tendon may induce ischemic changes [18].

An examination under anesthesia should be performed prior to initiation of the procedure as the affected shoulder can be compared to the contralateral extremity and can elucidate subtle pathology that was not evident with a conscious patient. While supine, the patient's shoulder should be taken through a full range of motion. Increased external rotation in adduction when compared to the contralateral shoulder suggests interval laxity, while excessive external rotation at 45 degrees of abduction suggests laxity of the middle glenohumeral ligament (MGHL) [22]. A load-shift test with varying degrees of abduction will help determine which portions of the anterior capsule are not functional.

It is the senior author's preference to operate in the lateral decubitus position, as this helps facilitate glenoid exposure through glenohumeral distraction and has been shown to lessen recurrence rate [23]. The patient is carefully positioned laterally on a beanbag with all bony prominences carefully padded, and the patient is placed in a slight posterior tilt as to allow the glenoid of the operative extremity to be parallel to the floor. The arm is hung in 30–45 degrees of abduction and 15 degrees of forward flexion, and 5 pounds of traction is initially utilized. If needed, up to 15 pounds of traction can be used in order to increase visualization [24].

Three arthroscopic portals are used during a remplissage procedure (Fig. 13.7); the posterior portal is usually established first, with optimal location being approximately 2 cm inferior and 2 cm medial to the posterolateral edge of the acromion. This is the "soft spot" and can be palpated with the thumb while grasping the shoulder with remaining fingers anteriorly. This portal is used as the primary viewing portal as well as a working portal during anchor placement. The anterolateral portal is created next right off the anterolateral corner of the acromion and is established just anterior to the leading edge of the supraspinatus. This will be the primary viewing

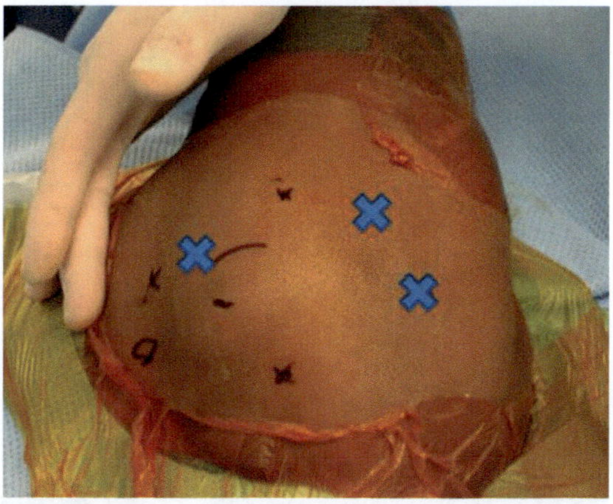

Fig. 13.7 Portals for execution of remplissage

portal during remplissage and Bankart repair. When the arthroscope is placed in this portal, it affords a superb "room with a view" of both the humeral head and the labrum. This portal generally renders an excellent view of the Hill-Sachs lesion, although on rare occasion a 70-degree scope is necessary to fully view the humeral head defect. This portal is thus used to assess the adequacy or inadequacy of the posterior portal for anchor placement in the Hill-Sachs lesion. Rarely, for more superior lesions, a more proximal posterior portal will be necessary. On many occasions, when more than one anchor is necessary for remplissage, a proximal anchor may be placed through the more proximal posterior portal, while distal anchors are inserted through the standard posterior portal.

Lastly, the standard anterior portal is established approximately 2 cm lateral to the coracoid process and can be localized with a spinal needle. It will ideally begin just cephalad to the subscapularis tendon with the cannula directed proximally just over the leading subscapularis tendon edge. The anterior portal can be used as a working portal during diagnostic arthroscopy and for labral anchor insertion and suture shuttling.

After all portals have been placed, a diagnostic arthroscopy is ensured, examining the labrum circumferentially to look for pathology around the face of the glenoid, with care to recognize any concealed posterior inferior labral tears [25]. After examining the labrum, glenoid, and humeral head chondral surfaces for any lesions, attention is turned to the biceps tendon and rotator cuff insertion. After the comprehensive diagnostic arthroscopy, humeral head pathology can be identified and classified as engaging (large and medial) or non-engaging (small and lateral) in the abducted and externally rotated position. At this point, one may remove the limb from traction and position the humerus in "90–90" of abduction and external rotation to confirm engagement arthroscopically, although this is clearly not necessary.

If both a remplissage and Bankart repair are to be undertaken, which is usually the case, the senior author believes that the anterior glenoid should be prepared first, in preparation for the Bankart repair, for two major reasons. Firstly, remplissage is a tenodesis of the infraspinatus into the humeral head defect, which causes a posterior shift of the humeral head relative to the glenoid. This affords much better access to the anterior glenoid. The tails of the remplissage anchor may be left long in order to retract the humeral head posteriorly during execution of the anterior capsulolabral repair. Secondly, by virtue of the posterior force vector that remplissage affords, a tight capsulolabral repair has the risk of losing tension if performed *before* remplissage.

For initiation of the remplissage after the labral preparation, viewing is done from the anterosuperolateral portal, and a shaver is introduced posteriorly. Using the shaver, the defect is gently abraded followed by a curette until the bleeding bone is exposed throughout the entire defect. A microfracture awl can also be introduced to further ensure a bleeding boney bed. After the preparation is completed, a decision is made as to how many anchors are to be used, which is proportionate to the size of the Hill-Sachs lesion. As a general rule, one anchor is placed per 1 cm of defect width. If two anchors are used, the inferior one is typically placed first as to not obscure visualization of placement of the second anchor. A small metal cannula is placed through the posterior portal, and a loaded anchor is then placed through the portal and into the defect, ensuring that the trajectory remains perpendicular the entire time. The posterior por-

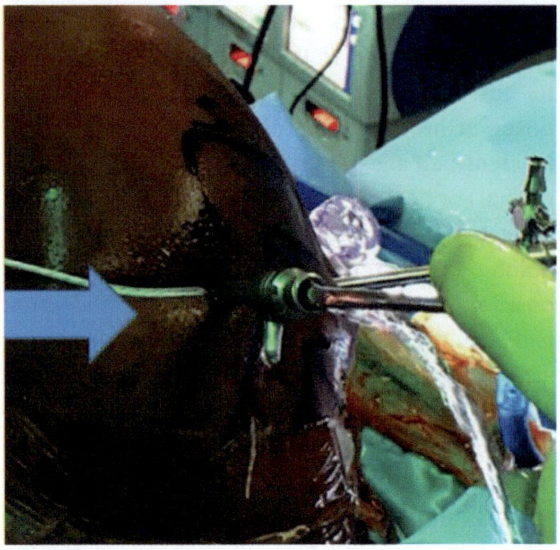

Fig. 13.8 Sutures outside of cannula after the first anchor insertion

tal can sometimes be too medial to maintain the correct trajectory, if this occurs an additional portal can be established more distally and laterally to the initial posterior portal. Furthermore, as stated above, a more proximal portal is necessary for expansive lesions. After the anchor is placed, a switching stick is placed into the metal cannula, and the cannula is removed and then immediately replaced over the switching stick, allowing the suture to be on the outside of the cannula (Fig. 13.8). The second anchor is placed in identical fashion, but superiorly to the first anchor and as close to the articular margin of the Hill-Sachs lesion as possible (Fig. 13.9). A perpendicular trajectory for the second anchor is again important, and if trouble is encountered with the existing portals, another portal can be made more proximally. The sheath is then removed and the ends of the sutures are clamped with a hemostat.

A posterolateral retrieving portal is established next, typically at least 1 cm lateral to the posterolateral aspect of the acromion. This portal allows for the sutures to be passed through the "safe zone" of the infraspinatus tendon as described by Garcia et al., and not through muscle belly (Fig. 13.10) [26]. It is important that the sutures pass more laterally in the tendon, as the suture anchors will have much greater purchase in tendon than in muscle. It is also important because a lateral tenodesis will confer significantly less loss of rotational motion as compared to a more medially based tenodesis [27]. A spinal needle can help establish this portal under direct visualization, followed by a stab incision with an 11-blade scalpel. A 6-mm cannula with a blunt obturator is then inserted to gain access to the subacromial space. The obturator is swept throughout the subacromial space to prevent the bursal tissue from becoming interposed between the suture knots and the infraspinatus tendon.

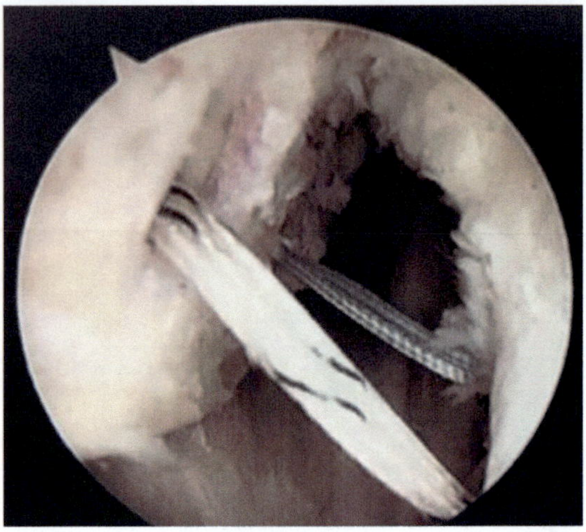

Fig. 13.9 Remplissage anchors placed near articular margin

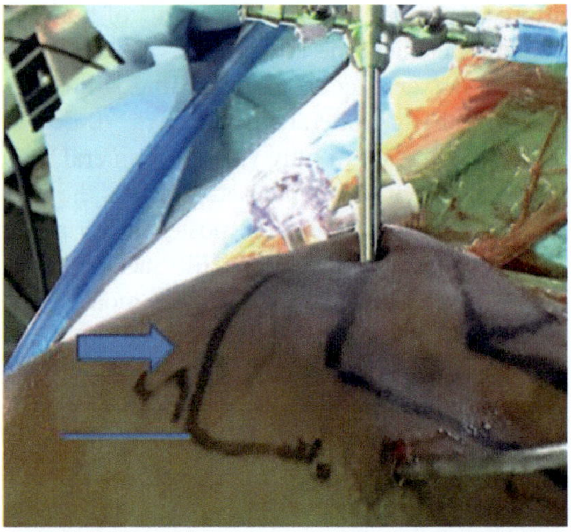

Fig. 13.10 Safe Zone for Portal Placement to avoid muscle in Remplissage

Once the retrieving portal has been established, the sutures are then passed through the infraspinatus tendon, approximately 1 cm medial to the tendinous insertion. The inferior/distal anchor's sutures are addressed first, ensuring that enough tissue is taken to allow for a stout repair. A penetrating-type retriever that is sturdy is helpful as tendon tissue may be rather thick. The sutures are retrieved through the cannula, and tension is applied to each limb of the distal anchor's sutures, which are then placed on the distal edge of the cannula. Attention is then turned to the proximal/superior sutures, which are passed in a similar fashion 1 cm from the insertion site of the infraspinatus tendon. Once all sutures have been passed through, tying should commence, with the distal sutures being tied prior to the proximal sutures. During tying, a gentle, posteriorly directed force should be applied to the humerus to allow for an anatomic reduction (Fig. 13.11). The senior author has recently transitioned to knotless anchors but still recommends practitioners should begin with the above technique as it is reproducible.

The capsulolabral repair is then performed, using a switching stick to re-establish the original posterior portal, which will be used for shuttling sutures during the Bankart repair.

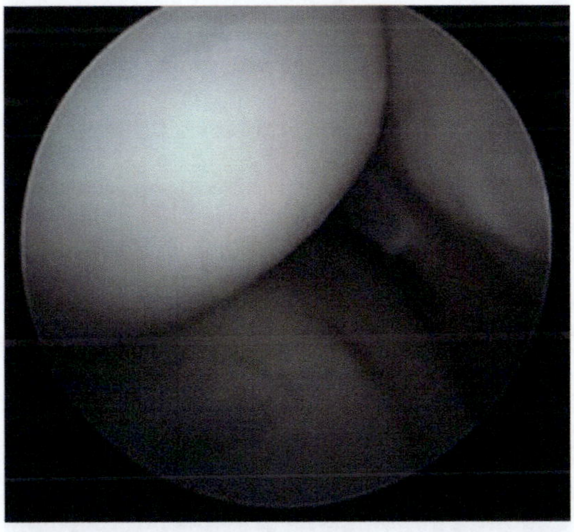

Fig. 13.11 Completed remplissage with anatomic reduction

Glenoid Grafting

For glenoid defects comprising more than 25–30% of the glenoid width, the senior author will often add cancellous bone to the anterior glenoid immediately prior to capsulolabral repair. This is in accordance with the work of Kitayama et al., who describe hypertrophy of smaller bony Bankart lesions repaired under tension [28]. A mosaicplasty harvester is used to retrieve a 6–7 mm x 15 mm cancellous bone plug at the site of remplissage anchor insertion (Fig. 13.12). This bone is gently delivered anterior to the glenoid rim (Fig. 13.13),

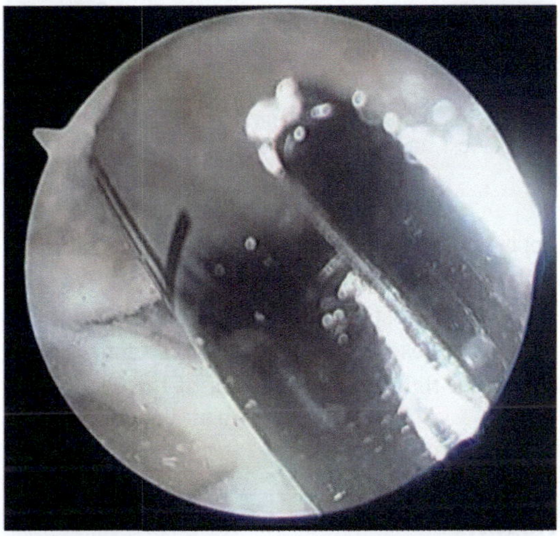

Fig. 13.12 Harvest of cancellous bone Hill-Sachs lesion

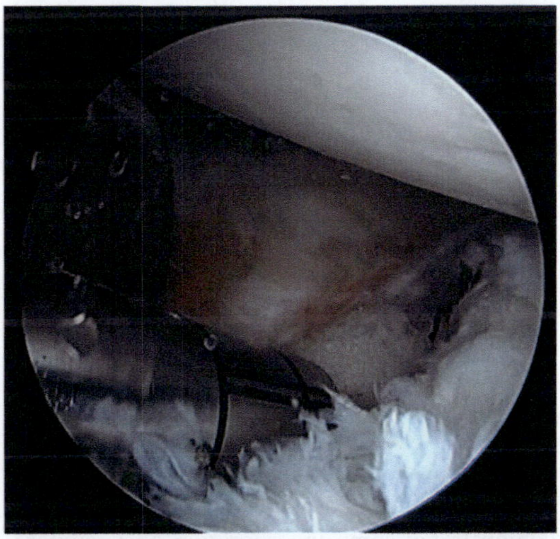

Fig. 13.13 Delivery of cancellous graft anteriorly

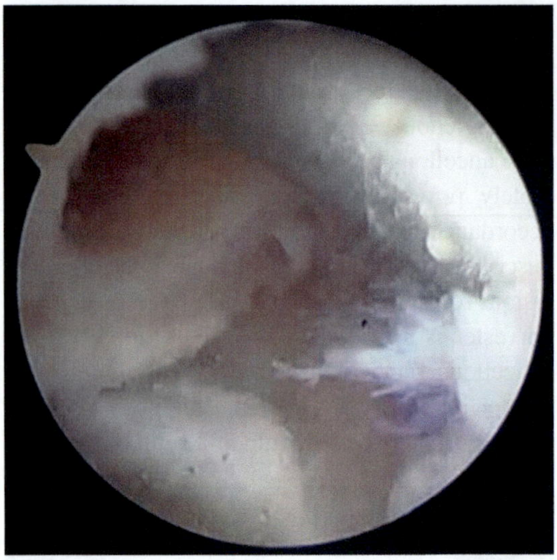

Fig. 13.14 Insertion of remplissage anchor into cancellous harvest site

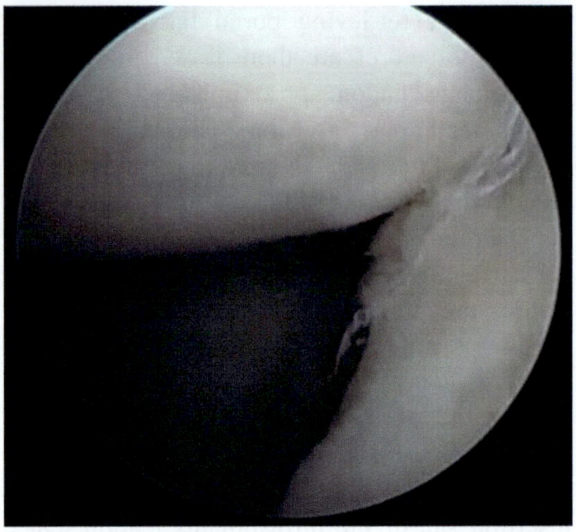

Fig. 13.15 Remplissage "recessed" into donor graft site

approximating the capsulolabral tissue immediately prior to glenoid anchor insertion.

Bone harvest confers an additional benefit in that it enables the infraspinatus to attain a deeper and more tightly applied "fill" of the Hill-Sachs lesion.

Results

Arthroscopic remplissage has emerged to be a most effective means of treating anterior shoulder instability [29–33]. Remplissage can be undertaken without adding significant operative time and, as stated above, may facilitate Bankart repair because the infraspinatus tenodesis directs the humeral head posteriorly and facilitates access to the anterior inferior glenoid. Park et al. has shown that the infraspinatus effectively integrates with the humeral head (Fig. 13.15), filling at least 75% of the lesion on postoperative MRI [34]. Fibrous-like tissue on imaging also raises the question of whether this viable tissue may undergo metaplastic changes in time and perhaps become more fibrocartilaginous. The senoir author's technique of anterior bone grafting has demonstrated some incorporation on postoperative MRI (Figs. 13.16 and 13.17).

Giles et al. evaluated the biomechanical stability of cadaveric shoulders subsequent to remplis-

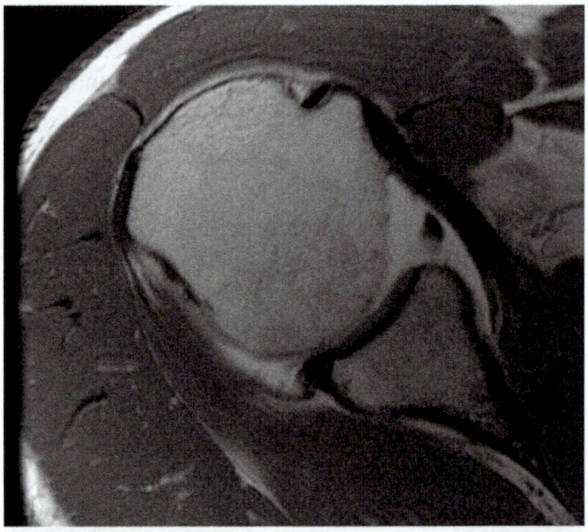

Fig. 13.16 Pre-op before glenoid grafting

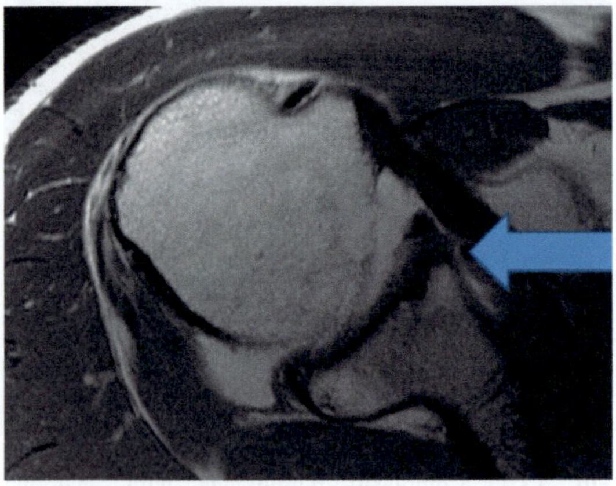

Fig. 13.17 Several months subsequent to glenoid bone grafting anterior glenoid. The blue arrow points to the incorporated graft

sage for Hill-Sachs defects of both 30% and 45% the diameter of the humeral head [35]. Remplissage effectively prevented engagement and dislocation for both lesion sizes [35]. Elkinson et al. also performed a cadaveric study that confirmed the previous study [27]. These investigators created Hill-Sachs defects of 15% and 30% of the diameter of the humeral head and subsequently tested the biomechanical stability of these specimens after a Bankart repair was performed, with and without a concomitant remplissage. In the 15% defect group, none of the shoulders were shown to dislocate when a Bankart repair alone was performed. In contrast, all shoulders with a 30% Hill-Sachs lesion dislocated with isolated Bankart repair. When a remplissage was added, none of the shoulders engaged or dislocated in full abduction and external rotation [27]. This study demonstrates in cadavers that large, engaging humeral head defects with minimal glenoid bone loss can be effectively addressed with a remplissage procedure added to a standard Bankart repair.

Since remplissage is in essence a tenodesis of the infraspinatus tendon, some studies have indicated that posterosuperior shoulder pain and loss of humeral external rotation may result [36, 37]. However, this has not been the senior author's experience and is supported by several other studies [14, 38–40]. In fact, we found that return to sport rates have been reported to range from 74% to 95% of patients following remplissage [39, 41].

When comparing a Latarjet procedure to Bankart plus remplissage, one study showed that there was no difference in recurrence between the two groups. However, the Latarjet group had an appreciably higher complication rate (14.3% for Latarjet versus 0% for Bankart plus remplissage) [42]. The two cohorts in this study appeared evenly matched with respect to both glenoid and humeral bone loss [42]. These findings were recently corroborated in a recent systematic review [43].

The senior author recently reviewed his cases with at least a 2-year follow-up and noted that of the 79 patients studied, only 3 experienced a recurrent instability event.

Summary

Arthroscopic remplissage is a highly effective adjunct for the treatment of anterior shoulder instability. It has stood the test of time and has proven to greatly reduce recurrence rates while subjecting the patient to minimal morbidity. It is a biologic tissue fill and if executed properly, confers only minimal effects on motion. Remplissage medializes the glenoid track by virtue of its posterior force vector and facilitates the performance of the anterior capsulolabral repair.

References

1. Burkhart SS, De Beer JF. Traumatic glenohumeral bone defects and their relationship to failure of arthroscopic Bankart repairs: significance of the inverted–pear glenoid and the humeral engaging Hill-Sachs lesion. Arthroscopy. 2000;16(7):677–94. https://doi.org/10.1053/jars.2000.17715.
2. Piasecki DP, Verma NN, Romeo AA, et al. Glenoid bone deficiency in recurrent anterior shoulder instability: diagnosis and management. J Am Acad Orthop Surg. 2009;17(8):482–93.
3. Yamamoto N, et al. Contact between the glenoid and the humeral head in abduction, external rotation, and horizontal extension: a new concept of glenoid track. J Shoulder Elb Surg. 2007;16(5):649–56.
4. Walia P, Patel RM, Gottschalk L, et al. The reduction in stability from combined humeral head and glenoid bony defects is influenced by arm position. Am J Sports Med. 2016;44(3):715–22.
5. Ratner D, Backes J, Tokish JM. Arthroscopic reduction and balloon humeroplasty in the treatment of acute Hill-Sachs lesions. Arthrosc Tech. 2016;5(6):e1327–32.
6. Re P, Gallo RA, Richmond JC. Transhumeral head plasty for large Hill-Sachs lesions. Arthroscopy. 2006;22(7):798–e1.
7. Grondin P, Leith J. Combined large Hill–Sachs and bony Bankart lesions treated by Latarjet and partial humeral head resurfacing: a report of 2 cases. Can J Surg. 2009;52(3):249.
8. Plath JE, et al. Does the arthroscopic Latarjet procedure effectively correct "off-track" Hill-Sachs lesions? Am J Sports Med. 2018;46(1):72–8.
9. Calvo C, et al. Clinical relevance of persistent off-track Hill-Sachs lesion after arthroscopic Latarjet procedure. Am J Sports Med. 2021;49(8):2006–12.
10. Zhuo H, et al. Osteochondral allograft transplantation for large Hill-Sachs lesions: a retrospective case series with a minimum 2-year follow-up. J Orthop Surg Res. 2019;14(1):1–7.

11. Black LO, et al. Fresh osteochondral allograft to the humeral head for treatment of an engaging reverse Hill-Sachs lesion: technical case report and literature review. Orthop J Sports Med. 2016;4(11):2325967116670376.
12. Mook WR, et al. Clinical and anatomic predictors of outcomes after the Latarjet procedure for the treatment of anterior glenohumeral instability with combined glenoid and humeral bone defects. Am J Sports Med. 2016;44(6):1407–16.
13. Tokish J, et al. Critical bone loss in shoulder instability reconsidered: subcritical bone loss correlates to worse outcome in arthroscopic Bankart repair. Arthroscopy. 2014;30(6):e4.
14. Park MJ, et al. Arthroscopic remplissage with Bankart repair for the treatment of glenohumeral instability with Hill-Sachs defects. Arthroscopy: The Journal of Arthroscopic & Related Surgery. 2011;27(9):1187–94.
15. Buza JA III, et al. Arthroscopic Hill-Sachs remplissage: a systematic review. J Bone Joint Surg. 2014;96(7):549–55.
16. Bushnell BD, Creighton RA, Herring MM. The bony apprehension test for instability of the shoulder: a prospective pilot analysis. Arthroscopy. 2008;24(9):974–82.
17. James M, et al. Bony apprehension test for identifying bone loss in patients with traumatic anterior shoulder instability: a validation study. Am J Sports Med. 2022;50(6):1520–8.
18. Funakoshi T, et al. Remplissage using interconnected knotless anchors: superior biomechanical properties to a knotted technique? Arthroscopy. 2018;34(11):2954–9.
19. McQuivey KS, et al. Arthroscopic remplissage using knotless, all-suture anchors. Arthrosc Tech. 2022;11(4):e615–21.
20. Hirahara AM, Andersen WJ, Yamashiro K. Arthroscopic knotless remplissage for the treatment of Hill-Sachs lesions using the PASTA bridge configuration. Arthrosc Tech. 2019;8(3):e275–81.
21. Koo SS, Burkhart SS, Ochoa E. Arthroscopic double-pulley remplissage technique for engaging Hill-Sachs lesions in anterior shoulder instability repairs. Arthroscopy. 2009;25(11):1343–8.
22. Gerber C, Werner CM, Macy JC, et al. Effect of selective capsulorrhaphy on the passive range of motion of the glenohumeral joint. J Bone Joint Surg Am. 2003;85:48–55.
23. Frank RM, et al. Outcomes of arthroscopic anterior shoulder instability in the beach chair versus lateral decubitus position: a systematic review and meta-regression analysis. Arthroscopy. 2014;30(10):1349–65.
24. McHale KJ, Park MJ, Kelly JD IV. Arthroscopic remplissage for humeral head defects. Tech Orthop. 2015;30:39–41.
25. Kim S-H, et al. The Kim test: a novel test for posteroinferior labral lesion of the shoulder—a comparison to the jerk test. Am J Sports Med. 2005;33(8):1188–92.
26. Garcia GH, Degen RM, Liu JN, et al. Accuracy of suture passage during arthroscopic remplissage—what anatomic landmarks can improve it? A cadaveric study. Orthop J Sports Med. 2016;4:2325967116663497. (online).
27. Elkinson I, Giles JW, Boons HW. The shoulder remplissage procedure for Hill-Sachs defects: does technique matter? J Shoulder Elb Surg. 2013;22:835–41.
28. Kitayama S, et al. Clinical outcome and glenoid morphology after arthroscopic repair of chronic osseous Bankart lesions: a five to eight-year follow-up study. J Bone Joint Surg. 2015;97(22):1833–43.
29. Alkaduhimi H, et al. Remplissage with Bankart repair in anterior shoulder instability: a systematic review of the clinical and cadaveric literature. Arthroscopy. 2019;35(4):1257–66.
30. Garcia GH, et al. Outcomes of the remplissage procedure and its effects on return to sports: average 5-year follow-up. Am J Sports Med. 2016;44(5):1124–30.
31. Hurley ET, et al. Remplissage for anterior shoulder instability with Hill-Sachs lesions: a systematic review and meta-analysis. J Shoulder Elb Surg. 2020;29(12):2487–94.
32. Rashid MS, et al. Arthroscopic "Remplissage" for shoulder instability: a systematic review. Knee Surg Sports Traumatol Arthrosc. 2016;24(2):578–84.
33. Gracitelli MEC, et al. Results from filling "remplissage" arthroscopic technique for recurrent anterior shoulder dislocation. Revista Brasileira de Ortopedia (English Edition). 2011;46(6):684–90.
34. Park MJ, Garcia G, Malhotra A, Major N, Tjoumakaris FP, Kelly JD IV. The evaluation of arthroscopic remplissage by high-resolution magnetic resonance imaging. Am J Sports Med. 2012;40:2331–6.
35. Giles JW, Elkinson I, Ferreira LM, et al. Moderate to large engaging Hill-Sachs defects: an in vitro biomechanical comparison of the remplissage procedure, allograft humeral head reconstruction, and partial resurfacing arthroplasty. J Shoulder Elb Surg. 2012;21:1142–51.
36. Nourissat G, Kilinc AS, Werther JR, et al. A prospective, comparative, radiological, and clinical study of the influence of the "remplissage" procedure on shoulder range of motion after stabilization by arthroscopic Bankart repair. Am J Sports Med. 2011;39:2147–52.
37. Deutsch AA, Kroll DG. Decreased range of motion following arthroscopic remplissage. Orthopedics. 2008;31:492.

38. Haviv B, Mayo L, Biggs D. Outcomes of arthroscopic "remplissage": capsulotenodesis of the engaging large Hill-Sachs lesion. J Orthop Surg Res. 2011;6:29.
39. Garcia GH, Wu HH, Liu JN, Huffman GR, Kelly JD IV. Outcomes of the remplissage procedure and its effects on return to sports: average 5-year follow-up. Am J Sports Med. 2016;44:1124–30.
40. Zhu YM, Lu Y, Zhang J, et al. Arthroscopic Bankart repair combined with remplissage technique for the treatment of anterior shoulder instability with engaging Hill-Sachs lesion: a report of 49 cases with a minimum 2-year follow-up. Am J Sports Med. 2011;39:1640–7.
41. Davis WH, et al. Arthroscopic Remplissage combined with Bankart repair results in a higher rate of return to sport in athletes compared with Bankart repair alone or the Latarjet procedure: a systematic review and meta-analysis. Am J Sports Med. 2023;51:03635465221138559.
42. Cho NS, Yoo JH, Rhee YG. Management of an engaging Hill–Sachs lesion: arthroscopic remplissage with Bankart repair versus Latarjet procedure. Arthroscopy. 2016;24:3793–800.
43. Haroun HK, Sobhy MH, Abdelrahman AA. Arthroscopic Bankart repair with remplissage versus Latarjet procedure for management of engaging Hill-Sachs lesions with subcritical glenoid bone loss in traumatic anterior shoulder instability: a systematic review and meta-analysis. J Shoulder Elb Surg. 2020;29(10):2163–74.

Treatment of Subcritical Bone Loss: The Distal Clavicle Autograft

14

John M. Tokish and James S. Shaha

Introduction

Shoulder instability in the glenohumeral joint remains a treatment challenge. This is further complicated with associated anterior-inferior glenoid bone loss as critical bone loss has been shown to compromise the outcome of an isolated Bankart repair [1–4]. This concern for bone loss has led to a lower threshold of subcritical bone loss >13.5% being established as predictive of a poorer clinical outcome [5, 6]. Given that the diameter of the inferior glenoid averages 24–26 mm, bone loss of as little as 3–4 mm can portend a poor outcome [7, 8]. More recently, the glenoid track has been assessed and clinically validated [9, 10]. Shaha et al. found that the presence of an off-track lesion predicted a significantly higher failure rate and a poorer subjective outcome following Bankart repair, even if the patient did not suffer recurrent instability. Thus, if the lesion is off track with subcritical bone loss or if there is critical glenoid bone loss irrespective of track status, a bony augmentation should be considered.

There are many bony options available including coracoid transfer, iliac crest autograft, and osteochondral allograft transfer [11–15]. An additional graft option is distal clavicle autograft. Tokish et al. first reported on the use of this graft in 2014 [16]. Since that time, others, including Boileau et al., have similarly reported on its use for reconstruction of a deficient anterior glenoid [17].

There are several advantages to the use of distal clavicle compared to alternative graft choices. First, the graft is nearly always available, avoiding the cost and logistical challenges of an allograft. Second, the graft is osteochondral, allowing for cartilage matching to the native glenoid [18, 19]. Third, the distal clavicle has been shown to appropriately match the contour of the glenoid, restore the articular arc, and approximate the contact area and pressures of a coracoid transfer [8, 20, 21]. Fourth, the graft is able to restore a significant amount of the glenoid articular cartilage with reports of restoration of up to 44% of the glenoid with articular cartilage thickness similar to that of the native glenoid (Image 14.1) [8, 20]. Finally, there is minimal donor site morbidity, as the distal clavicle is routinely resected for acromioclavicular arthritis (minimizing morbidity) with removal of up to 1.5 cm, yielding satisfactory results without injury to the coracoclavicular ligaments.

J. M. Tokish (✉)
Orthopedic Surgery, Mayo Clinic, Scottsdale, AZ, USA
e-mail: Tokish.John@Mayo.edu

J. S. Shaha
Pioneer Peak Orthopedics, Palmer, AK, USA

© The Author(s), under exclusive license to Springer Nature Switzerland AG 2026
R. M. Frank, J. M. Tokish (eds.), *Management of Shoulder Instability*,
https://doi.org/10.1007/978-3-032-18089-6_14

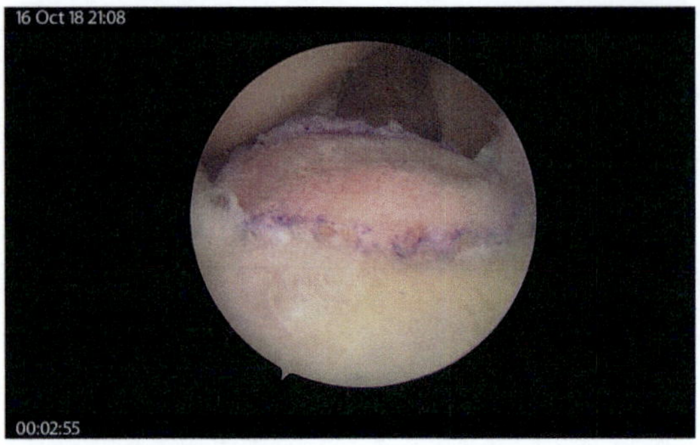

Image 14.1 The distal clavicle is shown here to restore the articular arc of the glenoid in settings with up to 40% glenoid bone loss

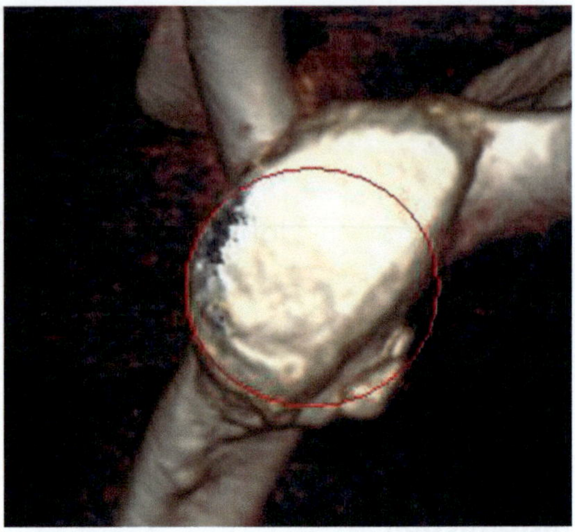

Image 14.2 A perfect circle is placed over a 3D CT reconstruction and demonstrates subcritical glenoid bone loss of 18%

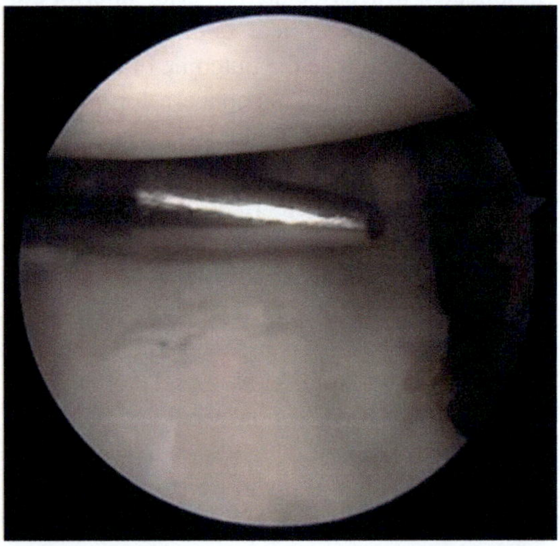

Image 14.3 The patient is in the lateral position and this is his left shoulder. The switching stick points to the deficient anterior glenoid with obvious loss of normal contour

Illustrative Clinical Case

This patient is a 19-year-old Division 1 football player with a history of a dislocation while attempting to make a tackle. The patient was closed reduced and placed in a sling. He was treated with closed reduction and attempted to return to play. He sustained two additional dislocations and was referred for treatment. The patient had radiographs and a CT scan. The CT scan (Image 14.2) demonstrated subcritical bone loss. The patient, being at high risk as a young male collision athlete with subcritical glenoid bone loss, was contraindicated for an isolated arthroscopic Bankart and, after a discussion of multiple options, was selected for distal clavicle autograft augmentation.

Intraoperative photographs demonstrate the anterior glenoid bone loss with obviously abnormal morphology (Image 14.3). Following completion of a standard diagnostic arthroscopy, the glenoid is prepared for the distal clavicle graft. The offset guide is placed along the articular surface through a widened posterior portal (Image 14.4). Care is taken to ensure that the guide is flat along the glenoid surface as this dictates the trajectory of the pins which can be visualized on the anterior glenoid. The pins are then overdrilled and the retrograde reamer is introduced. The reamers are then used to plane the glenoid in preparation for the distal clavicle autograft (Image 14.5). This ensures that the recipient site is completely flush to allow an excellent fit with the donor graft.

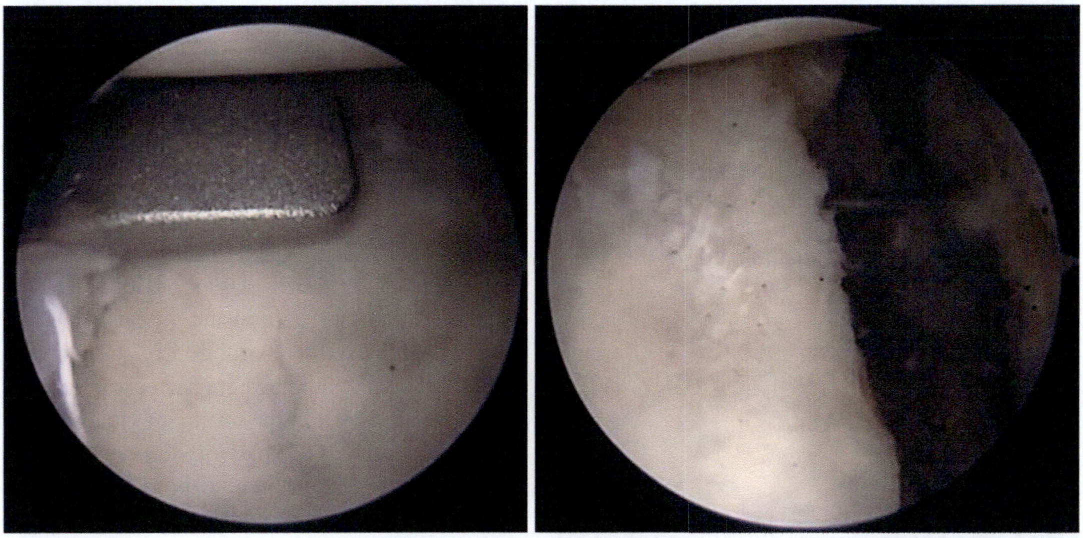

Image 14.4 The offset guide is placed through the posterior portal. Care is taken to keep the guide flat against the glenoid surface to ensure that the pins exit in an appropriate orientation as seen on the image on the right

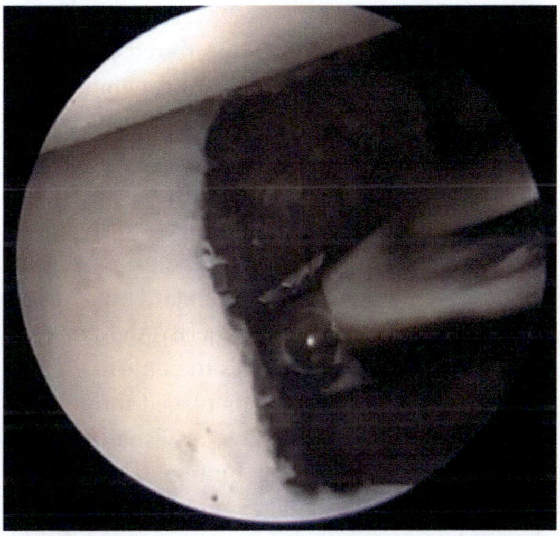

Image 14.5 The planed surface of the glenoid is visible here. The retrograde reamers have overlapped to allow for a smooth surface over the entire length of the recipient site

The distal clavicle is then harvested and prepared as described previously. This includes retrograde preplacement of two soft anchors with a self-locking mechanism. The graft is introduced into the shoulder through an enlarged midglenoid portal and reduced to the matching articular surface of the native glenoid (Image 14.6). The sutures from each anchor are passed through the knotless mechanism of the opposite anchor posteriorly and sequentially tightened. The graft is then tested with manual pressure to ensure that the graft is flush with the native glenoid and that the fixation is secure. Additional fixation can be added to the native labrum and/or to the native glenoid.

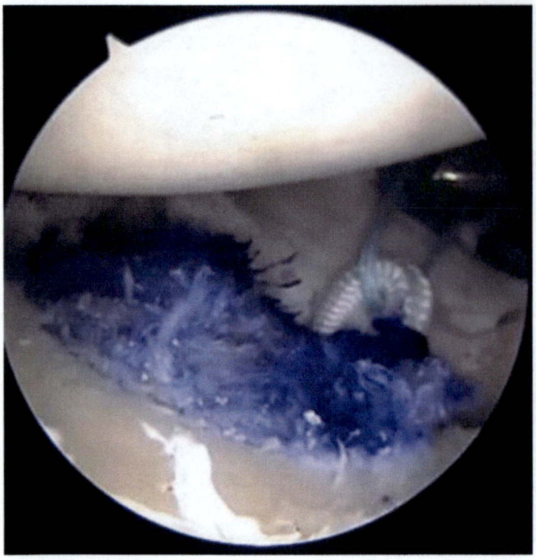

Image 14.6 The distal clavicle is slid into place. Note that the graft sits flush with the surface of the glenoid neck as well as with the articular surface

Etiology

The glenohumeral joint is uniquely structured to allow for a wide range of motion. However, to allow for significant motion, the joint is particularly vulnerable to episodes of instability [22–29]. This instability is defined as either a subluxation or a dislocation with resultant pain, loss of function, apprehension, and/or a sensation of slipping [24, 30, 31]. The loss of the synergistic action of the bones, ligaments, and muscles to provide dynamic and static stability is the root cause of this instability. The progressive episodes of instability have been shown, over time, to result in an erosive effect on the anteroinferior glenoid with resultant bone loss [32–36]. This resultant bone loss compromises the outcome of an isolated labral repair [5, 35].

Diagnosis/Imaging

Patients who present with glenohumeral instability undergo a standard history and physical. Care is taken to determine the frequency and direction of prior dislocations, energy required for dislocation, history of subluxations, and apprehension on exam. Care is taken when examining those with recurrent instability to avoid causing a dislocation while performing the exam.

Additionally, the patient obtains radiographs to include a true AP and axillary view. Further, an MRI scan and/or a CT scan is routine, especially in cases of recurrent dislocation or those with a suspicion of bone loss. Specific attention is directed to determining if glenoid bone loss is present. Using the sagittal cut of an MRI, CT scan, or a 3D CT reconstruction of the glenoid, bone loss is calculated using a perfect circle technique (Image 14.2). In the setting of glenoid bone loss compromising the patient's outcome with a labral repair (>13.5% glenoid bone loss at high risk for failure, off-track lesion), the decision is made to proceed with bony augmentation.

Surgical Technique

For the senior author's [JT] preferred technique, the patient is placed in the lateral decubitus position with all bony prominences well padded. An examination under anesthesia is performed. A posterior portal is used to start with anteroinferior and anterosuperior portals subsequently established, as generally done during routine shoulder arthroscopy. A standard diagnostic arthroscopy is performed to verify the presence of labral pathology as well as to confirm glenoid bone loss. The arthroscope is placed through the anterosuperior portal to allow for visualization of the glenoid defect during biologic preparation. The preparation includes a wide release of the glenoid labrum to allow for adequate mobility. A traction suture is placed through the labrum and withdrawn through a percutaneous portal made inferior to the anteroinferior portal. This allows for capsular retraction to better access the anterior glenoid for preparation and graft passage without concern for suture entanglement.

The posterior portal is then widened slightly to allow for introduction of a glenoid drill guide with 4 to 6 mm of offset (Parallel Drill Guide, Arthrex, Naples, FL) (Image 14.7). Two wires are placed from posterior-to-anterior and exit medial to the glenoid articular surface matching offset based on the guide. The wires are measured viewing from the anterosuperior portal with a measurement probe placed through the midglenoid portal to ensure that the wires exit at the desired offset from the glenoid surface. Wires that are misplaced will compromise the ultimate match of the native glenoid with the graft. Once the wires are confirmed in the correct position, they are overdrilled with a 2.4-mm drill bit. Leaving the drill bit in place, a 3.5 stepped ratchet drill sleeve (Arthrex, Naples FL) is advanced over the drill and tapped into the posterior glenoid until the stepped portion fully engages the posterior glenoid. The 2.4-mm drill is removed, and a 3.5 mm × 13 mm FlipCutter (Arthrex, Naples, FL) is advanced until it is visualized at the anterior glenoid defect. The FlipCutter is then flipped to where the cutting blade is perpendicular to the shaft and pulled posteriorly. This results in the FlipCutter acting as a router, creating a flush cut perfect circle on the native glenoid. This procedure is repeated over the superior pin, and because the two circles are overlapping, the result is an oval shaped flush cut that will accept a 20–25-mm-long graft (Image 14.8). Once the reaming is completed, the FlipCutters are removed, and a shuttling suture is passed with the looped end brought out the antero-inferior cannula. Care is taken to keep the inferior

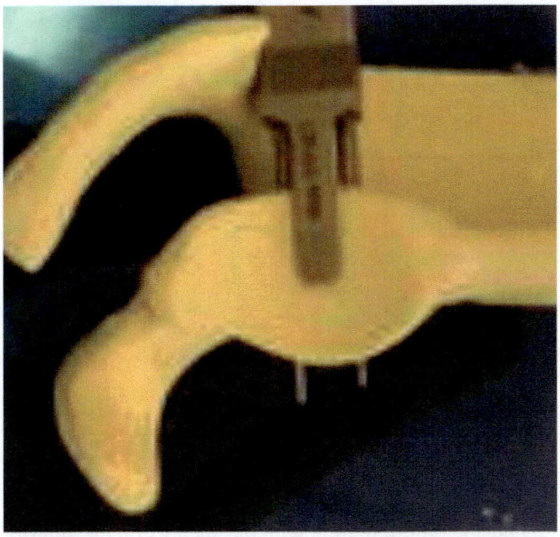

Image 14.7 An offset guide is introduced posterior into the shoulder with the guide placed flush on the articular surface. Visible are the two K-wires that are passed through the glenoid and below the articular surface in preparation for overdrilling

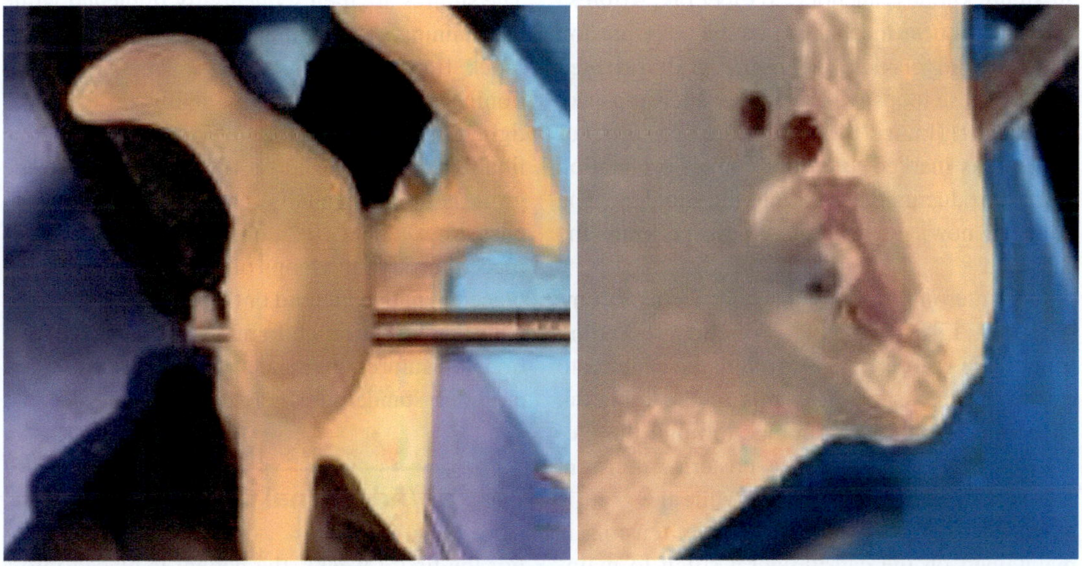

Image 14.8 The retrograde reamer is visible entering through the inferior hole. The eroded portion of the glenoid is planed using the reamer through both holes to provide a flat recipient site for the distal clavicle autograft. The planing effect of the retrograde reamer is easily visible in the image on the right. The inferior hole is reamed back until flush with overlap with the superior hole retrograde reamer ensuring that there is a completely flat recipient site for the graft

suture directed inferiorly and the superior suture directed superiorly to avoid suture entanglement. The portal through the midglenoid portal is exchanged for a larger cannula to allow easy passage of the graft.

Attention is then turned to the distal clavicle harvest. A single 3-cm horizontal incision is made over the AC joint along the clavicular axis. Full-thickness flaps are raised to expose the periosteum. A single, full-thickness periosteal flap is raised to expose the distal clavicle and AC joint. The distal clavicle is marked using electrocautery at 12 mm to allow for harvest. A 1-cm-wide saw blade is then used to remove the distal clavicle with soft tissues being released from the bone to allow for removal. The wound is irrigated and the periosteal flap is closed with nonabsorbable suture. The remainder of the incision is closed in standard fashion at completion of the case.

The distal clavicle is then prepared. Two holes are drilled from the undersurface of the clavicle to the superior surface centered using the same offset guide (generally 6 mm) to ensure that the articular surfaces of the distal clavicle and the glenoid align. A suture passer is used to pass an all-suture knotless anchor (2.6 FiberTak, Arthrex) with the knotless mechanism on the outer portion of the distal clavicle (with the graft oriented in vivo, these loops will be on the anterior aspect of the graft) (Image 14.9). The superior aspect of the graft is marked to ensure correct orientation when introducing the graft into the shoulder. The graft is now prepared for passage into the shoulder.

The anteroinferior portal is widened to accommodate a 17-mm cannula. Prior to proceeding further, the graft is passed through the cannula to ensure easy passage. The tails of the FiberTak anchors are shuttled retrograde through the glenoid and retrieved from the posterior incision. The sutures are then tensioned while the graft is advanced into the shoulder, while tension is maintained on the capsulolabral stitch to maintain open space for the graft. Once appropriately positioned, the working stitch of the inferior anchor is passed through the knotless mechanism of the superior anchor. The same is then done with the superior stitch and the inferior anchor.

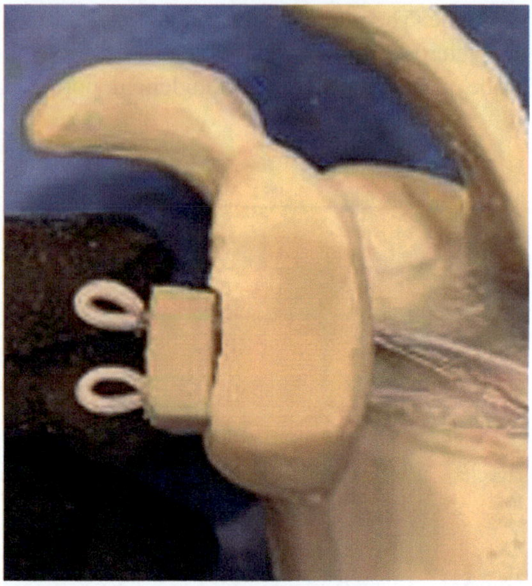

Image 14.9 This sawbones demonstration shows a distal clavicle representation with the anchors on the anterior surface of the bone block, before the sutures are tightened. The sutures are passed through the glenoid using shuttling sutures. The superior suture is passed through the inferior knotless mechanism. The inferior suture is passed through the superior knotless mechanism

The sutures are then sequentially tightened while maintaining alignment and reduction of the bone block. Because the tensioning is "one-way," positioning of the graft can be fine-tuned during the tightening process. Once the graft is flush, the final tension is placed on the construct, and the graft is then manually probed and loaded to ensure excellent fixation. Additional stitches placed through the loops of the FiberTaks can be placed in native glenoid or through the labrum for additional fixation and soft tissue reapproximation. All sutures are then cut and the incisions are closed in standard fashion.

Post-op/Additional Considerations

For the first 2 weeks, the patient is placed into a sling at all times except when showering. No active range of motion is allowed. Pendulums are allowed only for the first 4 weeks. The patient weans the sling and increases passive motion from weeks 4 to 6 with discontinuation at week 6.

Active-assisted motion is initiated as full passive motion is progressively achieved at this point. Beginning at week 8, active motion is initiated with a focus on balanced and rhythmic motion. This is continued until week 10 at which point the patient enters the strengthening phase. Overhead activities are initiated at 4–5 months as tolerated. Clearance for resumption of pre-injury activity is at the discretion of the treating surgery with a goal of 6–8 months.

References

1. Boileau P, et al. Risk factors for recurrence of shoulder instability after arthroscopic Bankart repair. J Bone Joint Surg Am. 2006;88(8):1755–63.
2. Itoi E, et al. The effect of a glenoid defect on anteroinferior stability of the shoulder after Bankart repair: a cadaveric study. J Bone Joint Surg Am. 2000;82(1):35–46.
3. Lo IK, Parten PM, Burkhart SS. The inverted pear glenoid: an indicator of significant glenoid bone loss. Arthroscopy. 2004;20(2):169–74.
4. Yamamoto N, et al. Effect of an anterior glenoid defect on anterior shoulder stability: a cadaveric study. Am J Sports Med. 2009;37(5):949–54.
5. Shaha JS, et al. Redefining "critical" bone loss in shoulder instability: functional outcomes worsen with "subcritical" bone loss. Am J Sports Med. 2015;43(7):1719–25.
6. Kane GG, Wilson K, Lesniak B, Lin R. Combined subcritical thresholds of glenoid and humeral sided bone loss are predictive of failure after arthroscopic Bankart repair. Orthop J Sports Med. 2020;8(7 suppl6):2020.
7. Gerber C, Nyffeler RW. Classification of glenohumeral joint instability. Clin Orthop Relat Res. 2002;400:65–76.
8. Kwapisz A, et al. Distal clavicular osteochondral autograft augmentation for glenoid bone loss: a comparison of radius of restoration versus latarjet graft. Am J Sports Med. 2018;46(5):1046–52.
9. Shaha JS, et al. Clinical validation of the glenoid track concept in anterior glenohumeral instability. J Bone Joint Surg Am. 2016;98(22):1918–23.
10. Di Giacomo G, Itoi E, Burkhart SS. Evolving concept of bipolar bone loss and the Hill-Sachs lesion: from "engaging/non-engaging" lesion to "on-track/off-track" lesion. Arthroscopy. 2014;30(1):90–8.
11. Helfet AJ. Coracoid transplantation for recurring dislocation of the shoulder. J Bone Joint Surg Br. 1958;40-B(2):198–202.
12. Hutchinson JW, Neumann L, Wallace WA. Bone buttress operation for recurrent anterior shoulder dislocation in epilepsy. J Bone Joint Surg Br. 1995;77(6):928–32.
13. Latarjet M. Treatment of recurrent dislocation of the shoulder. Lyon Chir. 1954;49(8):994–7.
14. Provencher MT, et al. Anatomic osteochondral glenoid reconstruction for recurrent glenohumeral instability with glenoid deficiency using a distal tibia allograft. Arthroscopy. 2009;25(4):446–52.
15. Warner JJ, et al. Anatomical glenoid reconstruction for recurrent anterior glenohumeral instability with glenoid deficiency using an autogenous tricortical iliac crest bone graft. Am J Sports Med. 2006;34(2):205–12.
16. Tokish JM, et al. Arthroscopic distal clavicular autograft for treating shoulder instability with glenoid bone loss. Arthrosc Tech. 2014;3(4):e475–81.
17. Boileau P, Baring T, Greco V. Arthroscopic distal clavicular autograft for congruent glenoid reconstruction. Arthrosc Tech. 2021;10(11):e2389–95.
18. Harris RI, et al. Anatomic variance of the coracoclavicular ligaments. J Shoulder Elb Surg. 2001;10(6):585–8.
19. Novak PJ, et al. Surgical resection of the distal clavicle. J Shoulder Elb Surg. 1995;4(1 Pt 1):35–40.
20. Hudson PW, et al. Distal clavicle autograft for anterior-inferior glenoid augmentation: a comparative cadaveric anatomic study. Shoulder Elbow. 2020;12(6):404–13.
21. Petersen SA, et al. Autologous distal clavicle versus autologous coracoid bone grafts for restoration of anterior-inferior glenoid bone loss: a biomechanical comparison. J Shoulder Elb Surg. 2016;25(6):960–6.
22. Apostolakos JM, et al. Anterior glenohumeral instability: current review with technical pearls and pitfalls of arthroscopic soft-tissue stabilization. World J Orthop. 2021;12(1):1–13.
23. Apostolakos JY, Hoberman A, Shoji M, Weinreb J, Voss A, DiVenere J, Mazzocca A. Glenoid Labrum. In: G. I. Bain E, Di Giacomo G, Sugaya H, editors. Normal and pathological anatomy of the shoulder. Springer; 2015. p. 83–91.
24. Cameron KL, et al. History of shoulder instability and subsequent injury during four years of follow-up: a survival analysis. J Bone Joint Surg Am. 2013;95(5):439–45.
25. Frank RM, Romeo AA. Arthroscopic soft tissue reconstruction in anterior shoulder instability. Orthopade. 2018;47(2):121–8.
26. Kroner K, Lind T, Jensen J. The epidemiology of shoulder dislocations. Arch Orthop Trauma Surg. 1989;108(5):288–90.
27. Owens BD, et al. Incidence of glenohumeral instability in collegiate athletics. Am J Sports Med. 2009;37(9):1750–4.

28. Owens BD, Campbell SE, Cameron KL. Risk factors for anterior glenohumeral instability. Am J Sports Med. 2014;42(11):2591–6.
29. Owens BD, et al. The incidence and characteristics of shoulder instability at the United States military academy. Am J Sports Med. 2007;35(7):1168–73.
30. Dumont GD, Russell RD, Robertson WJ. Anterior shoulder instability: a review of pathoanatomy, diagnosis and treatment. Curr Rev Musculoskelet Med. 2011;4(4):200–7.
31. Mutlu S, et al. Anterior Glenohumeral instability: classification of pathologies of Anteroinferior Labroligamentous structures using MR arthrography. Adv Orthop. 2013;2013:473194.
32. Edwards TB, Boulahia A, Walch G. Radiographic analysis of bone defects in chronic anterior shoulder instability. Arthroscopy. 2003;19(7):732–9.
33. Piasecki DP, et al. Glenoid bone deficiency in recurrent anterior shoulder instability: diagnosis and management. J Am Acad Orthop Surg. 2009;17(8):482–93.
34. Provencher MT, et al. Recurrent shoulder instability: current concepts for evaluation and management of glenoid bone loss. J Bone Joint Surg Am. 2010;92(Suppl 2):133–51.
35. Rabinowitz J, Friedman R, Eichinger JK. Management of Glenoid Bone Loss with anterior shoulder instability: indications and outcomes. Curr Rev Musculoskelet Med. 2017;10(4):452–62.
36. Taylor DC, Arciero RA. Pathologic changes associated with shoulder dislocations. Arthroscopic and physical examination findings in first-time, traumatic anterior dislocations. Am J Sports Med. 1997;25(3):306–11.

The Open Bankart with a Lateral Capsular Shift

15

Antonio Cusano and Robert A. Arciero

Introduction

Glenohumeral instability is a common problem with an annual incidence of 0.08 per 1000 person-years in the United States [1, 2]. Certain at-risk populations, such as military personnel and collision athletes, are particularly affected, with reported incidences of 1.69 per 1000 person-years and rates as high as 3% per year [1, 2]. Anterior shoulder dislocations classically result in capsulolabral injuries. Although Bankart originally characterized the labral tear as the main contributor to glenohumeral instability in these settings, the reality is that a spectrum of injuries can occur depending on the direction and degree of applied force to the extremity at the time of injury, the integrity of dynamic shoulder stabilizers, and the bony anatomy [3]. Associated capsular and ligamentous injuries classically include capsular deformation of the inferior glenohumeral ligament (IGHL) and, less commonly, humeral avulsions of the glenohumeral ligaments (HAGL) and capsular rupture; bony deficiencies can occur from attritional glenoid bone loss and can involve fractures to the glenoid (bony Bankart) and humeral head (Hill-Sachs) and less frequently to the coracoid, greater, and lesser tuberosities [4–6].

A. Cusano (✉) · R. A. Arciero
Department of Orthopaedic Surgery, University of Connecticut, Farmington, CT, USA
e-mail: acusano@uchc.edu; arciero@uchc.edu

The open Bankart repair has historically been the gold standard surgical approach for management of anterior shoulder instability in that it allows for direct visualization of the glenohumeral joint and associated pathology and for a large capsular shift with complete repair of the anteroinferior capsulolabral tissue [7–11]. Over the past 20 years, however, arthroscopic approaches have gained popularity. A recent study found that the arthroscopic Bankart repair was the most commonly utilized shoulder instability procedure from 2010 to 2019, increasing by 4.3% in annual usage compared to the open Bankart which declined by 6.9% annually [12]. Arthroscopic procedures allow for shorter operative times using smaller incisions and decreased patient morbidity, provide an opportunity to address concomitant intra-articular pathology, and do not violate the subscapularis tendon [9, 13, 14]. While initial failure rates were alarmingly high, recent technical advancements, including the utilization of three or more anchors, operating in the lateral decubitus position [15], and refined patient selection have led to more predictable outcomes [15]. Further, the use of a Bankart repair combined with Hill-Sachs remplissage, or infraspinatus transfer, has led to improved patient satisfaction and recurrent instability rates [16]. Still, the presence of glenoid or humeral head bone loss can lead to early failure, with rates reported up to 67% [17]. This is further magnified in the setting of recurrent instability,

© The Author(s), under exclusive license to Springer Nature Switzerland AG 2026

R. M. Frank, J. M. Tokish (eds.), *Management of Shoulder Instability*,
https://doi.org/10.1007/978-3-032-18089-6_15

where glenoid and Hill-Sachs lesions can be present with rates up to 72% and 88%, respectively [18].

Despite improvements in technique and surgical indications, there are still reports of suboptimal recurrence and reoperation rates and persistent capsular laxity following arthroscopic repair in higher-risk patients [7, 19, 20]. As such, it is possible that the open Bankart procedure may have a larger role in select clinical scenarios.

Case #1: The Young Contact Athlete

Case Presentation

A 17-year-old competitive multisport collision athlete (football, wrestling) presented to the clinic for evaluation of shoulder instability, with reports of multiple self-reducible dislocation events, one of which occurred while asleep and the others while at practice. His first dislocation event occurred approximately 1 week prior to presentation and was followed by almost 10 separate events thereafter. On evaluation, he described feelings of both anterior and posterior instability with symptoms that were refractory to bracing and activity modifications. Physical examination was notable for pain-free forward flexion and abduction to 170 and 160 degrees, respectively, with a fully intact rotator cuff on strength testing. The patient had a mild sulcus sign upon inferior stress of the extremity, positive apprehension relocation, and a 2+ shift on both anterior and posterior load testing done while in the supine position. Radiographs did not reveal any obvious glenohumeral joint subluxation or acute fracture/dislocation although there was question of a possible chronic, healed anterior rim fracture (Fig. 15.1a). Follow-up magnetic resonance imaging (MRI) showed a nondisplaced undersurface tear of the anterior/anteroinferior labrum with periosteal elevation, no significant bone loss, and a minimally depressed Hill-Sachs lesion (Fig. 15.1b). Given that he was at an elevated risk for recurrent instability with arthroscopic repair due to his young age and engagement in contact sport with overhead activity, he was surgically indicated for an open Bankart repair with capsulorrhaphy.

An examination under anesthesia again demonstrated a 2+ anterior load-and-shift test. Notable intraoperative findings included an anteroinferior labral tear extending between the 2 and 6 o'clock positions on the glenoid face, which was repaired using three double-loaded suture anchors affixed to the glenoid rim and secured utilizing horizontal mattress sutures. Pertinent negative findings included the absence of any humeral head or glenoid bony disruption, any HAGL lesions, and a normal-appearing rotator cuff.

Literature Review

Collision athletes are at increased risk for recurrent dislocation following Bankart procedures, with reported postoperative subluxation/dislocation rates of 11% to 16.5% at 3-year follow-up [21]. They are at risk of two and three times higher recurrence rates following open and arthroscopic Bankart repair, respectively [22], compared to their noncontact counterparts. To that end, a review of 48 shoulders with known instability (46 collision athletes) found that 25% of patients treated arthroscopically reported postoperative subluxation or dislocation events compared to 12.5% in those treated with open procedures [21]. Cho et al. [23] reported a high recurrence rate (17.2%) among athletes treated with arthroscopic stabilization procedures, with a 28.6% failure rate in the collision group compared to 6.7% in the non-collision group. In a final study of 67 competitive teenage overhead or contact sport athletes treated with arthroscopic capsulolabral repair, Castagna et al. [24] found a 21% failure rate that directly correlated with type of sport.

Younger age at time of first dislocation and male sex have also been identified as an independent risk factors for recurrent instability events [25–27], with males being 1.25 times more likely to develop recurrent instability following arthroscopic Bankart repair. This risk, however,

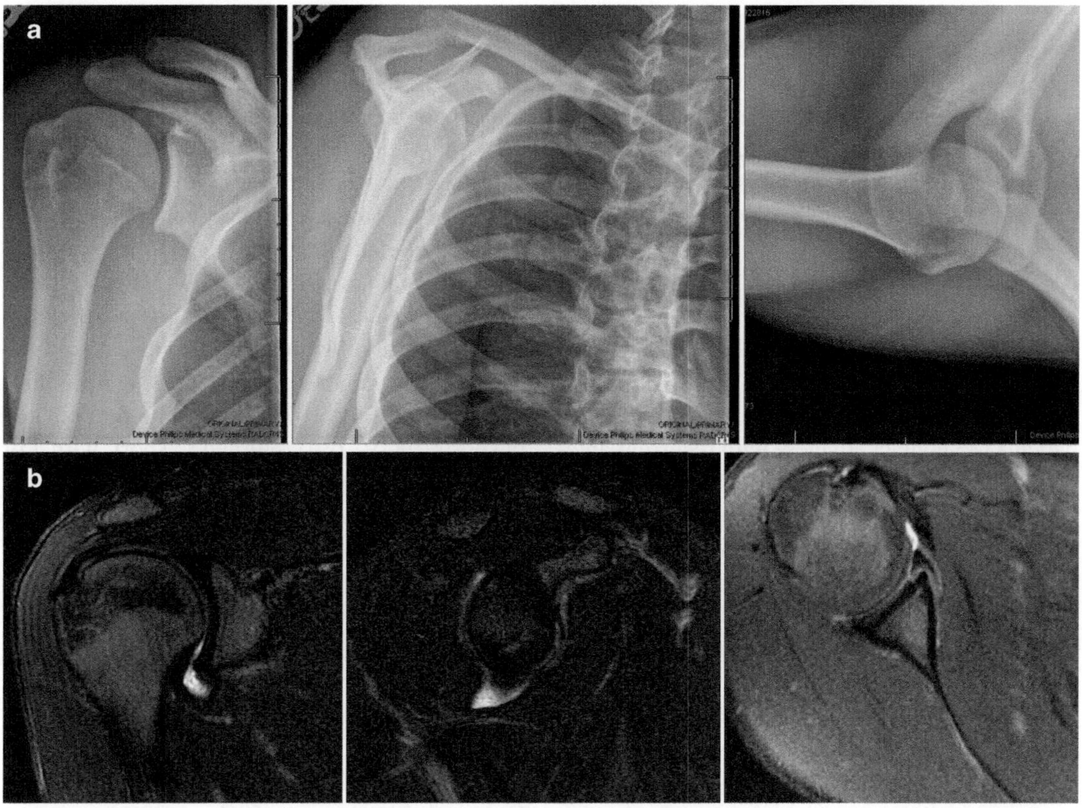

Fig. 15.1 (**a**) Anteroposterior, scapular Y, and axillary imaging show no obvious glenohumeral joint subluxation or acute fracture/dislocation although there was question of a possible chronic, healed anterior rim fracture. (**b**) Coronal, sagittal, and axial MRI images demonstrate a nondisplaced undersurface tear of the anterior/anteroinferior labrum with periosteal elevation, no significant bone loss, and a minimally depressed Hill-Sachs lesion

was not appreciated when open Bankart or Latarjet procedures were included. Nakagawa et al. [28] reported a 2-year 20.4% postoperative recurrent instability rate following arthroscopic Bankart repair without additional reinforcement procedures in 115 competitive athletes, including those with large glenoid defects. These rates differed based on type of sport (33.3% in rugby, 17.2% American football, 14.3% contact sports, 12.5% overhead sports, and 11.1% other collision sports), and multivariate analysis found that younger age and the presence of a preoperative glenoid defect with small or no bone fragment significantly influenced recurrent instability rates among competitive athletes. Similarly, a recent retrospective review of Irish collision sport athletes with a mean age of 19.9 years treated with arthroscopic Bankart stabilization showed a high rate of recurrent dislocation (21%). Although one's risk for recurrent instability is certainly complex and multifactorial, attempts have been made to create a simple scoring system to identify those patients at a higher risk for recurrent instability following an arthroscopic Bankart repair. To that end, a 2007 prospective case-control study by Balg and Boileau [29] found that age under 20 years at time of surgery, involvement in competitive contact sports or those involving forced overhead activity, shoulder hyperlaxity, and the presence of a Hill-Sachs lesion on an anteroposterior radiograph of the shoulder in external rotation and/or loss of the sclerotic inferior glenoid contour were associated with higher recurrent instability rates. The authors integrated these factors into a 10-point preoperative instability severity index (ISI) score and found that those who scored over six points were at an unacceptable recurrence risk of 70% and would be better suited with a Bristow-Latarjet procedure. A more recent follow-up systematic review by Rosenberg et al. [30], however, has since found that perhaps a lower score threshold of less than four may provide a better predictor of failure.

The high reported recurrent instability rates following arthroscopic stabilization have supported the use of the open Bankart as a reasonable approach to managing this high-risk patient population. In his case series of 119 consecutive patients (83 contact athletes) with recurrent anterior shoulder instability treated with an open stabilization procedure, Pagnani et al. [31] reported a 2% recurrence rate, all of which occurred in patients with Hill-Sachs lesions. Interestingly, bony defects of the glenoid or humeral head did not correlate with a statistically significant increase in recurrence risk, as had previously been shown with arthroscopic techniques. When contact athletes were isolated as a population, there were also no statistically significant increases in recurrence. A separate retrospective review [32] of 21 teenage patients with recurrent instability treated with open Bankart repair found no recurrences of instability at 2-year follow-up. In their retrospective review of 60 patients aged 15 to 20 years who underwent unilateral or bilateral open stabilization for recurrent anterior glenohumeral instability over a 7-year period, Crua et al. [33] found 92% return to sport rate. The redislocation rate was 13% (8/60), with 87.5% (7/8) of them occurring in traumatic setting upon return to high-impact sporting events. A similar review by Hickey et al. found high rates of patient-reported satisfaction, excellent functional outcomes, and high return to play rates (88.2%) in the medium term (5.8 ± 2.2 months) among young collision athletes aged 18 years or less who underwent an open Bankart repair for anterior shoulder instability.

Outside of its protective advantage against recurrent instability in the athletic population, the open Bankart repair has shown favorable outcomes with return to sport and work. A recent systematic review by AlSomali et al. [34] found an 87% postoperative return to sport and work rate in 563 high-demand patients (mean age of 27.4 years) treated with an open Bankart repair at a mean 11.5-year follow-up. Ninety-one percent had good to excellent outcomes as per patient-reported measures, and the recurrent instability rate was low (8.5%). Neviaser et al. [35] reviewed 127 patients at a mean follow-up of 17.1 years following open Bankart repair and found 0.8% recurrent dislocation and subluxation rates. Of the 107 patients who participated in sports, 98 (91.6%) returned to sport, with 7 of the remaining 9 discontinuing for reasons other than the shoulder itself. Lastly, Murphy et al. [36] recently performed a systematic review of 822 shoulders treated with arthroscopic Bankart stabilization across nine studies. The authors found that at a mean follow-up of 12 years, arthroscopic stabilization was associated with a 31% instability rate, as well as a lower return to sport and work rates compared to their open Bankart counterparts (87% vs. 77%). Osteoarthritic changes (59% vs. 33%) and revision rates (17% vs. 1%) were also higher in the included arthroscopic studies.

Case #2: The Revision Setting

Case Presentation

A 26-year-old, right-hand dominant, female athletic trainer and former collegiate softball player presented to our clinic with complaints of recurrent shoulder pain and instability. She had sustained a right shoulder dislocation 10 years prior while diving into a base with outstretched arms and subsequently underwent an arthroscopic debridement and anterior capsulorrhaphy with intact labrum. She had done well for 3 years after this index procedure until she ultimately redislocated during throwing drills. She underwent a revision arthroscopic capsulorrhaphy where the labrum was noted to be somewhat diminutive but intact. Following this second procedure, she never felt like she returned to her baseline condition and continued to have problems with painful popping/clicking with throwing and overhead motion as well as occasional episodes of instability. As a result of these persistent symptoms, she ultimately underwent a third procedure in the form of an arthroscopic labral repair and posterior capsulorrhaphy. In addition to the aforementioned dislocation events, she also had an isolated episode where she awoke to find her right shoulder dislocated and managed to self-reduce it. Her pain and instability were now affecting her activities of daily living, such that she was having subluxation events while at work when carrying or lifting an empty cooler or moving exercise equipment.

On examination, she had full and symmetric shoulder range of motion with a fully intact rotator cuff on strength testing. Instability testing was notable for a positive apprehension-relocation test and 2+ load shift. Radiographs showed a concentric glenohumeral joint with no obvious fracture or significant bone loss (Fig. 15.2a). CT imaging showed postoperative changes of the anteroinferior glenoid in accordance with her previous labral repair but otherwise showed no acute fractures or Hill-Sachs lesions (Fig. 15.2b). Similarly, an MRI was obtained which showed hyperlaxity with a patulous inferior capsule, less than 10% glenoid bone loss, and no significant Hill-Sachs lesion (Fig. 15.2c). In light of the patient's previous failed arthroscopic procedures and instability events sustained during activities

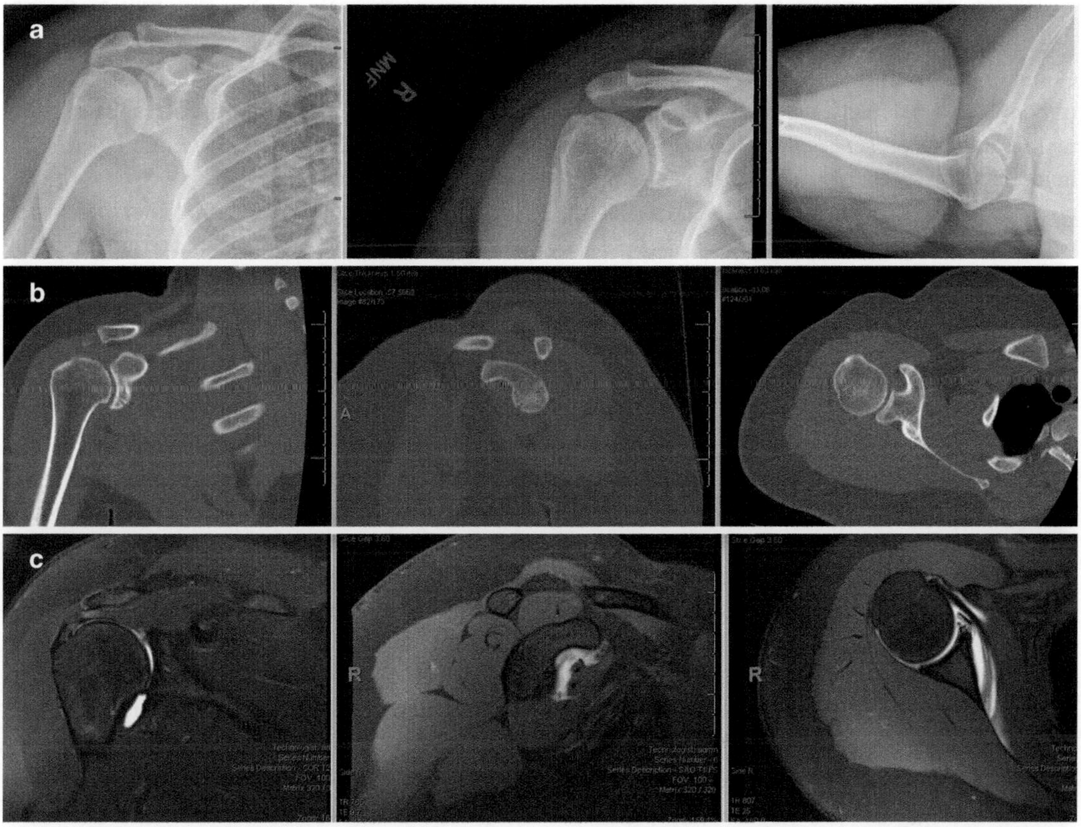

Fig. 15.2 (**a**) Three-view radiographs demonstrate a concentric glenohumeral joint with no obvious fracture or significant bone loss. (**b**) Representative select CT cuts are consistent with postoperative changes of the anteroinferior glenoid in accordance with patient's previous labral repair but otherwise showed no acute fractures or Hill-Sachs lesion. (**c**) Representative coronal, sagittal, and axial MRI cuts demonstrate a patulous inferior capsule suggestive of hyperlaxity, less than 10% glenoid bone loss, and no significant Hill-Sachs lesion

of daily living or sleep, recommendations were made for an open Bankart and capsulorrhaphy.

Intraoperatively, the patient was found to have degenerative thinning of the central glenoid cartilage, a diminutive but intact anteroinferior labrum, a patulous anterior inferior capsule, and several large knots of suture material along the junction of the posterior labrum joint surface stemming from her previous surgical attempts. Postoperatively, the patient did well. The patient had full active range of motion and rotator cuff strength. She had successfully completed physical therapy and was allowed to return to work and physical activities without restrictions.

Literature Review

An open Bankart can be useful in the revision setting following failed arthroscopic repair. Common reasons for failure include the presence of bony glenoid defects, generalized ligamentous laxity, and the presence and size of Hill-Sachs humeral lesions. Open procedures have traditionally been accepted as the gold standard in the revision setting.

Nonetheless, arthroscopic revisions have become increasingly more popular, with proponents of this approach advocating for improved visualization, less patient morbidity, and the ability to simultaneously address intra-articular pathology. Still, the literature has varied in terms of success rates for arthroscopic revision stabilization procedures. In a retrospective review of 22 patients who underwent arthroscopic capsuloplasty following a failed primary arthroscopic stabilization, De Giorgi et al. [37] reported a 36.4% failure rate, including frank dislocations, subluxations, and apprehension that significantly inhibited patients' quality of lives. Based on their outcomes, the authors recommended against arthroscopic revision procedures following failed instability surgery. A separate retrospective review by Neri et al. [38] of 12 arthroscopic revision Bankart repairs on patients with recurrent unidirectional shoulder instability found a 27% recurrent postoperative instability rate, with only 73% of patients reporting good to excellent results. Similar results were seen by Zabinski et al. [39] and Creighton et al. [40]

More recent studies have also shown mixed results with arthroscopic capsulolabral revisions. In a case series of 56 patients with recurrent anterior shoulder instability following a previous open or arthroscopic repair, Bartl et al. [41] found an 11% recurrent instability rate following arthroscopic repair using a minimum of three anchors with 86% of patients rating their postoperative results as good to excellent. A separate retrospective review [42] of 63 shoulders (62 patients) reported a 19% recurrent instability rate in those treated with arthroscopic stabilization with the number of prior surgeries and baseline hyperlaxity being independent risk factors and predictors for failure. Some of the lowest recurrent instability rates following revision arthroscopic repair were reported by Stein [43] (4.3%) and Imhoff et al. [44] (0%) although these studies were limited by their retrospective study design and small sample sizes. That being said, several other studies have published unfavorable results. In a retrospective review of consecutive patients treated with either a revision arthroscopic Bankart or open Latarjet following a failed primary arthroscopic repair, Elamo et al. [45] found a 43% recurrent instability rate. Similarly, Slaven et al. [46] reported a 36% failure rate following revision arthroscopic stabilization in a young, active duty military population with less than 20% bone loss. Interestingly, glenoid bone loss was similar in the successful and failure groups, with a mean loss of 7.8 ± 8.0%. In the revision setting, however, some data has suggested that traditional open procedures may offer more predictable outcomes. Cho et al. [47] presented a case series of 26 shoulders (mean age of 24 years) that underwent a traditional open Bankart repair as revision surgery after a failed arthroscopic Bankart procedure for traumatic anterior shoulder instability. The authors reported an 11.5% redislocation rate, all of which occurred in shoulders with an engaging Hill-Sachs and associated hyperlaxity (≥2+ on sulcus sign). At last follow-up, the mean Rowe score was 81 points with 88.5% of patients with good or excellent results.

Open Versus Arthroscopic Bankart Stabilization

The historic utilization of the open Bankart procedure has allowed for long-term examination of its outcomes. In one of the first longitudinal studies on open Bankart stabilization, Rowe et al. [48] reported early return of motion and resumption of athletic activities in patients treated over a 30-year period. Of the 161 shoulders included in the analysis, 77% had Hill-Sachs lesions and 73% had bony disruption of the anterior glenoid rim (including fracture). Still, 98% of patients rated their outcomes as good to excellent, 69% had full range of motion, and only 2% experienced another dislocation. In a similar study of 49 patients (50 shoulders) who underwent an open Bankart stabilization, at a mean of 28 years follow-up, Fabre et al. [49] reported only 8 recurrent dislocations, each of which was preceded by a new traumatic event (6 while playing rugby, 2 of which required reoperation). Of the contact athlete cohort which accounted for 73% of all patients, 82% of them returned to their previous level of sports activities. A separate study by Berendes et al. [50] showed good long-term results in 31 patients treated with an open modified Bankart procedure as at a mean follow-up of 11 years, all patients had returned to work and 94% had resumed their preoperative occupation and level of activity. Recurrence rates varied between 6.7 and 9.7% as two patients had a significant new injury at 1 and 9 years postoperatively, respectively. Further, in their review of 30 patients treated with an open Bankart procedure, Pelet et al. [51] showed 100% recovery to pretraumatic levels of sporting and professional activities and a 10% (3 of 30 patients) recurrent dislocation rate (one requiring reoperation) at a mean follow-up of 29 years. Lastly, a more recent review [52] that followed 47 patients without bone loss treated with an open Bankart for a minimum of 20 years between 1989 and 1994 showed a 97.5% satisfied to very satisfied rate and a 17.5% recurrence rate (five dislocations, two subluxations in seven patients), with six of seven patients developing instability after being symptom-free for at least 8 years.

There have also been several studies looking at long-term outcomes in the setting of arthroscopic Bankart stabilization with varying results. Owens et al. reported a 37.5% recurrent instability rate (subluxations, dislocations) at a mean follow-up of 11.7 years in 39 first-time dislocators (40 shoulders) treated acutely with an arthroscopic Bankart repair. In a retrospective case series of 30 patients (31 shoulders) treated arthroscopically, Castagna et al. [24] reported 22.6% recurrence and 84% patient satisfaction rates at a mean 10.9 years. Similarly, Kavaja et al. reported a 22.9% recurrent instability rate at a minimum of 11 years following arthroscopic repair, with a 75% extremely satisfied to satisfied patient rating. In addition, Privitera et al., in a retrospective review of 20 consecutive patients treated with an arthroscopic Bankart repair at a minimum 10-year follow-up, showed a 35% recurrence rate (three out of seven patients requiring reoperation), with 25% of shoulders failing after recurrent dislocation and 10% with signs of anterior instability on examination at a mean 4.2 years postoperatively. Outside of recurrent instability rates, multiple studies have also reported high return to sport rates following arthroscopic Bankart repair. A recent systematic review on 34 studies by Memon et al. [53] found an 81% return to sport rate. Similar findings were seen in a separate review by Kasik et al. [54] who reported an 81.5% return to sport to preinjury levels at an average of 5 months postoperative in 461 adolescent athletes (mean age of 15.7 years). Lastly, Abdul-Rassoul et al. [55] found a 97.5% return to sport rate following arthroscopic Bankart at a mean 5.9 months postoperative across 16 studies. Nonetheless, wide variation across published studies with respect to return to sport criteria and consideration of the athlete's psychological state certainly confound these outcomes [56].

More recently, there has been an emergence of direct comparison studies between arthroscopic and open Bankart procedures in an effort to establish clinical equivalence. In a prospective, randomized multicenter study of 56 patients (30 arthroscopy, 26 open), Sperber et al. [57] demonstrated a trend toward more redislocations in the arthroscopic group at 2-year follow-up (23% vs. 12%) although this did not achieve statistical significance. Similarly, Bottoni's [58] randomized controlled trial of 64 consecutive patients found a statistically significant improvement in Single Assessment Numeric Evaluation (SANE) scores in both arthroscopic and open groups with similar recurrence rates. These results were comparable to those published in another randomized controlled trial by Fabbriciani et al. [59] which showed no recurrent dislocations in either group and similar improvements in Constant and Rowe scores at 2-year follow-up.

A more recent review of 48 shoulders in 46 collision athletes by Rhee et al. [21], however, found that while open and arthroscopic procedures experienced similar postoperative improvements in visual analog, Rowe, and Constant scores, the number of shoulders with postoperative subluxation or dislocation events following stabilization was markedly higher in the arthroscopically-treated cohort compared to open treatment (25% vs. 12.5%). Similarly, in their 2007 systematic review of 18 published studies, Lenters et al. [20] found that arthroscopic repairs were associated with significantly higher risks of recurrent instability (relative risk (RR): 2.37), recurrent dislocation (RR: 2.74), and reoperation (RR: 2.32). They, too, were less effective than open procedures at returning patients to work and/or sports (RR: 0.87). When considered alone, arthroscopic suture anchor techniques resulted in higher risks of recurrent dislocation and instability. In a separate prospective, randomized clinical trial by Mohtadi et al. [60], open repair had a statistically lower risk of recurrence although similar patient-reported outcomes in terms of Western Ontario Shoulder Instability (WOSI) and American Shoulder and Elbow Surgeons (ASES) scores at 2-year follow-up. Retrospective reviews by Gaunche [61] and Virk et al. [11] found a 0% recurrence rate following open Bankart (compared to 33% in those done arthroscopically) and a significantly shorter time to recurrent instability following arthroscopic repair, respectively. A separate meta-analysis [62] reported higher rates of recurrent dislocation (12.4% vs. 3.4%) and total recurrence (dislocation or subluxation, 20.3% vs. 10.3%), as well as a lower proportion of patients with excellent or good postoperative Rowe scores following arthroscopic stabilization versus open repair. Similarly, a recent prospective review by Uchiyama et al. [63] of patients with recurrent anterior shoulder instability found that an open Bankart plus inferior capsular shift had lower instability rates (0%) compared to arthroscopic repair (26.6%) although this was at the expense of greater limitations in external rotation, external rotation at 90 degrees abduction, and horizontal extension. Lastly, a smaller retrospective review [64] of 15 patients at over 7 years follow-up found that for patients with up to 30% glenoid bone defect and Hill-Sachs lesion, the open Bankart surgery with anteroinferior capsular shift provided desirable results in terms of shoulder function (final mean VAS: 0.4/10; mean Activity of Daily Living Score: 28.97; mean ASES: 96.1 1 mean CMS 93.9) and recurrence rate (3.3% recurrent dislocation, 13.4% recurrent subluxation).

Nonetheless, the advent of newer technology and refined techniques have shown improving results with arthroscopic repair. A 2007 systematic review of published literature from 1985 to 2006 found that arthroscopic anterior stabilization using the most effective surgical techniques had similar recurrent instability rates for open versus arthroscopic repair (10.2% vs. 12.8%, respectively). Similarly, a separate systematic review of 11 studies by Ng et al. [65] found open and arthroscopic stabilization to be equally effective in managing traumatic anterior glenohumeral instability. However, poor methodological quality, clinical heterogeneity, and variable definitions of recurrent instability and outcome measures limit the interpretation of these results. A 2012 controlled trial [66] comparing 42 patients randomized to either open or arthroscopic Bankart repair found that both modalities were effective. Although arthroscopic techniques showed a lower index of functional limitation of the upper limb as per the Disabilities of the Arm, Shoulder, and Hand (DASH) questionnaire, this did not reach clinical significance. Lastly, a recent systematic review looked at the temporal association between literature publication dates and clinical authors and found that newer studies published after 2000 were associated with more favorable arthroscopic outcomes [67].

Further research is warranted to better discern outcome differences between open and arthroscopic Bankart repair, particularly in higher-risk patient populations and as arthroscopy technique continues to develop. The author's indications for an open Bankart repair include high-risk or collision male athletes aged less than 25 years old with an intact subscapularis, revisions of well-done arthroscopic procedures with minor bone loss, "intermediate bone loss" (characterized as 10% to 20% of glenoid bone loss), and instability events sustained during activities of daily living or sleep. Support of these management decisions are depicted in the following case presentations and literature reviews.

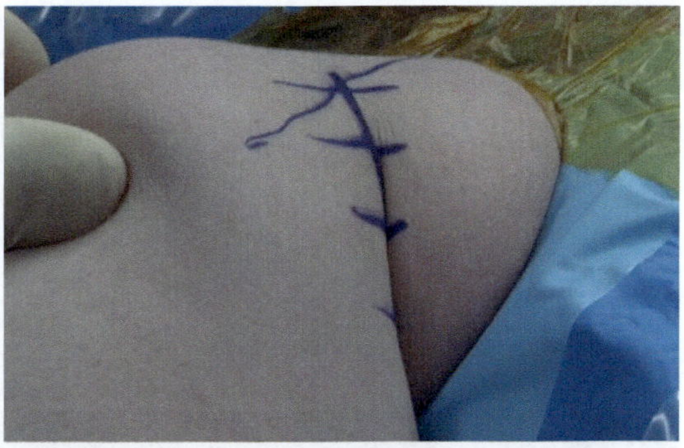

Fig. 15.3 Representative intraoperative image outlining standard anterior axillary incision from the coracoid to the axilla following Langer's lines

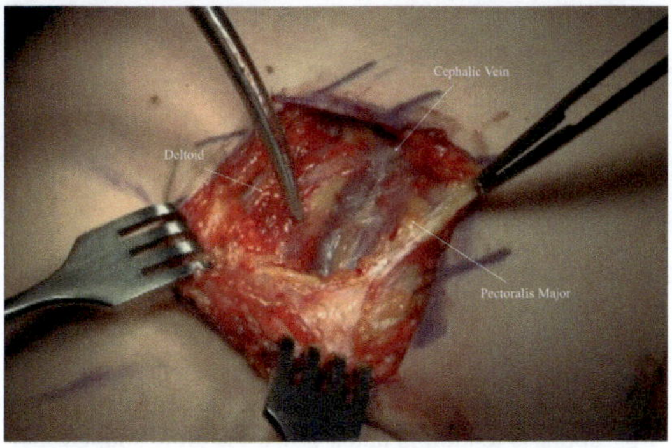

Fig. 15.4 Intraoperative photo highlighting the deltopectoral interval and the cephalic vein, which is taken laterally so as to not disrupt any collateral vessels from the deltoid

Our Technique

A formal examination under anesthesia is carried out in order to determine load-shift grading, concomitant posterior or multidirectional instability, or engagement with a Hill-Sachs lesion. The patient is subsequently placed in a modified beach-chair position with the scapula bumped to protract it forward.

A standard anterior axillary incision from the coracoid to the axilla following Langer's lines is carried out (Fig. 15.3). A combination of sharp and blunt dissection and needle-tip electrocautery are utilized to get down to the level of the deltopectoral fascia and cephalic vein, which is taken laterally so as to not disrupt any feeder vessels from the deltoid (Fig. 15.4). A self-retaining or link retractor is utilized to retract the deltoid laterally and the pectoralis major muscle medially. The clavipectoral fascia is incised longitudinally just lateral to the coracobrachialis and extended superiorly and inferiorly to the coracoacromial and falciform ligaments, respectively. The retractors are advanced deeper into the wound so as to retract the deltoid laterally and the conjoint tendon medially.

Attention is then given to identifying the superior and inferior extents of the subscapularis tendon with respect to the adjacent bicipital groove, anterior humeral circumflex vessels, and lesser tuberosity. Typically, three to four heavy, nonabsorbable tagging stitches are placed approximately 1.5 to 2.0 cm medial to the lesser tuberosity (Fig. 15.5a). The subscapularis is taken down via an L-shaped incision with the vertical limb made just lateral to the tagging sutures (Fig. 15.5b) and extending from the rotator interval to a point just proximal to the anterior humeral circumflex vessels, and the horizontal limb carried medially so as to avoid injuring the axillary nerve. Careful blunt dissection is carried out to separate the subscapularis tendon from the

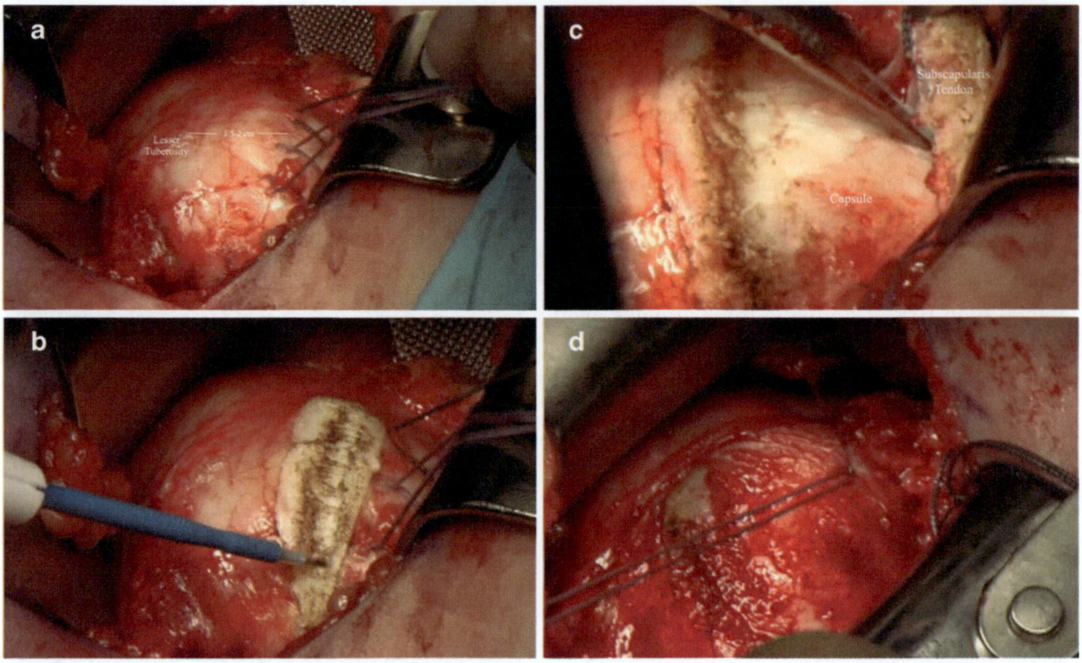

Fig. 15.5 (**a**) The superior and inferior extents of the subscapularis tendon, anterior humeral circumflex vessels, and lesser tuberosity are identified. Three to four heavy, nonabsorbable tagging sutures are placed approximately 1.5–2.0 cm medial to the lesser tuberosity. (**b**) The subscapularis tendon is taken down via an L-shaped incision, with the vertical limb made just lateral to the tagging sutures. (**c**) Utilizing careful blunt and scissor dissection, the subscapularis tendon is freed off from the underlying shoulder capsule. This interval is typically most easily appreciated along the inferomedial corner of the subscapularis. (**d**) A suture is placed laterally within the rotator interval in order to provide additional stability, particularly in patients with notable inferior laxity

underlying shoulder capsule (Fig. 15.5c). From a technical standpoint, this interval is typically most easily found along the inferomedial corner of the subscapularis.

Once this interval is fully identified, a suture is placed laterally within the rotator interval to provide additional stability, particularly in patients with inferior laxity (Fig. 15.5d). With the arm externally rotated to 45°, a nonabsorbable suture is placed to close the lateral 1 to 1.5 cm of the rotator interval. Next, with the patient's arm placed in 30° of external rotation, a T-capsulotomy is performed, with the vertical limb made laterally at the level of the humeral neck (Fig. 15.6a). Two tagging sutures are placed along the superior and inferior borders of the cut capsule. A horizontal limb is made at the midglenoid level and extended medially in between the two tagging sutures (Fig. 15.6b), thereby creating superior and inferior leaflets (Fig. 15.6c). Retractors are placed to allow for visualization of the glenoid and Bankart lesion. Specifically, a Fukuda is used to retract the humeral head and a capsular or Batman retractor is put around the glenoid neck medially and a spiked Hohmann deep to the Bankart lesion.

With the anterior glenoid now fully exposed, care is given to repairing the Bankart lesion (Fig. 15.7a). A bony bed is made in preparation for suture anchor placement and any existing fibrous or poor-appearing tissue is removed via a combination of rongeur and burr. Anchors are placed at the glenoid articular surface, typically in at least the 5 o'clock or 7 o'clock position in right and left shoulders, respectively. The authors prefer to utilize three to four double-loaded suture anchors, separated approximately 5 mm apart from one another so as to avoid any potential anchor failure or pullout. If needed, a double-row construct can be made medially on the

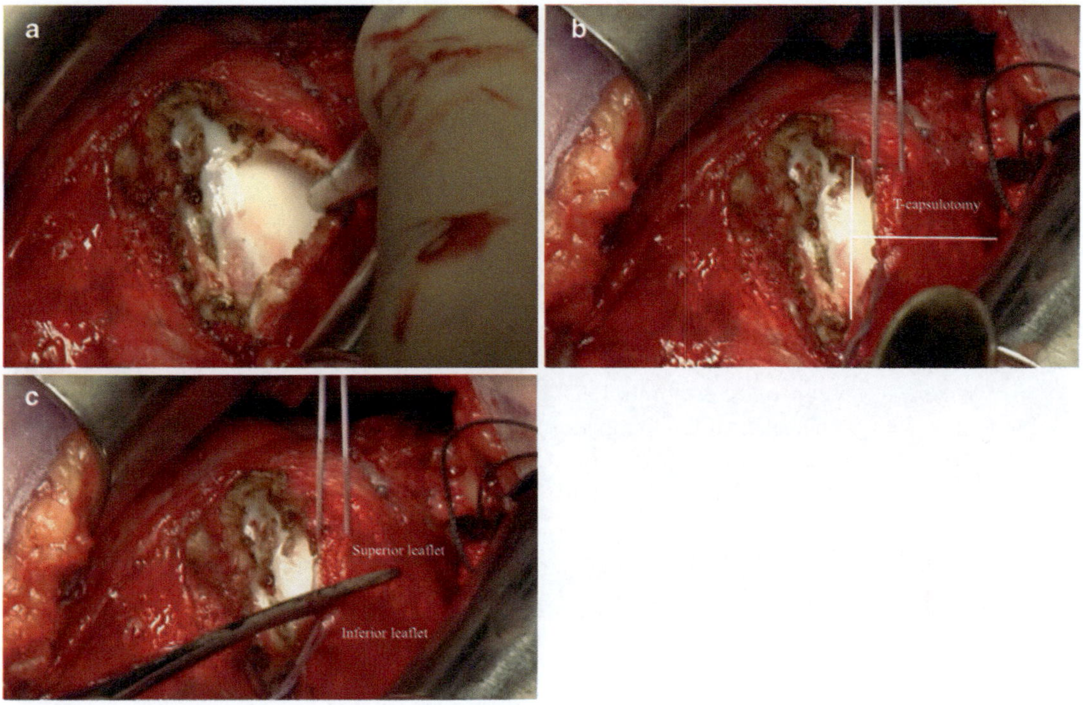

Fig. 15.6 (**a**) With the patient's arm placed in 30° external rotation, a T-capsulotomy is made with the vertical limb placed laterally at the level of the humeral neck. (**b**) Two tagging sutures are placed along the superior and inferior borders of the cut capsule. (**c**) The horizontal limb of the T-capsulotomy is made at the midglenoid level and extended medially in between the tagging sutures, thereby creating superior and inferior leaflets

glenoid neck in patients with larger Bankart lesions (Fig. 15.7b). After the anchors have been placed, the spiked Hohmann is removed, and sutures are passed in a horizonal mattress fashion from inferior to superior through the torn capsulolabral tissue (Fig. 15.7c). After all sutures have been passed, they are sequentially tied from inferior to superior (Fig. 15.7d).

Next, a capsular shift is performed (Fig. 15.8a). First, a high-strength, nonabsorbable suture is used as a reefing stitch to close the horizontal limb of the capsulotomy. A separate high-strength, nonabsorbable suture is used to tension the leaflets via an outside-in, outside-in approach for the superior limb and inside-out, inside-out technique for the inferior limb. Two double-loaded anchors are then placed along the superolateral and inferolateral aspects of the lesser tuberosity, just medial to the subscapularis insertion site. The inferior leaflet is tensioned toward the superolateral anchor and secured in place with horizontal mattress sutures from the anchor (Fig. 15.8b). Similarly, the superior leaflet is tensioned toward the inferolateral anchor and secured in a similar fashion to complete the capsular shift (Fig. 15.8c).

Lastly, the subscapularis tendon is repaired by passing the previously placed subscapularis tendon sutures into the remaining stump on the lesser tuberosity in a horizontal mattress fashion tied from superior to inferior. The repair is oversewn with No. 1 Vicryl suture from superior to inferior (Fig. 15.9). The arm is taken through range of motion and stability testing. Closure of the deltopectoral interval and skin is left at the discretion of the operating surgeon.

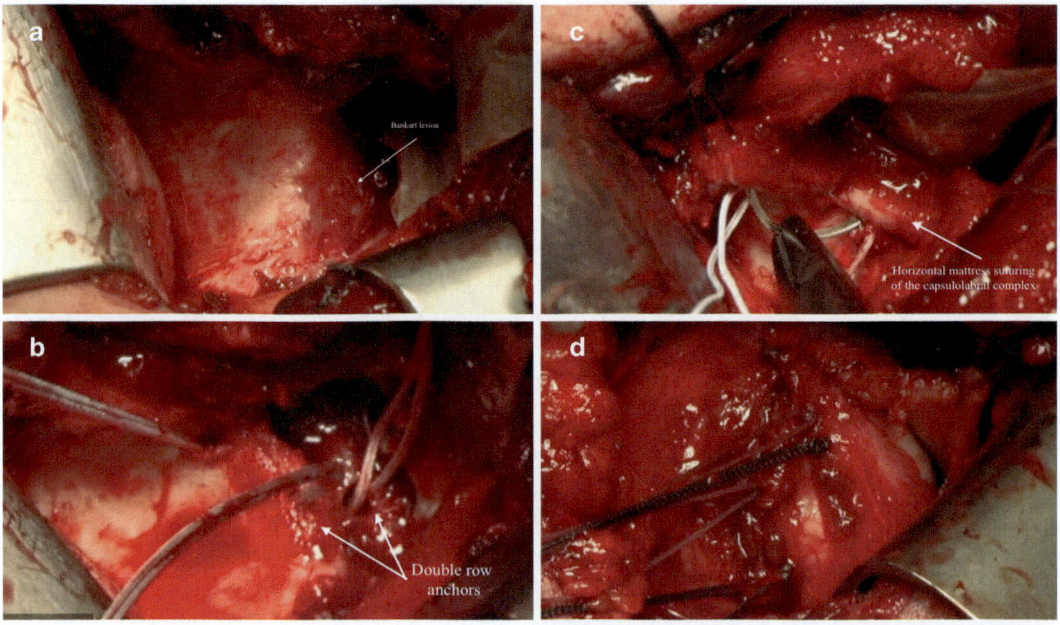

Fig. 15.7 (**a**) With the anterior glenoid fully exposed, the Bankart lesion can be easily visualized. (**b**) A bony bed is made in preparation for suture anchor placement, and a combination of rongeur and burr are utilized to remove any existing fibrous or malappearing tissue. Anchors are placed along the glenoid articular surface, typically in at least the 5 o'clock and 7 o'clock positions on right and left shoulders, respectively. For patients with larger Bankart lesions, a double-row construct can be made medially on the glenoid neck, as depicted here. (**c**) Sutures are passed in a horizontal mattress fashion from inferior to superior through the torn capsulolabral tissue. (**d**) After all sutures have been passed, they are sequentially tied from inferior to superior to complete the labral repair

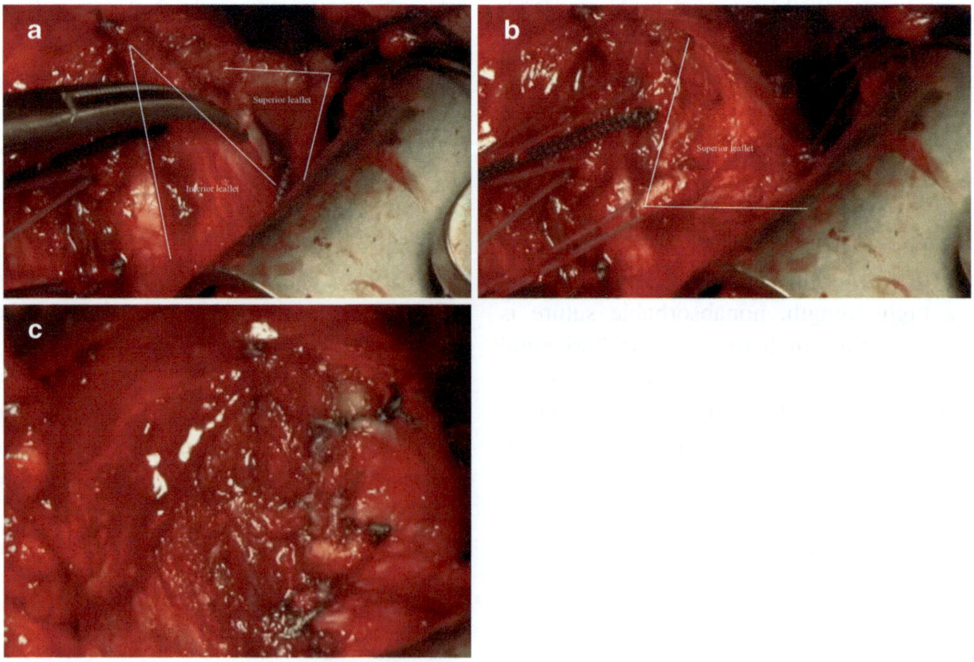

Fig. 15.8 (**a**) A capsular shift is then planned, utilizing the previously made superior and inferior leaflets. (**b**) The inferior leaflet is tensioned toward the superolateral anchor and secured in placed with horizontal mattress sutures from the anchor. The superior leaflet can then be tensioned toward the inferolateral anchor and secured in a similar fashion. (**c**) Completed capsular shift

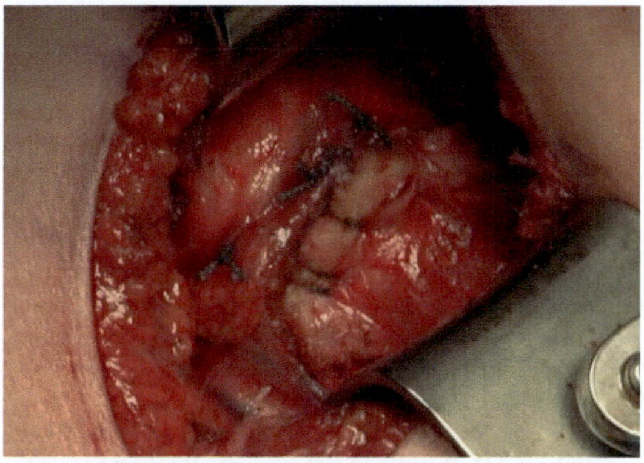

Fig. 15.9 The subscapularis tendon is then repaired by passing the previously placed subscapularis tendon sutures into the remaining stump on the lesser tuberosity in a horizontal mattress fashion. This is tied from superior to inferior. The repair is oversewn with absorbable suture from superior to inferior

Conclusion

The open Bankart repair has historically been regarded as the gold standard surgical approach for management of anterior shoulder instability. Although arthroscopic approaches have gained increasing popularity, high recurrence/reoperation rates and persistent capsular laxity have called into question its efficacy in higher-risk patients. Further research is needed to better determine outcome differences between open and arthroscopic Bankart repairs, particularly in this patient population. The author's indications for an open Bankart repair include high-risk or collision male athletes aged less than 25 years old with an intact subscapularis; revisions of well-done arthroscopic procedures with minor bone loss; 10% to 20% of glenoid bone loss, so called "intermediate bone loss"; and instability events sustained during activities of daily living or sleep. As technology continues to improve and surgical techniques become more refined, future research is warranted to better discern open versus arthroscopic outcomes.

References

1. Owens BD, Dawson L, Burks R, Cameron KL. Incidence of shoulder dislocation in the United States military: demographic considerations from a high-risk population. J Bone Joint Surg Am. 2009;91(4):791–6. https://doi.org/10.2106/jbjs.H.00514.
2. Waterman B, Owens BD, Tokish JM. Anterior shoulder instability in the military athlete. Sports Health. 2016;8(6):514–9. https://doi.org/10.1177/1941738116672161.
3. Bankart A. The pathology and treatment of recurrent dislocation of the shoulder joint. Br J Surg. 1938;26(101):23–9.
4. HA Hill MS. The grooved defect of the humeral head. Radiology. 1940;35(6):690–700.
5. Verma N, Chahar D, Chawla A, Sreenivasan R, Pankaj A. Recurrent anterior instability of the shoulder associated with coracoid fracture - an unusual presentation. J Clin Orthop Trauma. 2016;7(Suppl 1):99–102. https://doi.org/10.1016/j.jcot.2016.05.009.
6. Wintzell G, Haglund-Akerlind Y, Tengvar M, Johansson L, Eriksson E. MRI examination of the glenohumeral joint after traumatic primary anterior dislocation. A descriptive evaluation of the acute lesion and at 6-month follow-up. Knee Surg Sports Traumatol Arthrosc. 1996;4(4):232–6. https://doi.org/10.1007/bf01567969.
7. Boileau P, Villalba M, Héry JY, Balg F, Ahrens P, Neyton L. Risk factors for recurrence of shoulder instability after arthroscopic Bankart repair. J Bone Joint Surg Am. 2006;88(8):1755–63. https://doi.org/10.2106/jbjs.E.00817.
8. Chen L, Xu Z, Peng J, Xing F, Wang H, Xiang Z. Effectiveness and safety of arthroscopic versus open Bankart repair for recurrent anterior shoulder dislocation: a meta-analysis of clinical trial data. Arch Orthop Trauma Surg. 2015;135(4):529–38. https://doi.org/10.1007/s00402-015-2175-0.
9. Coughlin RP, Crapser A, Coughlin K, Coughlin LP. Open Bankart revisited. Arthrosc Tech. 2017;6(1):e233–7. https://doi.org/10.1016/j.eats.2016.09.027.
10. Mohtadi NG, Bitar IJ, Sasyniuk TM, Hollinshead RM, Harper WP. Arthroscopic versus open repair for traumatic anterior shoulder instability: a meta-analysis. Arthroscopy. 2005;21(6):652–8. https://doi.org/10.1016/j.arthro.2005.02.021.
11. Virk MS, Manzo RL, Cote M, Ware JK, Mazzocca AD, Nissen CW, et al. Comparison of time to recurrence of instability after open and arthroscopic

Bankart repair techniques. Orthop J Sports Med. 2016;4(6):2325967116654114. https://doi.org/10.1177/2325967116654114.
12. Haskoor J, Wang KY, Best MJ, Agarwal AR, Mikula JD, Sharma S, et al. Trends in utilization and patient demographics for shoulder instability procedures from 2010 to 2019. J Shoulder Elbow Surg. 2022; https://doi.org/10.1016/j.jse.2021.12.020.
13. van der Linde JA, van Kampen DA, Terwee CB, Dijksman LM, Kleinjan G, Willems WJ. Long-term results after arthroscopic shoulder stabilization using suture anchors: an 8- to 10-year follow-up. Am J Sports Med. 2011;39(11):2396–403. https://doi.org/10.1177/0363546511415657.
14. Zhang AL, Montgomery SR, Ngo SS, Hame SL, Wang JC, Gamradt SC. Arthroscopic versus open shoulder stabilization: current practice patterns in the United States. Arthroscopy. 2014;30(4):436–43. https://doi.org/10.1016/j.arthro.2013.12.013.
15. Leroux TS, Saltzman BM, Meyer M, Frank RM, Bach BR Jr, Cole BJ, et al. The influence of evidence-based surgical indications and techniques on failure rates after arthroscopic shoulder stabilization in the contact or collision athlete with anterior shoulder instability. Am J Sports Med. 2017;45(5):1218–25. https://doi.org/10.1177/0363546516663716.
16. Boileau P, McClelland WB Jr, O'Shea K, Vargas P, Pinedo M, Old J, et al. Arthroscopic Hill-Sachs Remplissage with Bankart repair: strategy and technique. JBJS Essent Surg Tech. 2014;4(1):e4-e4. https://doi.org/10.2106/JBJS.ST.M.00033.
17. Burkhart SS, De Beer JF. Traumatic glenohumeral bone defects and their relationship to failure of arthroscopic Bankart repairs: significance of the inverted-pear glenoid and the humeral engaging Hill-Sachs lesion. Arthroscopy. 2000;16(7):677–94. https://doi.org/10.1053/jars.2000.17715.
18. Nakagawa S, Iuchi R, Hanai H, Hirose T, Mae T. The development process of bipolar bone defects from primary to recurrent instability in shoulders with traumatic anterior instability. Am J Sports Med. 2019;47(3):695–703. https://doi.org/10.1177/0363546518819471.
19. Kim SH, Ha KI, Cho YB, Ryu BD, Oh I. Arthroscopic anterior stabilization of the shoulder: two to six-year follow-up. J Bone Joint Surg Am. 2003;85(8):1511–8. Published 2003/08/20.
20. Lenters TR, Franta AK, Wolf FM, Leopold SS, Matsen FA 3rd. Arthroscopic compared with open repairs for recurrent anterior shoulder instability. A systematic review and meta-analysis of the literature. J Bone Joint Surg Am. 2007;89(2):244–54. https://doi.org/10.2106/jbjs.E.01139.
21. Rhee YG, Ha JH, Cho NS. Anterior shoulder stabilization in collision athletes: arthroscopic versus open Bankart repair. Am J Sports Med. 2006;34(6):979–85. https://doi.org/10.1177/0363546505283267.
22. Yamamoto N, Kijima H, Nagamoto H, Kurokawa D, Takahashi H, Sano H, et al. Outcome of Bankart repair in contact versus non-contact athletes. Orthop Traumatol Surg Res. 2015;101(4):415–9. https://doi.org/10.1016/j.otsr.2015.03.008.
23. Cho NS, Hwang JC, Rhee YG. Arthroscopic stabilization in anterior shoulder instability: collision athletes versus noncollision athletes. Arthroscopy. 2006;22(9):947–53. https://doi.org/10.1016/j.arthro.2006.05.015.
24. Castagna A, Delle Rose G, Borroni M, Cillis BD, Conti M, Garofalo R, et al. Arthroscopic stabilization of the shoulder in adolescent athletes participating in overhead or contact sports. Arthroscopy. 2012;28(3):309–15. https://doi.org/10.1016/j.arthro.2011.08.302.
25. Aboalata M, Plath JE, Seppel G, Juretzko J, Vogt S, Imhoff AB. Results of arthroscopic Bankart repair for anterior-inferior shoulder instability at 13-year follow-up. Am J Sports Med. 2017;45(4):782–7. https://doi.org/10.1177/0363546516675145.
26. Goodrich E, Wolf M, Vopat M, Mok A, Baker J, Bernard C, et al. Sex-specific differences in outcomes after anterior shoulder surgical stabilization: a meta-analysis and systematic review of literature. JSES Int. 2022;6(1):123–31. https://doi.org/10.1016/j.jseint.2021.10.002.
27. Shymon SJ, Roocroft J, Edmonds EW. Traumatic anterior instability of the pediatric shoulder: a comparison of arthroscopic and open bankart repairs. J Pediatr Orthop. 2015;35(1):1–6. https://doi.org/10.1097/bpo.0000000000000215.
28. Nakagawa S, Mae T, Sato S, Okimura S, Kuroda M. Risk factors for the postoperative recurrence of instability after arthroscopic Bankart repair in athletes. Orthop J Sports Med. 2017;5(9):2325967117726494. https://doi.org/10.1177/2325967117726494.
29. Balg F, Boileau P. The instability severity index score. A simple pre-operative score to select patients for arthroscopic or open shoulder stabilisation. J Bone Joint Surg. 2007;89(11):1470–7. https://doi.org/10.1302/0301-620x.89b11.18962.
30. Rosenberg SI, Padanilam SJ, Pagni BA, Tjong VK, Sheth U. A lower instability severity index score threshold may better predict recurrent anterior shoulder instability after arthroscopic Bankart repair: a systematic review. J Isakos. 2021;6(5):295–301. https://doi.org/10.1136/jisakos-2020-000584.
31. Pagnani MJ. Open capsular repair without bone block for recurrent anterior shoulder instability in patients with and without bony defects of the glenoid and/or humeral head. Am J Sports Med. 2008;36(9):1805–12. https://doi.org/10.1177/0363546508316284.
32. Hatch MD, Hennrikus WL. The open Bankart repair for traumatic anterior shoulder instability in teenage athletes. J Pediatr Orthop. 2018;38(1):27–31. https://doi.org/10.1097/bpo.0000000000000744.
33. Crua E, Gatenby GC, Walsh AJ, Monk AP, Stanley JC, Rosenfeldt MP, et al. Clinical outcomes following open anterior shoulder stabilisation for glenohumeral instability in the young collision athlete. J Shoulder Elbow Surg. 2022; https://doi.org/10.1016/j.jse.2021.12.013.

34. AlSomali K, Kholinne E, Van Nguyen T, Cho C-H, Kwak J-M, Koh K-H, et al. Outcomes and return to sport and work after open Bankart repair for recurrent shoulder instability: a systematic review. Orthop J Sports Med. 2021;9(10):23259671211026907. https://doi.org/10.1177/23259671211026907.
35. Neviaser RJ, Benke MT, Neviaser AS. Mid-term to long-term outcome of the open Bankart repair for recurrent traumatic anterior dislocation of the shoulder. J Shoulder Elbow Surg. 2017;26(11):1943–7. https://doi.org/10.1016/j.jse.2017.04.013.
36. Murphy AI, Hurley ET, Hurley DJ, Pauzenberger L, Mullett H. Long-term outcomes of the arthroscopic Bankart repair: a systematic review of studies at 10-year follow-up. J Shoulder Elbow Surg. 2019;28(11):2084–9. https://doi.org/10.1016/j.jse.2019.04.057.
37. De Giorgi S, Garofalo R, Tafuri S, Cesari E, Rose GD, Castagna A. Can arthroscopic revision surgery for shoulder instability be a fair option? Muscles Ligaments Tendons J. 2014;4(2):226–31. Published 2014/10/22.
38. Neri BR, Tuckman DV, Bravman JT, Yim D, Sahajpal DT, Rokito AS. Arthroscopic revision of Bankart repair. J Shoulder Elbow Surg. 2007;16(4):419–24. https://doi.org/10.1016/j.jse.2006.05.016.
39. Zabinski SJ, Callaway GH, Cohen S, Warren RF. Revision shoulder stabilization: 2- to 10-year results. J Shoulder Elbow Surg. 1999;8(1):58–65. https://doi.org/10.1016/s1058-2746(99)90057-5.
40. Creighton RA, Romeo AA, Brown FM Jr, Hayden JK, Verma NN. Revision arthroscopic shoulder instability repair. Arthroscopy. 2007;23(7):703–9. https://doi.org/10.1016/j.arthro.2007.01.021.
41. Bartl C, Schumann K, Paul J, Vogt S, Imhoff AB. Arthroscopic capsulolabral revision repair for recurrent anterior shoulder instability. Am J Sports Med. 2011;39(3):511–8. https://doi.org/10.1177/0363546510388909.
42. Frank RM, Mellano C, Shin JJ, Feldheim TF, Mascarenhas R, Yanke AB, et al. Clinical outcomes following revision anterior shoulder stabilization: arthroscopic revision stabilization versus Latarjet. Orthop J Sports Med. 2015;3(7 suppl2):2325967115S2325900048. https://doi.org/10.1177/2325967115S00048.
43. Stein T, Buckup J, Mehling AP, Hoffmann R, Efe T, von Eisenhart-Rothe R, et al. Restoration of joint congruency and the glenoidal labrum after arthroscopic revision Bankart repair: a MRI match-paired analysis comparing primary Bankart repair and the uninjured labrum. Arch Orthop Trauma Surg. 2014;134(8):1121–34. https://doi.org/10.1007/s00402-014-1990-z.
44. Imhoff AB, Ansah P, Tischer T, Reiter C, Bartl C, Hench M, et al. Arthroscopic repair of anterior-inferior glenohumeral instability using a portal at the 5:30-o'clock position: analysis of the effects of age, fixation method, and concomitant shoulder injury on surgical outcomes. Am J Sports Med. 2010;38(9):1795–803. https://doi.org/10.1177/0363546510370199.
45. Elamo S, Selänne L, Lehtimäki K, Kukkonen J, Hurme S, Kauko T, et al. Bankart versus Latarjet operation as a revision procedure after a failed arthroscopic Bankart repair. JSES Int. 2020;4(2):292–6. https://doi.org/10.1016/j.jseint.2020.01.004.
46. Slaven SE, Tardif R, Foley K, Cameron KL, Posner MA, Dickens JF. Revision arthroscopic Bankart repair in the military. Orthop J Sports Med. 2020;8(3_suppl2):2325967120S2325900119. https://doi.org/10.1177/2325967120S00119.
47. Cho NS, Yi JW, Lee BG, Rhee YG. Revision open Bankart surgery after arthroscopic repair for traumatic anterior shoulder instability. Am J Sports Med. 2009;37(11):2158–64. https://doi.org/10.1177/0363546509339015.
48. Rowe CR, Patel D, Southmayd WW. The Bankart procedure: a long-term end-result study. J Bone Joint Surg Am. 1978;60(1):1–16. Published 1978/01/01.
49. Fabre T, Abi-Chahla ML, Billaud A, Geneste M, Durandeau A. Long-term results with Bankart procedure: a 26-year follow-up study of 50 cases. J Shoulder Elbow Surg. 2010;19(2):318–23. https://doi.org/10.1016/j.jse.2009.06.010.
50. Berendes TD, Wolterbeek R, Pilot P, Verburg H, te Slaa RL. The open modified Bankart procedure: outcome at follow-up of 10 to 15 years. J Bone Joint Surg. 2007;89(8):1064–8. https://doi.org/10.1302/0301-620x.89b8.19280.
51. Pelet S, Jolles BM, Farron A. Bankart repair for recurrent anterior glenohumeral instability: results at twenty-nine years' follow-up. J Shoulder Elbow Surg. 2006;15(2):203–7. https://doi.org/10.1016/j.jse.2005.06.011.
52. Moroder P, Odorizzi M, Pizzinini S, Demetz E, Resch H, Moroder P. Open Bankart repair for the treatment of anterior shoulder instability without substantial osseous glenoid defects: results after a minimum follow-up of twenty years. J Bone Joint Surg Am. 2015;97(17):1398–405. https://doi.org/10.2106/jbjs.N.01214.
53. Memon M, Kay J, Cadet ER, Shahsavar S, Simunovic N, Ayeni OR. Return to sport following arthroscopic Bankart repair: a systematic review. J Shoulder Elbow Surg. 2018;27(7):1342–7. https://doi.org/10.1016/j.jse.2018.02.044.
54. Kasik CS, Rosen MR, Saper MG, Zondervan RL. High rate of return to sport in adolescent athletes following anterior shoulder stabilisation: a systematic review. J Isakos. 2019;4(1):33–40. https://doi.org/10.1136/jisakos-2018-000224.
55. Abdul-Rassoul H, Galvin JW, Curry EJ, Simon J, Li X. Return to sport after surgical treatment for anterior shoulder instability: a systematic review. Am J Sports Med. 2019;47(6):1507–15. https://doi.org/10.1177/0363546518780934.

56. Rossi LA, Pasqualini I, Tanoira I, Ranalletta M. Factors that influence the return to sport after arthroscopic Bankart repair for glenohumeral instability. Open Access J Sports Med. 2022;13:35–40. https://doi.org/10.2147/oajsm.S340699.
57. Sperber A, Hamberg P, Karlsson J, Swärd L, Wredmark T. Comparison of an arthroscopic and an open procedure for posttraumatic instability of the shoulder: a prospective, randomized multicenter study. J Shoulder Elbow Surg. 2001;10(2):105–8. https://doi.org/10.1067/mse.2001.112019.
58. Bottoni CR, Smith EL, Berkowitz MJ, Towle RB, Moore JH. Arthroscopic versus open shoulder stabilization for recurrent anterior instability: a prospective randomized clinical trial. Am J Sports Med. 2006;34(11):1730–7. https://doi.org/10.1177/0363546506288239.
59. Fabbriciani C, Milano G, Demontis A, Fadda S, Ziranu F, Mulas PD. Arthroscopic versus open treatment of Bankart lesion of the shoulder: a prospective randomized study. Arthroscopy. 2004;20(5):456–62. https://doi.org/10.1016/j.arthro.2004.03.001.
60. Mohtadi NGH, Chan DS, Hollinshead RM, Boorman RS, Hiemstra LA, Lo IKY, et al. A randomized clinical trial comparing open and arthroscopic stabilization for recurrent traumatic anterior shoulder instability: two-year follow-up with disease-specific quality-of-life outcomes. JBJS. 2014;96(5):353–60. https://doi.org/10.2106/jbjs.L.01656.
61. Guanche CA, Quick DC, Sodergren KM, Buss DD. Arthroscopic versus open reconstruction of the shoulder in patients with isolated Bankart lesions. Am J Sports Med. 1996;24(2):144–8. https://doi.org/10.1177/036354659602400204.
62. Freedman KB, Smith AP, Romeo AA, Cole BJ, Bach BR Jr. Open Bankart repair versus arthroscopic repair with transglenoid sutures or bioabsorbable tacks for recurrent anterior instability of the shoulder: a meta-analysis. Am J Sports Med. 2004;32(6):1520–7. https://doi.org/10.1177/0363546504265188.
63. Uchiyama Y, Handa A, Shimpuku E, Omi H, Hashimoto H, Imai T, et al. Open Bankart repair plus inferior capsular shift versus arthroscopic Bankart repair without augmentations for traumatic anterior shoulder instability: a prospective study. J Orthop Surg. 2017;25(3):2309499017727947. https://doi.org/10.1177/2309499017727947.
64. Amroodi MN, Jafari D, Kousari AA. Results of open Bankart surgery for recurrent anterior shoulder dislocation with glenoid bone defect and Concomitant Hill-Sachs lesion. Arch Bone Jt Surg. 2018;6(3):212–8. https://pubmed.ncbi.nlm.nih.gov/29911138; https://www.ncbi.nlm.nih.gov/pmc/articles/PMC5990709/.
65. Ng C, Bialocerkowski A, Hinman R. Effectiveness of arthroscopic versus open surgical stabilisation for the management of traumatic anterior glenohumeral instability. Int J Evid Based Healthc. 2007;5(2):182–207. https://doi.org/10.1111/j.1479-6988.2007.00064.x.
66. Archetti Netto N, Tamaoki MJ, Lenza M, dos Santos JB, Matsumoto MH, Faloppa F, et al. Treatment of Bankart lesions in traumatic anterior instability of the shoulder: a randomized controlled trial comparing arthroscopy and open techniques. Arthroscopy. 2012;28(7):900–8. https://doi.org/10.1016/j.arthro.2011.11.032.
67. Gao B, DeFroda S, Bokshan S, Ready LV, Sullivan K, Etzel C, et al. Arthroscopic versus open Bankart repairs in recurrent anterior shoulder instability: a systematic review of the association between publication date and postoperative recurrent instability in systematic reviews. Arthroscopy. 2020;36(3):862–71. https://doi.org/10.1016/j.arthro.2019.10.022.

16 The Open Bankart Repair with a Medial Capsular Shift: Indications and Technical Tips

Matthew S. Fury and David W. Altchek

History

In 1923, Arthur Sidney Blundell Bankart described the anatomic lesion responsible for recurrent anterior instability of the shoulder—the detachment of the fibrous capsule and the fibrocartilaginous glenoid ligament (labrum) from the anterior glenoid rim. Unlike the purely capsular injury, which Bankart felt tended to heal spontaneously, he proposed that the capsulolabral injury adjacent to the glenoid rim demonstrated no tendency to heal. This defect allowed the humeral head to freely translate anteriorly over the glenoid rim with "the slightest provocation." In fact, in his original description, Bankart demonstrated great nuance regarding the role of the capsule as well as the trade-off between stability and motion. He noted that the shoulder capsule is normally a lax structure, and he felt that an attempt at capsular imbrication without addressing the critical lesion would simply draw the capsulolabral junction away from the glenoid rim and fail to restore stability unless a significant reduction in capsular volume was obtained. However, this stability would not be obtained by restoration of anatomy but by the compromise of free joint motion [1].

Despite the technological advancements and the proliferation of data surrounding shoulder instability since 1923, the initial open Bankart description contains fundamental steps that are largely preserved in the modern techniques of labral repair. Bankart's procedure was performed in the supine position through a deltopectoral approach. The coracoid was osteotomized to reflect the conjoint tendon inferiorly, and a subscapularis tenotomy was performed to expose the anterior glenoid and scapular neck. The labral injury was identified, and the glenoid rim was prepared with an osteotome in order to encourage a healing response. Sutures were passed around the labrum through glenoid bone tunnels in a horizontal mattress fashion, and the sutures were tied inferiorly to superiorly. The subscapularis tenotomy and coracoid osteotomy were repaired with suture, and the patient was immobilized in neutral for 4 weeks before beginning shoulder motion with a goal of full motion restoration [1]. Although his initial description reported the outcomes of only 4 patients, Bankart's colleagues later published a series of 50 patients in 1957. Two patients (4%) demonstrated recurrence, and the average loss of external rotation was 20° compared to the contralateral side. In fact, 50% of patients had less than a 10° motion deficit [2].

Although Bankart emphasized the importance of recognizing and addressing the capsulolabral injury in preventing recurrence, the concept of capsular insufficiency as a risk factor for recurrent instability has also been long-standing. Sir Harry Platt and Vittorio Putti independently

M. S. Fury · D. W. Altchek (✉)
Sports Medicine and Shoulder Service, Hospital for Special Surgery, New York, NY, USA
e-mail: altchekd@hss.edu

© The Author(s), under exclusive license to Springer Nature Switzerland AG 2026
R. M. Frank, J. M. Tokish (eds.), *Management of Shoulder Instability*,
https://doi.org/10.1007/978-3-032-18089-6_16

described the Putti-Platt procedure, a stabilizing procedure that involved shortening the subscapularis tendon and anterior capsule by double breasting them over one another. By Sir Harry Platt's account, this procedure was developed after noting that some cases of recurrent shoulder instability had no identifiable Bankart lesion [3, 4]. In 1980, Dr. Charles Neer published his results of the inferior capsular shift as a treatment for involuntary inferior and multidirectional instability (MDI), and this article was practice-changing within the orthopedic community for its evaluation of capsular laxity and its role in glenohumeral instability as well as its description of an effective treatment option for a challenging patient presentation [5]. Dr. Neer's technique involved a deltopectoral approach and a subscapularis tenotomy. A T-shaped opening was made in the anterior capsule, comprising of a transverse cut between the middle and inferior glenohumeral ligaments and a vertical incision at the humeral attachment of the capsule. The inferior flap was mobilized superiorly to eliminate the inferior capsular pouch, and the superior flap was sutured over the top in order to act as a reinforcement of the anterior capsule [5].

Dr. David Altchek and Dr. Russell Warren described a modification of the inferior capsular shift in 1991. In their description, a transverse incision was made in the mid-capsule anteriorly, but the vertical incision was made just medial to the glenoid margin. This medially-based capsular shift allowed for easier evaluation and repair of the glenoid labrum as failure to repair a Bankart lesion was considered a risk factor for failed stabilization [6].

Key Principles

Indications

Despite the proliferation of arthroscopic procedures as well as the increasing incidence of bone-block reconstructions performed for recurrent shoulder instability, the open Bankart repair with medial capsular shift still serves a vital role in the treatment algorithm for shoulder instability. The modern indications for this procedure are:

- Recurrent anterior shoulder instability with capsular insufficiency but minimal bone loss
- Multidirectional instability with a primary anterior component
- Collision-athlete with recurrent anterior instability but without glenoid bone loss or a Hill-Sachs lesion to the humerus

Case Presentation

An 18-year-old female dancer presented to clinic with the insidious onset of left shoulder instability. She denied a history of shoulder trauma, and she had never experienced a dislocation event. She had completed a course of physical therapy with an emphasis on scapular rhythm as well as periscapular and rotator cuff strengthening, but she remained symptomatic.

On physical examination, she had 170° of forward flexion and 80° of external rotation bilaterally. She had marked apprehension of the left shoulder while in abduction and internal rotation, and her symptoms improved with a relocation force. She had a 2+ anterior load and shift and a 2+ posterior load and shift, but she had no pain with a posterior jerk test. She demonstrated a 3+ sulcus that mildly improved with external rotation. Of note, her asymptomatic shoulder demonstrated mild laxity both anteriorly and posteriorly without pain. She had a Beighton score of 7 out of 9, indicating a generalized hyperlaxity.

Her MRI evaluation demonstrated a dysplastic anterior labrum with a tear in the anterior-inferior quadrant (Figs. 16.1 and 16.2). No bone loss was appreciated on the sagittal series (Fig. 16.3). There was no evidence of superior or posterior labral tear, rotator cuff pathology, or loose body.

The history, physical exam, and radiographic images were consistent with anterior-predominant multidirectional instability with a torn, dysplastic glenoid labrum in the setting of generalized liga-

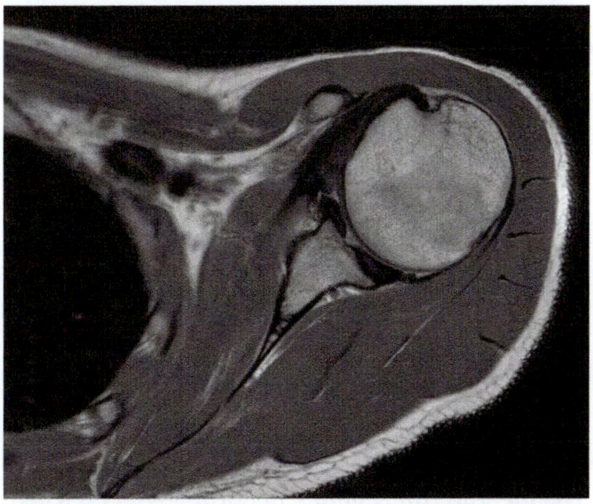

Fig. 16.1 Axial proton-density MRI demonstrating dysplasia of the anterior glenoid labrum

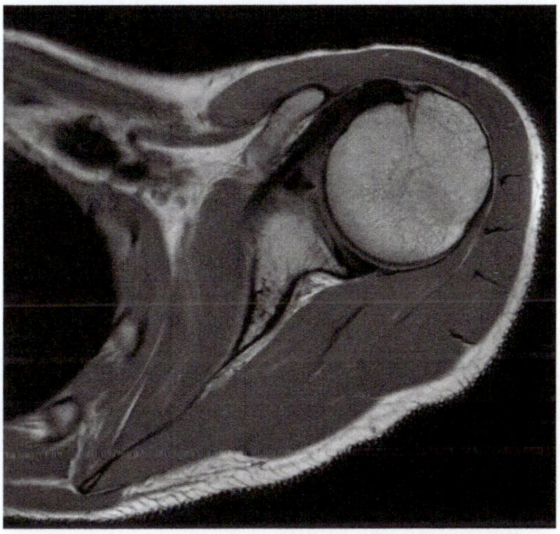

Fig. 16.2 Axial proton-density MRI demonstrating a tear in the anterior-inferior labrum with displacement off the medial aspect of the glenoid rim

mentous laxity. Therefore, she was indicated for left shoulder arthroscopy, open Bankart repair with a glenoid-based inferior capsular shift.

On the day of surgery, an examination under anesthesia was consistent with the findings from the office visit. Left shoulder arthroscopy was

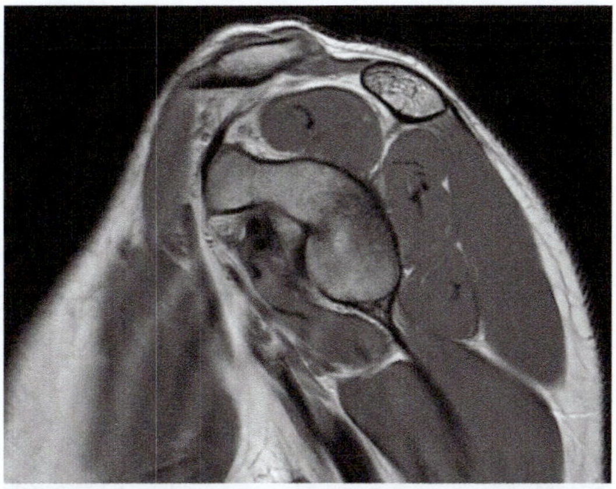

Fig. 16.3 Sagittal proton-density MRI demonstrating no anterior glenoid bone loss

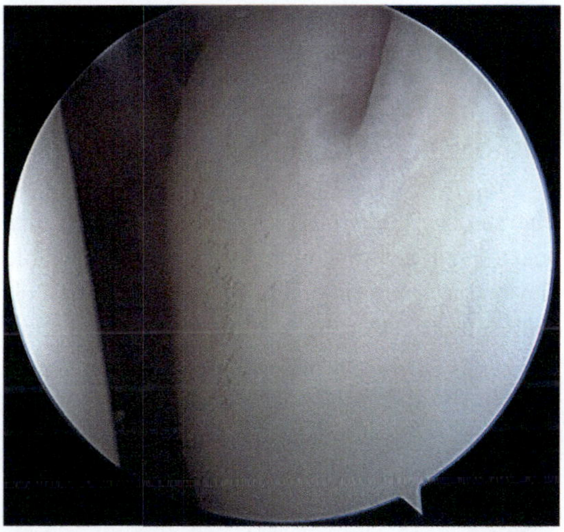

Fig. 16.4 Arthroscopic image of the anterior glenoid from the posterior viewing portal demonstrating dysplasia of the chondrolabral junction

performed demonstrating a dysplastic glenoid labrum that was torn and recessed off of the glenoid margin (Fig. 16.4), and the inferior axillary pouch was patulous with thin-appearing capsular tissue but no discrete tear (Fig. 16.5). Given these findings, an open Bankart repair with glenoid-based inferior capsular shift was performed.

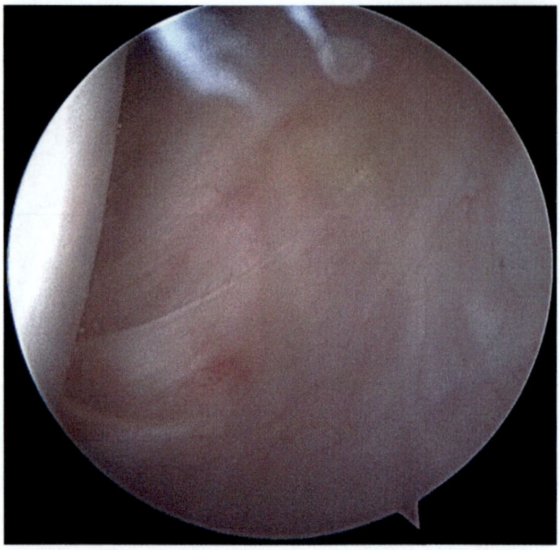

Fig. 16.5 Arthroscopic image of the axillary pouch from the posterior viewing portal demonstrating inferior capsular laxity without a discrete capsule or ligamentous tear

Authors' Preferred Technique

The senior author performs the procedure in a beach-chair position with the back of the table elevated to approximately 45°. An inflatable bolster is placed under the medial border of the scapula in order to allow for the scapula to fall posteriorly and present the glenoid rim in line with the surgical field. The authors frequently perform an expeditious diagnostic shoulder arthroscopy to ensure there is no concomitant pathology that may require intervention, but operative time and additional portals are minimized in order to prevent unnecessary fluid extravasation into the surrounding tissues.

An 8 cm incision is made over the deltopectoral interval, and the cephalic vein is identified and retracted laterally. The clavipectoral fascia is incised just lateral to the conjoint tendon, and this tendon is retracted medially. The coracoacromial ligament is identified and partially released from the acromion as it is the senior author's experience that this release may prevent impingement during the early phases of rehabilitation when the rotator cuff is weak. The subscapularis is identified, and an oblique tenotomy is performed while taking care to avoid entering the joint capsule. The subscapularis is then meticulously dissected medially off of the anterior capsule to the glenoid margin and inferiorly until the 6 o'clock position of the capsule is reached.

Two capsulotomy incisions are made. The first incision is made vertically, just medial to the glenoid margin. A transverse capsular incision is then made at the midportion of the anterior capsule with care not to injure the labrum lying deep to the capsule. The anterior aspect of the glenoid margin should now be visualized. The labrum is mobilized from the glenoid neck until it can be reduced back to the glenoid rim without tension. The glenoid rim is gently decorticated with a rasp or a curette, but care is taken to not unnecessarily remove glenoid bone stock. A labral scorpion suture passer is used to pass suture tape around the glenoid labrum in a simple suture configuration, and this tape is loaded into a knotless 2.9 mm PEEK suture anchor. A pilot hole is drilled on the glenoid face adjacent to the rim, and the anchor is inserted with appropriate tension on the suture tapes. The arm is placed in 45° of abduction and 40° of external rotation. The inferior capsular leaflet is advanced superiorly in order to eliminate the laxity and redundancy of the inferior capsule, and it is advanced medially to restore appropriate tension while still allowing the desired amount of external rotation. The scorpion suture passer is used to pass sutures through the inferior leaflet in a horizontal mattress fashion while working inferiorly to superiorly. The suture limbs are loaded into knotless 2.9 mm PEEK suture anchors, and the anchors are placed into the glenoid neck to reduce the capsule to the bone. The superior capsular flap is advanced inferiorly and sutured to the inferior flap at the glenoid margin. Additional sutures are placed laterally along the transverse capsulotomy incision. This effectively reinforces the anterior capsule. Finally, the medial margin of the inferior flap is then folded back laterally and sutured to the medial margin of the superior flap to further reinforce the glenoid margin. The repair is evaluated, and anterior-inferior instability should be eliminated. External rotation should be preserved without excess tension on the repair.

After irrigation, the subscapularis tenotomy is closed with #2 Ethibond figure-of-8 stitches, and the deltopectoral interval is also closed with #2 Ethibond sutures. The skin is closed in a layered fashion with absorbable sutures, and a sterile dressing is applied.

Postoperatively, the patient is placed into a shoulder abduction immobilizer. The patient is encouraged to perform distal range of motion, scapular retraction exercises, and active-assisted forward elevation in the plane of the scapula up to 90° until formal physical therapy is begun at 3 weeks. External rotation is limited to 30° during the first 3 weeks. By 6 weeks, patients should have minimal pain and 60° of external rotation with 145° of forward flexion, and they should demonstrate good cuff activation. Weeks 6–12 are devoted to restoration of full shoulder motion, normal scapulothoracic mechanics, and near-normal rotator cuff strength. At week 14, plyometric exercises are initiated before transitioning to a return-to-sport progression as long as isokinetic internal and external rotation strength is symmetric to the contralateral side.

Technical Tips, Modifications, and Other Considerations

History taking remains the foundation of shoulder instability care. One should obtain an understanding of the patient's number of instability events as well as the recent injury mechanism as repeated events or decreasing energy requirement for dislocation may indicate progressive bone loss that should be addressed with a bony reconstruction procedure. A personal or family history of other joint instability may indicate a hereditary collagen disorder like Ehlers-Danlos syndrome, and this may raise suspicions for multidirectional instability or capsular insufficiency.

The physical exam provides critical information that can influence treatment decisions and postoperative outcomes. Scapular dyskinesis is common in patients with shoulder instability. Especially in the setting of MDI, one must ensure that a course of nonoperative management emphasizing scapular mechanics was diligently performed. Previous studies have demonstrated that rehabilitating scapular positioning can provide a meaningful benefit to patients with multidirectional instability [7, 8]. In conjunction with the patient's history, the load and shift examination can be used to determine if there is a predominant instability direction in patients with MDI. Although the inferior capsular shift decreases the global volume of the capsule, surgeons may opt for a posterior shift in patients with primarily posterior instability. It is also important to note the native motion of the contralateral shoulder, if asymptomatic, and compare this to the position of apprehension on the affected side. If a patient has hyperlaxity and externally rotates to 80° but they become apprehensive at 30° on the injured shoulder, one would consider tensioning the operative shoulder closer to 30°. Although some motion may be regained in the rehabilitation period, it may be prudent to counsel this patient on potential stiffness when compared to the contralateral shoulder.

Radiographic assessment of the patient with recurrent instability should include x-rays. In addition to evaluating the rotator cuff integrity, MRI is critical for assessing the integrity of the labrum as well as the presence of capsular injury or chondral defect that may further predispose to instability. Attritional bone loss can also be appreciated on MRI, but a CT scan with 3-dimensional reconstructions may improve bony assessment in equivocal cases. A Hill-Sachs lesion, or humeral-sided bone loss, may contribute to instability depending on its relationship to the glenoid track. The presence of an offtrack Hill-Sachs lesion may introduce the remplissage procedure into consideration as a treatment option.

Some surgeons may prefer to perform the Bankart repair arthroscopically before proceeding with the open capsular shift. Although possible, there are multiple pitfalls that require attention to avoid. First, arthroscopy time should be limited in order to prevent fluid extravasation into the soft tissues. The dissection between the subscapularis and anterior capsule can be challenging, and this may be further compromised by a distortion of normal tissue planes. Anterior portals should be minimized, and they should be repaired upon transitioning to the open procedure since they may impair appropriate tensioning of the capsule. When passing sutures around the labrum, care must be taken to ensure that capsule is not inadvertently captured as this will compromise the ability to perform an effective shift later in the case. When performing the open procedure, a free needle can be used to shuttle suture, but arthroscopic instruments may also prove helpful.

After the capsular shift is completed, glenohumeral stability should be reassessed. If anterior instability remains, the surgeon must determine if either an insufficient shift was performed or if limitations from capsular tissue quality exist. If an insufficient shift is responsible, the sutures can be removed and the inferior leaflet can be further advanced. In cases of compromised tissues, an Achilles allograft, hamstring allograft, or human acellular dermal allograft may be used to reconstruct the anterior capsule. However, in the senior author's experience, this is rarely required.

Outcomes

In the initial description of the open Bankart with glenoid-based inferior capsular shift, Altchek and Dines reported the outcomes of 42 shoulders in 40 patients. Twenty shoulders had preserved external rotation with the humeral adducted to the side while 22 shoulders had 5 to 25° of rotation deficit (mean 10°). Twenty-five shoulders had preserved external rotation with 90° of humeral abduction while 17 had a loss of 5 to 20° (mean 10°). All patients endorsed a reduction in preoperative shoulder pain, and all patients returned to sport at 6.5 months. However, all three throwing athletes demonstrated a loss in ball velocity. Four patients experienced recurrent instability postoperatively, and 95% of patients endorsed excellent satisfaction with the procedure. There were two cases of transient neuropraxia that spontaneously resolved and one case of a hematoma requiring drainage [6].

Rubenstein et al. presented their outcomes of 75 patients at an average of 39 months postoperatively. Seventy-two (96%) of patients were satisfied with the procedure, and 93% returned to the same preinjury level of competition. Interestingly, their cohort included 29 professional athletes of which 62% reported excellent results on the modified Rowe grading scale. Ten of 13 professional baseball pitchers (77%) returned to their previous competitive level. In the overall cohort, the average loss of external rotation in 90° of abduction was 2° (range 0–15) [9]. Since the publication of these initial results, recent reviews have synthesized the literature and reaffirmed the role of the open Bankart procedure with inferior capsular shift [10].

Conclusion

The open Bankart with medial capsular shift remains an effective intervention for patients with recurrent instability. The procedure is associated with high likelihood of return to sport with low rates of recurrent instability or complication.

References

1. Blundell Bankart AS. Recurrent or habitual dislocation of the shoulder-joint. Br Med J [Internet]. 1923 [cited 2023 Jan 17];2:1132–3. Available from: https://pubmed.ncbi.nlm.nih.gov/20771383/
2. Dickson JW, Devas MB. Bankart's operation for recurrent dislocation of the shoulder. J Bone Joint Surg Br [Internet]. 1957 [cited 2023 Jan 17];39-B:114–9. Available from: https://pubmed.ncbi.nlm.nih.gov/13405954/
3. Rashid MS, Arner JW, Millett PJ, Sugaya H, Emery R. The Bankart repair: past, present, and future. J Shoulder Elbow Surg [Internet]. 2020 [cited 2023 Jan 17];29:e491–8. Available from: https://pubmed.ncbi.nlm.nih.gov/32621981/
4. Osmond-Clarke H. Habitual dislocation of the shoulder; the Putti-Platt operation. J Bone Joint Surg Br. 1948;30B:19–25.
5. Neer CS, Foster CR. Inferior capsular shift for involuntary inferior and multidirectional instability of the shoulder. A preliminary report. J Bone Joint Surg Am. 1980;62:897–908.
6. Altchek DW, Warren RF, Skyhar MJ, Ortiz G. T-plasty modification of the Bankart procedure for multidirectional instability of the anterior and inferior types. J Bone Joint Surg Am. 1991;73:105–12.

7. Watson L, Balster S, Lenssen R, Hoy G, Pizzari T. The effects of a conservative rehabilitation program for multidirectional instability of the shoulder. J Shoulder Elbow Surg [Internet]. 2018 [cited 2023 Jan 17];27:104–11. Available from: https://pubmed.ncbi.nlm.nih.gov/28947382/
8. Warby SA, Ford JJ, Hahne AJ, Watson L, Balster S, Lenssen R, et al. Comparison of 2 exercise rehabilitation programs for multidirectional instability of the glenohumeral joint: a randomized controlled trial. Am J Sports Med [Internet]. 2018 [cited 2023 Jan 17];46:87–97. Available from: https://pubmed.ncbi.nlm.nih.gov/29048942/
9. Rubenstein DL, Jobe FW, Glousman RE, Kvitne RS, Pink M, Giangarra CE. Anterior capsulolabral reconstruction of the shoulder in athletes. J Shoulder Elbow Surg [Internet]. 1992 [cited 2023 Jan 17];1:229–37. Available from: https://pubmed.ncbi.nlm.nih.gov/22959195/
10. Haratian A, Yensen K, Bell JA, Hasan LK, Shelby T, Yoshida B, et al. Open stabilization procedures of the shoulder in the athlete: indications, techniques, and outcomes. Open Access J Sports Med [Internet]. 2021 [cited 2023 Jan 17];12:159–69. Available from: https://pubmed.ncbi.nlm.nih.gov/34754248/

The Open Bankart: Through a Subscapular Split

17

Bonnie P. Gregory and John E. Conway

Introduction

Traumatic shoulder dislocations are a common occurrence, with a rate of 23.9 per 100,000 persons per year in the United States, 90% of which are anteroinferior [1]. However, the true incidence may be higher as many anterior instability events self-reduce and therefore never present to the emergency department. One study of a military population found that 85% of anterior shoulder instability events in the course of a year were subluxations with self-reduction, and only 15% were frank dislocations [2].

The nonoperative management of these injuries in young, active patients leads to high recurrent instability rates; as such, operative management is common [3–5]. The optimal surgical management of patients who experience anterior shoulder instability remains controversial. Age, timing of the injury, the presence of a bony lesion, and patient involvement in contact sports all influence treatment decision-making. The open approach to anterior stabilization was long considered the gold standard [6]. However, advances in arthroscopic technology in the past three decades coupled with concerns about weakness, development of secondary osteoarthritis, and loss of glenohumeral motion, particularly external rotation, have led to an increasing number of arthroscopic stabilizations performed [7–9]. Recently, reports have shown that 87 to 89% of shoulder stabilizations are arthroscopic, indicating a transition away from open repair [10–12]. This increase is likely fueled not only by improved arthroscopic techniques and implants in the past several decades but also an emphasis in arthroscopic versus open techniques in the training of younger surgeons.

Many techniques for open stabilization have been described including largely historical procedures (Putti-Platt, Magnuson-Stack), anterior bone grafting procedures (iliac crest allograft or autograft, Latarjet, Bristow, distal tibial allograft), anatomic reconstruction (open Bankart repair, capsular shift), and those that address humeral-sided lesions (humeral head bone grafting, remplissage) [13]. In its modern iteration, open anterior labral repair/capsulorrhaphy has shown consistently favorable outcomes in terms of recurrent dislocation rates and patient outcomes [14]. Additionally, several studies have shown relatively high redislocation and reoperation rates with arthroscopic repairs, especially in young, athletic populations [15–17]. In addition to younger age, several other risk factors for recurrence have been identified and include the instability severity score (ISIS), which provides indications for open stabilization over

B. P. Gregory · J. E. Conway (✉)
Department of Orthopaedic Surgery, University of Texas Health Science Center at Houston/ McGovern Medical School, Houston, TX, USA
e-mail: bonnie.p.gregory@uth.tmc.edu; john.e.conway@uth.tmc.edu

© The Author(s), under exclusive license to Springer Nature Switzerland AG 2026

R. M. Frank, J. M. Tokish (eds.), *Management of Shoulder Instability*,
https://doi.org/10.1007/978-3-032-18089-6_17

arthroscopic [18]. Additionally, open Bankart can avoid potential morbidity and complication of bone-block procedures. Finally, open Bankart has shown reliable results for the management of failed prior stabilization procedures [19]. In this chapter, we will delve into the open Bankart repair, discussing diagnosis, indications, surgical technique, rehabilitation, return to sport, and complications as every shoulder surgeon should have this procedure in their armamentarium.

Clinical Case Presentation

The case presented is that of a 20-year-old, right-hand dominant, male, multisport athlete who presented 2 years after an initial shoulder dislocation event while playing soccer, with one subsequent anterior dislocation and multiple subluxation events. At presentation, he complained of persistent pain and apprehension despite completing physical therapy after both instability events. He denied any neurologic symptoms currently or following any instability event.

Clinical examination demonstrated no tenderness to palpation about the shoulder girdle and near full, symmetric range of motion but with a lack of 15 degrees of external rotation secondary to apprehension and pain compared to uninjured shoulder. Strength was full and symmetric throughout rotator cuff testing. Provocative maneuvers were positive for pain with Whipple, circumduction, dynamic labral shear, and passive ABER. Speeds, O'Brien's, Jobe's/empty can, and biceps load were not painful. Instability testing revealed moderate apprehension, 1+ anterior load and shift, and 1 to 2+ posterior load and shift. Neurovascular examination was normal.

Radiographic examination including plain radiographs, MRI without contrast, and CT with 3D reconstructions was remarkable for approximately 14% glenoid bone loss with associated soft tissue and bony Bankart lesion (14 by 3 mm), an 18 by 20 mm posterior humeral head Hill-Sachs lesion which was noted to be on-track, several chondral loose bodies in the inferior recess, and an intact rotator cuff (Figs. 17.1a, b). Surgical options were discussed at length with the patient, and he was indicated for a shoulder arthroscopy with glenohumeral debridement, removal of loose fragments, capsular mobilization, posterior augmentation with either a remplissage capsular tenodesis or posterior humeral head allograft reconstruction, and an open capsulorrhaphy with Bankart repair.

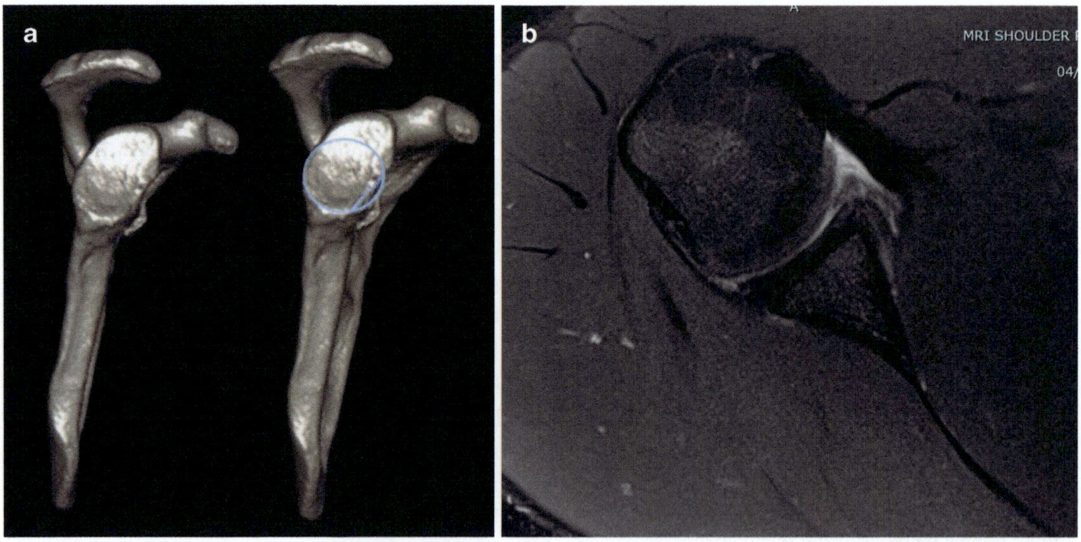

Fig. 17.1 (**a**) Preoperative 3D CT scan demonstrating anteroinferior glenoid rim fracture (bony Bankart lesion) representing 10% glenoid bone loss. (**b**) Representative axial MRI scan demonstrating anteroinferior labral tear (Bankart lesion)

The Open Bankart

The "essential lesion" of recurrent glenohumeral instability was first described by Bankart in 1923. Before this, recurrent anterior instability was thought to be a function of capsular laxity and muscular weakness. Now known as a "Bankart lesion," this tearing of the capsulolabral attachment is present in 85 to 90% of traumatic anterior shoulder dislocations [2, 20, 21]. After Bankart's initial description, which indicated a split of the subscapularis in line with its fibers, anatomic repair of the anterior labrum and inferior glenohumeral ligament (IGHL) remained the central goal of stabilization surgery for decades. Over the twentieth century, the surgical exposure evolved from one of subscapularis splitting to a tenotomy and peel-back method for improved visualization [6].

In the classic description of the open Bankart procedure by Rowe et al., a redislocation rate of 3.9% was reported in 142 of 164 patients with a mean follow-up of 6 years [6]. Rowe et al. used a subscapularis splitting approach to drill holes through the anterior glenoid and tie down the avulsed labrum. In a later report, however, Rowe et al. found residual Bankart lesions in 84% of instability repairs that required revision [22]. At the time, appropriate anatomic landmarks and fixation methods were not yet fully understood, and as such, these repairs failed to restore appropriate IGHL tension. Surgeons began to explore nonanatomic solutions, only to return to arthroscopic and open anterior Bankart repair and stabilization procedures due to the continued risk of recurrence with many other nonanatomic techniques. In its modern iteration, which focuses on anatomic repair, the open Bankart reconstruction affords the surgeon the ability to perform a labral and/or glenoid fracture (or "bony Bankart") repair in addition to an open capsular shift. As such, the open Bankart is the standard against which all arthroscopic techniques are compared.

Multiple meta-analyses and systematic reviews have attempted to address the controversy of arthroscopic versus open Bankart repair [9, 23–29]. All of these studies demonstrated at least equivalent postoperative stability between arthroscopic and open repair. The majority of these studies found lower rates of recurrent instability and overall improved outcomes with open repair [9, 23–25].

In another recent systematic review, authors compared open and arthroscopic Bankart repair with the Latarjet procedure in a total of 705 patients. In similar cohorts with no significant heterogeneity noted, they found significantly lower rates of recurrent instability in the Latarjet group (11.6%) compared to the Bankart group (21.1%; $p = 0.0009$), as well as to open and arthroscopic Bankart repairs individually ($p = 0.01$ and $p = 0.03$, respectively). Further, the Rowe score was significantly higher in the Latarjet group (85.4 vs 79.0; $p < 0.001$), and mean loss in external rotation was also significantly reduced. There was no significant difference in complications, revision surgeries, or return to function [30]. Another recent study showed no significant differences in complication rates between arthroscopic and open Bankart, with both having less complications than open Latarjet procedures [31].

Further, in another recent systematic review, authors found studies published from 1995 through 2004 demonstrated significant differences ($P = 0.015$) in recurrence rates favoring open surgery. In contrast, no significant differences ($P = 0.09$) in recurrence rates were observed for studies published from 2005 through 2015. The pooled estimate for all studies in both groups demonstrated significant differences ($P = 0.001$) in external rotation deficits between open and arthroscopic shoulder stabilization favoring arthroscopic surgery [28]. Additionally, in a 2015 systematic review, authors reported no significant difference in failure rates between open and arthroscopic stabilization for anterior instability [32]. However, another meta-analysis looked at results based on publication date and showed newer studies reported more favorable outcomes with arthroscopic stabilization [33].

One meta-analysis looked at sex-specific differences in anterior stabilization surgeries in published studies from 1960 to 2022 and found a significantly higher rate of recurrent instability in males than in females who underwent arthroscopic Bankart repair (risk ratio [RR] = 0.25; 95% confidence interval [CI] = (1.03, 1.52); $P = 0.0239$) [34].

Another study reported outcomes at 20-year follow-up on 47 patients who underwent primary open Bankart repair for recurrent instability without associated significant glenoid defects. Authors described significant decreases in abduction (4°; $p = 0.009$), internal rotation (two vertebral levels; p = 0.003), and external rotation in neutral (7°; $p < 0.001$) and 90° of abduction (7°; $p = 0.04$). They described good postoperative subjective outcomes scores but reported a 17.5% rate of recurrent instability [35].

There are some criticisms of the open technique regarding increased operative time, concern for subscapularis failure or insufficiency, and loss of external rotation when compared to arthroscopic stabilization [6, 36–39]. However, long-term clinical outcomes between arthroscopic and open stabilization groups are comparable in many of these studies [36]. The sum of the presented literature suggests that open anterior stabilization may provide improved stability over arthroscopic stabilizations but may result in a modest loss of motion.

Indications and Contraindications

In many settings, a successful surgery and result can be achieved with either arthroscopic or open anterior stabilization, with appropriate history, physical examination, and review of diagnostic imaging guiding decision-making. In particular, consideration of age, sports participation, number of prior dislocations, bone loss, and associated injuries help guide surgical indications. Additionally, there is a role for nonsurgical treatment in the form of activity modification, physical therapy, and bracing for anterior glenohumeral instability in the setting of minimal bone loss, absence of neurologic injury, and presence of dynamic stability with brief rehabilitation. In particular, nonsurgical management may be offered for in-season first-time dislocators, patient over the age of 25, non-collision athletes, or nonathletes.

Controversy remains regarding arthroscopic versus open treatment options for first-time anterior glenohumeral dislocations, but the following considerations can help guide treatment. As mentioned, there may be a role for nonsurgical management in in-season athletes; however, if any glenoid bone loss or a central on-track Hill-Sachs lesion is present, these authors advocate for surgical intervention. Similarly, early surgical intervention is offered for young (less than 25 years of age), out-of-season, male, collision athletes, with any degree of glenoid bone loss (Table 17.1).

Open stabilization has also been advocated by some surgeons in the primary setting for management of significant glenoid bone loss, engaging

Table 17.1 Anterior dislocation algorithm

First-time dislocation
In-season vs out-of-season
- Ok to RTP if minimal bone loss, no nerve injury, and dynamically stable with brief rehabilitation.
- Prefer early surgery if out-of-season, any glenoid bone loss, > central on-track Hill-Sachs
Less than 25 vs over 25 years old
- More inclined to offer early surgery in younger patient
Collison vs non-collision vs OH athlete
- More inclined to offer open surgery repair and remplissage for collision athlete
- More inclined to offer arthroscopic repair and posterior HH allograft for OH athlete.
Glenoid bone loss.
- Less than 10%: arthroscopic or open repair based on sport
~ Remplissage for peripheral on-track and just off-track Hill Sachs (not far off-track)
- 10–15%: prefer open repair
~ Remplissage for peripheral on-track and just off-track Hill-Sachs (not far off-track)
~ HH allograft OAT for OH athlete and far off-track Hill Sachs
- 15–25%: prefer Latarjet reconstruction
~ Posterior augmentation based on Hill-Sachs defect size.
* None vs remplissage vs HH OAT.
- Greater than 25%: prefer DTA.
~ Posterior augmentation based on Hill-Sachs defect size.
~ None vs remplissage vs HH OAT
Open capsulorrhaphy
- Primarily indicated for 5–15% glenoid bone loss, especially in collision athlete

Hill-Sachs lesions, HAGL lesions, associated subscapularis tears, and patients with an Instability Severity Index Score (ISIS) greater than seven [18]. The factors comprising ISIS and indicating increased risk of recurrence after arthroscopic Bankart include patients younger than 20 years of age, participation in contact or competitive sports, hyperlaxity, Hill-Sachs lesions visible on AP external rotation radiographs, and loss of glenoid contour on AP radiographs. In 2000, Burkhart and De Beer echoed these findings, reporting a recurrence rate of 4% after arthroscopic Bankart repair for anterior instability in patients without significant bone deficiency, whereas the rate of recurrence was 67% in the presence of bony deficiency. They described significant glenoid bone loss as an "inverted pear glenoid," signifying greater than 25% loss of the inferior glenoid diameter.

Less controversy exists in the role of open stabilization in addressing instability in the revision setting. Traumatic anterior instability may recur following surgical stabilization, especially with continued participation in high-risk activity. Sometimes, a technical error such as inadequate mobilization or tissue tensioning, minimal fixation, poor anchor position, or insufficient knot security can be identified as contributing factors. Alternatively, unrecognized pathology at initial intervention, significant humeral or glenoid bone loss, poor tissue quality, patient noncompliance, and/or inadequate rehabilitation can be contributing factors for failure [40, 41]. With technical errors and minimal bone loss, revision arthroscopic anterior capsulolabral reconstruction can be considered. However, even in these cases, open stabilization provides reliable, consistent results. Regardless of the reason for failure, revision open stabilization has shown good results with low rates of recurrence [6, 19, 41]. In addition, any concomitant HAGL lesion repair, revision bony Bankart reduction and fixation, or primary failure of the subscapularis can be addressed with an open approach.

Authors' indications for open capsulorrhaphy include failed prior arthroscopic Bankart repair, 5 to 15% glenoid bone loss, and participation in contact and non-throwing sports. Management of associated central and peripheral on-glenoid track Hill-Sachs lesions is determined by the associated glenoid bone loss. For 0 to 10% glenoid bone loss, remplissage is used, and for 10 to 15% glenoid bone loss, fresh humeral head allograft is used. For off-glenoid track Hill-Sachs lesions, fresh humeral head allograft is also used (see Table 17.1).

Contraindications for open stabilization are limited to voluntary instability, psychological disease, or the presence of large humeral head or glenoid bone defects requiring bone grafting. Additionally, overhead athletes are preferentially treated with arthroscopic stabilization due to concern over any loss of external rotation or subscapularis insufficiency [6, 42, 43]. Otherwise, open stabilization is an acceptable alternative to arthroscopic intervention in most cases based on surgeon preference.

Surgical Technique

The author's technique for open anterior capsulolabral repair is as follows. After the induction of general anesthesia, a complete examination of both shoulders is performed to assess the extent of native laxity and acquired instability in the operative shoulder. The patient is then rolled into the lateral decubitus position on a Vac-Pac bean bag and secured with the bean bag and a vertical table post behind the shoulder, positioned at about the level of the axilla. The legs are well padded beneath and between. An axillary roll is placed, the head is supported, and the cervical spine is aligned to diminish traction on the brachial plexus. The shoulder and arm are suspended with 7 to 10 pounds of balanced traction though a shoulder holder (Fig. 17.2). The shoulder is prepped and draped in the routine manner. A standard posterior arthroscopic portal is created, and the arthroscope is introduced. A 1 o'clock anterior-superior portal is created using an outside-inside method with an 18-gauge needle for localization and alignment. A complete inspection of the glenohumeral joint space and contents is performed.

When open anterior capsule labrum repair is planned, the anterior capsule and labrum, as well as any anteroinferior glenoid fracture fragments, are fully mobilized from the anterior glenoid rim and neck arthroscopically using an arthroscopic elevator (Figs. 17.3a, b) This step will facilitate the open approach to the anterior glenoid and protect the capsule and labrum for repair. Any concomitant indicated procedures—debridement, superior labrum repair, posterior labrum repair, and/or posterior humeral head remplissage capsulotenodesis—are performed arthroscopically. Additionally, if indicated, posterior humeral head allograft reconstruction is performed through an open technique while still in the lateral decubitus position.

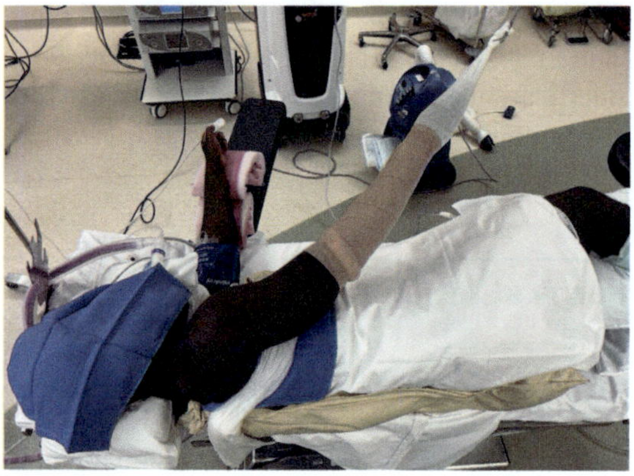

Fig. 17.2 Patient setup in lateral decubitus with bean bag, axillary roll, bony prominences padded, and 10 lb. of balanced axial traction

The arthroscopic portals and wounds are closed, a temporary dressing is applied, and the patient is returned to the supine position in preparation for the open capsule labrum repair. The arm is rested on two arm boards, and the shoulder and arm are re-prepped and draped in the routine manner. A vertical saber incision is made in the axillary line and carried down to the muscle fascia. While less cosmetic, and not typically necessary, a deltopectoral incision may be employed (Fig. 17.4).

The deltopectoral interval is defined and developed, typically retracting the cephalic vein with the deltoid. Goulet retractors, or conversely Richardson retractors or a self-retaining Kölbel retractor, is placed beneath the deltoid and pectoralis major muscle margins. This provides a clear view of the conjoined tendon and lateral humeral head. The clavipectoral fascia along the lateral margin of the conjoined tendon is divided proximally to the coracoid and distally to the superior margin of the pectoralis major, taking care to identify and protect the musculocutaneous nerve if exposed. The axillary nerve can typically be palpated at this time, beneath the conjoined tendon and below the subscapularis inferior muscle

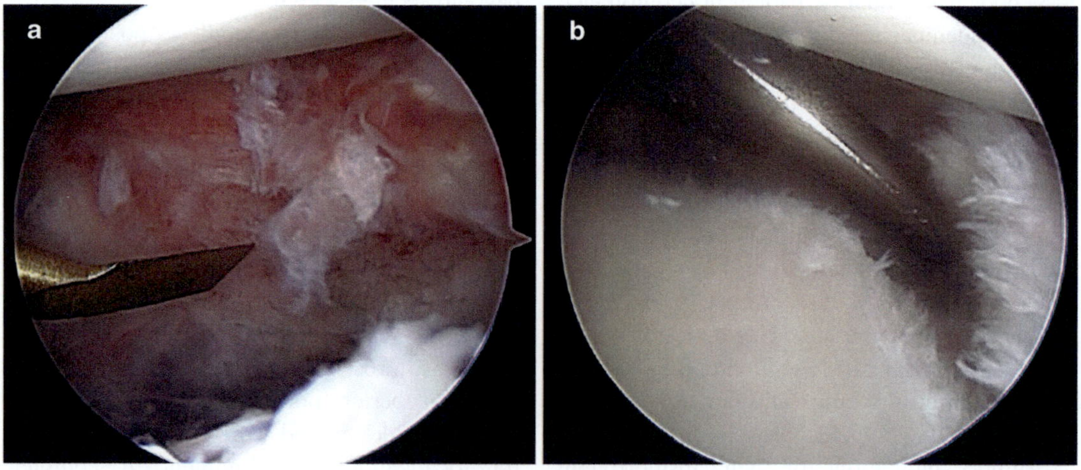

Fig. 17.3 (**a**) View with arthroscope in posterior portal demonstrating anteroinferior glenoid fragment and capsulolabral tissue "floating" after elevation with arthroscopic elevator. (**b**) View from 1 o'clock anterosuperior portal once again demonstrating anteroinferior glenoid fragment and capsulolabral tissue after elevation

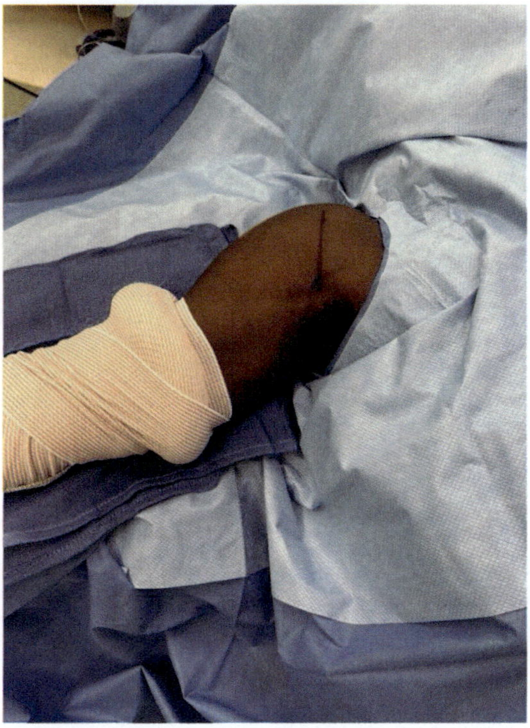

Fig. 17.4 Vertical saber incision: made in axillary line

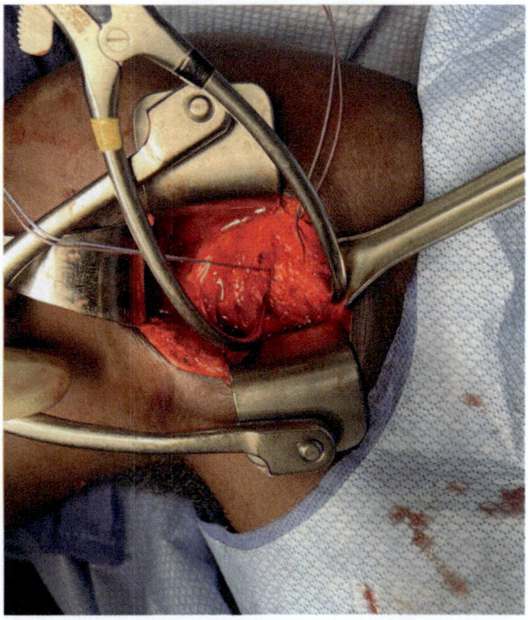

Fig. 17.5 The tendon-capsule interval is visually apparent laterally and easily developed with a small and then a large Cobb elevator, completely developing the capsule tendon interval inferiorly. Tag sutures are placed in the split tendon margins and a right-angle deep blunt-tipped Gelpi retractor is placed for exposure of the capsule

margin, heading into the axillary recess. A long, right-angle retractor is placed beneath the conjoined tendon providing a complete view of the entire subscapularis muscle tendon and muscle tendon junction. Some may choose to reposition the Kölbel retractor beneath the conjoined tendon, but caution must be exercised to avoid injury to the musculocutaneous nerve.

The subscapularis tendon is divided at the junction of the superior two-thirds and inferior one-third, beginning laterally and progressing medially, with care to avoid dividing the underlying capsule or dissecting too far medially to protect the subscapularis motor branches. The tendon-capsule interval is visually apparent laterally and easily developed with a small and then large Cobb elevator, completely developing the capsule tendon interval inferiorly. Tag sutures are placed in the split tendon margins, and a right-angle, deep, blunt-tipped Gelpi retractor is placed for exposure of the capsule (Fig. 17.5). The capsule is then split from lateral to medial, directed toward the 1 to 2 o'clock glenoid rim position, and then out onto the glenoid neck. As the capsule had been previously elevated from the glenoid rim and neck arthroscopically, the entire capsule-labrum-periosteum sleeve is typically easily defined and separated from the glenoid neck medially and inferiorly. A tag suture is placed at the superior capsule-labrum junction in the inferior flap. A broad, multiple fork-tipped glenoid neck retractor is placed followed by a Fukuda humeral head retractor. A narrow, single forked-tipped retractor is placed beneath the inferior glenoid rim, providing a complete view of the anterior glenoid rim and neck (Fig. 17.6).

In this setting, it is common for there to be 5 to 15% anterior glenoid bone loss, and the anterior labrum is often deficient. The remaining anterior glenoid rim and neck are prepared for suture anchor placement with a long handle, small Cobb retractor or a No. 3 to 4 long handle curette. Typically, four 2.4 mm Peek SutureTak suture anchors (or four to five 1.8 mm knotless FiberTak suture anchors) with No. 2 FiberWire are placed

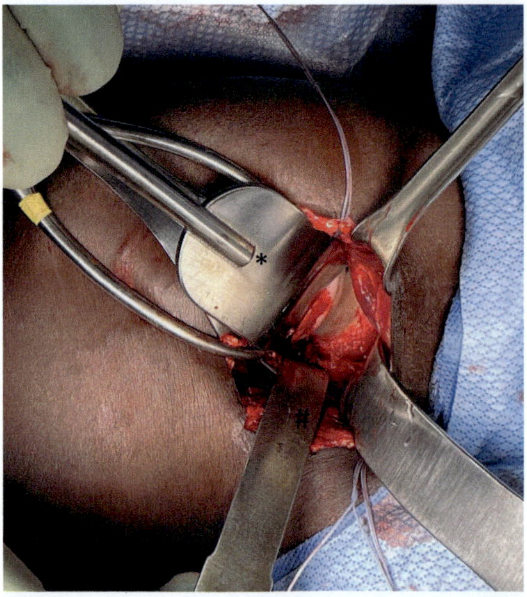

Fig. 17.6 View of the anterior glenoid neck after placing Fukuda retractor (*) and narrow, single forked-tipped retractor (#) beneath the inferior glenoid rim

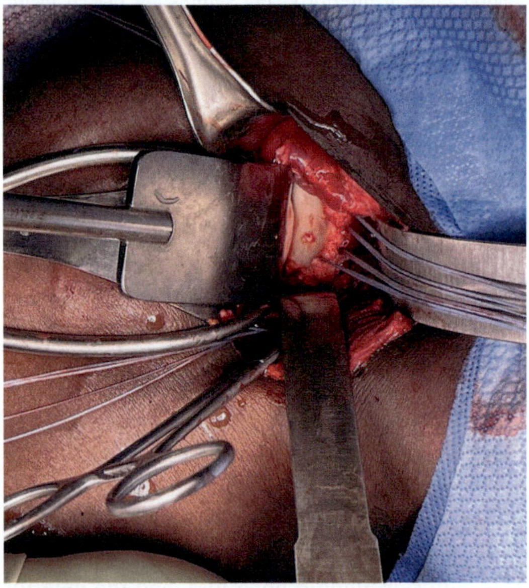

Fig. 17.7 View of anterior glenoid neck after placing four suture anchors along the glenoid rim

along the anterior glenoid rim (Fig. 17.7). The sutures are then passed from intra-articular to extracapsular through the remaining labrum and capsule under direct visualization, superiorly advancing the inferior and anterior capsule based on the intended extent of capsular shift (Fig. 17.8). The shoulder may be abducted and externally rotated during suture placement to determine the appropriate extent of superior capsular shift. The sutures are then tied (or the suture fixation loops are tensioned) from inferior to superior.

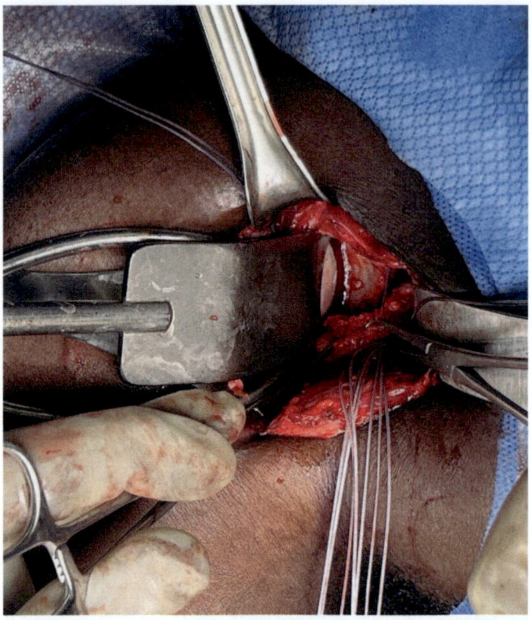

Fig. 17.8 View of anterior glenoid after suture pairs from anchors passed from intra-articular to extracapsular through the remaining labrum and capsule under direct visualization, superiorly advancing the inferior and anterior capsule based on the intended extent of capsular shift

In the case of a displaced but repairable anterior glenoid rim fracture fragment, the fragment is anatomically reduced, and suture anchor drill tunnels are made through the fragment, marking the appropriate anchor tunnel positions on the glenoid neck. The anchors are then placed into the glenoid neck, and sutures are passed from inside to outside through the drill tunnels in the fragment. Alternatively, if it is a smaller but still repairable piece, a cutting needle can be used to pass the sutures through the fragment. The sutures are then linked in inferior/superior pairs and tied using a double-anchor/double-pulley method, anatomically reducing and securing the fragment to the glenoid rim. As this is more common in an acute setting, it is uncommon to have significant residual capsule redundancy from traumatic capsular attenuation. Any redundancy encountered may be addressed with the mid-capsular longitudinal closure.

The retractors are removed, and the shoulder is examined for residual instability and preservation of shoulder motion. Any residual anterior instability may be addressed at this time using a vest-over-pants mattress repair of the mid-capsule longitudinal split using No. 2 FiberWire suture. The shoulder should be stable in all planes with preservation of full, or nearly full, abduction and external rotation. The mid subscapularis longitudinal split is closed side to side, the deltopectoral interval is closed, and a superficial closure is performed in routine fashion.

Postoperatively, the patient is placed into a sling with an abduction pillow and secured in neutral to slight internal rotation. A cryotherapy device is given to aid in pain control. The sling is maintained at all times for 4 weeks, with physical therapy initiated at 3 weeks postop. During the first phase of rehabilitation (protective, weeks one to four), motion is first passive, then actively assisted, and finally active as tolerated. During this phase, range of motion (ROM) is restricted to 90 degrees of forward flexion, 20 degrees of external rotation at the side, and internal rotation to the belly, with cross body adduction avoided. Isometrics are initiated during phase one, but resisted internal rotation is avoided due to subscapularis precautions.

At the beginning of phase two (restrictive, weeks four to eight) the sling is discontinued, and range of motion is increased. External rotation (ER) at the side is progressed to end range, but ER at 90 degrees of shoulder abduction does not exceed 90 degrees, focusing on very slow progression each week. Strengthening is advanced from isometrics to light bands, and strengthening begins for scapular stabilizers. However, resisted internal rotation continues to be avoided until 3 months.

During phase three (active, weeks 8 to 12), range of motion, including passive, is increased as tolerated in all planes. Additionally, strengthening is advanced as tolerated, and at 12 weeks, light resisted internal rotation is initiated. Phase four (return to function/sport, months 3 to 12) should see full restoration of range of motion and includes progressive strengthening. Sports-specific rehabilitation is begun between 3 and 4.5 months, a return to throwing program is initiated at 5.5 months, and progression back into contact activities starts at 6 months [44] (Table 17.2).

Table 17.2 PT protocol

	Range of motion	Sling	Therapeutic exercises
0–7 days	*No shoulder motion* Gentle active assisted elbow motion Full wrist and hand motion	Worn at all times	Follow home exercise program provided. Scapular retractions Supported pendulums
Phase 1 *1–4 weeks*	Restrict motion to 90° FF 20° ER at side IR to stomach No cross arm ADD *PROM → AAROM → AROM as tolerated*	Worn at all times	Isometrics in the sling NO IR
Phase 2 *4–8 weeks*	160° FF ER at neutral: 0°- end range ER at 90° Not to exceed 90° with slow approach of 5°–10° per week IR behind back to waist Cross body ADD at 6 wk.	D/C at 4 weeks	Strengthening (isometrics/light bands) within AROM limitations, horizontal abduction exercises Also start strengthening scapular stabilizers (traps/rhomboids/lev. scap/etc.) ****NO RESISTED IR for 3 months****
Phase 3 *8–12 weeks*	If ROM lacking, increase to full with gentle passive stretching at end ranges	None	Advance strengthening as tolerated ****At 12 weeks may begin light resisted IR strengthening****

(continued)

Table 17.2 (continued)

	Range of motion	Sling	Therapeutic exercises
Phase 4 *3–12 months*	Should have full ROM; if still lacking, continue with gentle passive stretching at end ranges	None	Only do strengthening 3×/week to avoid rotator cuff tendonitis Begin UE ergometer Begin sports-related rehab at 3–4.5 months, including advanced conditioning Begin eccentrically resisted motions, plyometric (e.g., weighted ball toss), proprioception (e.g., body blade), and closed chain exercises at 4.5 months. Return to throwing at 5½ months Throw from pitcher's mound at 6 months MMI is usually at 12 months

Return to Sport

As many traumatic anterior shoulder dislocations occur in the young, athlete population, consideration of not only subjective outcomes but also return to play rates for various treatment interventions is necessary. Although many early studies did not report extensive return to play data, several more recent reviews have discussed this outcome. A recent 7-year series of open Bankart stabilization in young collision sport athletes revealed excellent outcomes with 92% return to sport, low redislocation rate (13%), and a low revision rate (7%) [45]. Further, in a series of 21 teenage athletes with recurrent anterior instability and a minimum 2-year follow-up, no recurrence events, 100% excellent results based on the Rowe score, and 100% good to excellent results based on the UCLA shoulder score were observed, with all patients returning to preoperative high school sports (Hatch 2018). Finally, another recent study of medium-term outcomes of athletes 18 years or younger showed high rates of patient-reported satisfaction, excellent functional outcomes, and high rates of RTP (90%). However, there were high rates of recurrence (23.5%) with moderate rates of revision surgical stabilization (11.7%) in the medium term [46].

In a systematic review of return to play after open Bankart repair, a redislocation rate of 5.3% with an average return to play at 23.2 weeks was reported, with contact and throwing athletes requiring more time [47]. Another recent systematic review evaluated return to play in adolescent athletes (age 10 to 19 years) and found an 81.5% rate of return to preinjury levels of sport at an average of 5 months following surgery. However, the mean rate of recurrent instability in the adolescent population was 18.5%, and revision surgery was 12.1% [48]. In a systematic review of 563 patients (566 shoulders), with 82% male patients, average age at the time of surgery of 27.4 years, and a mean follow-up of 11.5 years (range, 2.5–29 years), authors showed good to excellent results (mean, 88.5 points). The overall recurrent instability rate in this study, including dislocation and subluxation as a postoperative complication, was 8.5%. A total of 87% of patients were able to return to sport and work postoperatively. Overall, OA changes were reported in 33% of the patients, and the overall revision rate was 1% [49]. Finally, a systematic review comparing return to play rates after various surgical options for the management of anterior instability showed an 86.1% return to sport rate. [50]

Complications

Historically, complications of open stabilization have been reported in upwards of 25% of cases, including neurovascular injury, infection, wound complications, hematoma formation, stiffness, hardware-related failures, bony rim fractures, and humeral fractures [30, 51, 52]. However, with modern techniques, complication rates have been much lower. In one recent study reviewing

NSQIP data from 2005 to 2014, open Bankart stabilization was shown to have a 1% 30-day complication rate, comparted to 5.5% with Latarjet and 0.6% with arthroscopic Bankart procedures [31]. Another NSQIP database study showed a major complication rate of 0.6% and minor complication rate of 0.3% in open Bankart stabilizations [12]. A systematic review looking at complications and redislocations of various anterior shoulder stabilization procedures found open soft tissue repair had a complication rate of 6.2% [53]. In another study, compared to other open stabilization procedures, open Bankart also had the lowest 1-year postoperative complication rates at 10.8% versus 19.2% for bony augmentation procedures [54].

Regarding the most commonly referenced concerns with open Bankart, subscapularis dysfunction has been noted to have a reoperation rate as high as 4.5% [24, 37, 55, 56]. However, similar to other historical concerns, the advent of modern techniques, including a subscapularis split versus takedown, have lessened this concern.

Though rare, neurologic complications have been noted with open stabilization. Anatomic studies have demonstrated that the axillary nerve is located just 1 to 1.5 cm below the inferior glenohumeral capsule, and the sensory branch lies close to the glenoid rim. Further, the musculocutaneous nerve may penetrate the coracobrachialis muscle belly just 5 cm distal to the coracoid process. [57]. Neurologic complications have been reported in 0 to 10% of open stabilization procedures [58].

Recurrent instability is the most common and concerning complication following shoulder stabilization procedures. Most studies demonstrate a recurrence rate after open Bankart repair of less than 5%, even in contact athletes [6, 19, 41, 43]. Additionally, several meta-analyses have shown lower recurrence rates with open stabilization versus arthroscopic stabilization [9, 23–25]. However, one long-term (16- to 26-year follow-up) study showed a 23% subluxation or apprehension rate, as well as 51% rate of osteoarthritis [59].

Conclusions

Despite advances in arthroscopic shoulder technology and emphasis on arthroscopic management of shoulder pathologies, in general, the open Bankart repair continues to be a powerful tool in the shoulder surgeon's toolbox, in particular for the care of young, contact athletes and in revision scenarios. The literature supports the use of open stabilization techniques for these cases as recurrence rates seem to be lower in these high-risk patient cohorts. Although the complication profile of open stabilization is inherently elevated compared to arthroscopic stabilization, surgeons can mitigate these risks with knowledge of the anatomy, refined surgical techniques, and appropriate rehabilitation and return to sport protocols.

References

1. Zacchilli MA, Owens BD. Epidemiology of shoulder dislocations presenting to emergency departments in the United States. J Bone Joint Surg Am. 2010;92(3):542–9. https://doi.org/10.2106/JBJS.I.00450. PMID: 20194311.
2. Owens BD, Duffey ML, Nelson BJ, DeBerardino TM, Taylor DC, Mountcastle SB. The incidence and characteristics of shoulder instability at the United States Military Academy. Am J Sports Med. 2007;35(7):1168–73. https://doi.org/10.1177/0363546506295179. PMID: 17581976.
3. Hovelius L. Anterior dislocation of the shoulder in teen-agers and young adults. Five-year prognosis. J Bone Joint Surg Am. 1987;69(3):393–9. PMID: 2434509.
4. Arciero RA, Wheeler JH, Ryan JB, McBride JT. Arthroscopic Bankart repair versus nonoperative treatment for acute, initial anterior shoulder dislocations. Am J Sports Med. 1994;22(5):589–94. https://doi.org/10.1177/036354659402200504. PMID: 7810780.
5. Postacchini F, Gumina S, Cinotti G. Anterior shoulder dislocation in adolescents. J Shoulder Elb Surg. 2000;9(6):470–4. https://doi.org/10.1067/mse.2000.108385. PMID: 11155298.
6. Rowe CR, Patel D, Southmayd WW. The Bankart procedure: a long-term end-result study. J Bone Joint Surg Am. 1978;60(1):1–16. PMID: 624747.
7. Malhotra A, Freudmann MS, Hay SM. Management of traumatic anterior shoulder dislocation in the 17- to 25-year age group: a dramatic evolution of practice.

J Shoulder Elb Surg. 2012;21(4):545–53. https://doi.org/10.1016/j.jse.2011.01.006. Epub 2011 Mar 30. PMID: 21454100.

8. Owens BD, Duffey ML, Deberardino TM, Cameron KL. Physical examination findings in young athletes correlate with history of shoulder instability. Orthopedics. 2011;34(6):460. https://doi.org/10.3928/01477447-20110427-21. PMID: 21661678.
9. Wang L, Liu Y, Su X, Liu S. A meta-analysis of arthroscopic versus open repair for treatment of Bankart lesions in the shoulder. Med Sci Monit. 2015;21:3028–35. https://doi.org/10.12659/MSM.894346. PMID: 26446430; PMCID: PMC4603609.
10. Riff AJ, Frank RM, Sumner S, Friel N, Bach BR Jr, Verma NN, Romeo AA. Trends in shoulder stabilization techniques used in the United States based on a large private-payer database. Orthop J Sports Med. 2017;5(12):2325967117745511. https://doi.org/10.1177/2325967117745511. PMID: 29318175; PMCID: PMC5753960.
11. Bonazza NA, Liu G, Leslie DL, Dhawan A. Trends in surgical management of shoulder Instability. Orthop J Sports Med. 2017;5(6):2325967117712476. https://doi.org/10.1177/2325967117712476. PMID: 28695137; PMCID: PMC5495509.
12. Eberlin CT, Varady NH, Kucharik MP, Naessig SA, Best MJ, Martin SD. Comparison of perioperative complications following surgical treatment of shoulder instability. JSES Int. 2022;6(3):355–61. https://doi.org/10.1016/j.jseint.2022.01.001. PMID: 35572454; PMCID: PMC9091785.
13. Levy DM, Cole BJ, Bach BR Jr. History of surgical intervention of anterior shoulder instability. J Shoulder Elb Surg. 2016;25(6):e139–50. https://doi.org/10.1016/j.jse.2016.01.019. Epub 2016 Apr 8. PMID: 27066962.
14. Coughlin RP, Crapser A, Coughlin K, Coughlin LP. Open Bankart revisited. Arthrosc Tech. 2017;6(1):e233–7. https://doi.org/10.1016/j.eats.2016.09.027. PMID: 28409106; PMCID: PMC5382355.
15. Porcellini G, Campi F, Pegreffi F, Castagna A, Paladini P. Predisposing factors for recurrent shoulder dislocation after arthroscopic treatment. J Bone Joint Surg Am. 2009;91(11):2537–42. https://doi.org/10.2106/JBJS.H.01126. PMID: 19884424.
16. Wasserstein D, Dwyer T, Veillette C, Gandhi R, Chahal J, Mahomed N, Ogilvie-Harris D. Predictors of dislocation and revision after shoulder stabilization in Ontario, Canada, from 2003 to 2008. Am J Sports Med. 2013;41(9):2034–40. https://doi.org/10.1177/0363546513492952. Epub 2013 Jun 20. PMID: 23788683.
17. Lee SH, Lim KH, Kim JW. Risk factors for recurrence of anterior-inferior instability of the shoulder after arthroscopic Bankart repair in patients younger than 30 years. Arthroscopy. 2018;34(9):2530–6. https://doi.org/10.1016/j.arthro.2018.03.032. PMID: 30173793.
18. Balg F, Boileau P. The instability severity index score. A simple pre-operative score to select patients for arthroscopic or open shoulder stabilisation. J Bone Joint Surg Br. 2007;89(11):1470–7. https://doi.org/10.1302/0301-620X.89B11.18962. PMID: 17998184.
19. Neviaser AS, Benke MT, Neviaser RJ. Open Bankart repair for revision of failed prior stabilization: outcome analysis at a mean of more than 10 years. J Shoulder Elb Surg. 2015;24(6):897–901. https://doi.org/10.1016/j.jse.2014.11.036. Epub 2014 Dec 10. PMID: 25498480.
20. Taylor DC, Arciero RA. Pathologic changes associated with shoulder dislocations. Arthroscopic and physical examination findings in first-time, traumatic anterior dislocations. Am J Sports Med. 1997;25(3):306–11. https://doi.org/10.1177/036354659702500306. PMID: 9167808.
21. Owens BD, Agel J, Mountcastle SB, Cameron KL, Nelson BJ. Incidence of glenohumeral instability in collegiate athletics. Am J Sports Med. 2009;37(9):1750–4. https://doi.org/10.1177/0363546509334591. Epub 2009 Jun 25. PMID: 19556471.
22. Rowe CR, Zarins B, Ciullo JV. Recurrent anterior dislocation of the shoulder after surgical repair. Apparent causes of failure and treatment. J Bone Joint Surg Am. 1984;66(2):159–68. PMID: 6693441.
23. Freedman KB, Smith AP, Romeo AA, Cole BJ, Bach BR Jr. Open Bankart repair versus arthroscopic repair with transglenoid sutures or bioabsorbable tacks for Recurrent Anterior instability of the shoulder: a meta-analysis. Am J Sports Med. 2004;32(6):1520–7. https://doi.org/10.1177/0363546504265188. Epub 2004 Jul 20. PMID: 15310581.
24. Mohtadi NG, Bitar IJ, Sasyniuk TM, Hollinshead RM, Harper WP. Arthroscopic versus open repair for traumatic anterior shoulder instability: a meta-analysis. Arthroscopy. 2005;21(6):652–8. https://doi.org/10.1016/j.arthro.2005.02.021. PMID: 15944618.
25. Lenters TR, Franta AK, Wolf FM, Leopold SS, Matsen FA 3rd. Arthroscopic compared with open repairs for recurrent anterior shoulder instability. A systematic review and meta-analysis of the literature. J Bone Joint Surg Am. 2007;89(2):244–54. https://doi.org/10.2106/JBJS.E.01139. PMID: 17272436.
26. Petrera M, Patella V, Patella S, Theodoropoulos J. A meta-analysis of open versus arthroscopic Bankart repair using suture anchors. Knee Surg Sports Traumatol Arthrosc. 2010;18(12):1742–7. https://doi.org/10.1007/s00167-010-1093-5. Epub 2010 Mar 17. PMID: 20237768.
27. Owens BD, Williams AE, Wolf JM. Risk factors for surgical complications in rotator cuff repair in a veteran population. J Shoulder Elb Surg. 2015;24(11):1707–12. https://doi.org/10.1016/j.jse.2015.04.020. Epub 2015 Jul 9. PMID: 26164483.

28. Hohmann E, Tetsworth K, Glatt V. Open versus arthroscopic surgical treatment for anterior shoulder dislocation: a comparative systematic review and meta-analysis over the past 20 years. J Shoulder Elb Surg. 2017;26(10):1873–80. https://doi.org/10.1016/j.jse.2017.04.009. Epub 2017 Jul 5. PMID: 28688936.
29. Miura K, Tsuda E, Tohyama H, Iwahori Y, Mae T, Mochizuki Y, Nakagawa K, Nakamae A, Nakamura T, Takao M, Uchida S, Muneta T, Ochi M. Can arthroscopic Bankart repairs using suture anchors restore equivalent stability to open repairs in the management of traumatic anterior shoulder dislocation? A meta-analysis J Orthop Sci. 2018;23(6):935–41. https://doi.org/10.1016/j.jos.2018.06.016. Epub 2018 Jul 26. PMID: 30057323.
30. An VV, Sivakumar BS, Phan K, Trantalis J. A systematic review and meta-analysis of clinical and patient-reported outcomes following two procedures for recurrent traumatic anterior instability of the shoulder: Latarjet procedure vs. Bankart repair J Shoulder Elbow Surg. 2016;25(5):853–63. https://doi.org/10.1016/j.jse.2015.11.001. Epub 2016 Jan 19. PMID: 26809355.
31. Bokshan SL, DeFroda SF, Owens BD. Comparison of 30-Day morbidity and mortality after arthroscopic Bankart, open Bankart, and Latarjet-Bristow procedures: a review of 2864 cases Orthop J Sports Med. 2017;5(7):2325967117713163. https://doi.org/10.1177/2325967117713163. PMID: 28781973; PMCID: PMC5518960.
32. Chalmers PN, Mascarenhas R, Leroux T, Sayegh ET, Verma NN, Cole BJ, Romeo AA. Do arthroscopic and open stabilization techniques restore equivalent stability to the shoulder in the setting of anterior glenohumeral instability? A systematic review of overlapping meta-analyses. Arthroscopy. 2015;31(2):355–63. https://doi.org/10.1016/j.arthro.2014.07.008. Epub 2014 Sep 10. PMID: 25217207.
33. Gao B, DeFroda S, Bokshan S, Ready LV, Sullivan K, Etzel C, Owens BD. Arthroscopic versus open Bankart repairs in recurrent anterior shoulder instability: a systematic review of the association between publication date and postoperative recurrent instability in systematic reviews. Arthroscopy. 2020;36(3):862–71. https://doi.org/10.1016/j.arthro.2019.10.022. Epub 2019 Dec 20. PMID: 31870747.
34. Goodrich E, Wolf M, Vopat M, Mok A, Baker J, Bernard C, Tarakemeh A, Vopat B. Sex-specific differences in outcomes after anterior shoulder surgical stabilization: a meta-analysis and systematic review of literature. JSES Int. 2021;6(1):123–31. https://doi.org/10.1016/j.jseint.2021.10.002. PMID: 35141686; PMCID: PMC8811409.
35. Moroder P, Odorizzi M, Pizzinini S, Demetz E, Resch H, Moroder P. Open Bankart repair for the treatment of anterior shoulder instability without substantial osseous glenoid defects: results after a minimum follow-up of twenty years. J Bone Joint Surg Am. 2015;97(17):1398–405. https://doi.org/10.2106/JBJS.N.01214. PMID: 26333734; PMCID: PMC7535105.
36. Bottoni CR, Smith EL, Berkowitz MJ, Towle RB, Moore JH. Arthroscopic versus open shoulder stabilization for recurrent anterior instability: a prospective randomized clinical trial. Am J Sports Med. 2006;34(11):1730–7. https://doi.org/10.1177/0363546506288239. Epub 2006 May 30. PMID: 16735589.
37. Greis PE, Dean M, Hawkins RJ. Subscapularis tendon disruption after Bankart reconstruction for anterior instability. J Shoulder Elb Surg. 1996;5(3):219–22. https://doi.org/10.1016/s1058-2746(05)80010-2. PMID: 8816343.
38. Sachs RA, Williams B, Stone ML, Paxton L, Kuney M. Open Bankart repair: correlation of results with postoperative subscapularis function. Am J Sports Med. 2005;33(10):1458–62. https://doi.org/10.1177/0363546505275350. Epub 2005 Jul 11. PMID: 16009981.
39. Scheibel M, Tsynman A, Magosch P, Schroeder RJ, Habermeyer P. Postoperative subscapularis muscle insufficiency after primary and revision open shoulder stabilization. Am J Sports Med. 2006;34(10):1586–93. https://doi.org/10.1177/0363546506288852. Epub 2006 Jun 26. PMID: 16801689.
40. Waterman B, Owens BD, Tokish JM. Anterior shoulder instability in the military athlete. Sports Health. 2016;8(6):514–9. https://doi.org/10.1177/1941738116672161. Epub 2016 Oct 1. PMID: 27694151; PMCID: PMC5089361.
41. Cho NS, Yi JW, Lee BG, Rhee YG. Revision open Bankart surgery after arthroscopic repair for traumatic anterior shoulder instability. Am J Sports Med. 2009;37(11):2158–64. https://doi.org/10.1177/0363546509339015. Epub 2009 Sep 23. PMID: 19776342.
42. Hattrup SJ, Cofield RH, Weaver AL. Anterior shoulder reconstruction: prognostic variables. J Shoulder Elb Surg. 2001;10(6):508–13. https://doi.org/10.1067/mse.2001.118417. PMID: 11743527.
43. Levine WN, Flatow EL. The pathophysiology of shoulder instability. Am J Sports Med. 2000;28(6):910–7. https://doi.org/10.1177/03635465000280062501. PMID: 11101119.
44. Lloyd G, Day J, Lu J, Lincoln A, Attanasio S, Svoboda S. Postoperative rehabilitation of anterior glenohumeral joint instability surgery: a systematic review. Sports Med Arthrosc Rev. 2021;29(2):54–62. https://doi.org/10.1097/JSA.0000000000000305. PMID: 33972482.
45. Monk AP, Crua E, Gatenby GC, Walsh AJ, Stanley JC, Rosenfeldt MP, Twaddle BC, Walsh SJ. Clinical outcomes following open anterior shoulder stabilization for glenohumeral instability in the young collision athlete. J Shoulder Elb Surg. 2022;31(7):1474–8. https://doi.org/10.1016/j.jse.2021.12.013. Epub 2022 Jan 17. PMID: 35051538.

46. Hickey IPM, Davey MS, Hurley ET, Gaafar M, Delaney RA, Mullett H. Return to play following open Bankart repair in collision athletes aged 18 years or less. J Shoulder Elb Surg. 2022;31(6S):S8–12. https://doi.org/10.1016/j.jse.2021.11.001. Epub 2021 Dec 11. PMID: 34906680.
47. Stone GP, Pearsall AW 4th. Return to play after open Bankart repair: a systematic review. Orthop J Sports Med. 2014;2(2):2325967114522960. https://doi.org/10.1177/2325967114522960. PMID: 26535302; PMCID: PMC4555624.
48. Kasik CS, Rosen MR, Saper MG, Zondervan RL. High rate of return to sport in adolescent athletes following anterior shoulder stabilisation: a systematic review. J ISAKOS. 2019;4(1):33–40. https://doi.org/10.1136/jisakos-2018-000224. Epub 2018 Nov 10. PMID: 31044093; PMCID: PMC6487304.
49. AlSomali K, Kholinne E, Van Nguyen T, Cho CH, Kwak JM, Koh KH, Jeon IH. Outcomes and return to sport and work after open Bankart repair for recurrent shoulder instability: a systematic review. Orthop J Sports Med. 2021;9(10):23259671211026907. https://doi.org/10.1177/23259671211026907. PMID: 34660820; PMCID: PMC8511924.
50. Abdul-Rassoul H, Galvin JW, Curry EJ, Simon J, Li X. Return to sport after surgical treatment for anterior shoulder instability: a systematic review. Am J Sports Med. 2019;47(6):1507–15. https://doi.org/10.1177/0363546518780934. Epub 2018 Jun 27. PMID: 29949383.
51. Allain J, Goutallier D, Glorion C. Long-term results of the Latarjet procedure for the treatment of anterior instability of the shoulder. J Bone Joint Surg Am 1998;80(6):841–52. https://doi.org/10.2106/00004623-199806000-00008. PMID: 9655102.
52. Kang RW, Frank RM, Nho SJ, Ghodadra NS, Verma NN, Romeo AA, Provencher MT. Complications associated with anterior shoulder instability repair. Arthroscopy. 2009;25(8):909–20. https://doi.org/10.1016/j.arthro.2009.03.009. PMID: 19664511.
53. Williams HLM, Evans JP, Furness ND, Smith CD. It's not all about redislocation: a systematic review of complications after anterior shoulder stabilization surgery. Am J Sports Med. 2019;47(13):3277–83. https://doi.org/10.1177/0363546518810711. Epub 2018 Dec 10. PMID: 30525905.
54. Kowalski TJ, Khan AZ, Cohen JR, Lord EL, Ishmael C, Soohoo NF, McAllister DR, Gulotta LV, Wang JC, Petrigliano FA. Open shoulder stabilization: current trends and 1-year postoperative complications. JSES Open Access. 2017;1(2):72–8. https://doi.org/10.1016/j.jses.2017.07.001. PMID: 30675543; PMCID: PMC6340864.
55. Hiemstra LA, Sasyniuk TM, Mohtadi NG, Fick GH. Shoulder strength after open versus arthroscopic stabilization. Am J Sports Med. 2008;36(5):861–7. https://doi.org/10.1177/0363546508314429. Epub 2008 Mar 4. PMID: 18319347.
56. Hatch MD, Hennrikus WL. The open Bankart repair for traumatic anterior shoulder instability in teenage athletes. J Pediatr Orthop. 2018;38(1):27–31. https://doi.org/10.1097/BPO.0000000000000744. PMID: 26945245.
57. Loomer R, Graham B. Anatomy of the axillary nerve and its relation to inferior capsular shift. Clin Orthop Relat Res. 1989;243:100–5. PMID: 2721048.
58. Shah AA, Butler RB, Romanowski J, Goel D, Karadagli D, Warner JJ. Short-term complications of the Latarjet procedure. J Bone Joint Surg Am. 2012;94(6):495–501. https://doi.org/10.2106/JBJS.J.01830. PMID: 22318222.
59. Berendes T, Mathijssen N, Verburg H, Kraan G. The open-modified Bankart procedure: long-term follow-up 'a 16-26-year follow-up study'. Arch Orthop Trauma Surg. 2018;138(5):597–603. https://doi.org/10.1007/s00402-017-2866-9. Epub 2018 Jan 3. PMID: 29299668.

Glenoid Bone Loss: The Latarjet, the Open Approach

18

Christopher M. Loftis and T. Bradley Edwards

Case Example

The case example is a 33-year-old male patient who has had a 10-year history of recurrent dislocations of the left shoulder. His instability began 10 years prior with a traumatic dislocation. He underwent arthroscopic capsulolabral repair 10 years ago followed by a revision capsulolabral repair 1 year ago due to continued instability. Despite these measures, he continued with instability of the left shoulder multiple times in the last year, many of which he was able to reduce himself. His physical exam at initial presentation was significant for a positive apprehension in abduction and external rotation as well as a positive relocation test. He also had 2+ anterior translation. Fig. 18.1 shows the patient's preoperative radiographs. There is noted blunting of the anterior glenoid on the Bernageau view of the left shoulder compared to the right. Given the patient's history of failed Bankart repair and loss of anterior glenoid bone, the authors felt he was indicated for an open stabilization procedure in the form of an open Latarjet procedure.

The patient underwent a Latarjet procedure without complication. He was placed in a sling for 2 weeks and allowed to undergo gentle shoulder range of motion exercises on his own. By 3 months postoperatively, the patient was allowed to resume all activities as tolerated. Fig. 18.2 shows the patient's radiographs at 1 year postoperatively showing a healed coracoid graft to the anterior glenoid. At time of final follow-up at 1 year, the patient had full range of motion with 170 degrees of forward flexion, 160 degrees of abduction, and 90 degrees of external rotation at 90 degrees of abduction and could internally rotate to T12. He had no anterior translation on exam, and he had a negative apprehension and relocation test. He had no episodes of recurrent instability at 1 year postoperatively.

C. M. Loftis (✉)
Tennessee Orthopaedic Alliance, Columbia, TN, USA

Tennessee Orthopeaedic Alliance, Center for Research and Education Foundation, Nashville, TN, USA
e-mail: loftiscm@toa.com

T. B. Edwards
Fondren Orthopedic Group, Houston, TX, USA

Texas Orthopedic Hospital, Houston, TX, USA

Fondren Orthopedic Research Institute, Houston, TX, USA
e-mail: bemd@fondren.com

© The Author(s), under exclusive license to Springer Nature Switzerland AG 2026
R. M. Frank, J. M. Tokish (eds.), *Management of Shoulder Instability*,
https://doi.org/10.1007/978-3-032-18089-6_18

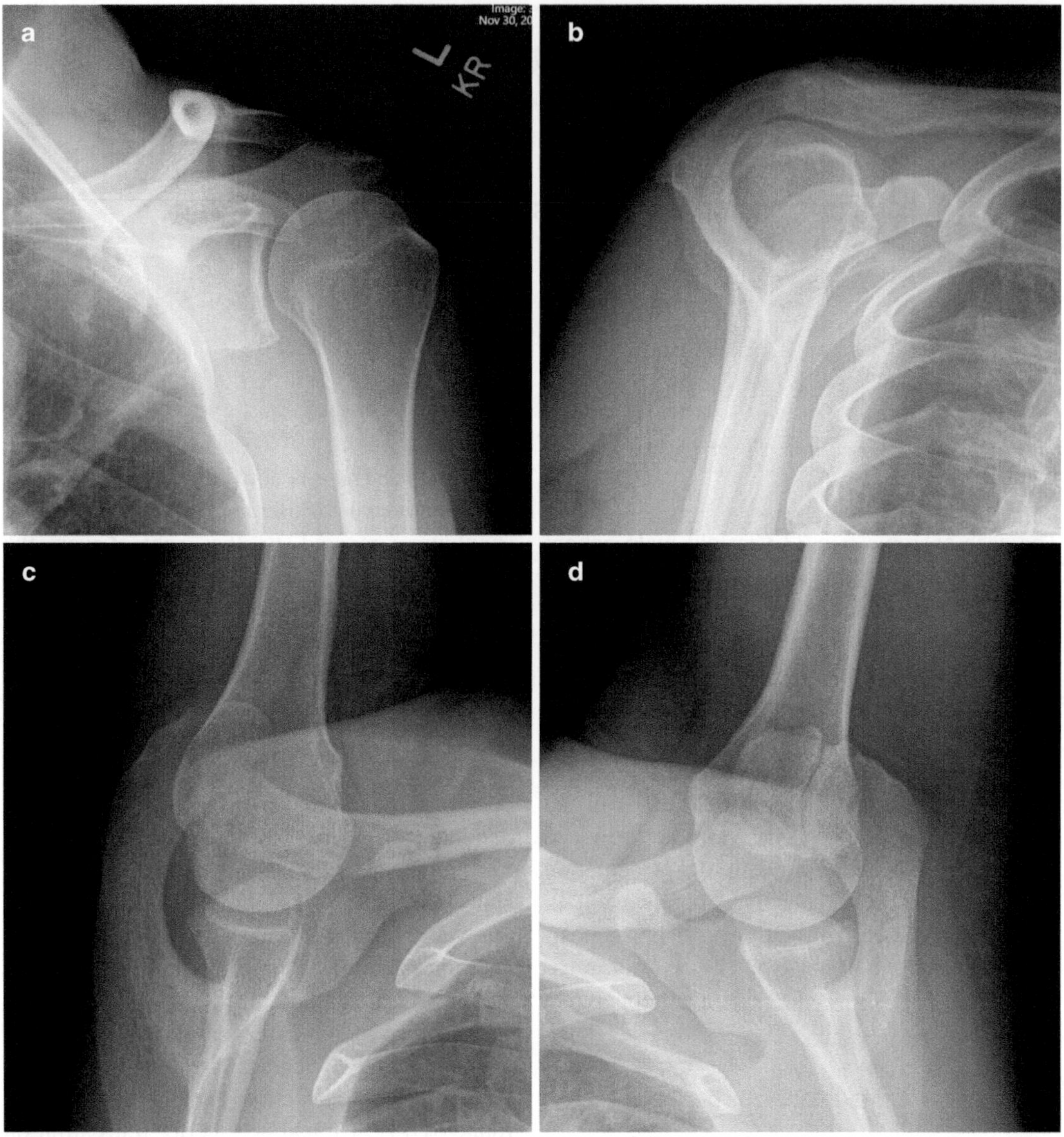

Fig. 18.1 Preoperative radiographs including Grashey view (**a**), scapulary-Y view (**b**), and Bernageau view of the affected side (**c**) and unaffected side (**d**)

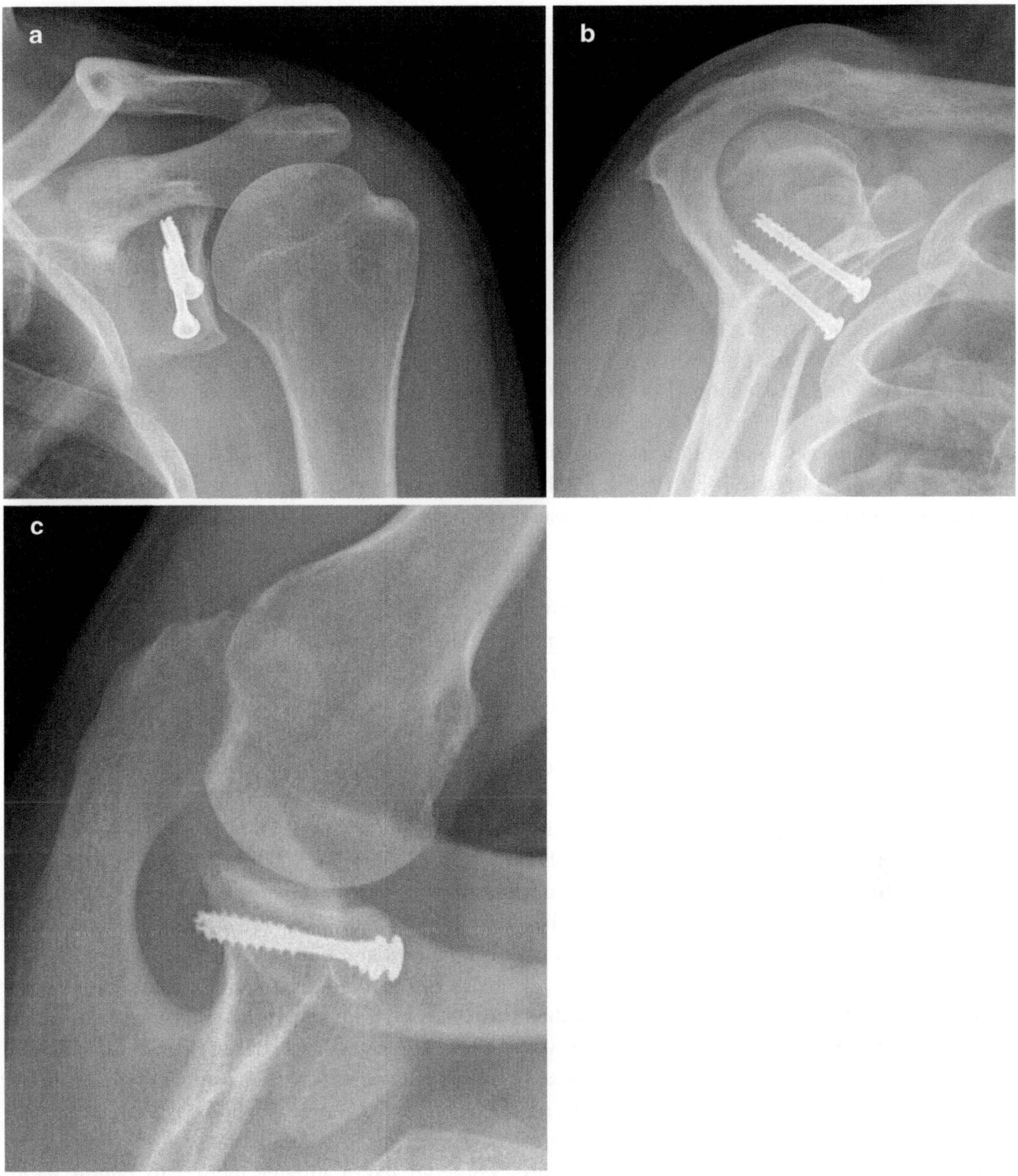

Fig. 18.2 Radiographs at 1 year postoperatively including Grashey (**a**), scapulary-Y view (**b**), and Bernageau view (**c**)

History of the Coracoid Transfer

In 1918, Rudolf Eden first described his technique of augmenting the anterior glenoid with use of an autograft, corticocancellous bone block from the tibia [1]. This is the first reported use of bone graft augmentation of the glenoid for patients with anterior instability of the glenohumeral joint and is later referenced by Latarjet when he describes his technique [2]. Eden's technique is intended to extend the anterior buttress of the glenoid and prevent dislocation of the humeral head. In 1932, Samuel Hybbinette published a similar technique in using the iliac crest as an autograft augmentation of the anterior glenoid [3]. His work along with Eden's original technique gave rise to the Eden-Hybbinette procedure which was popular for shoulder stabilization. Its modification even remains in use today as a salvage operation following failed Latarjet procedures.

The coracoid became an interest for potential utility in stabilizing the glenohumeral joint in 1924 when Oudard published his technique. It involved osteotomizing the coracoid and interposing a tibial graft while repositioning the coracoid inferiorly forming a "canopy" anterior to the glenohumeral joint. This helped to stabilize the anterior glenohumeral joint following plication of the subscapularis muscle [4]. In 1954, Michel Latarjet described his technique in which he osteotomized the coracoid, and rather than make an anterior canopy for the glenohumeral joint, he described moving the coracoid to the anteroinferior glenoid, referencing back to Eden's technique utilizing the tibial graft for anteroinferior glenoid augmentation [5]. In 1958, Latarjet published a detailed description of the procedure, in which he utilized a tenotomy of the subscapularis muscle and screw fixation of his coracoid graft. It should also be noted that in 1954, Arthur Trillat also described a similar procedure to Latarjet, but rather than use a subscapularis tenotomy to gain access to the anterior glenoid, he advised utilizing a retractor to move the subscapularis out of the way and keep its insertion intact [6].

The work of Arthur Helfet was also published in 1958. He described a procedure in which the coracoid tip was osteotomized and passed through the subscapularis tendon to the anterior neck of the glenoid. He named his procedure after one of his mentors, W. Rowley Bristow, who is said to have first described the technique to Helfet. His procedure differed from Latarjet in that only the coracoid tip was moved to the anterior glenoid and that it was originally secured with suture [7], though later modifications to the technique opted for a single screw fixation instead. While his bony augmentation was not as substantial as the Latarjet procedure, he described the effect of the soft tissue augmentation that the conjoined tendon provided, particularly in abduction and external rotation, to the anteroinferior capsule of the glenohumeral joint, which has become known as the "sling effect." Both the Bristow and the Latarjet procedures provided solutions for problems with glenohumeral instability, utilizing both bone augmentation and soft tissue reinforcement. The procedures are at times referred to synonymously as the Bristow-Latarjet procedure though the differences should be noted.

The authors prefer the classic Latarjet procedure as the increased size of the coracoid bone graft better reinforces the anteroinferior glenoid. In 1980, Patte described the rationale of the Latarjet procedure as the "triple blocking" effect [8]. He summarized that stability was regained through the procedure firstly by the coracoid bone graft increasing the bone stock of the glenoid anteriorly to prevent dislocation, secondly by the "sling effect" of the conjoined tendon reinforcing the anteroinferior soft tissues when the arm is brought into abduction and external rotation (Fig. 18.3), and thirdly by the repair of the coracoacromial ligament stump to the humeral capsule to reconstruct the anterior capsule of the glenohumeral joint.

The Latarjet procedure has since had some modifications made to the original described technique. Burkhart and De Beer have published on their "congruent arc" technique in which the coracoid is rotated 90 degrees before being fixed to the anteroinferior glenoid. By doing so, the authors contend that the inferior coracoid more closely resembles the curvature of the glenoid, and therefore, the graft will have a smoother transition to the glenoid surface. Additionally, the coracoid has a greater medial to lateral width than a superior to inferior depth, and this technique may allow for greater glenoid bone defects to be grafted [10]. Another innovation of the procedure has been the introduction the arthroscopic Latarjet procedure which was described by Lafosse and Boileau [11–13]. While the utility of the arthroscopic Latarjet is likely to continue to grow, the authors prefer the open Latarjet for the efficiency of the procedure.

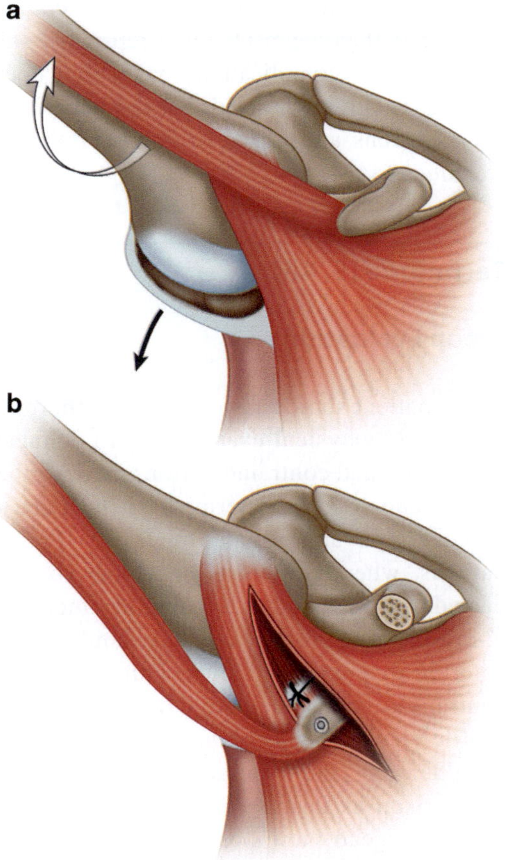

Fig. 18.3 Illustration rendering of the unstable shoulder in abduction and external rotation (**a**) and the "sling effect" of the conjoined tendon following a Latarjet procedure when the arm is brought into abduction and external rotation (**b**). (Modified from Edwards et al. 2012 [9])

Indications and Contraindications

The indications for the Latarjet procedure have typically been reserved for patients with glenohumeral instability in the setting of glenoid bone loss and/or failure of previous capsulolabral repair. Bankart repair, both open and arthroscopic, have shown utility in being able to restore glenohumeral stability in many patients with a reported failure rate of <5% [14] in some studies, but others reporting higher failure rates of 16–21% at long-term follow-up [15, 16]. Patient factors do play a role in the risk of recurrence of instability events even after Bankart repair. These factors are glenoid bone loss [17–21], presence of a Hill-Sachs lesion [22, 23], patient age [22–28] and activity level (i.e., participant in a collision sport, overhead throwing) [23, 28–34], ligament quality [22, 35], and number of previous dislocations [27].

Attempts have been made to take these factors into account when counseling patients on their risk of recurrence preoperatively prior to a Bankart repair, but also to advocate for open procedures, like the Latarjet, in lieu of a capsulolabral repair. Balg and Boileau published their scoring system called the instability severity index score (ISIS) in 2007 which takes into account the patient's age, level of sports participation (competitive or recreational), type of sport (contact/force overhead or other), presence of hyperlaxity, presence of a Hill-Sachs lesion, and loss of inferior glenoid contour [36]. Current literature suggests that a patient with an ISIS score > 3 has a high likelihood of failing a capsulolabral repair [37]. In this setting, the authors advocate for an open bone augmentation procedure, like the Latarjet, to address the patient's instability. However, multiple recent studies have found no correlation in the ISIS and prediction of failure of a Bankart repair [23, 37, 38]. More recently, the glenoid track instability management score (GTIMS) has been proposed and it replaces the XR imaging scores of the ISIS with CT imaging "on-track" or "off-track" scoring into the system [39]. While there is promising data on this scoring tool, further studies will need to be done on its validity.

While there may eventually be a scoring system to help the surgeon delineate which patients will benefit from a soft tissue repair vs. those who need an open bone augmentation procedure, it is our opinion that currently this decision must be made on a patient-by-patient basis taking into account the following:

1. Recurrent anterior instability.
2. Participation in collision sports.
3. Suboptimal patient compliance.
4. Glenoid insufficiency.
5. Failed Bankart repair.

In our practice, we consider recurrent anterior instability or a failed previous Bankart repair as absolute indications for a Latarjet procedure. Contact or collision athletes, poor patient compliance, or glenoid insufficiency are all relative indications as these patients have a high rate of recurrence if given either nonoperative management or Bankart repair [31–33]. We do not necessarily consider the Latarjet as a purely salvage procedure for failed Bankart repairs as we also know that there is a risk of inferior results after a Latarjet procedure performed following a failed Bankart repair [40]. The importance of identifying the patients at risk of failing both nonoperative management and Bankart repair is essential, and the above criteria have served our practice well. The authors also stress several contraindications to the procedure as well. They are as follows:

1. Stiffness.
2. Subscapularis tear.
3. Multidirectional instability (MDI).
4. Habitual dislocators.
5. Loss of >1/3 of the glenoid articular surface.
6. Age > 40.

Patients with stiffness prior to a Latarjet are likely to have a further loss of range of motion and have a suboptimal result. MDI and habitual dislocators are usually best managed nonoperatively. In cases in which there is loss of more than 1/3 of the articular surface, the coracoid transfer procedures will not have sufficient bone to reconstruct the glenoid. In such cases, open reduction and internal fixation of the fracture fragment should be attempted first. If this is not possible, then reconstruction of the glenoid should be performed with use of either distal tibial allograft or iliac crest autograft. In the authors' experience, older patients generally have worse outcomes following a Latarjet procedure, with increased stiffness and worse function. Because of these outcomes, we do not offer the procedure to patients over the age of 40.

The decision to proceed with a Latarjet should involve extensive discussion with the patient as it is known to carry a higher complication rate than a capsulolabral repair [41–43]. Though these complications have been documented, it is hypothesized that the majority of complications are related to improper surgical technique [44, 45].

Technique [9, 46]

Preop Evaluation

Every patient should have a full and thorough history and physical examination to delineate indications and contraindications, as described above, and to help determine if the Latarjet procedure is appropriate treatment. For all patients where shoulder instability is suspected, imaging studies are obtained including X-ray imaging of the affected shoulder with anterior to posterior views with the arm in neutral, external, and internal rotation. Glenoid profile views are also obtained of the affected shoulder and the contralateral shoulder for comparison as described by Bernageau [47]. The Bernageau view's reliability and validity in identifying glenoid bone loss compared to computed tomography scan has been shown [48], and, in the authors' practice, both the Grashey and Bernageau view show a glenoid rim lesion 85% of the time and a Hill-Sachs lesion 75% of the time [49]. The computerized tomography scan is not routinely utilized in the preoperative evaluation of shoulder instability.

Figures 18.4 and 18.5 show the routine imaging studies of a 23-year-old male with history of right recurrent glenohumeral instability. Figure 18.2 shows the Grashey view of the affected shoulder and Fig. 18.5 shows the comparison of the Bernageau views between the affected and unaffected shoulders. Figure 18.6 shows the approximate bone loss by inverting and overlaying the unaffected image over the affected image and highlighting the area of lost bone.

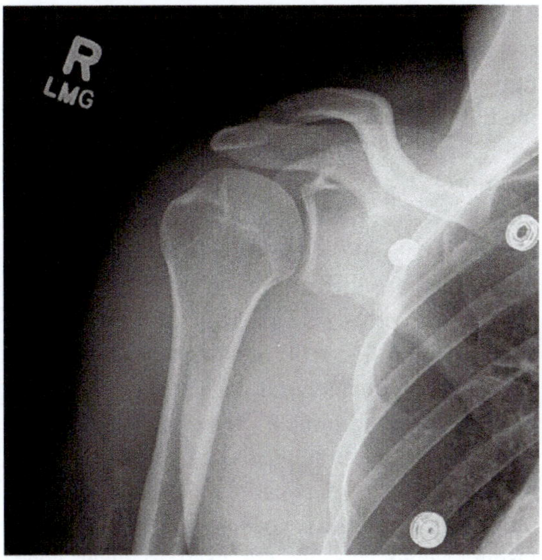

Fig. 18.4 The Grashey AP view of the right shoulder in a 23-year-old patient with a history of recurrent right shoulder glenohumeral instability

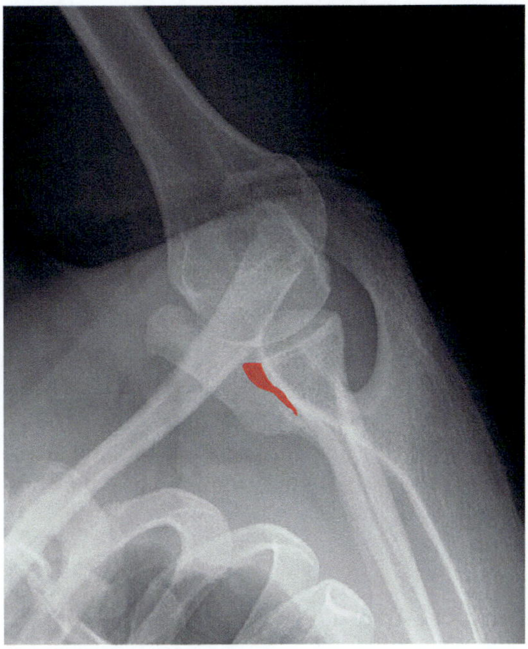

Fig. 18.6 The red outline shows the approximate bone loss based on comparison to this patient's unaffected left side, via inverting and overlaying the radiograph of the unaffected side over the affected side

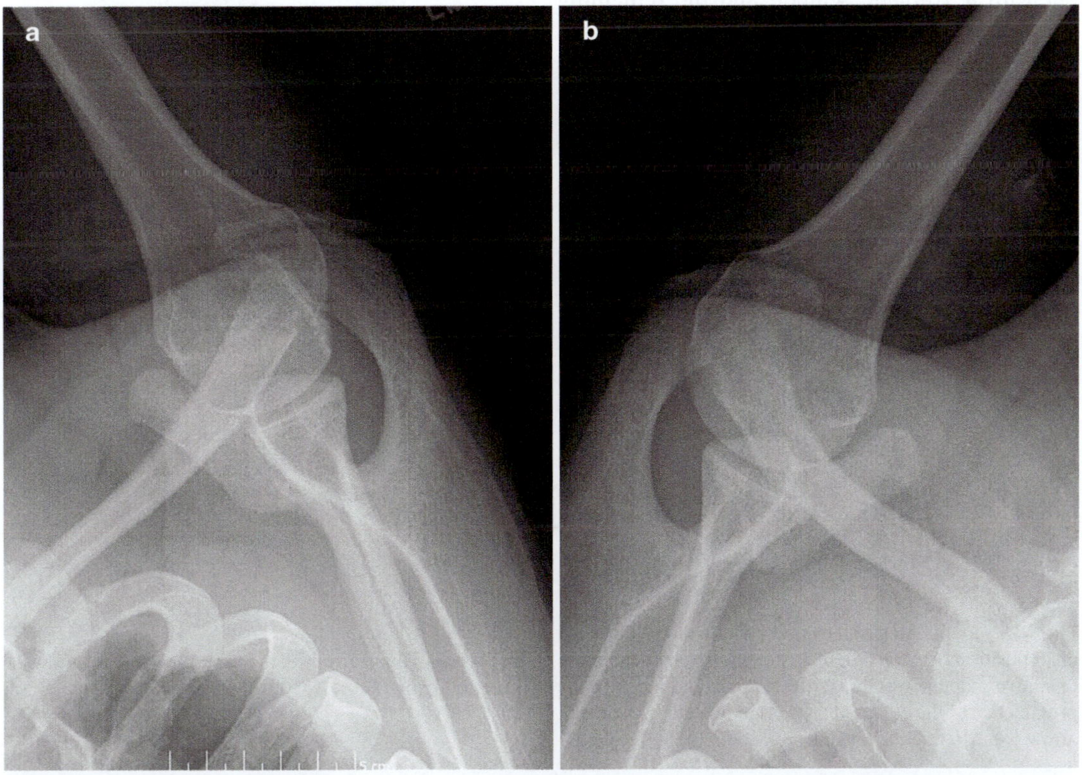

Fig. 18.5 Comparison of right (**a**) and left (**b**) Bernageau views. The right side is the affected side with recurrent episodes of glenohumeral instability. (**a**) shows loss of the anterior glenoid when compared to (**b**) (the unaffected left side)

Positioning

The shoulder girdle is shaved, and the patients are told to shower with an antibacterial soap the night prior to surgery. The patient is given an interscalene block by the anesthesia service. General anesthesia is then administered. We position the patient in the modified beach chair position with the patient torso moved toward the operative side of the bed until the lateral shoulder is even with edge of the bed. We do not move the patient so far laterally that the arm hangs off the operative table. A 1-cm thick folded sheet is then placed under the operative scapula to stabilize the scapula and increase the prominence of the coracoid process (Fig. 18.7).

Surgical Approach

The skin incision is marked from the tip of the coracoid process superiorly proceeding inferiorly toward the axillary fold and is about 5 cm in length (Fig. 18.8). The epidermis and dermis are cut with a 10-blade scalpel, and the remaining subcutaneous tissue is divided with use of an electrocautery. Meticulous hemostasis is maintained throughout the procedure. Superiorly and medially in the incision, the deltopectoral interval is exposed by first identifying the area devoid of muscle between the deltoid and pectoralis major. The cephalic vein is then identified and retracted laterally while the intermuscular plane is developed with use of right-angle retractors. Frequently, crossing branches of the cephalic vein are identified within the deltopectoral interval. These are cauterized with electrocautery or, in cases of prominent vessels, ligated with braided absorbable suture. A self-retaining retractor is then placed between the deltoid and pectoralis major muscle exposing the clavipectoral fascia. Mayo scissors are used to clear space superiorly to the coracoid process, which should now be readily palpable. The Mayo scissors are removed and a Hohman retractor is placed over the coracoid process, thus obtaining full exposure of the coracoid process (Fig. 18.9).

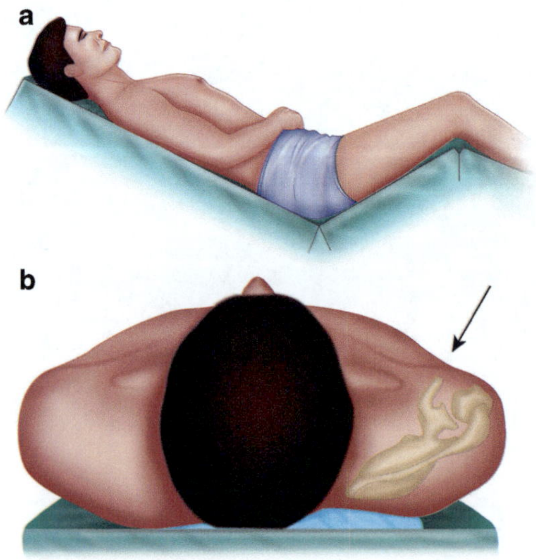

Fig. 18.7 Positioning of the patient in the modified beach chair position (**a**). A 1-cm thick sheet is placed behind the operative scapula to stabilize the scapula and increase the prominence of the coracoid process indicated by the black arrow (**b**). Modified from Edwards et al. 2012 [9]

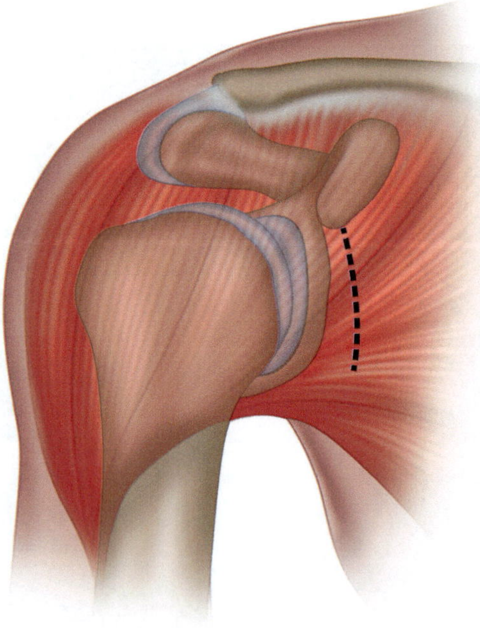

Fig. 18.8 Illustration of the skin incision for an open Latarjet procedure. (Modified from Edwards et al. 2012 [9])

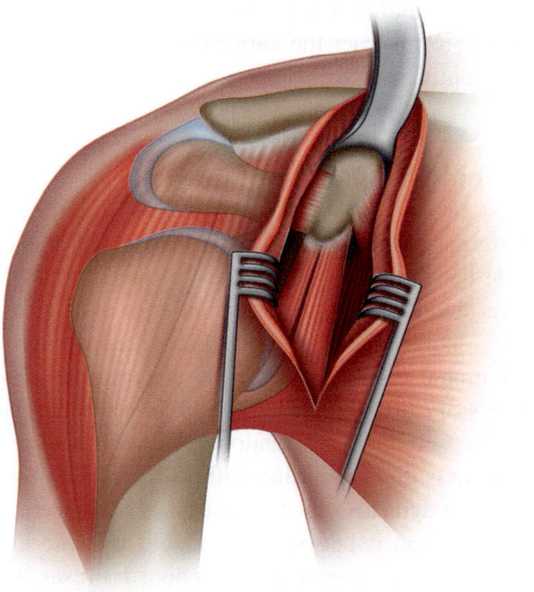

Fig. 18.9 Illustration of the full exposure of the coracoid process. (Modified from Edwards et al. 2012 [9])

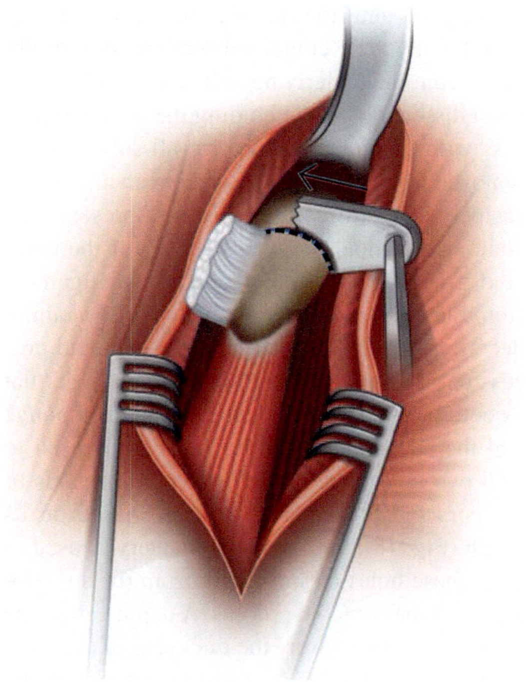

Fig. 18.10 The coracoid osteotomy is performed with a 90-degree reciprocating saw from medial to lateral in order to protect vital neurovascular structures. (Modified from Edwards et al. 2012 [9])

Coracoid Graft Harvest and Preparation

With the arm abducted and externally rotated, the leading edge of the coracoacromial ligament is identified. The coracoacromial ligament is followed to its insertion on the acromion and is released off of the acromion with electrocautery. At least 1 cm of coracoacromial ligament is necessary for reconstruction of the anterior glenohumeral capsule at the end of the procedure. The arm is then brought back into an adducted and internally rotated position to expose the medial aspect of the coracoid. Fibers of the pectoralis minor tendon are identified on the medial aspect of the coracoid. The pectoralis minor tendon is released with electrocautery from the coracoid, but care should be taken to avoid the blood supply of the coracoid process which typically enters at the distal aspect of the coracoid. At this point, a periosteal elevator is utilized to clear the soft tissue from the medial coracoid posteriorly to the level of the flexure of the coracoid process. This elevator is used to retract the tissues medially to the coracoid while a micro sagittal saw equipped with a 90-degree blade is inserted down to the flexure of the coracoid. The periosteal elevator is then removed, and two hands are used to control the saw (Fig. 18.10). The saw is used to osteotomize the coracoid from medial to lateral. At times, it may be necessary to complete the osteotomy with a periosteal elevator. Lahey grasping forceps are then used to grasp the coracoid and the arm is abducted and externally rotated. Finally, the coracohumeral ligament is released from the inferolateral aspect of the coracoid, thus freeing the coracoid process.

The arm is returned to the adducted and internally rotated position, and a gauze sponge is then placed over the distal portion of the incision to protect the skin distally during coracoid preparation. The coracoid process is then everted toward the surgeon until the inferior surface is pointing superficially. The conjoined tendon is carefully freed from the underlying soft tissue with use of blunt dissection. While holding the coracoid process with the grasping forceps, all soft tissue is removed from the inferior surface with a 10-blade scalpel while still being mindful to preserve the conjoined tendon, the blood supply of the coracoid process, and the coracoacromial ligament stump laterally. The saw is then utilized again to decorticate the undersurface of the coracoid process until a flat surface is obtained. A wide, flat osteotome is placed between the gauze sponge and the coracoid. A 3.2 mm drill bit is used to drill two holes perpendicular to the long axis of the coracoid process and centered based on its width (Fig. 18.11). The electrocautery is used to clear these holes of soft tissue from the superior aspect of the coracoid process. A depth gauge can then be used to measure the thickness of the coracoid process. The gauze sponge and osteotome are removed, and the coracoid process is then placed behind the medial arm of the self-retaining retractor holding the pectoralis major muscle so as not to obstruct the surgical view of the subscapularis muscle.

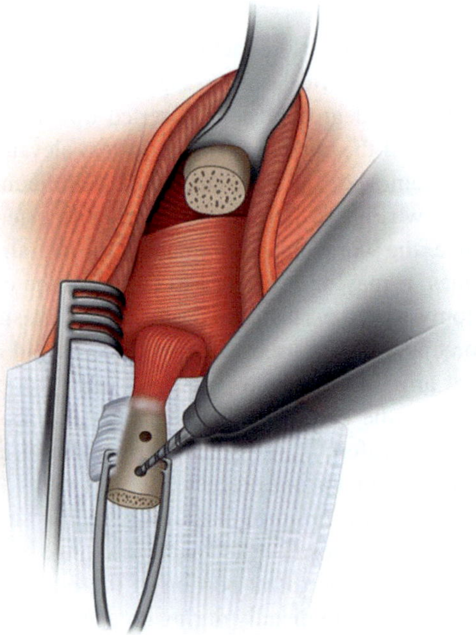

Fig. 18.11 The osteotomized coracoid process is inverted onto a gauze sponge and a 3.2 mm drill is used to pre-drill screw holes into the coracoid bone block. (Modified from Edwards et al. 2012 [9])

Glenoid Exposure

External rotation with the arm adducted at the side better facilitates exposure of the subscapularis tendon. The superior and inferior margins of the tendon are then identified. Occasionally, additional dissection with the electrocautery is necessary distally to identify the inferior margin of the subscapularis tendon. The subscapularis muscle is divided in line with its fibers with use of the mayo scissors. In most cases, the level of this division is between the middle and inferior thirds of the subscapularis tendon; however, in hyper lax patients, this level can be moved superiorly to the junction of the superior and middle thirds of the tendon to maximize the effect of the conjoined tendon sling. After a horizontal split is made in the muscle, the mayo scissors are then turned and spread in order to separate the subscapularis muscle fibers and expose the underlying joint capsule (Fig. 18.12). A gauze sponge is then packed into the subscapularis fossa between the anterior scapula and subscapularis muscle belly. This elevates the subscapularis off of the anterior joint capsule. A Hohman retractor is then placed deep to the gauze sponge on the anterior scapula to retract the medial soft tissues. Another Hohman retractor is placed along the inferior glenoid neck to retract the inferior portion of the subscapularis. A 10-blade scalpel is used to further split the subscapularis muscle and tendon laterally though care should be taken not to violate the joint capsule deep to the tendon. The joint line of the glenohumeral joint is then palpated. A 1 cm vertical capsulotomy is then made with a 10-blade scalpel, and the articular cartilage of the humeral head should be visualized (Fig. 18.13). A humeral head retractor is then placed into the glenohumeral joint to aid in posterior retraction of the humeral head (we prefer a Trillat retractor). The superior portion of the subscapularis muscle is then retracted superiorly and held there by placement of a large Steinmann pin into the

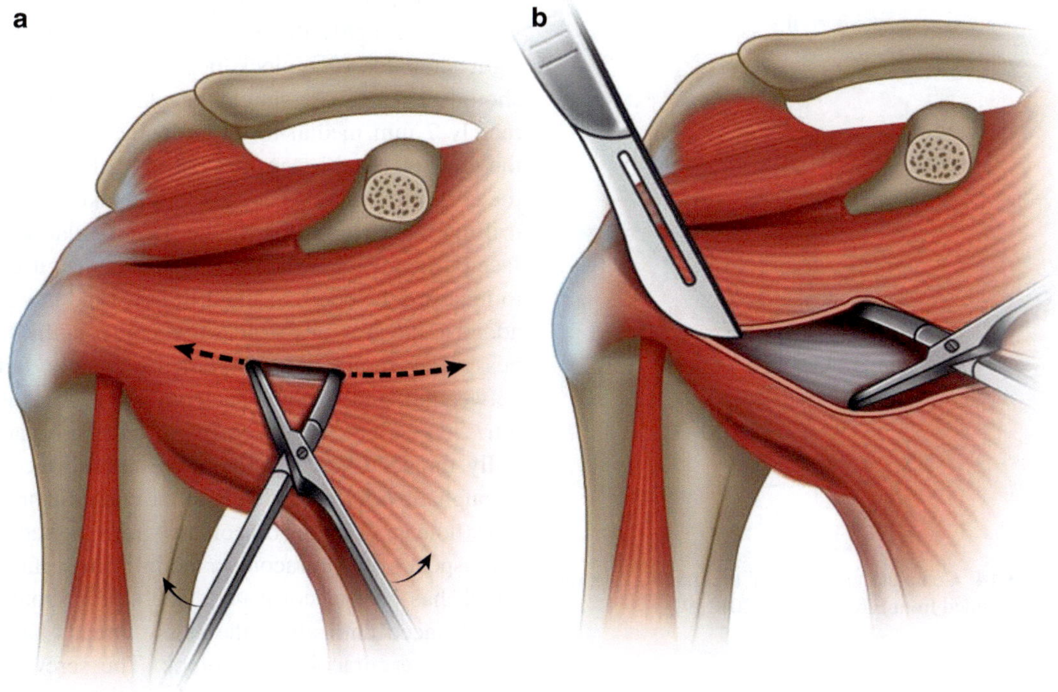

Fig. 18.12 (**a**) A longitudinal split is made in the subscapularis muscle belly at one-half to two-thirds of the width of the muscle belly. (**b**) The muscle fibers are separated to expose the underlying joint capsule, and a scalpel is used to longitudinally split the subscapularis tendon to its insertion on the lesser tuberosity. (Modified from Edwards et al. 2012 [9])

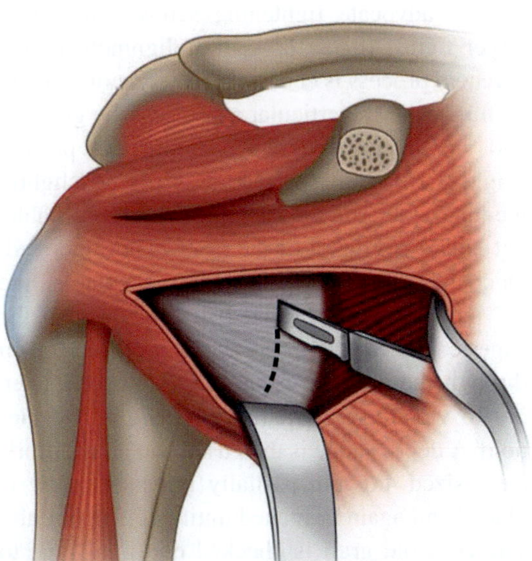

Fig. 18.13 A vertical capsulotomy is made with a scalpel. (Modified from Edwards et al. 2012 [9])

base of the coracoid or surgical neck of the scapula taking care that this pin does not violate the glenoid articular surface. The medial Hohman retractor is then replaced by a Bankart retractor, completing the exposure of the anterior glenoid (Fig. 18.14).

Preparation of the Anterior Glenoid and Graft Fixation

The anteroinferior glenoid labrum is transected with use of electrocautery starting laterally and extending medially about 2 cm past the articular surface. Care should be taken not to damage the articular cartilage of the glenoid. The soft tissue is then incised superiorly about 3 cm and then back laterally, again being careful to avoid damage to the articular cartilage (Fig. 18.15). The labral tissue and periosteum are then retracted medially with Metzenbaum scissors and an

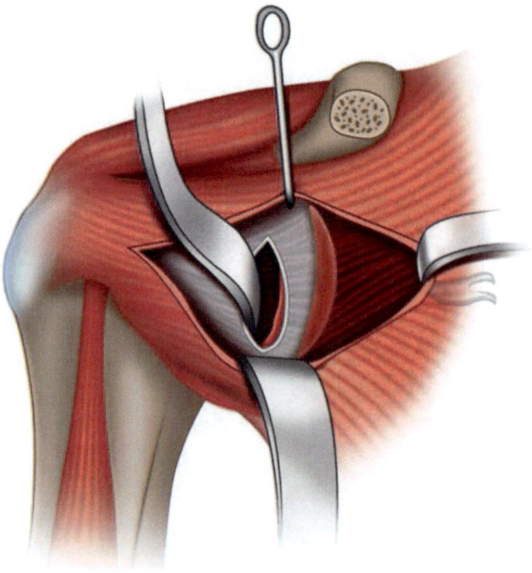

Fig. 18.14 Complete exposure of the anterior glenoid rim. (Modified from Edwards et al. 2012 [9])

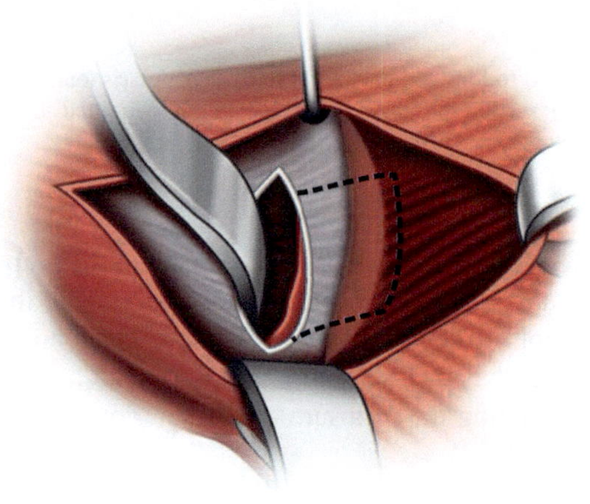

Fig. 18.15 The anterior glenoid capsulolabral complex is outlined. This is removed and the bone prepared for bone graft placement. (Modified from Edwards et al. 2012 [9])

osteotome is used to prepare the anteroinferior glenoid and detach the labrum and periosteum previously incised. The soft tissue components of the Bankart lesion are then removed. An osteotome or rongeur are then further utilized to roughen the anterior scapula to stimulate healing of the coracoid process. A 3.2 mm drill bit is then used to drill and anterior to posterior hole in the scapula at roughly the 5 o'clock position in the right shoulder (7 o'clock position for the left shoulder). The hole should be placed approximately 7 mm medial to the articular surface of the glenoid, but this can vary based on the size of the coracoid process. Care should be taken when drilling this hole not to violate the articular surface of the glenoid. The depth gauge is then used to measure the depth of the drill hole, and this is added to the previously measured coracoid thickness. The summed measurements usually fall between 30 and 40 mm. The coracoid process is retrieved with the Lahey grasping forceps. A partially threaded 4.0 mm screw is then advanced through the inferior drill hole of the coracoid process (hole nearest the coracoid tip) from the superior aspect of the coracoid to the inferior surface which has been decorticated. The screw should be advanced until all of the screw threads have cleared the coracoid bone block. The screw is then placed into the drilled hole in the anterior glenoid neck and advanced utilizing forceps to control the orientation of the coracoid process until it is secured to the anterior glenoid. Care should be taken not to overtighten the screw to avoid fracturing the coracoid bone graft. The authors advocate tightening screws until two-finger tight. At this time, the alignment of the coracoid process is checked. The coracoid should be flush with the articular surface of the glenoid, and no lateral overhang should be present (Fig. 18.16). If the coracoid is placed slightly medial to the articular surface, this is acceptable, but lateral overhang of the graft is not tolerated. Once the coracoid position is acceptable, the 3.2 mm drill bit is utilized to drill through the superior hole in the coracoid graft and then through the scapula. Again, care must be taken not to violate the articular cartilage of the glenoid. A depth gauge is then used and an appropriately sized 4.0 mm partially threaded screw is placed and again tightened until two-finger tight. The coracoid graft is checked one final time to ensure acceptable position.

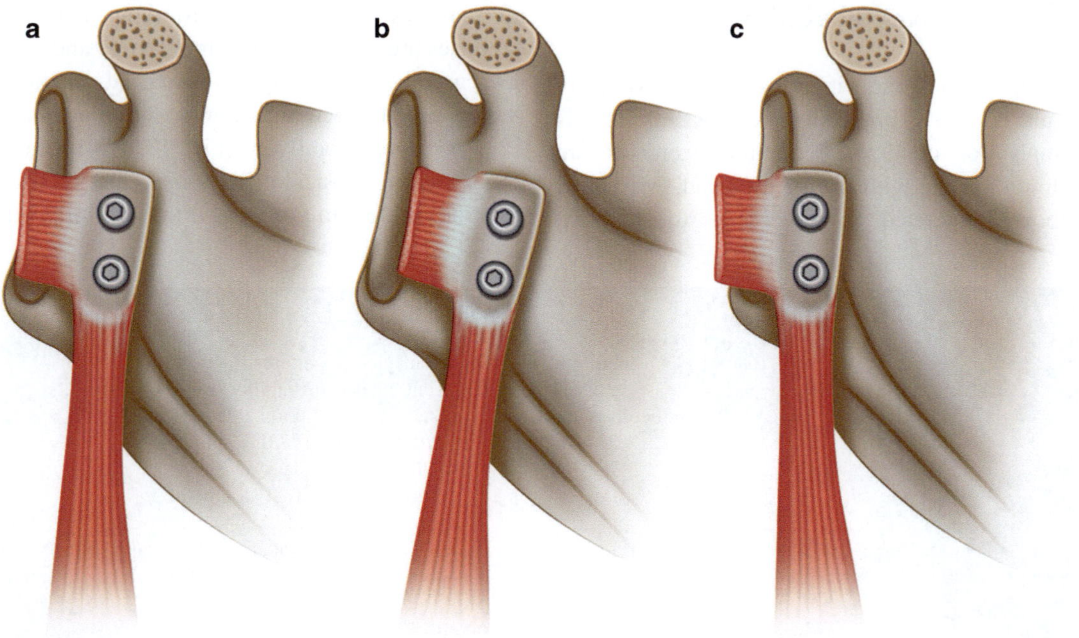

Fig. 18.16 (**a**) proper coracoid graft placement. (**b**) Graft placement too medial increasing the risk of recurrent instability. (**c**) Graft placement too lateral increasing the risk of graft-induced arthrosis of the glenohumeral joint. (Modified from Edwards et al. 2012 [9])

Anterior Capsule Reconstruction and Closure

A number 0 nonabsorbable suture is then passed through the stump of the coracoacromial ligament. The humeral head retractor is removed and the arm is brought into external rotation. The suture is then passed through the anterior capsule and inferior glenohumeral ligament of the humerus. The position of the arm in this step is important to avoid overtightening the shoulder postoperatively. The same suture is then utilized to pass a second stitch superior to the first stitch to further repair the coracoacromial ligament stump to the anterior capsule of the humerus and complete the technical aspects of the Latarjet procedure (Fig. 18.17). The medial Bankart retractor is removed and the sponge from the subscapularis fossa is then removed. The Steinmann pin and remaining retractors are removed. We do not repair the split in the subscapularis. The wound is thoroughly irrigated and is closed in layers.

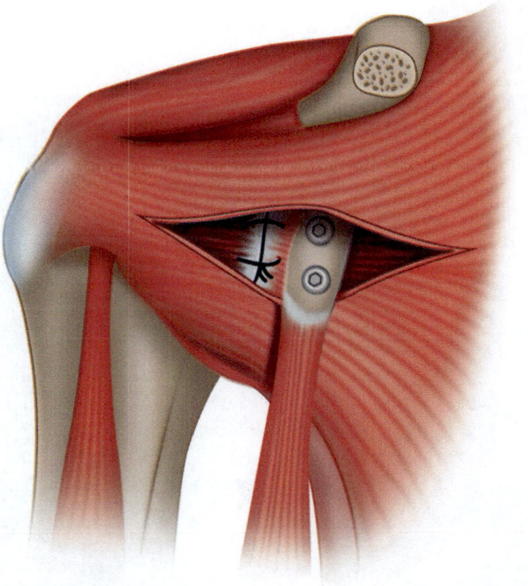

Fig. 18.17 Final repair construct with repair of the CA ligament stump to the humeral capsular insertion. (Modified from Edwards et al. 2012 [9])

Postoperative Rehabilitation

Postoperatively, the patient's operative extremity is placed into a simple sling for 2 weeks. This is simply for comfort. Pendulum exercises are allowed, along with use of the hand, wrist, and elbow as tolerated. By 6 weeks postoperatively, all activities of daily living are allowed. Home exercises are utilized focusing on active and passive mobility including full external rotation. X-rays are obtained at follow-up visits at 6 and 12 weeks postoperatively (Fig. 18.18). In most cases, formal physical therapy is not used, but if a patient is slow to progress, it may be initiated.

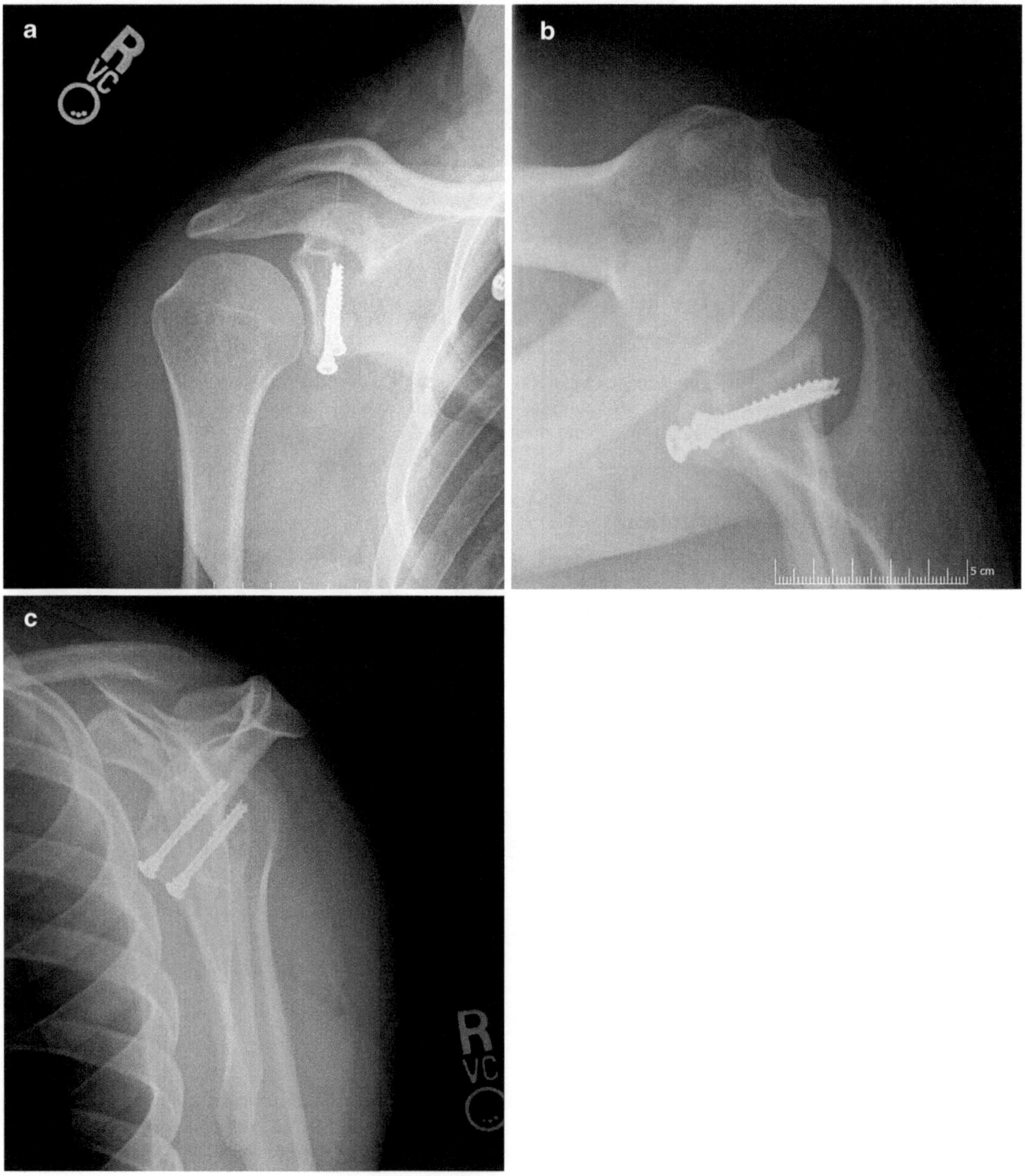

Fig. 18.18 Postoperative radiographs following right-sided Latarjet procedure, including Grashey (**a**), axillary (**b**), and scapular Y (**c**)

Return to sports has been reported in the literature from 3 to 9 months postoperatively [50–52]. It is the authors' experience that most patients are able to be released back to full participation in sports, including contact sports, at 3 months postoperatively.

Results

Several studies have been recently published evaluating patient satisfaction, return to play, and recurrence rates among patients who have undergone an open Latarjet procedure. Ialenti et al. published a systematic review and metanalysis of open Latarjet vs. open Bankart repair vs. arthroscopic Bankart repair. They found that in their analysis of 1036 patients in total, 353 underwent an open Latarjet procedure. Patients who had an arthroscopic Bankart repair or an open Latarjet returned to sport at significantly higher rates, 71% and 73% respectively, compared to open Bankart repair. In terms of recurrency of instability, the open Latarjet outperformed the other two procedures with a recurrence rate of 3.5% [53]. Ranalletta et al. published a cohort of 50 collision sport athletes who underwent an open Latarjet with the congruent arc modification without anterior capsular reconstruction with at least 2 years of follow-up. They found no significant change in postoperative ROM compared to preop. All patients had significant increases in their ROWE, VAS, and ASOSS scores. The rate of return to previous level of play was 93.7%. They had no patients who report recurrence [54]. Periera et al. published a metanalysis of eight studies examining the open Latarjet in collision athletes. They found that the return to sport rate varied between studies from 67% to 100%. They also found that patients reported high satisfaction rates from 93% to 100% [55]. Hurley et al. published a systematic review of return to play following an open Latarjet procedure. They ultimately evaluated 2134 cases and found an overall 88% return to play rate with 72% feeling they returned to the same level. When the patients were broken down by type of sport, they found that collision athletes had an 88% return to play with 69.5% feeling they returned to the same level. Overhead athletes had a 90% return to sport and 80% felt they returned to the same level [56].

Overall, the authors feel that the procedure has had success in their practices and have reported previously a 96% rate of return to sport in a cohort of 26 athletes treated with the procedure as well as a 3.5% rate of recurrence following the procedure [57].

Complications

The rate of complications following the Latarjet procedure has been reported in the literature between 5% and 30% [41, 58]. They can be divided into intraoperative complications or postoperative complications. Intraoperative complications include graft malposition, graft fracture, nerve injury, and vascular injury. Postoperative complications include hematoma, infection, neuropraxia, nonunion, osteolysis, and arthritis [44]. It is the authors' belief that the vast majority of complications seen following the Latarjet procedure are secondary to improper surgical technique.

Graft malposition has long been known to cause suboptimal outcomes from a Latarjet procedure. The most significant of which is if the graft is positioned too lateral, as this leads to the development of arthritis and can be a devastating complication in a young active individual [59, 60]. If a graft is placed too superiorly, the suprascapular nerve is at risk from the superior screw. Additionally, there is a loss of some tension of the conjoined tendon over the subscapularis which leads to some loss of the "sling effect" leading to higher rates of recurrent instability. The graft should be placed below the equator of the glenoid [61]. When the graft is placed too far inferiorly, there is a danger of loss of fixation of the inferior screw. When this occurs, there is a risk of failure of fixation or nonunion. Single screw fixation constructs have higher rates of these complications [62]. Finally, if the graft is placed too medially, there is a loss of some of the bone block effect and some increase in rate of recurrence [60]. The optimal position of the coracoid bone graft should be even with the subchondral bone medial to lateral, and the proximal coracoid should be at the level of the equator of the glenoid. Graft fracture is also a complication that can significantly alter the outcomes following a Latarjet or make a straightforward operation very difficult to salvage. The overall graft fracture rate is about 1.5% [41], but avoiding drilling holes in the coracoid larger than 3.2 mm can lower this rate. Additionally, care must be taken when tightening screws. Use of the two-finger tightening technique will help to avoid graft fracture intraoperatively [44].

Nerve injury intraoperatively has been widely reported from 1.5% to 20% following a Latarjet procedure [41, 42, 45, 58]. The axillary nerve has been most commonly reported as the nerve being injured, followed by the musculocutaneous and the suprascapular nerve. Our own reported incidence of nerve injury was 13 (3.1%) in a cohort of 416 Latarjet procedures. Of these 13 nerve injuries, 11 recovered in the immediate postoperative period [58]. Delaney et al. utilized intraoperative neuromonitoring during their open Latarjet procedures and found a 20% incidence of nerve injury, all of which resolved. The neuropraxias correlated with an increase in operative time [45]. These findings are extremely important and demonstrate the importance of efficiency in the operating room to minimize the amount of time retractors are being used to retract neurovascular structures. Vascular injuries have also been reported with the procedure with an incidence of 1.4% [41].

The complications of postoperative hematoma and infection have been reported in the literature. Hematoma risk can be lowered through meticulous hemostasis maintained throughout the procedure. Superficial infection has been reported as high as 6% [42]. Nonunion and osteolysis have also been reported as high as 9.1% and 59.5%, respectively. Interestingly, both of these complications appear to only be found on imaging and have no clinical implications [41, 60, 63]. Arthritis is a complication of the procedure and, as discussed above, is usually related to improper graft placement. Long-term follow-up from the procedure has shown development of arthrosis over time. At 15 years, Hovelius et al. reported a 14% development of moderate arthrosis and a 35% development of mild arthrosis in 118 shoulders [64]. Their group then followed their results out to 33 to 35 years of follow-up in 31 shoulders and found 23% mild arthrosis, 27% moderate arthrosis, and 11% severe arthrosis. All patients said they were either satisfied or very satisfied with the procedure [65]. Mizuno et al. reported a 20% rate of arthritis at 20 years following the procedure [66]. The authors' own cohort of patients have shown a development of 14% mild arthrosis, 5% moderate arthrosis, and 0.4% severe arthrosis at an average of 6.5 years following a Latarjet procedure when the patients had no preoperative findings of arthritis [67].

Conclusions

Glenohumeral instability is a complex problem for patients. Its cause is likely multifactorial, and so there are a host of options to treat patients with instability of the glenohumeral joint. Currently, the preferred algorithm for the authors' practice in treating glenohumeral instability is to use an arthroscopic technique to perform a Bankart repair in cases where there is minimal or no bone loss and there is sufficient soft tissue to repair. In cases where there is significant bone loss, greater than 10% in our practice, or loss of the capsulolabral complex, we prefer the open Latarjet to address glenohumeral instability. The biggest exception to this algorithm is the overhead throwing athlete with involvement of the dominant arm. For this patient, we prefer an arthroscopic Bankart repair and use the open Latarjet as a salvage as return to high-level throwing following a Latarjet is unpredictable. We have rarely seen the need to add a remplissage to our cases of glenohumeral instability. Our patients with engaging lesions almost always have glenoid bone loss which is addressed with an open Latarjet. In doing so, these "off-track" lesions are converted to "on-track" lesions without addressing the Hill-Sachs lesion.

The utility of arthroscopic procedures will continue to grow in the future. As we have seen in the past moving from open rotator cuff repair to arthroscopic rotator cuff repair and moving from open Bankart repair to arthroscopic Bankart repair, it stands to reason that perhaps we will move to an arthroscopic Latarjet in the future. Currently, however, the data shows outcomes to be equivalent between the arthroscopic and open Latarjet. The arthroscopic Latarjet has been shown to be technically challenging, have a steep learning curve, and be more expensive than the open Latarjet [68–71]. In our hands, the open Latarjet is efficient and effective in addressing glenohumeral instability. While the arthroscopic Latarjet's utilization may increase in the future, we still advocate for a thorough understanding of the open approach to address glenoid bone loss prior to attempting to address glenoid bone loss arthroscopically.

References

1. Eden R. Zur Operation der habituellen Schulterluxation unter Mitteilung eines neuen verfahrens bei Abriß am inneren Pfannenrande. Deutsche Zeitschrift f Chirurgie. 1918;144(3–4):269–80.
2. van der Linde JA, van Wijngaarden R, Somford MP, van Deurzen DFP, van den Bekerom MPJ. The Bristow–Latarjet procedure, a historical note on a technique in comeback. Knee Surg Sports Traumatol Arthrosc 2016;24(2):470–478.
3. Hybbinette S (r). De la transplantation d'un fragment osseux pour remédier aux luxations récidivantes de l'épaule: Constatations et résultats opératoires. Acta Chir Scand 1932;71(411–445):26.
4. Oudard P. La Luxation Recidivante de L' paule (Variet6 Antero Interne). Proc Operatoire J Chi (Paris) 1924;23:13–25.
5. Latarjet M. Treatment of recurrent dislocation of the shoulder. Lyon Chir. 1954;49(8):994–7.
6. Trillat A. Treatment of recurrent dislocation of the shoulder; technical considerations. Lyon Chir. 1954;49(8):986–93.
7. Helfet AJ. Coracoid transplantation for recurring dislocation of the shoulder. J Bone Joint Surg Br. 1958;40-B(2):198–202.
8. Patte D, Debeyre J. Luxations récidivantes de l'épaule. Encycl Med Chir Paris-Technique chirurgicale. 1980;44265(4)
9. Edwards TB, Walch G. The Latarjet procedure for recurrent anterior shoulder instability: rationale and technique. Oper Tech Sport Med. 2012;20(1):57–64.
10. Burkhart SS, De Beer JF. Traumatic glenohumeral bone defects and their relationship to failure of arthroscopic Bankart repairs: significance of the inverted-pear glenoid and the humeral engaging Hill-Sachs lesion. Arthroscopy. 2000;16(7):677–94.
11. Lafosse L, Boyle S. Arthroscopic Latarjet procedure. J Shoulder Elb Surg. 2010;19(2):2–12.
12. Lafosse L, Lejeune E, Bouchard A, Kakuda C, Gobezie R, Kochhar T. The arthroscopic Latarjet procedure for the treatment of anterior shoulder instability. Arthroscopy. 2007;23(11):1242.e1–5.
13. Boileau P, Bicknell RT, El Fegoun AB, Chuinard C. Arthroscopic Bristow procedure for anterior instability in shoulders with a stretched or deficient capsule: the "belt-and-suspenders" operative technique and preliminary results. Arthroscopy. 2007;23(6):593–601.
14. Gill TJ, Micheli LJ, Gebhard F, Binder C. Bankart repair for anterior instability of the shoulder. Long-term outcome. J Bone Joint Surg Am. 1997;79(6):850–7.
15. Castagna A, Markopoulos N, Conti M, Delle Rose G, Papadakou E, Garofalo R. Arthroscopic Bankart suture-anchor repair: radiological and clinical outcome at minimum 10 years of follow-up. Am J Sports Med. 2010;38(10):2012–6.
16. Plath JE, Aboalata M, Seppel G, Juretzko J, Waldt S, Vogt S, et al. Prevalence of and risk factors for dislocation arthropathy: radiological long-term outcome of arthroscopic Bankart repair in 100 shoulders at an average 13-year follow-up. Am J Sports Med. 2015;43(5):1084–90.
17. Rhee YG, Lim CT. Glenoid defect associated with anterior shoulder instability: results of open Bankart repair. Int Orthop. 2007;31(5):629–34.
18. Kim SH, Ha KI, Cho YB, Ryu BD, Oh I. Arthroscopic anterior stabilization of the shoulder: two to six-year follow-up. J Bone Joint Surg Am. 2003;85(8):1511–8.
19. Itoi E, Lee SB, Berglund LJ, Berge LL, An KN. The effect of a glenoid defect on anteroinferior stability of the shoulder after Bankart repair: a cadaveric study. J Bone Joint Surg Am. 2000;82(1):35–46.
20. Churchill RS, Moskal MJ, Lippitt SB, Matsen FA. Extracapsular Anatomically Contoured Anterior Glenoid Bone Grafting for Complex Glenohumeral Instability. Tech Shoulder Elbow Surg. 2001;2(3):210–8.
21. Chen AL, Hunt SA, Hawkins RJ, Zuckerman JD. Management of bone loss associated with recurrent anterior glenohumeral instability. Am J Sports Med. 2005;33(6):912–25.
22. Voos JE, Livermore RW, Feeley BT, Altchek DW, Williams RJ, Warren RF, et al. Prospective evaluation of arthroscopic Bankart repairs for anterior instability. Am J Sports Med. 2010;38(2):302–7.
23. Dekker TJ, Peebles LA, Bernhardson AS, Golijanin P, Di Giacomo G, Provencher MT. Limited predictive value of the instability severity index score: evaluation of 217 consecutive cases of recurrent anterior shoulder instability. J Shoulder Elb Surg. 2021;30(7):e414.

24. Bacilla P, Field LD, Savoie FH. Arthroscopic bankart repair in a high demand patient population. Arthroscopy: The Journal of Arthroscopic & Related Surgery. 1997;13(1):51–60.
25. Flinkkilä T, Hyvönen P, Ohtonen P, Leppilahti J. Arthroscopic Bankart repair: results and risk factors of recurrence of instability. Knee Surg Sports Traumatol Arthrosc. 2010;18(12):1752–8.
26. Gartsman GM, Roddey TS, Hammerman SM. Arthroscopic treatment of anterior-inferior Glenohumeral instability: two to five-year follow-up. J Bone Joint Surg. 2000;82(7):991.
27. Kandziora F, Jäger A, Bischof F, Herresthal J, Starker M, Mittlmeier T. Arthroscopic labrum refixation for post-traumatic anterior shoulder instability: suture anchor versus transglenoid fixation technique. Arthroscopy. 2000;16(4):359–66.
28. Pagnani MJ, Warren RF, Altchek DW, Wickiewicz TL, Anderson AF. Arthroscopic shoulder stabilization using transglenoid sutures: a four-year minimum followup. Am J Sports Med. 1996;24(4):459–67.
29. An VVG, Sivakumar BS, Phan K, Trantalis J. A systematic review and meta-analysis of clinical and patient-reported outcomes following two procedures for recurrent traumatic anterior instability of the shoulder: Latarjet procedure vs. Bankart repair. J Shoulder Elb Surg. 2016;25(5):853–63.
30. Galvin JW, Ernat JJ, Waterman BR, Stadecker MJ, Parada SA. The epidemiology and natural history of anterior shoulder instability. Curr Rev Musculoskelet Med. 2017;10(4):411–24.
31. Kasik CS, Rosen MR, Saper MG, Zondervan RL. High rate of return to sport in adolescent athletes following anterior shoulder stabilisation: a systematic review. J ISAKOS. 2019 Jan;4(1):33–40.
32. Ranalletta M, Rossi LA, Alonso Hidalgo I, Sirio A, Puig Dubois J, Maignon GD, et al. Arthroscopic stabilization after a first-time dislocation: collision versus contact athletes. Orthop J Sports Med. 2017;5(9):232596711772932.
33. Rossi LA, Tanoira I, Gorodischer T, Pasqualini I, Ranalletta M. Recurrence and revision rates with arthroscopic Bankart repair compared with the Latarjet procedure in competitive Rugby players with Glenohumeral instability and a glenoid bone loss <20. Am J Sports Med. 2021;49(4):866–72.
34. Torrance E, Clarke CJ, Monga P, Funk L, Walton MJ. Recurrence after arthroscopic labral repair for traumatic anterior instability in adolescent Rugby and contact athletes. Am J Sports Med. 2018;46(12):2969–74.
35. Kempf JF, Lacaze F, Hila A. Anterior instability and hyperlaxity of the shoulder. Rev Chir Orthop Reparatrice Appar Mot. 2000;86(Suppl 1):132–7.
36. Balg F, Boileau P. The instability severity index score. A simple pre-operative score to select patients for arthroscopic or open shoulder stabilisation. J Bone Joint Surg Br. 2007;89(11):1470–7.
37. Verweij LPE, van Spanning SH, Grillo A, Kerkhoffs GMMJ, Priester-Vink S, van Deurzen DFP, et al. Age, participation in competitive sports, bony lesions, ALPSA lesions, >1 preoperative dislocations, surgical delay and ISIS score>3 are risk factors for recurrence following arthroscopic Bankart repair: a systematic review and meta-analysis of 4584 shoulders. Knee Surg Sports Traumatol Arthrosc. 2021;29(12):4004–14.
38. Ruiz Ibán MA, Asenjo Gismero CV, Moros Marco S, Ruiz Díaz R, del Olmo Hernández T, del Monte Bello G, et al. Instability severity index score values below 7 do not predict recurrence after arthroscopic Bankart repair. Knee Surg Sports Traumatol Arthrosc. 2019;27(12):3905–11.
39. Weber SC. The instability severity index score in arthroscopic instability surgery (ISIS): failure to validate its predictive value in the selection of arthroscopic instability surgery. J Shoulder Elb Surg. 2014;23(9):e231.
40. Di Giacomo G, Peebles LA, Pugliese M, Dekker TJ, Golijanin P, Sanchez A, et al. Glenoid track instability management score: radiographic modification of the instability severity index score. Arthroscopy. 2020;36(1):56–67.
41. Flinkkilä T, Knape R, Nevalainen M, Sirniö K, Ohtonen P, Leppilahti J. Previous arthroscopic Bankart repair is an independent risk factor for an inferior outcome after Latarjet procedure. Orthop Traumatol Surg Res. 2019;105(8):1481–5.
42. Griesser MJ, Harris JD, McCoy BW, Hussain WM, Jones MH, Bishop JY, et al. Complications and reoperations after Bristow-Latarjet shoulder stabilization: a systematic review. J Shoulder Elb Surg. 2013;22(2):286–92.
43. Shah AA, Butler RB, Romanowski J, Goel D, Karadagli D, Warner JJP. Short-term complications of the Latarjet procedure. J Bone Joint Surg Am. 2012;94(6):495–501.
44. Longo UG, Loppini M, Rizzello G, Ciuffreda M, Berton A, Maffulli N, et al. Remplissage, humeral osteochondral grafts, weber osteotomy, and shoulder arthroplasty for the management of humeral bone defects in shoulder instability: systematic review and quantitative synthesis of the literature. Arthroscopy. 2014;30(12):1650–66.
45. Gupta A, Delaney R, Petkin K, Lafosse L. Complications of the Latarjet procedure. Curr Rev Musculoskelet Med. 2015;8(1):59–66.
46. Delaney RA, Freehill MT, Janfaza DR, Vlassakov KV, Higgins LD, Warner JJP. 2014 Neer award paper: neuromonitoring the Latarjet procedure. J Shoulder Elb Surg. 2014;23(10):1473–80.
47. Edwards TB, Walch G. The latarjet procedure for recurrent anterior shoulder instability: rationale and technique. Operat Tech Sport Med. 2002;10(1):25–32.
48. Bernageau J, Patte D, Debeyre J, Ferrane J. Value of the glenoid profile in recurrent luxations of the shoulder. Rev Chir Orthop Reparatrice Appar Mot. 1976;62(2 suppl):142–7.
49. Pansard E, Klouche S, Billot N, Rousselin B, Kraus TM, Bauer T, et al. Reliability and validity assess-

ment of a glenoid bone loss measurement using the Bernageau profile view in chronic anterior shoulder instability. J Shoulder Elb Surg. 2013;22(9):1193–8.
50. Edwards TB, Boulahia A, Walch G. Radiographic analysis of bone defects in chronic anterior shoulder instability. Arthroscopy. 2003;19(7):732–9.
51. Bohu Y, Abadie P, van Rooij F, Nover L, Société Française de Traumatologie du Sport, Kany J, et al. Latarjet procedure enables 73% to return to play within 8 months depending on preoperative SIRSI and Rowe scores. Knee Surg Sports Traumatol Arthrosc 2021;29(8):2606–2615.
52. Colegate-Stone TJ, van der Watt C, de Beer JF. Evaluation of functional outcomes and complications following modified Latarjet reconstruction in athletes with anterior shoulder instability. Shoulder Elb. 2015 Jul;7(3):168–73.
53. Gowd AK, Liu JN, Polce EM, Agarwalla A, Garcia GH, Nicholson GP, et al. Return to sport following Latarjet glenoid reconstruction for anterior shoulder instability. J Shoulder Elb Surg. 2021;30(11):2549–59.
54. Ialenti MN, Mulvihill JD, Feinstein M, Zhang AL, Feeley BT. Return to play following shoulder stabilization: a systematic review and meta-analysis. Orthop J Sports Med. 2017;5(9):232596711772605.
55. Ranalletta M, Rossi LA, Bertona A, Tanoira I, Hidalgo IA, Maignon GD, et al. Modified Latarjet without Capsulolabral repair in Rugby players with recurrent anterior Glenohumeral instability and significant glenoid bone loss. Am J Sports Med. 2018;46(4):795–800.
56. Paulino Pereira NR, van der Linde JA, Alkaduhimi H, Longo UG, van den Bekerom MPJ. Are collision athletes at a higher risk of re-dislocation after an open Bristow-Latarjet procedure? A systematic review and meta-analysis. Shoulder Elb. 2018;10(2):75–86.
57. Hurley ET, Montgomery C, Jamal MS, Shimozono Y, Ali Z, Pauzenberger L, et al. Return to play after the Latarjet procedure for anterior shoulder instability: a systematic review. Am J Sports Med. 2019;47(12):3002–8.
58. Cerciello S, Edwards TB, Walch G. Chronic anterior glenohumeral instability in soccer players: results for a series of 28 shoulders treated with the Latarjet procedure. J Orthopaed Traumatol. 2012;13(4):197–202.
59. Gartsman GM, Waggenspack WN, O'Connor DP, Elkousy HA, Edwards TB. Immediate and early complications of the open Latarjet procedure: a retrospective review of a large consecutive case series. J Shoulder Elb Surg. 2017;26(1):68–72.
60. Cassagnaud X, Maynou C, Mestdagh H. Clinical and computed tomography results of 106 Latarjet-Patte procedures at mean 7.5 year follow-up. Rev Chir Orthop Reparatrice Appar Mot. 2003;89(8):683–92.
61. Allain J, Goutallier D, Glorion C. Long-term results of the Latarjet procedure for the treatment of anterior instability of the shoulder. J Bone Joint Surg Am. 1998;80(6):841–52.
62. Hovelius L, Körner L, Lundberg B, Akermark C, Herberts P, Wredmark T, et al. The coracoid transfer for recurrent dislocation of the shoulder. Technical aspects of the Bristow-Latarjet procedure. J Bone Joint Surg Am. 1983;65(7):926–34.
63. Weppe F, Magnussen RA, Lustig S, Demey G, Neyret P, Servien E. A biomechanical evaluation of bicortical metal screw fixation versus absorbable interference screw fixation after coracoid transfer for anterior shoulder instability. Arthroscopy. 2011;27(10):1358–63.
64. Di Giacomo G, Costantini A, de Gasperis N, De Vita A, Lin BKH, Francone M, et al. Coracoid graft osteolysis after the Latarjet procedure for anteroinferior shoulder instability: a computed tomography scan study of twenty-six patients. J Shoulder Elb Surg. 2011;20(6):989–95.
65. Hovelius L, Sandström B, Saebö M. One hundred eighteen Bristow-Latarjet repairs for recurrent anterior dislocation of the shoulder prospectively followed for fifteen years: study II-the evolution of dislocation arthropathy. J Shoulder Elb Surg. 2006;15(3):279–89.
66. Gordins V, Hovelius L, Sandström B, Rahme H, Bergström U. Risk of arthropathy after the Bristow-Latarjet repair: a radiologic and clinical thirty-three to thirty-five years of follow-up of thirty-one shoulders. J Shoulder Elb Surg. 2015;24(5):691–9.
67. Mizuno N, Denard PJ, Raiss P, Melis B, Walch G. Long-term results of the Latarjet procedure for anterior instability of the shoulder. J Shoulder Elb Surg. 2014;23(11):1691–9.
68. Buscayret F, Edwards TB, Szabo I, Adeleine P, Coudane H, Walch G. Glenohumeral arthrosis in anterior instability before and after surgical treatment: incidence and contributing factors. Am J Sports Med. 2004;32(5):1165–72.
69. Hurley ET, Lim Fat D, Farrington SK, Mullett H. Open versus arthroscopic Latarjet procedure for anterior shoulder instability: a systematic review and meta-analysis. Am J Sports Med. 2019;47(5):1248–53.
70. Randelli P, Fossati C, Stoppani C, Evola FR, De Girolamo L. Open Latarjet versus arthroscopic Latarjet: clinical results and cost analysis. Knee Surg Sports Traumatol Arthrosc. 2016;24(2):526–32.
71. Zhu Y, Jiang C, Song G. Arthroscopic versus open Latarjet in the treatment of recurrent anterior shoulder dislocation with marked glenoid bone loss: a prospective comparative study. Am J Sports Med. 2017;45(7):1645–53.

The Arthroscopic Latarjet: Technical Tips and Keys to Success

19

Pascal Boileau, Juan David Lacouture, and Camilo Andres Estrada Cely

Introduction

Anterior dislocation of the glenohumeral joint is a common injury that affects patients across a wide range of age and levels of activity, with an increased frequency "in younger patients". It represents about 95% of shoulder dislocations, being the traumatic origin, the main cause [28]. The natural history demonstrates that patients younger than 22 years who initially are treated nonoperatively are likely to develop recurrent anterior glenohumeral instability (AGHI) in 67% of the cases. Of these populations, 40% eventually undergo stabilization surgery within 25 years follow-up [28].

Currently, it is possible to identify preopera tively those patients with an elevated risk of failure with the performance of Bankart surgery using the ISI score [3]. It has been demonstrated that those patients with an ISI score equal to or greater than 3 points have a high risk of failure with Bankart surgery. Perhaps one of the most important factors in the risk assessment is the definition of the bone defect (glenoid or humeral) that accompanies glenohumeral instability; it is clear that glenoid bone defects are present in up to 90% of cases of recurrent instability and that they may be associated with a posterosuperior humeral defect (Hill-Sachs) between 80% and 90% of cases [14, 23, 35, 53]. In those cases of a severe bone defect, a Bankart surgery has been shown to fail at an unacceptably high level [64].

The beauty of the Latarjet procedure resides in the fact that it allows the simultaneous treatment of two pathologies: The transferred coracoid bone block solves the problem of the glenoid deficiency (static, bony effect), whereas the lowered and medialized conjoined tendon, by lowering the inferior portion of the subscapularis muscle, solves the problem of the capsular deficiency. The coracoid process is a vascularized bone graft, located in situ, inside the shoulder; it is a combined graft (bony and tendinous) allowing a solution to complex instability cases with bony and capsular deficiency. The Latarjet procedure is superior to the iliac crest bone graft with less morbidity (avoiding second site surgery) and better efficiency to stabilize the shoulder (bony effect and sling or "seatbelt" effect provided by the conjoined tendon and lowered subscapularis).

The arthroscopic Latarjet procedure has been in the literature since 2007 [37]. Since then, the author (PB) has worked constantly to improve all possible technical aspects of the

P. Boileau (✉)
ICR-Institut de Chirurgie Réparatrice—Groupe KANTYS, Institute for Sports and Reconstructive Surgery, Nice, France
e-mail: pr.boileau@icr-nice.com

J. D. Lacouture · C. A. E. Cely
Orthopedics and Traumatology, Hospital Serena del Mar, Cartagena de Indias, Provincia de Cartagena, Bolívar, Colombia

© The Author(s), under exclusive license to Springer Nature Switzerland AG 2026

R. M. Frank, J. M. Tokish (eds.), *Management of Shoulder Instability*,
https://doi.org/10.1007/978-3-032-18089-6_19

arthroscopic technique, systematize it, and demonstrate its clinical and radiological effectiveness over all these years. Previously, he has raised the need to put into practice the arthroscopic technique, convinced that with appropriate training, including a cadaver performance and a surgical observation, this complex surgery is widely applicable [12].

Clinical Case

A 19-year-old male, right-handed, practicing sports (football) at a competitive level, 2 years ago has the first anterior dislocation episode during abduction and external rotation (ABER) movement in a football match that required reduction of the dislocation in the field by a physician, after the first dislocation has not presented new dislocation but referred 15 episodes of subluxation during the last year initially in movements of ABER in sports and after in these movements in daily life, at the moment stop competition in football because of his shoulder.

At the clinical examination, its identified hyperlaxity was defined by more than 90° of external rotation with the arm at the side (ER1) in the left and right shoulder as shown in Fig. 19.1, in specific maneuvers modified hyperabduction test (HAT) with more than 20° of difference between both shoulders in abduction and also the presence of soft end in the right shoulder (Fig. 19.2) with the presence of apprehension in 90° abduction and external rotation and also apprehension and relocation positive in the clinical examination (Fig. 19.3).

In the initial shoulder x-ray (Fig. 19.4), there is identified loss of contour of the inferior glenoid, no engaging Hill-Sachs defect, and no frac-

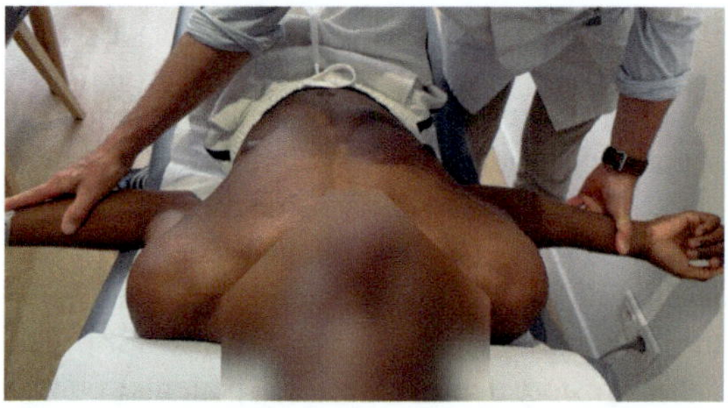

Fig. 19.1 Hyperlaxity was defined by more than 90° of external rotation with the arm at the side (ER1) in the left and right shoulder

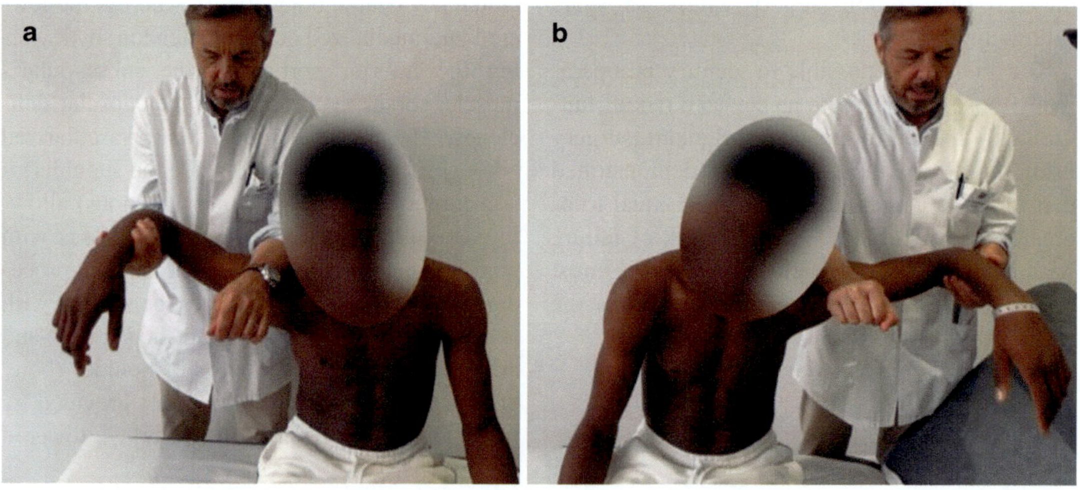

Fig. 19.2 Modified hyperabduction test (HAT) with more than 20° of difference between right (**a**) and left (**b**) shoulder

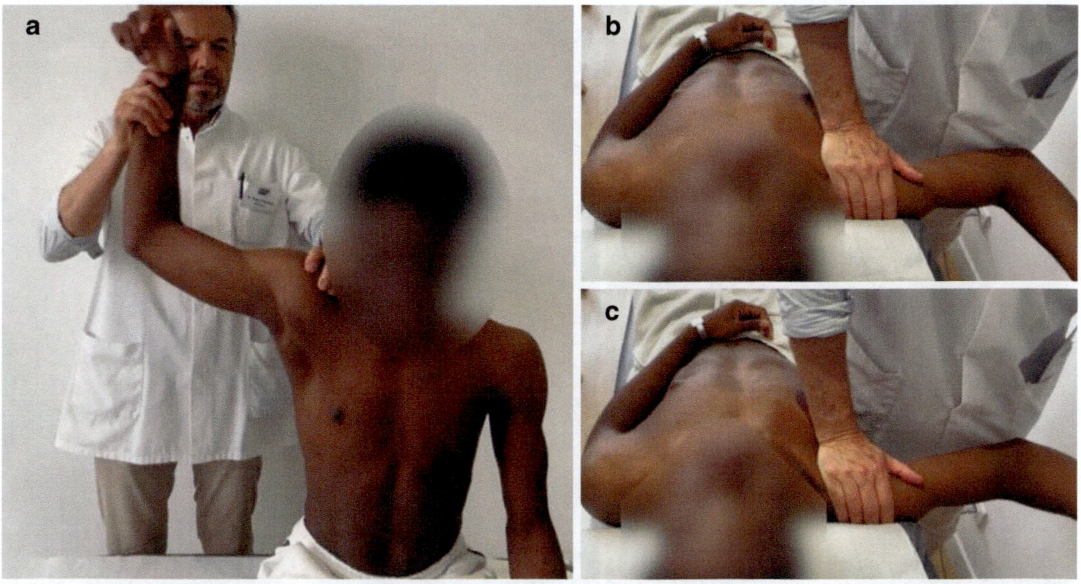

Fig. 19.3 Apprehension in 90° abduction and external rotation (**a**) and apprehension and relocation positive in the clinical examination (**b** and **c**)

Fig. 19.4 Shoulder x-ray. (**a**) AP projection with loss of glenoid contour in the inferior part. (**b**) Scapulohumeral projection

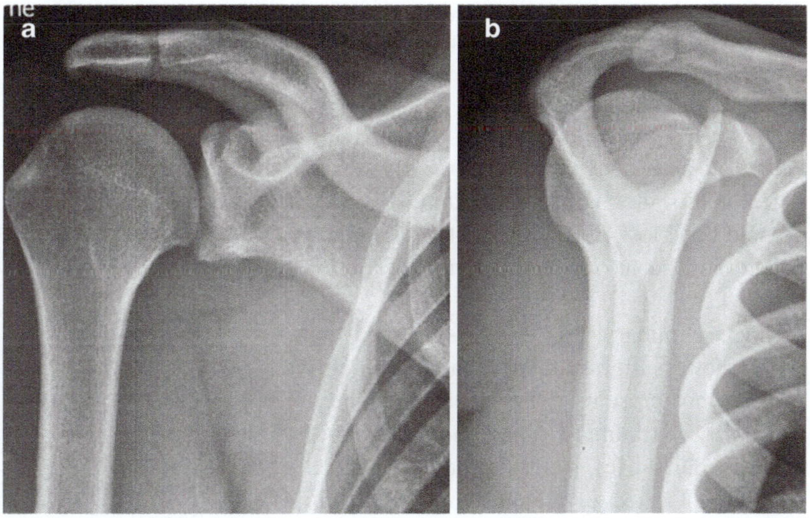

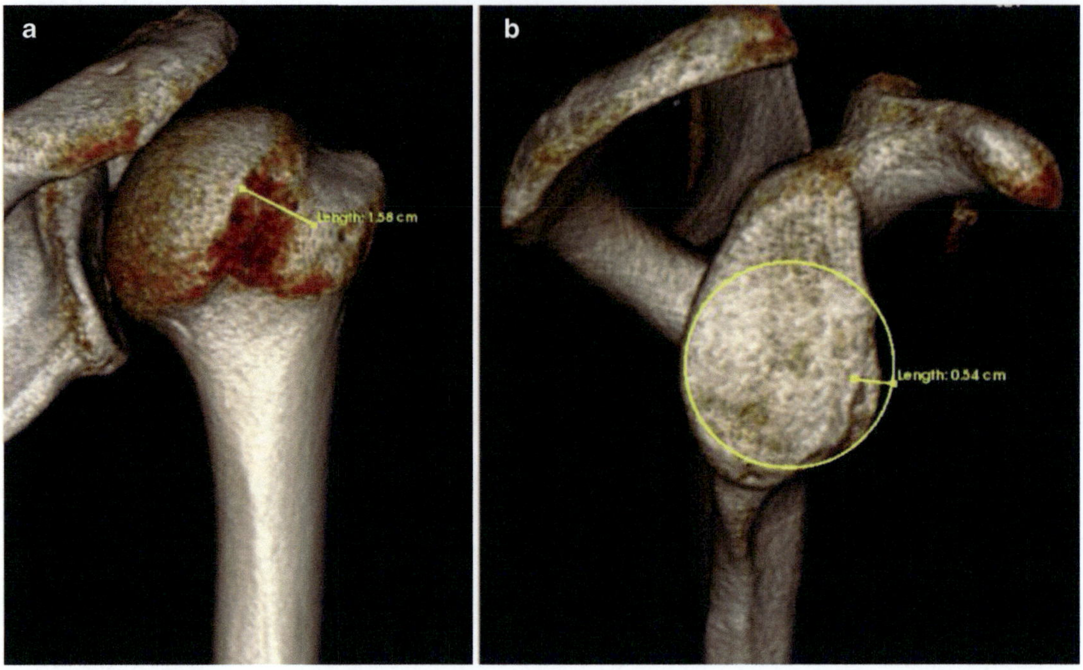

Fig. 19.5 Bone defect determined in 3D reconstruction CT scan. (**a**) Hill-Sachs lesion measured and determined on-track. (**b**) Glenoid bone loss measured best fit circle determined 20%. It is identified a medially healed bony Bankart lesion

ture. Posteriorly in CT scan imaging, it is described as a bony Bankart medially consolidated, and in the 3D reconstruction, it is a 20% glenoid bone loss (GBL) (best-fit circle method) and a Hill-Sachs lesions determined on-track (Fig. 19.5).

So in summary, this is a 19-year-old male, who practices high-risk sports at a competitive level, who presents with recurrent anterior instability (1 traumatic dislocation +15 subluxation in daily life), with shoulder hyperlaxity (ER1 > 90°), loss of glenoid contour in initial x-ray in which is considered an initial ISI score of 8/10 (Table 19.1), and posteriorly identified in CT scan a GBL of 20% with a medial consolidated bony Bankart and an on-track Hill-Sachs lesion. Due to the high risk of failure of a soft tissue procedure, a guided Latarjet is considered the best option with suture button fixation and Bankart repair.

Table 19.1 ISI score, highlighted the positive findings in the patient with a total score of 8/10

Age at surgery	
</= 20	2
> 20	0
Degree of sports participation	
Competitive	2
Recreational	0
Type of sport	
Contact or forced overhead	1
Other	0
Shoulder hyper-laxity	
Antero-inferior	1
Normal	0
Hill Sachs lesion	
Visible on ER view	2
Not visible on ER	0
Glenoid loss of contour	
Loss of contour	2
No lesion	0
Total	8/10

Etiology

To successfully treat shoulder instability, it is imperative to first understand the mechanism by which the humeral head is held reduced in the glenoid fossa. This is a complex biomechanical relationship among the osseous architecture, the static soft tissue stabilizers, and the dynamic soft tissue stabilizers. The glenoid itself serves as a pedestal on which the humeral head must balance. The native glenoid is larger in the inferior-superior direction than it is in the anteroposterior direction. This renders the shoulder particularly susceptible to instability in the axial plane. Even small derangements of its shape and bone stock have important consequences for stability, and the amount of "critical" bone loss remains controversial at this time [40].

In this regard, Burkhart et al. described the resulting changes to bone defects related to episodes of instability. In this aspect, Burkhart describes how the containment of the humeral head in the glenoid is due to two geometric variables: The first variable is the "deepening effect" of a wider glenoid due to the longer arc of its concave surface, especially the anterior glenoid rim which acts as a buttress. This typical morphology of the glenoid contributes to deepening it and, in this way, increases the resistance to the shear displacement forces exerted by the humeral head on it. In this sense, the loss of the osseous surface of the glenoid decreases the depth of the glenoid and the resistance to the shear forces that are associated with the episodes of luxation. The second variable described is the so-called effect of glenoid arc length, which explains how the vertical forces exerted by the humeral head are resisted by the surface of the glenoid, but once the vector of the forces changes, taking an orientation that exceeds the osseous edge, the forces are going to be concentrated on the bone-ligament union and the labrum, being able to generate a Bankart lesion. In the case of an osseous glenoid defect, the area of the glenoid that acts resisting the vertical forces of the humeral head decreases ("the safe arc"), increasing the concentration of loads exerted on the soft structures, mainly the labrum. In other words, it could be said that as there is a glenoid bone defect, the width of the glenoid track decreases and thereby increases the transmission of loads over adjacent soft tissues [15].

In the scenario of bone defects of the humeral head (Hill-Sachs), even in cases where there is no associated Bankart lesion, a phenomenon similar to subluxation may occur due to the lack of a joint segment of the humeral head, where the humeral defect can engage the anterior glenoid ridge. This phenomenon is known as the arc deficit joint [15].

Burkhart and Di Giacomo [20] described the behavior of simultaneous bone defects (glenoid and humeral), known as bipolar defects, and reinforced the initial description of engaging and nonengaging lesions, which is complemented by the concept of the glenoid track, described by Yamamoto et al. In this regard, the senior author (PB) argues that all bipolar bone defects are by definition engaging, whereas the mechanical explanation for the formation of the Hill-Sachs lesion in the context of glenohumeral dislocation indicates that there was an engagement and that subsequently, with a force applied large enough, the engagement mechanism will be reproduced.

Quantitative studies of images have confirmed the changes in soft tissues, secondary to repetitive episodes of luxation, especially the effect on the joint capsule as it elongates, being a contributing factor to instability due to the resulting functional insufficiency of the lower glenohumeral ligament, due to its disinsertion in the glenoid. Urayama et al. reported that the capsule undergoes a process of elongation in its anteroinferior and inferior portions, on average of 19% (from 2.6 to 6.7 mm) in shoulders with recurrent anterior dislocation [58]. Recent studies have confirmed these findings, associating other alterations in the capsular insertion on the glenoid, being much more frequent find in the insertion of capsular glenohumeral type III (in the classification of Moseley), which means a capsular insertion into a more medial position following the scapular neck. In addition, the authors found that patients with recurrent shoulder dislocations showed a greater postoperative increase in capsular length and capsular cross-sectional area [34, 45].

It is important to mention the role of hyperlaxity as a determining factor in the natural evolution of recurrent shoulder dislocation and as a decisive prognostic factor in surgical treatment. In this regard, it is necessary to consider possible associations between ligament hyperlaxity and anatomical variations in the morphology of coracoids and glenoids as predisposing factors of instability. Concerning the morphology of the glenoid, the mechanical factors described above allow us to understand its relevance and the anatomy of the coracoid; its importance lies in the fact that it is a soft tissue insertion point that acts as a buttress that prevents the anterior displacement of the glenoid, while the conjoined tendon acts as a seatbelt containing the anterior translation of the humeral head [50, 57]. Additionally, coracoid morphology can alter the line of pull of the subscapularis, which is an important anterior shoulder stabilizer [39]. In this sense, Owens et al. described anatomical variables related to increased risk of instability such as tall and thin glenoids, compared with short and wide glenoids and the coracohumeral distance as an independent risk factor for traumatic anterior instability (for each increase of 1 mm in the coracohumeral distance, the risk of instability increases by 20%) [48]. More recently, Jacxsens et al. corroborate this information from the results of their study, where they find that coracoid, acromial, and glenoid morphology differ between individuals with and without recurrent traumatic anterior shoulder instability, specifically in the following aspects: (1) shorter coracoid process angled more superomedially, (2) more vertically oriented acromion from a scapular spine, and (3) more anteriorly tilted glenoid that was flatter in the AP direction with a shape approximating an ellipse rather than a pear [32].

Indications

Boileau et al. established the most relevant clinical factors related to prognosis and the risk of recurrent instability after an arthroscopic Bankart procedure, becoming a practical tool to guide the type of treatment for each patient. The clinical factors were grouped within a score: The Instability Severity Index Score (ISI) includes patients aged under 20 years at the time of surgery, involvement in competitive or contact sports or those involving forced overhead activity, shoulder hyperlaxity, a Hill-Sachs lesion present on an anteroposterior radiograph of the shoulder in external rotation, and/or loss of the sclerotic inferior glenoid contour. From this, the close relationship between recurrent glenohumeral instability and patient-specific factors such as age and glenohumeral hyperlaxity as well as injury-related factors such as associated bone defects (bony Bankart and Hill-Sachs) was established [3, 5]. It was possible to establish a numerical relationship between the presence of these factors and the sum of points assigned for each one, with the result that the presence of 6 or more points in the evaluation is associated with a probability of recurrence of instability of 70% if only Bankart surgery is performed. Subsequently, the ISI score and the presence of bone lesions in the glenoid or humerus were established as parameters to define the type of surgery to be performed. An ISI score of 3 points was established as a cutoff. Patients with 3 or more points will require different interventions, depending on the presence of associated bone lesions [52]: (1) In the case of glenoid defects greater than 15%, it would be contraindicated to perform only interventions on soft tissues. For this, it is necessary to perform arthroscopic Latarjet + Bankart surgery. (2) In the case of presenting Hill-Sachs lesions with bone lesions less than 15% in glenoid, arthroscopic Bankart + remplissage should be performed. In combined lesions (glenoid bone lesion >15% and Hill-Sachs), Latarjet + remplissage + arthroscopic Bankart should be performed. Patients with less than 3 points without bone injury in the glenoid, benefit from arthroscopic Bankart surgery, however, in the presence of ligament hyperlaxity, the possibility of performing additional Trillat surgery should be evaluated. It is worth mentioning at this point that for some authors, the cutoff point that defines glenoid bone loss is 13.5%, especially in populations with high levels of physical activity [56].

It is necessary to consider the risk factors of recurrence for Latarjet surgery, within the evaluation and selection process of the patients for surgery. In this regard, Di Giacomo described the following: (1) atraumatic mechanism of primary shoulder dislocation (5 times greater risk of recurrence), (2) patients with bilateral shoulder instability (4 times greater), and (3) female patients (3 times) [21, 46].

Arthroscopic Latarjet

General Considerations

The transfer of the coracoid process with the attached conjoined tendon to the anteroinferior aspect of the glenoid rim for treatment of recurrent anterior dislocation of the shoulder was first described by Michel Latarjet in 1954 [38]. Four years later, Helfet described the Bristow procedure, which used only the tip of the coracoid process through a vertical split in the myotendinous junction of the subscapularis [27]. Since then, Gilles Walch popularized the "open Bristow-Latarjet procedure" [59] by transferring the coracoid process and the conjoined tendon onto the anterior neck of the glenoid. This procedure not only restores the glenoid bone defect but also reinforces the weak and definitively stretched anteroinferior capsule, with a mean follow-up of 20 years and a recurrence rate of 5.9%. The Latarjet procedure is an effective treatment option for recurrent anterior shoulder instability in patients with severe glenoid bone loss and capsular deficiency [13, 44]. Subsequently, the procedure was performed by arthroscopy which provides good visualization of the glenohumeral joint, facilitating accurate placement of the transferred coracoid bone block and in an extra-articular position, allowing secure labral repair and repair of associated lesions if needed (Hill-Sachs) [13]. The first description of an all-arthroscopic Latarjet procedure was by Lafosse et al. in 2007. They performed a coracoid transfer to the anteroinferior glenoid rim through a subscapularis split after complete resection of the anterior labrum and the joint capsule while achieving fixation with two cannulated screws [37].

The technique described is a complex procedure and requires a degree of experience and expertise. It is a reproducible technique, but it is reported that 20 arthroscopic Latarjet procedures were needed to achieve equal operating time to the open technique. The learning curve is important but the rate of adverse events reported in this arthroscopic series is similar to that reported with the traditional open Latarjet [24]. The safety, 90-day complication, and readmission profile of arthroscopic Latarjets are similar to open Latarjet procedure. That's why with appropriate training, the arthroscopic Latarjet procedure can be effective for the management of patients with complex shoulder instability [2, 16, 18, 31, 37].

Triple Blocking Effect

Lafosse et al. resected the anterior labrum and capsule in their arthroscopic Latarjet procedure, with the hypothesis that the anterior capsule regenerated after its resection but resulted in fibrous scar tissue that loses all proprioceptive capacity. Better results have been reported for stability when the Bristow-Latarjet procedure was associated with a capsular repair using suture anchors [29, 37].

Because of this concept, Boileau et al. (2010) described the arthroscopic Bankart-Bristow-Latarjet procedure (2B3), which combines a coracoid transfer fixed with a screw and the reattachment of the capsule and labrum to the native glenoid, rendering the bone graft extra-articular. The technical modification of adding a Bankart repair to the Bristow-Latarjet procedure stabilizes the shoulder by the so-called "triple blocking effect," as described by Patte and De-Beyre: (1) the "bony effect" of the transferred coracoid bone block; (2) the "bumper effect" of the capsulolabral repair (Bankart repair), which protects the humeral head from direct contact with the coracoid bone graft and theoretically reduces the risk of future glenohumeral osteoarthritis; and (3) the "sling effect," which is the main stabilizing mechanism of the Bristow-Latarjet procedure [9, 10, 13, 49] (Fig. 19.6).

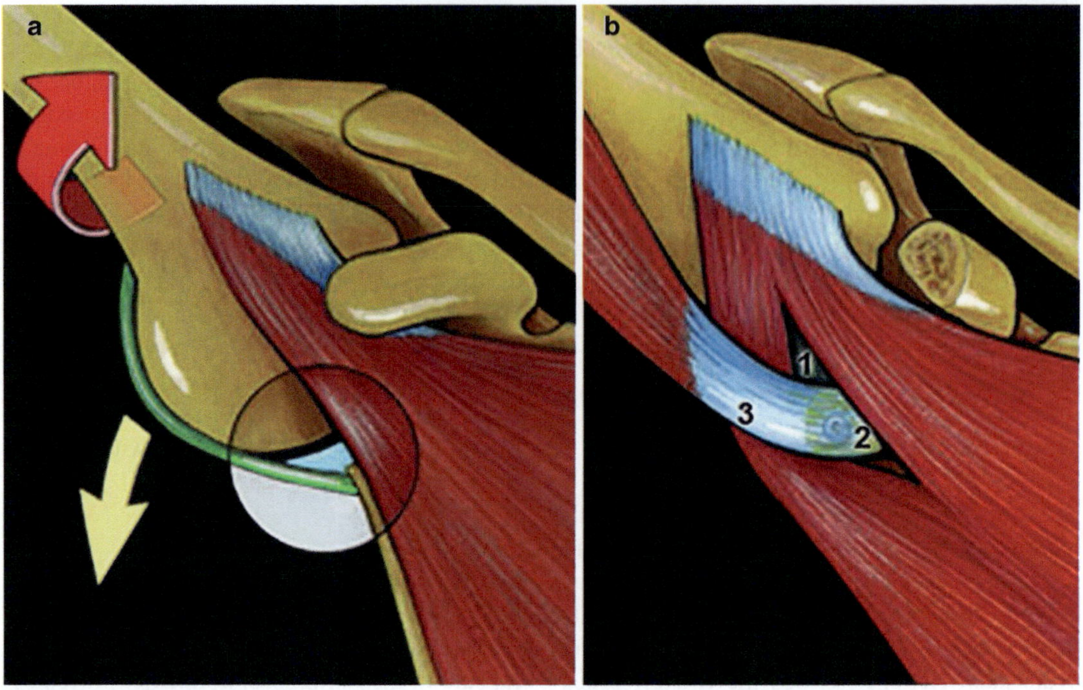

Fig. 19.6 The benefits of the Bristow-Latarjet-Bankart procedure are illustrated. (**a**) In the throwing position (abduction external rotation), the subscapularis slides over the equator, leaving only the weak detached anteroinferior labrum and stretched capsule to stabilize the humeral head. The 5 o'clock point is truly the vulnerable point of the glenoid rim. (**b**) By performing two procedures (Bankart + Latarjet), a triple blocking of the shoulder is obtained. (1) Bumper (Bankart), (2) bony effect (bone block), and (3) belt (or biceps) effect. (Reproduced from Boileau et al. [9, 10])

Guided Fixation Device

With improvements in arthroscopic techniques, the arthroscopic Latarjet procedure is becoming increasingly popular [6, 9, 10, 13, 36, 37, 47]. However, based on the literature and our experience, there are at least three drawbacks to arthroscopic techniques.

First, arthroscopic *positioning of the bone block* flush and the screws parallel to the glenoid surface is technically difficult. Many complications related to this procedure are attributed to graft malposition [1, 30, 60, 63]. The obliquity of the scapula on the thorax makes it challenging to place the screws strictly parallel to the glenoid surface [13, 43]. Excessive screw obliquity may cause impingement with the humeral head, leading to rapid-onset arthropathy [44, 54, 60, 62].

Second, although fixation of the graft with two bicortical metal screws is the recommended method of fixation [1, 44, 60, 61], it is also recognized as the main source of intraoperative and postoperative complications [5, 13, 55, 63, 65]. There are several potential disadvantages of the screw fixation: screw pullout or loosening, bending or breakage, bone block fracture, nonunion, resorption (3–28%), and graft migration (4–11%) [1, 60]. Some of these complications may be serious and symptomatic enough to warrant reoperation [13, 55, 63, 65].

Godenèche et al. [25] described the outcomes of 461 shoulders treated for anterior instability using open Latarjet and described that 4.6% had unexplained pain without recurrence of instability, and each underwent reoperation to remove the two screws used to fix their bone blocks.

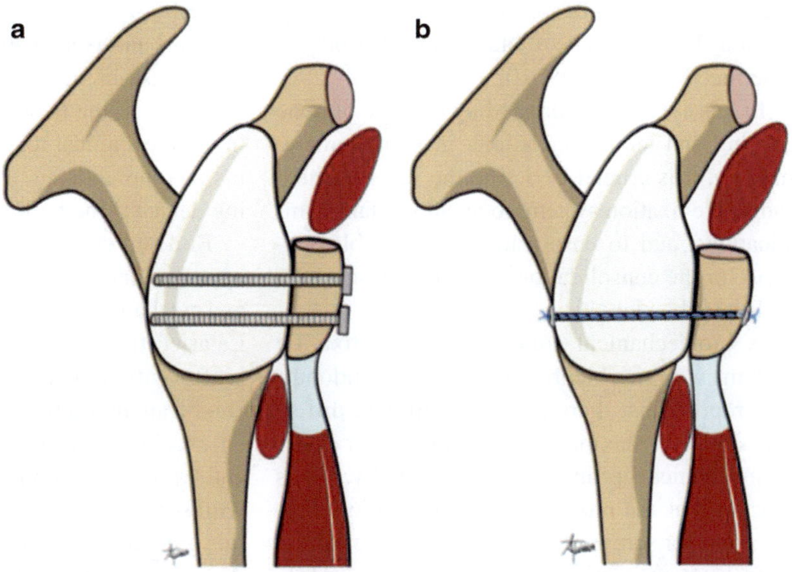

Fig. 19.7 Illustration of the Bristow-Latarjet procedure performed through a subscapularis split using two screws (**a**) and a suture-button construct (**b**) for fixation. (Reproduced from Lemmex et al. [40] published in JBJS Reviews)

Screw removal alleviated pain completely in 67% and reduced pain in the remaining 33%.

Third, the proximity of the brachial plexus (especially axillary and musculocutaneous nerves) means that any drilling or screw insertion performed arthroscopically anteriorly is potentially dangerous [9, 10, 19, 63, 65]. Posteriorly, there is also a risk of suprascapular nerve injury if the drill and screws are too medially oriented [41–43]. Laederman et al. [41] reported that in the axial plane, the screws were not in contact with the suprascapular nerve if the angle relative to the glenoid was less than or equal to 10°. Determining the safe zone, we should consider also when using screws as the fixation method (Fig. 19.7).

Fixation Device Biomechanically Buttons Versus Screws

In the mechanical and anatomical considerations related to recurrent instability, it is necessary to define the role of the anteroinferior labrum and glenoid bone stock, within the transmission of compressive loads and shear forces, by the humeral head. The progressive deterioration or loss of the labrum (especially the anteroinferior labrum), with each luxation episode, leads to an approximate decrease of 7–15% of the contact surface area, generating an 8–20% increase in contact pressure. If glenoid bone loss is greater than 30%, the contact area decreases by about 41%, while contact pressures increase by 100–400%, mainly in the anteroinferior quadrant [26]. From this information, it is understood as the progressive decrease of the contact area associated with an increase in peak pressures and may lead to a failure in repairs with Bankart surgery, especially in cases with significant bone defects, being pressure overload at the labrum repair site, the main responsible for this. If a major Hill-Sachs injury is added, the probability of failure is greater, so it is necessary to consider the repair of the humeral defect simultaneously [11].

Understanding the leading role of Latarjet surgery in the management of glenohumeral instability, it is important to understand the so-called triple blocking effect [9, 10]. This theory is supported by publications such as that of Di Giacomo, who evaluates by tomography, the behavior of the bone graft that has been fixed by two bicortical screws, and describes how an important part of the graft suffers osteolysis (mean percentage 59.5%), especially in the more proximal and superficial zone, probably concerning Wolff's law by the lower transmission of loads at this site, so that the effect of bone blockage is not the main factor in glenohumeral stabilization but the set of stabilizing factors as described by Boileau [9, 10].

In this context, understanding the role of bone grafting and tendon insertions in glenohumeral stability, it is crucial to define the most suitable and stable fixation system, to avoid implant complications, and to ensure the best possible scenario for the consolidation and integration of the graft into the glenoid.

A biomechanical study comparing fixation systems with two bicortical screws and endobuttons reports that there are no significant differences in the maximal load-to-failure or other biomechanical properties. Additionally, it is described as the most frequent mechanical failure point for screws, the holes at the level of the bone graft generating a fracture of this, while for endobutton systems, the failure mechanism was a fracture at the level of the posterior glenoid. The results conclude that both fixation systems are biomechanically comparable for graft fixation [33]. These results are supported by other comparative biomechanical studies with similar results, describing the similarity in resistance to cyclic loads without a significant difference in ultimate load to failure between the screw and suture button fixation group [17, 51].

Outcomes

While two screws are traditionally used for coracoid bone block fixation, the use of 2-button (instead of 4-button) for coracoid bone block fixation is suggested, and the bone block healing rate is similar in both groups: 91% in group 4-button versus 95.5% in group 2-button. A 4-button fixation technique did not demonstrate any anatomic or clinical advantages when compared with a 2-button fixation technique, and a 2-button fixation is simple, safe, and sufficient to solidly fix the transferred coracoid bone block [4].

Is also important to mention that after transfer of the bone block on the anterior neck of the scapula, compression (100 N) was obtained with the help of a tensioning device (mechanical tensioning) and is also shown when compared with hand tensioning; the rate of bone block healing was 74% in the hand tensioning group and 94% in the mechanical tensioning group (P 0.043), so it's recommended to use the mechanical tensioning device if the buttons fixation device is used.

Boileau et al. described a guided surgical approach and novel fixation method with 2-button and mechanical tensioning device for arthroscopic Latarjet; the guided surgical approach optimizes graft positioning accuracy. Suture button fixation can be an alternative to screw fixation, obtaining an excellent rate of the bone union. Neurologic and hardware complications, classically reported with screw fixation, have not been observed with this guided technique and novel fixation method. A mean follow-up of 26 months (range, 24–47 months) presented 95% of graft healing and 95% flush positioning of the graft, with 3% of shoulder instability recurrence, and no neurologic complications or hardware failures were observed; no patients had secondary surgery for implant removal.

Surgical Technique

Latarjet Guiding System

A number of instruments have been designed and developed to improve the safety and accuracy of the arthroscopic Latarjet procedure (Latarjet Guiding System; Smith & Nephew Inc., Andover, MA, USA).

1. The *glenoid drill guide* has two functions. First, it ensures that the cortical button suture tunnel is almost parallel (10° angulation) and 5 mm medial to the anterior glenoid rim. Second, it allows intra-articular drilling from posterior to anterior that is limited by a drill stop to avoid neurovascular injury.
2. The *coracoid drill guide* ensures that the cortical button suture tunnel is perpendicular to the coracoid, equidistant from its margins (5 mm), and at a fixed distance from its tip.

3. Two purpose-designed 2.8-mm drill bits (RCG Drill, Smith & Nephew) comprising an inner K-wire and outer sleeve.
4. A pin puller for removal of the K-wires.
5. Two low-profile mechanical subscapularis spreaders. First, these split the subscapularis muscle along its fibers. Second, they protect the axillary and musculocutaneous nerves at the time of coracoid transfer.
6. An oscillating rasp to create two opposing flat osseous surfaces of anterior glenoid and coracoid undersurfaces.
7. An oscillating saw blade for safe and rapid coracoid osteotomy.
8. A pair of arthroscopic tissue retractors to improve safety and visualization: the curved (north) retractor to elevate the upper part of the subscapularis and the straight (south) retractor to protect the axillary and musculocutaneous nerves and pull down the inferior part of the subscapularis.
9. A cannulated awl and a K-wire can be used to create pilot holes and to insert a K-wire to improve visualization of the anterior glenoid neck (by lifting up the upper subscapularis).
10. A suture tensioner to obtain compression between the graft and the anterior glenoid.
11. A coracoid grasper to manipulate the bone block during fixation.
12. Two half-pipe cannulas (long and short) for atraumatic insertion of instruments: The short half-pipe is used to introduce intra-articular instruments; the long half-pipe is used to introduce instruments through the anteromedial transpectoral portal into the anterior subdeltoid space.

Scope

We use a 70° scope (in preference to a 30° scope) for the procedure as it offers superior visualization of the anterior neck of the scapula. Furthermore, the advantage of viewing around "acute angles" with a 70° scope obviates the need for additional portals and thereby eliminates the problem of instrument crowding.

Cortical Button Fixation Device

The fixation device consists of two circular metallic buttons, used with a No. 3–4 ultrahigh-molecular-weight polyethylene suture sling running through them. The coracoid (anterior) button is convex (to adapt to the coracoid's shape) and pegged to prevent suture cut-through of the bone during the period before bone union. The glenoid (posterior) button has one hole allowing suture passage. A specific sliding knot (nice knot) is tied posteriorly to obtain bone compression. Further bone compression is obtained with the help of the suture tensioner and three additional surgeon's knots to lock the construct.

Position

General anesthesia and interscalene block were used in all patients. Abduction of the arm is detrimental by bringing the axillary nerve in the operative field, and thus, we recommend performing this procedure in the beach chair position. Anyway, the position of the arm is important during the entire procedure; the arm is placed in a movable support (Spider Limb Positioner, Smith & Nephew) without traction. The shoulder is placed in 60° of flexion (to relax the anterior deltoid) and 30° of internal rotation (to increase the subcoracoid space and to relax the axillary nerve). The elbow is placed at 90° of flexion (to relax the conjoint tendon). Shoulder abduction is absolutely contraindicated as it brings the neurovascular structures laterally, in front of the scapular neck, putting them at risk. Shoulder extension is also contraindicated as it reduces the anterior subdeltoid space and puts the axillary nerve under tension.

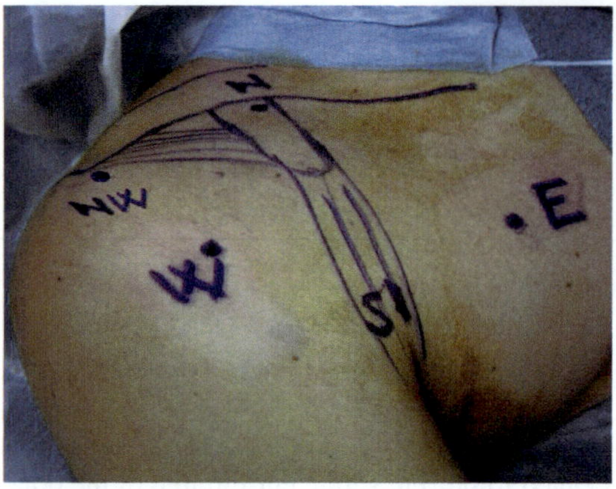

Fig. 19.8 Right shoulder of a patient in the beach chair position: proximal (north), distal (south), lateral (west), and medial (east) to the coracoid process. The north-west portal (located at the anterolateral corner of the acromion) is the rotator interval portal used to work inside the joint; the other four portals are used to work mainly extra-articularly. (Reproduced from Boileau et al.)

Portals

Northwest–Anterolateral corner of the acromion, this is the rotator interval portal used to work inside the joint
West–Two fingerbreadths lateral to the tip of the coracoid process
North–One fingerbreadths proximal and medial to the tip of the coracoid
South–Two fingerbreadths distal to the tip of the coracoid in axillary fold
East–Three fingerbreadths medial to the tip of the coracoid process (Fig. 19.8)

Through a standard posterior portal, a systematic inspection of the joint is performed. The first anterior (north-west) portal is used for intra-articular work; it is located on the skin at the anterolateral corner of the acromion. Four additional anterior portals are created as described, on each side of the tip of the coracoid. It is important to know the correct position and how to use the east portal. We explain in the following paragraph the technical tips for its realization safely.

Using the transpectoralis major portal, or "east" portal, requires detailed knowledge of the arthroscopic anatomy of the anterior shoulder and a mastery of the 70° arthroscope (although the procedure can be performed with a 30° scope). Our own clinical experience with the arthroscopic Latarjet over the last decade has shown us that the safety of the arthroscopic medial transpectoralis portal depends on four technical considerations:

1. The portal should always be established in an outside-in fashion from anterior to posterior.

   The inside-out technique that uses a switching stick to be placed from posterior to anterior through the subscapularis and out of the skin places the neurovascular structures at significant risk. This technique is constrained by the osseous anatomy of the patient's glenohumeral joint and eliminates the safety benefits of the transpectoralis portal. As such, we landmark our skin incision located 49.9 +/− 4.5 mm distal and 36.4 +/− 3.6 mm medial to the tip of the coracoid as Dunn et al. described [22].
2. The stick or half-pipe must be oriented 45° toward the tip of the coracoid.

   This relatively superficial trajectory allows us to work safely in the anterior extra-articular space of the shoulder.
3. Visual control of the anterior extra-articular subdeltoid space to end up lateral to the coracoid process.
4. Use the transpectoral portal as a protecting portal, not as a working portal.

   Once the coracoid has been osteotomized and the conjoint tendon retracted distally, all instruments passing through the transpectoral portal are directly in contact with the neurovascular structures. This is why working through the medial transpectoralis portal should be done only with the help of a cannula or half-pipe. Ideally, the transpectoral portal should not be used as a "working portal" but as a "protecting portal" instead, placing a stick or spreader to protect the neurovascular structures. The transpectoral portal makes the arthroscopic safe as it allows the introduction of a spreader to retract the subscapularis muscle and protect the neurovascular structures during transfer and fixation of the coracoid bone block.

For performing this procedure safely using the transpectoralis major portal, it's important to have a detailed knowledge of anterior arthroscopic shoulder anatomy, have familiarity with the use of a 70° arthroscope, and make a systematic identification of the axillary and musculocutaneous nerves, and a systematic use of specifically designed cannulas and/or retractors to protect the neurovascular structures after osteotomy of the coracoid in the way is described in the previous steps [8].

The technique comprises *four steps*, all performed arthroscopically, in addition to the Bankart repair.

Step 1: Coracoid Preparation, Drilling, and Osteotomy

The location of the posterior portal is crucial. It is located 1 cm inferior and medial to the posterior angle of the acromion. A spinal needle is used to make sure that the scope and instruments will be flush with the glenoid surface and at the level of the equator. With the arthroscope in the posterior portal, the first anterior (north-west) portal is created. A needle is used to ensure that instrumentation will be tangential to the anterior neck of the glenoid and to the undersurface of the coracoid. With use of electrocautery, the coracoid process is identified.

The 70° scope, being in the posterior portal, is pushed through the rotator interval. This allows release of the coracoacromial ligament from the lateral border of the acromion and identification of the conjoint tendon. The north portal is then created (medial to the coracoid process) with the help of the spinal needle. This allows release of the pectoralis minor from the medial border of the coracoid. The undersurface of the coracoid process is abraded with the motorized rasp (introduced through the north-west portal) to create a flat surface (Fig. 19.9a).The coracoid guide is introduced to grasp the coracoid perpendicular to its surface. This means that it must be tilted 45-medially (Fig. 19.9b). A first drill-tipped K-wire housed inside an outer sleeve is advanced through the guide and drilled until it exits the inferior surface of the coracoid. The hole is placed 5 mm from coracoid margins (Fig. 19.9b). The coracoid K-wire is replaced with a polydioxanone (PDS) suture, which is passed through the sleeve and the coracoid hole. The PDS suture is retrieved through the west portal. The coracoid guide and the sleeve are removed. The coracoid peg button (with the 4-strand suture) is pulled into place using the PDS suture as a shuttle (Fig. 19.9c). The coracoid is osteotomized with a motorized saw (introduced through the north-west portal), harvesting about 15–20 mm of bone (Fig. 19.9d). The north portal is closed with a clip to avoid losing water outside the shoulder.

Step 2: Glenoid Preparation and Drilling

The anterior labrum is completely detached (but preserved) to visualize the glenoid bone defect. A suture is passed through the labrum at the 5-o'clock position and retrieved through the west portal, allowing the labrum to be pulled away from the glenoid neck. The glenoid neck is abraded to a flatbed by use of the motorized rasp (Fig. 19.10). A glenoid anchor hole is drilled at 3 o'clock (through the west portal), and a suture anchor (SUTUREFIX, Smith & Nephew) is inserted; it will be used later for the labrum repair.

Using switching sticks, the scope is transferred to the north-west portal while a short half-pipe cannula is placed through the posterior portal. The glenoid drill guide is introduced inside the joint along the cannula. The guide is placed flush to the glenoid surface, at the 5-o'clock position, with the tip of the hook of the guide 5 mm medial to the glenoid rim (Fig. 19.10b). A switching stick is introduced through the west portal to retract the labrum and subscapularis. The second drill-tipped K-wire housed inside an outer sleeve is drilled from posterior to anterior through the guide. The hole in the glenoid must be located at the 5-o'clock position (in a right shoulder) and 5 mm medial to the glenoid rim.

The glenoid guide is removed, leaving the sleeve in place. The subscapularis spreader is inserted inside the joint and pushed through the subscapularis muscle (at 5 o'clock) to act as a landmark for the split.

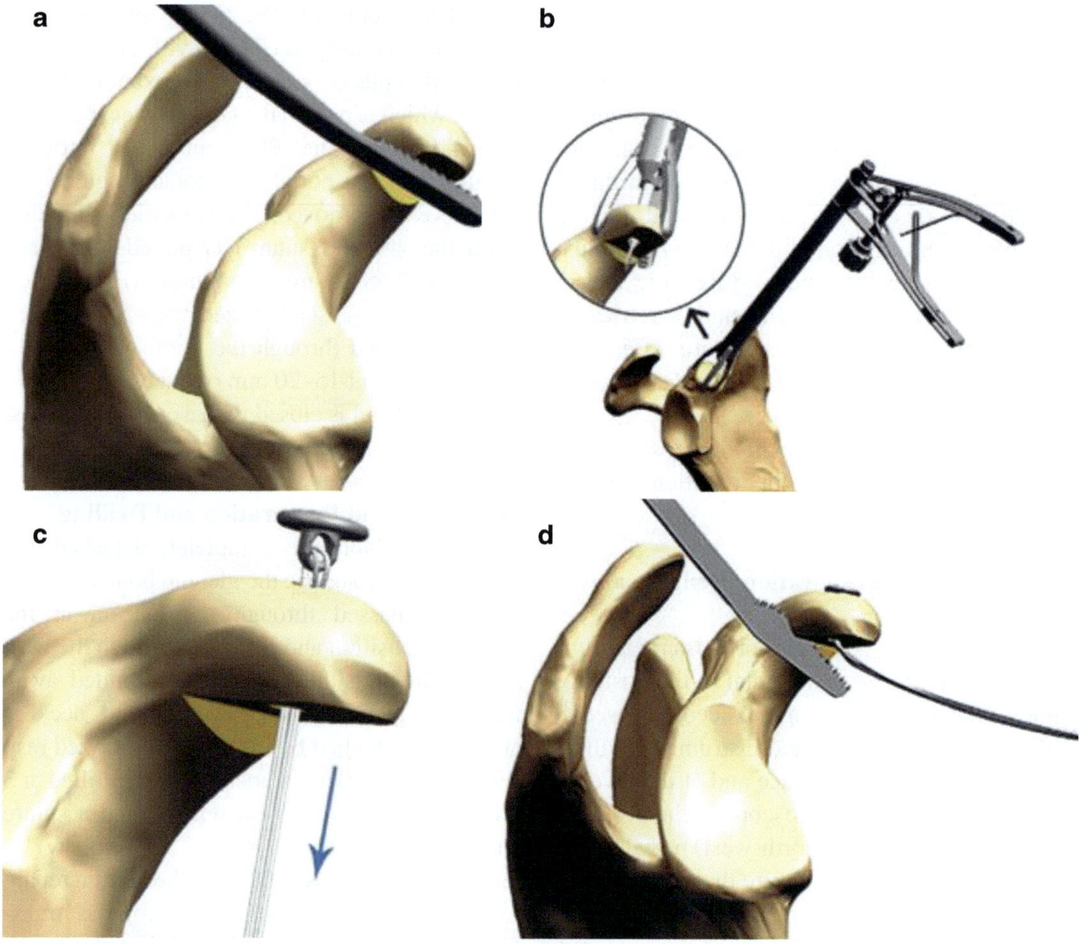

Fig. 19.9 Coracoid preparation, drilling, and osteotomy. (**a**) The coracoid graft site is abraded with a motorized rasp introduced from the north-west portal. (**b**) The coracoid guide is introduced through the north portal and used to grasp the coracoid and to drill a 2.8-mm hole strictly perpendicular to the coracoid process. (**c**) The peg cortical button is placed over the coracoid using a shuttle suture. (**d**) The coracoid osteotomy is performed with a motorized saw introduced from the north-west portal. (Reproduced from Boileau et al.)

Step 3: Subscapularis Splitting and Axillary Nerve Protection

With the arthroscope in the west portal and the shoulder in slight internal rotation, the axillary and musculocutaneous nerves must be clearly and systematically identified and protected. Following the anterior axillary vessels (the so-called three sisters) medially allows us to identify the two nerves (the so-called two brothers); hence, our saying, "The three sisters guide the surgeon to the two brothers." The straight blunt retractor, introduced through the south portal, is used to separate the conjoint tendon from the subscapularis muscle and to protect the nerves.

With the arm by the side and slightly externally rotated, the subscapularis muscle is fully exposed. The posterior spreader is gently pushed farther through the muscle in a lateral direction (Fig. 19.11a, b). The muscle belly is divided parallel with its fibers, at the superior $^{2}/3$ inferior $^{1}/3$ junction. While the spreader is opened, the cauterizing instrument is used to incise 1 cm longitudinally into the superficial tendon of the subscapularis; great care is taken to incise only the

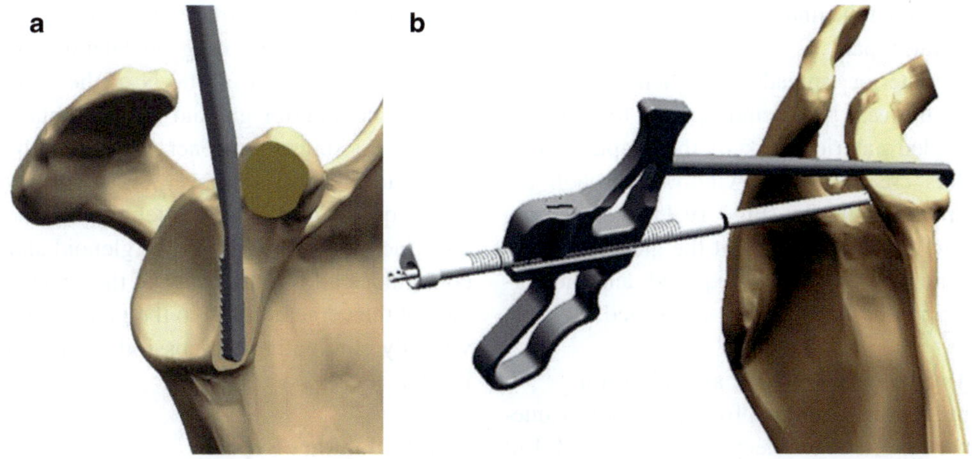

Fig. 19.10 Glenoid preparation and drilling. (**a**) The glenoid neck is abraded with a motorized rasp. (**b**) The glenoid guide (10- angulated) is introduced inside the shoulder with the help of a half-pipe cannula. It allows drilling of a 2.8-mm hole almost parallel to the glenoid surface, below the equator (at the 5 o'clock position) and 5 mm medial to the anterior glenoid rim. (Reproduced from Boileau et al.)

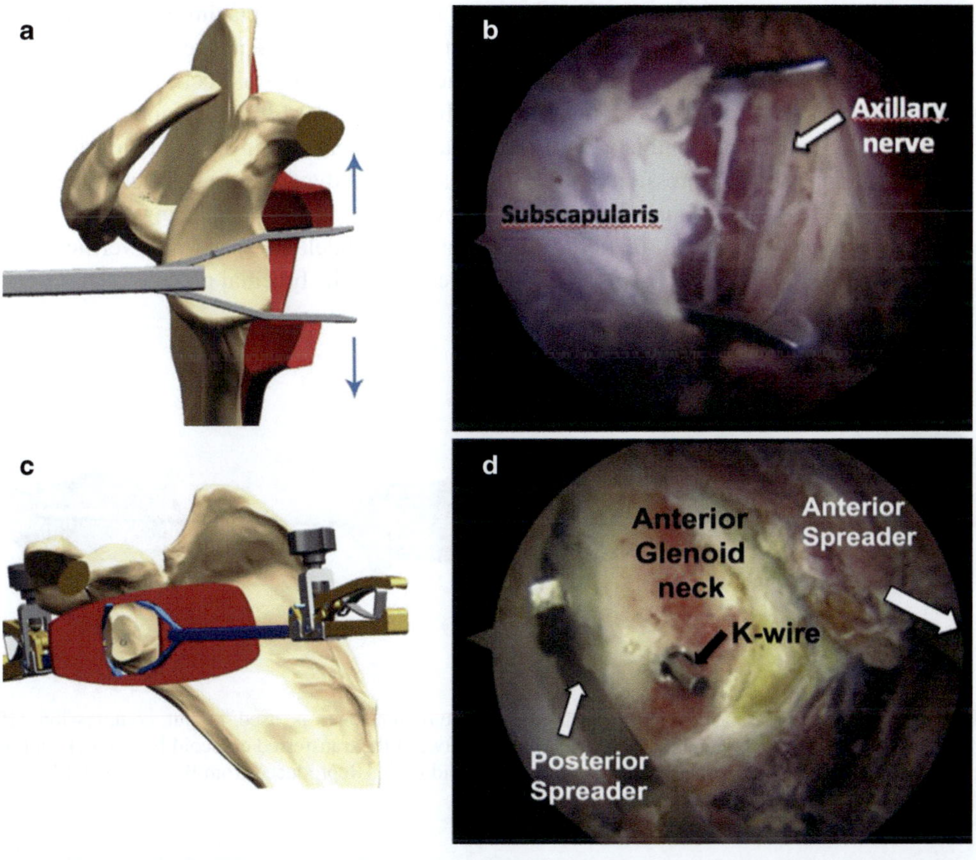

Fig. 19.11 Subscapularis split. After the axillary and musculocutaneous nerves have been located and protected with a retractor, the first (posterior) spreader is gently pushed through the subscapularis muscle (from posterior to anterior), staying lateral to the nerves, and opened (**a** and **b**). The second (anterior) spreader is placed in the split and opened. This allows the creation of a "safe window" through the muscle and protects the axillary and musculocutaneous nerves. The outer sleeve of the drill is seen and will be used to shuttle the suture in the back of the shoulder (**c** and **d**). (Reproduced from [7])

tendon and not the underlying capsule (used later for Bankart repair).

The anterior spreader is then introduced through the east portal and opened to visualize the abraded anterior neck of the scapula. Both spreaders create a "safe window" through the subscapularis muscle (Fig. 19.11c, d), giving access to the anterior neck of the glenoid, which should now be completely exposed, and the correct position of the K-wire is confirmed.

Step 4: Coracoid Transfer and Fixation

A suture retriever (passing from posterior to anterior through the outer sleeve of the glenoid drill piece) is used to catch the coracoid PDS suture, which is then retrieved posteriorly (Fig. 19.12a). The drill piece in the glenoid is retrieved, and the PDS suture is used to shuttle the suture of the cortical button and to transfer the graft with the conjoint tendon onto the glenoid neck. The four strands of suture are passed through the hole of the second (glenoid) cortical button, and a sliding-locking knot (nice knot) is then tied. The suture tensioner is put in place in the back of the shoulder, and a temporary compression of 25 N is first obtained. The scope is reintroduced inside the joint to control placement and rotation of the bone graft. The positioning and rotation of the coracoid graft are controlled with the help of the coracoid grasper, ensuring no lateral overhang. Further compression of 100 N of the bone graft against the anterior glenoid neck is obtained by use of the suture tensioner (Fig. 19.12b). The suture tensioner is removed. It is followed by three square knots tied to definitively lock the construct. Combined use of the glenoid and coracoid guides allows matching of the articular surface of the coracoid graft to the glenoid rim, thus virtually eliminating the possibility of an articular step.

Step 5: Bankart Repair

Visualization from the posterior portal and palpation with a probe confirm the absence of overhanging of the coracoid bone block and the stiffness of the construct (Fig. 19.13a). The remaining capsule and labrum are now reattached to the glenoid rim, placing the graft in an extra-articular position. The previously placed suture anchor (placed at 3 o'clock) is used to repair the labrum (Fig. 19.13b). Additional sutures can be placed to perform an anterior inferior capsulorrhaphy. The dynamic sling effect of the block can now be visualized by placing the scope in the anterior subdeltoid space and verified no compression of the brachial plexus.

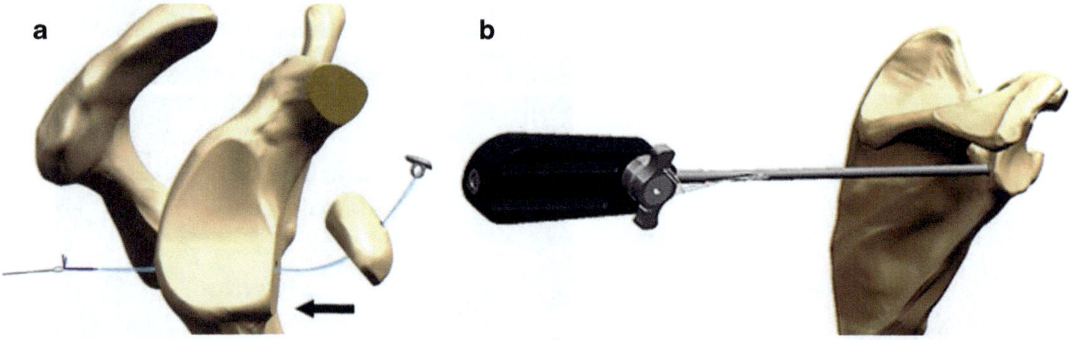

Fig. 19.12 Coracoid transfer and fixation. (**a**) The four-strand suture is shuttled through the glenoid, which brings the coracoid graft onto the anterior neck of the scapula. (**b**) After rotation of the bone block has been controlled, a suture tensioner is used to put compression (100 N) between the transferred coracoid bone block and the glenoid neck. (Reproduced from Boileau et al. [7])

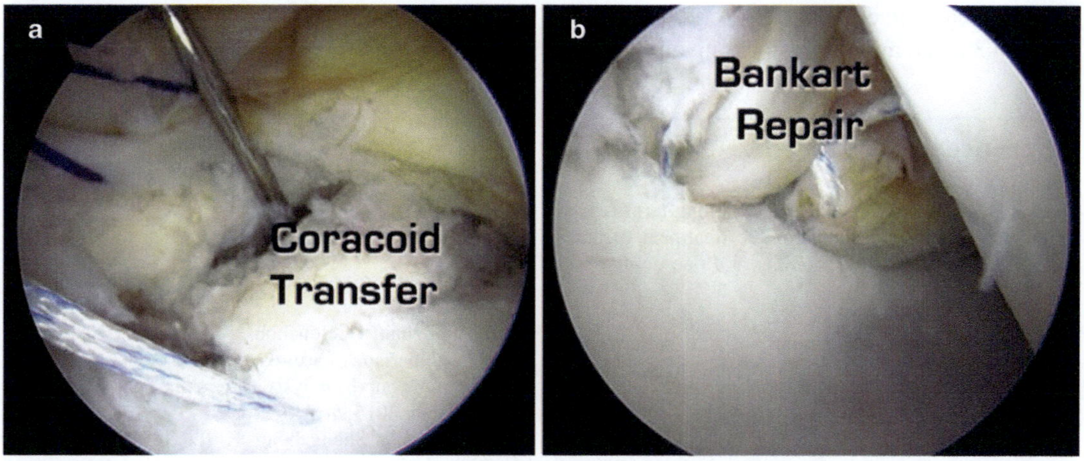

Fig. 19.13 Arthroscopic final view. Intra-articular views show (**a**) perfect positioning of the coracoid bone block and (**b**) capsulolabral repair producing the bumper effect (and placing the bone block in an extra-articular position). (Reproduced from Boileau et al. [7])

Five Steps: Guided Arthroscopic Latarjet with Button Fixation—Summary

Step 1: *Coracoid preparation*
- Coracoid dissection
- Coracoid abrasion
- Coracoid drilling
- Implant placement
- Suture management
- Coracoid osteotomy
- Final soft tissue release

Step 2: *Glenoid preparation*
- Labrum detachment
- Glenoid neck abrasion
- 3 o'clock anchor insertion
- Glenoid guide placement
- Glenoid drilling
- Posterior spreader placement

Step 3: *Subscapularis split*
- Anterior bursectomy
- Axillary nerve protection
- Lateral subscapularis split
- Medial subscapularis split

Step 4: *Coracoid transfer and fixation*
- Suture shuttling
- Coracoid transfer
- Posterior button placement and knot tightening
- Bone block rotation and compression

Step 5: *Bankart repair*
- Bankart repair
- Verified dynamic sling of transfer in the anterior subdeltoid space
- Verified no compression of the brachial plexus

Postop/Additional Considerations

Postoperative radiographs are taken to confirm the correct graft position. The patient is discharged from the hospital the same day or the day after surgery. The arm is strictly immobilized for 2 weeks in a neutral rotation sling; this allows healing of the conjoint tendon in the muscular part of the subscapularis muscle and avoids postoperative loss of external rotation. Pendulum exercises start after 2 weeks (5 times a day, 5 min each session). After 4 weeks, the sling is removed and formal rehabilitation with a physiotherapist is started. Swimming pool therapy is encouraged. No heavy lifting is allowed for the first 12 weeks. Return to all types of sports activities, including collision and contact-overhead sports, is allowed between 3 and 6 months postoperatively.

References

1. Allain J, Glorion C, Goutallier D. Long-term results of the Latarjet procedure for the treatment of anterior instability of the shoulder. J Bone Joint Surg. 1998;80:841–52.
2. Athwal GS, Favorito P, Getz C, Meislin R, Weinstein D. Short-term complications of the arthroscopic Latarjet procedure: a North American experience. Arthroscopy. 2016;32:1965–70.
3. Balg F, Boileau P. The instability severity index score. The Journal of Bone and Joint Surgery British volume. 2007;89-B:1470–7.
4. Barret H, Boileau P, Chelli M, Langlais T, Van Der Meijden O. Arthroscopic Latarjet: 2 or 4 cortical buttons for coracoid fixation? A case-control comparative study. Am J Sports Med. 2022;50:311–20.
5. Boileau P, Ahrens P, Balg F, Héry J-Y, Neyton L, Villalba M. Risk factors for recurrence of shoulder instability after arthroscopic Bankart repair. J Bone Joint Surg. 2006;88:1755–63.
6. Boileau P, Bicknell RT, Chuinard C, El Fegoun AB. Arthroscopic Bristow procedure for anterior instability in shoulders with a stretched or deficient capsule: the "belt-and-suspenders" operative technique and preliminary results. Arthroscopy. 2007;23:593–601.
7. Boileau P, Gendre P, Baba M, Thélu CÉ, Baring T, Gonzalez JF, Trojani C. A guided surgical approach and novel fixation method for arthroscopic Latarjet. J Shoulder Elbow Surg. 2016;25:78–89. https://doi.org/10.1016/j.jse.2015.06.001. Open Access. Copyright: © 2016 The Authors. Published by Elsevier Inc
8. Boileau P, Lemmex DB. Editorial commentary: the shoulder transpectoralis portal for arthroscopic Latarjet: medial to the coracoid can also be a safe side! Arthroscopy. 2021;37:477–9.
9. Boileau P, Mercier N, Old J. Arthroscopic Bankart-Bristow-Latarjet (2B3) procedure: how to do it and tricks to make it easier and safe. Orthop Clin N Am. 2010a;41:381–92.
10. Boileau P, Mercier N, Old J, Roussanne Y, Thélu C-É. Arthroscopic Bankart-Bristow-Latarjet procedure: the development and early results of a safe and reproducible technique. Arthroscopy. 2010b;26:1434–50.
11. Boileau P, Old J, O'Shea K, Pinedo M, Vargas P, Zumstein M. Anatomical and functional results after Arthroscopic Hill-Sachs Remplissage. J Bone Joint Surg. 2012;94:618–26.
12. Boileau P, Saliken D. Editorial commentary: the wake of the dragon: will the orthopaedic community adopt the shoulder arthroscopic Latarjet procedure as we adopted the arthroscopic rotator cuff repair? Arthroscopy. 2017;33:2139–43.
13. Boileau P, Carles M, Houghton-Clemmey R, Mercier N, Thélu C-É, Ohl X, Trojani C. Arthroscopic Bristow-Latarjet combined with Bankart repair restores shoulder stability in patients with glenoid bone loss. Clin Orthop Relat Res. 2014;472:2413–24.
14. Bois AJ, Fening SD, Jones MH, Miniaci A, Polster J. Quantifying glenoid bone loss in anterior shoulder instability. Am J Sports Med. 2012;40:2569–77.
15. Burkhart SS, De Beer JF. Traumatic glenohumeral bone defects and their relationship to failure of arthroscopic Bankart repairs. Arthroscopy. 2000;16:677–94.
16. Cunningham G, Benchouk S, Kherad O, Lädermann A. Comparison of arthroscopic and open Latarjet with a learning curve analysis. Knee Surg Sports Traumatol Arthrosc. 2015;24:540–5.
17. Daqiang L, Shengzheng K (2020) Biomechanical comparative analysis of screw fixation and cortical endo-button fixation in Latarjet procedure for anterior dislocation of shoulder joint. Chin J Reparative Reconstruct Surg 15;34(5):602-607.
18. Dauzère F, Bonnevialle N, Faraud A, Faruch M, Lebon J, Mansat P. Is the Latarjet procedure risky? Analysis of complications and learning curve. Knee Surg Sports Traumatol Arthrosc. 2016;24:557–63.
19. Delaney RA, Freehill MT, Higgins LD, Janfaza DR, Vlassakov KV, Warner JJP. 2014 neer award paper: Neuromonitoring the latarjet procedure. J Shoulder Elb Surg. 2014;23:1473–80.
20. Di Giacomo G, Burkhart SS, Itoi E. Evolving concept of bipolar bone loss and the hill-sachs lesion: from "engaging/non-engaging" lesion to "on-track/off-track" lesion. Arthroscopy: The Journal of Arthroscopic & Related Surgery. 2014;30:90–8.
21. Di Giacomo G, de Gasperis N, Midtgaard KS, Peebles LA, Provencher CPTM, Scarso P. Risk factors for recurrent anterior glenohumeral instability and clinical failure following primary Latarjet procedures. J Bone Joint Surg. 2020;102:1665–71.
22. Dunn ASM, Petterson SC, Plancher KD. The shoulder trans-pectoralis arthroscopic portal is a safe approach to the arthroscopic Latarjet procedure: a cadaveric analysis. Arthroscopy. 2021;37:470–6.
23. Edwards TB, Boulahia A, Walch G. Radiographic analysis of bone defects in chronic anterior shoulder instability. Arthroscopy. 2003;19:732–9.
24. Ekhtiari S, Ayeni OR, Bedi A, Horner NS, Khan M. The learning curve for the Latarjet procedure: a systematic review. Orthop J Sports Med. 2018;6:232596711878693.
25. Godenèche A, Delgrande D, Le Chatelier M, Merlini L, Roulet S, Saffarini M. Screw removal can resolve unexplained anterior pain without recurrence of shoulder instability after open Latarjet procedures. Am J Sports Med. 2020;48:1450–5.
26. Greis PE, Bachus KN, Burks RT, Mohr A, Scuderi MG. Glenohumeral articular contact areas and pressures following labral and osseous injury to the anteroinferior quadrant of the glenoid. J Shoulder Elb Surg. 2002;11:442–51.

27. Helfet AJ. Coracoid transplantation for recurring dislocation of the shoulder. The Journal of Bone and Joint Surgery British volume. 1958;40-B:198–202.
28. Hovelius L, Augustini BG, Fredin H, Johansson O, Norlin R, Thorling J. Primary anterior dislocation of the shoulder in young patients. A ten-year prospective study*. J Bone Joint Surg. 1996;78:1677–84.
29. Hovelius L, Rahme H. Primary anterior dislocation of the shoulder: long-term prognosis at the age of 40 years or younger. Knee Surg Sports Traumatol Arthrosc. 2016;24:330–42.
30. Hovelius L, Olofsson A, Rahme H, Sandström B, Svensson O. The effect of capsular repair, bone block healing, and position on the results of the Bristow-Latarjet procedure (study III): long-term follow-up in 319 shoulders. J Shoulder Elb Surg. 2012;21:647–60.
31. Hurley ET, Jazrawi LM, Jia NW, Manjunath AK, Matache BA, Virk M. No difference in 90-day complication rate following open versus arthroscopic Latarjet procedure. Knee Surg Sports Traumatol Arthrosc. 2020;29:2333–7.
32. Jacxsens M, Brady SE, Chalmers PN, Elhabian SY, Henninger HB, Tashjian RZ. Coracoacromial morphology: a contributor to recurrent traumatic anterior glenohumeral instability? J Shoulder Elbow Surg. 2019; https://doi.org/10.1016/j.jse.2019.01.009.
33. Kazum E, Chechik O, Dolkart O, Morag G, Mozes G, Pritsch T. Biomechanical evaluation of suture buttons versus cortical screws in the Latarjet–Bristow procedure: A fresh-frozen cadavers study. Arch Orthop Trauma Surg. 2019;139:1779–83.
34. Kim DH, Choi HY, Kim DY, Lee YH, Oh JH, Park JS. Assessment of capsular insertion type and of capsular elongation in patients with anterior shoulder instability and it's correlation with surgical outcome: a quantitative assessment with computed tomography arthrography. Clinic Shoulder Elbow. 2016;19:155–62.
35. Kodali P, Fening SD, Jones MH, Miniaci A, Polster J. Accuracy of measurement of hill-Sachs lesions with computed tomography. J Shoulder Elb Surg. 2011;20:1328–34.
36. Lafosse L, Boyle S, Gutierrez-Aramberri M, Meller R, Shah A. Arthroscopic latarjet procedure. Orthop Clin N Am. 2010;41:393–405.
37. Lafosse L, Bouchard A, Gobezie R, Kakuda C, Kochhar T, Lejeune E. The arthroscopic Latarjet procedure for the treatment of anterior shoulder instability. Arthroscopy. 2007; https://doi.org/10.1016/j.arthro.2007.06.008.
38. Latarjet M. Treatment of recurrent dislocation of the shoulder. Lyon Chir. 1954;1954(49(8)):994–7.
39. Lee S-B, An K-N, Kim K-J, Morrey BF, O'Driscoll SW. Dynamic Glenohumeral stability provided by the rotator cuff muscles in the mid-range and end-range of motion. J Bone Joint Surg. 2000;82:849–57.
40. Lemmex D, Boileau P, Cárdenas G, Chelli M, Ricks M, Woodmass J. Arthroscopic management of anterior glenoid bone loss. JBJS Rev. 2020; https://doi.org/10.2106/jbjs.rvw.19.00049.
41. Lädermann A, Burkhart SS, Denard PJ. Injury of the suprascapular nerve during Latarjet procedure: An anatomic study. Arthroscopy. 2012;28:316–21.
42. Maquieira GJ, Gerber C, Schneeberger AG. Suprascapular nerve palsy after the Latarjet procedure. J Shoulder Elb Surg. 2007; https://doi.org/10.1016/j.jse.2006.04.001.
43. Meyer DC, Ek ETH, Gerber C, Moor BK. Accurate coracoid graft placement through use of a drill guide for the latarjet procedure. J Shoulder Elb Surg. 2013;22:701–8.
44. Mizuno N, Denard PJ, Melis B, Raiss P, Walch G. Long-term results of the Latarjet procedure for anterior instability of the shoulder. J Shoulder Elb Surg. 2014;23:1691–9.
45. Moseley HF. Recurrent dislocation of the shoulder. Postgrad Med. 1962;31:23–9.
46. Moya D, Aydin N, Robles PP, Simone JP, Tytherleigh-Strong G, Yamamoto N. Current concepts in anterior glenohumeral instability: diagnosis and treatment. SICOT-J. 2021;7:48.
47. Nourissat G, Debet-Mejean A, Dumontier C, Nedellec G, O'Sullivan NA, Sautet A. Mini-open arthroscopically assisted Bristow-Latarjet procedure for the treatment of patients with anterior shoulder instability: a cadaver study. Arthroscopy. 2006;22:1113–8.
48. Owens BD, Cameron KL, Campbell SE. Risk factors for anterior glenohumeral instability. Am J Sports Med. 2014;42:2591–6.
49. Patte D. Recurrent dislocation of the shoulder. Encycl Med Chir Paris Technique Chirurgical Orthopedie. 1980;44265:44–02.
50. Provencher CDRM, Bach BR, Bhatia S, Ghodadra NS, Grumet RC, Romeo AA. Recurrent shoulder instability: current concepts for evaluation and management of glenoid bone loss. J Bone Joint Surg. 2010;92:133–51.
51. Provencher MT, Aman ZS, Bernhardson AS, LaPrade CM, Moatshe G, Storaci HW. Biomechanical comparison of screw fixation versus a cortical button and self-tensioning suture for the Latarjet procedure. Orthop J Sports Med. 2018;6:232596711877784.
52. Rouleau DM, Djahangiri A, Balg F, Godbout V, Hébert-Davies J, Pelet S. Validation of the instability shoulder index score in a multicenter reliability study in 114 consecutive cases. Am J Sports Med. 2012;41:278–82.
53. Saito H, Itoi E, Minagawa H, Sugaya H, Tuoheti Y, Yamamoto N. Location of the glenoid defect in shoulders with recurrent anterior dislocation. Am J Sports Med. 2005;33:889–93.
54. Schmid SL, Catanzaro S, Gerber C, Farshad M. The Latarjet procedure for the treatment of recurrence of anterior instability of the shoulder after operative repair. J Bone Joint Surg. 2012; https://doi.org/10.2106/jbjs.k.00380.
55. Shah AA, Butler RB, Goel D, Romanowski J, Karadagli D, Warner JJP. Short-term complications of the Latarjet procedure. J Bone Joint Surg. 2012;94:495–501.

56. Shaha JS, Bottoni CR, Cook JB, Rowles DJ, Shaha SH, Song DJ. Redefining "critical" bone loss in shoulder instability. Am J Sports Med. 2015;43:1719–25.
57. Turkel SJ, Girgis FG, Marshall JL, Panio MW. Stabilizing mechanisms preventing anterior dislocation of the glenohumeral joint. J Bone Joint Surg. 1981;63:1208–17.
58. Urayama M, Itoi E, Sashi R, Sato K, Minagawa H. Capsular elongation in shoulders with recurrent anterior dislocation. Am J Sports Med. 2003;31:64–7.
59. Walch G, Boileau P. Latarjet-Bristow procedure for recurrent anterior instability. Tech Shoulder Elbow Surg. 2000;1:256–61.
60. Walch G, Dejour H, Trillat AG. Recurrent anterior luxation of the shoulder occurring after the age of 40. Rev Chir Orthop Reparatrice Appar Mot. 1987;73(8):609–16.
61. Weppe F, Demey G, Lustig S, Magnussen RA, Neyret P, Servien E. A biomechanical evaluation of bicortical metal screw fixation versus absorbable interference screw fixation after coracoid transfer for anterior shoulder instability. Arthroscopy. 2011;27:1358–63.
62. Young AA, Berhouet J, Maia R, Walch G. Open latarjet procedure for management of bone loss in anterior instability of the glenohumeral joint. J Shoulder Elbow Surg. 2011; https://doi.org/10.1016/j.jse.2010.07.022.
63. Young DC, Rockwood CA. Complications of a failed Bristow procedure and their management. J Bone Joint Surg Am. 1991;73(7):969–81.
64. Zimmermann SM, Gerber C, Catanzaro S, Farshad M, Rahm S, Scheyerer MJ. Long-term restoration of anterior shoulder stability: a retrospective analysis of arthroscopic Bankart repair versus open Latarjet procedure. J Bone Joint Surg. 2016;98:1954–61.
65. Zuckerman JD, Matsen FA. Complications about the glenohumeral joint related to the use of screws and staples. J Bone Joint Surg Am. 1984;66(2):175–80.

Glenoid Bone Loss: The Fresh Distal Tibial Allograft, Logistics, Graft Preparation, and Open Approach

20

Abdulaziz F. Ahmed, Daniel J. Stokes, and Rachel M. Frank

Introduction

Glenoid bone loss is a well-recognized cause of recurrent shoulder instability following primary dislocation [1–3]. A fracture or bony erosion changes normal shoulder biomechanics and decreases articulating surface area. Young male contact sport athletes are particularly susceptible to recurrent instability [4]. Subsequent dislocations significantly increase the rate for glenoid and humeral defects to develop or enlarge [5]. Therefore, surgery may be desirable to prevent recurrence and further structural damage [6–10].

Various surgical options are available to address a glenoid deficiency. However, it is imperative to consider the degree of bone loss. Though current recommendations support critical bone loss parameters defined as a 20–25% loss of the bony glenoid, recent literature suggests this number may be as low as 13.5% [9, 11, 12]. When glenoid bone loss reaches critical levels, arthroscopic and open Bankart procedures alone are associated with high failure rates [9, 11]. In these cases, bony procedures should be considered for glenoid reconstruction, including Latarjet or Bristow coracoid transfer versus an autograft or allograft procedure. Due to the broader radius of reconstruction, bone grafting procedures are preferred in cases with glenoid bone loss that exceeds the capacity of a coracoid graft [13].

Techniques designed to augment a deficient glenoid or revise a failed Latarjet include iliac crest autograft, distal clavicle autograft, and distal tibial allograft (DTA) [14–16]. Iliac crest and distal clavicle autografts have the advantages of earlier graft incorporation because the graft comes from the patient's tissue [15]. However, these patients are susceptible to donor-site morbidity. Iliac crest autografts provide easy shaping to restore the anatomic contour although they lack a chondral surface [16]. Distal clavicle autografts incorporate an osteochondral component but depend on a healthy AC joint without osteoarthritis [17].

DTA has the distinct advantage of providing a robust articular cartilage surface with graft curvature to restore the native glenoid surface and allow for humeral head congruency without donor-site morbidity [18]. The dense, bony composition of this graft has shown excellent integration with minimal graft resorption [14, 19–21]. DTA procedures can be performed open and arthroscopically. Open procedures have proven to be an effective and reliable treatment to restore stability and biomechanics, enabling a return to high-demand physical function [14, 22, 23]. This

A. F. Ahmed · D. J. Stokes
Department of Orthopaedic Surgery, Division of Sports Medicine, University of Colorado School of Medicine, Aurora, CO, USA

R. M. Frank (✉)
Orthopaedic Surgery, University of Colorado Anschutz Medical Center, Denver, CO, USA
e-mail: Rachel.Frank@cuanschutz.edu

© The Author(s), under exclusive license to Springer Nature Switzerland AG 2026
R. M. Frank, J. M. Tokish (eds.), *Management of Shoulder Instability*,
https://doi.org/10.1007/978-3-032-18089-6_20

chapter highlights glenoid reconstruction with fresh DTA, graft preparation, and execution utilizing an open approach.

Illustrative Clinical Case

A 32-year-old female presented with recurrent left shoulder instability in the setting of a prior arthroscopic Bankart repair that occurred 2 years before her current presentation. The patient reported initial improvement following surgery with subsequent return of symptoms. She denied shoulder pain but endorsed mechanical symptoms and instability, consisting of repeat episodes of subluxation with overhead activities. The patient completed several months of physical therapy and a home exercise program with no improvement. She is an active individual and enjoys recreational rock climbing.

On physical examination, the patient demonstrated shoulder range of motion (ROM) within normal limits and strength equivalent to the contralateral side. However, special testing revealed a positive anterior apprehension and relocation test. Generalized ligamentous laxity was assessed, and hyperlaxity was determined with a Beighton score of 7.

An imaging workup consisting of x-rays, magnetic resonance imaging (MRI), and computed tomography (CT) three-dimensional (3D) reconstruction was used to identify bone loss and assess for soft-tissue injury. No glenoid bone loss was evident on plain radiographs (Figs. 20.1 and 20.2). However, the MRI demonstrated an anteroinferior labrum tear (Fig. 20.3). In the 3D-CT reconstruction images, the linear-based method quantified 10.2% of anterior glenoid bone loss (Fig. 20.4).

Both operative and nonoperative treatment options were discussed with the patient. Given the continued dysfunction despite extensive physical therapy, we recommended operative treatment in the form of revision arthroscopic Bankart repair with a remplissage versus an anterior glenoid bone reconstruction procedure. Considering she participates in high-demand activities, such as rock climbing, and the presence of subcritical anterior glenoid bone loss in the setting of a prior failed soft-tissue stabilization procedure, we opted for a bone reconstruction procedure.

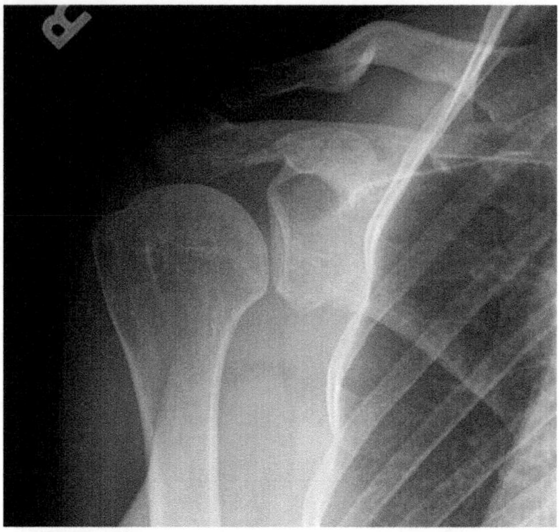

Fig. 20.1 A Grashey shoulder radiograph of the illustrated case without evidence of fractures, dislocation, or apparent bone loss

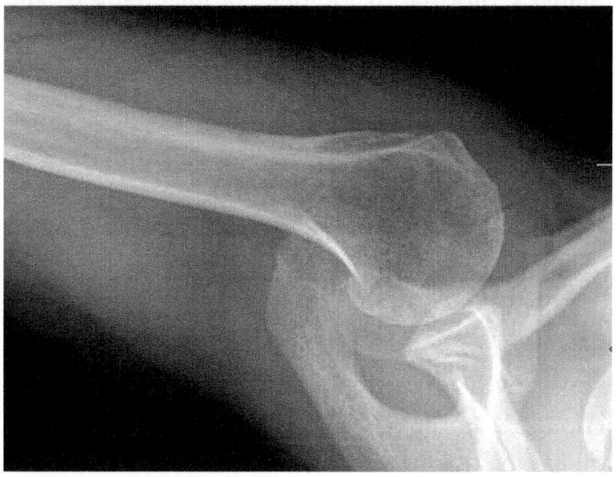

Fig. 20.2 An axillary shoulder radiograph of the illustrated case without evidence of fractures, dislocation, or apparent bone loss

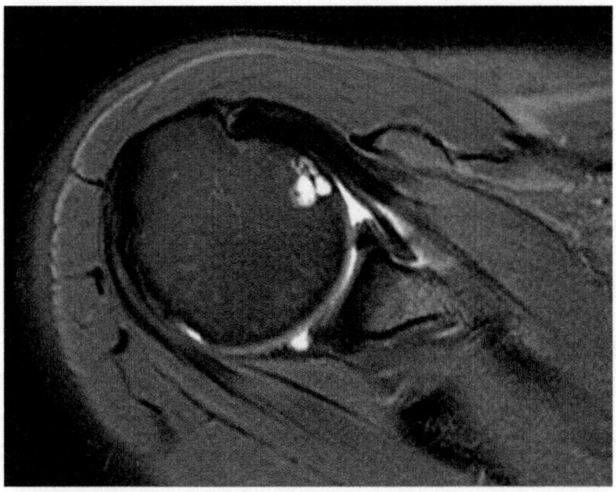

Fig. 20.3 An axial magnetic resonance image demonstrating an anteroinferior capsulolabral tear

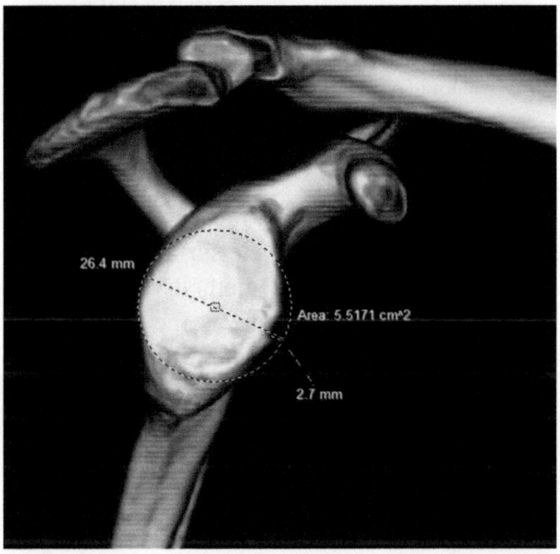

Fig. 20.4 An en face view of the glenoid computed tomography three-dimensional reconstruction image. The degree of anterior bone loss is measured with the linear method

Etiology

The most consistent risk factor for anterior glenoid bone loss in patients with shoulder instability is the number of instability events. In a prospective study of 714 patients with a history of shoulder dislocation, glenoid bone loss of 6.8% was found in first-time dislocators. However, in patients with recurrent shoulder instability, the quantity of anterior glenoid bone loss was significantly increased to 22.8% [24]. Another large cohort of 892 patients with anterior shoulder instability demonstrated that the predictors of any glenoid bone loss included (1) increasing age, (2) male sex, (3) contact athletes, and (4) the number of shoulder dislocations [25]. For patients with an anterior bone loss of more than 10%, the only risk factor was the number of shoulder dislocations [25].

History and Physical Examination

As with any shoulder instability patient, a thorough history is crucial to evaluate the parameters and risk factors predictive for recurrent instability, understand why a prior shoulder stabilization surgery has failed, and identify patients who are better suited for a bone reconstruction procedure. The history should include the patient's age, handedness, type of sports, level of competition, unilateral or bilateral shoulder instability, and an understanding of the initial traumatic event, including how the shoulder was dislocated and reduced, the number of instability events, the force required to recreate a dislocation, the presence of pain, the presence of mechanical symptoms, neurological symptoms, prior surgical procedures, and whether any complications have occurred.

Physical examination generally includes provocative and laxity tests. The anterior apprehension and relocation tests are easily elicited in patients with anterior glenoid bone loss. The load and shift test, sulcus test, and the Beighton criteria identify instability and laxity. Determining generalized ligamentous laxity or multidirectional shoulder instability is crucial as it can uncover systemic laxity due to a connective tissue disease and alter the treatment plan. Furthermore, one must evaluate for prior surgical incisions, including any potential signs of infection, and perform a thorough neurovascular examination.

Table 20.1 Anterior glenoid bone loss can be measured using the surface area, linear, and superimposed best-fit circle methods

Measuring glenoid bone loss		
Method	Description	Calculation
Surface area	1. Draw a best-fit circle on the inferior glenoid surface and the glenoid surface area is calculated (A) 2. Draw the area around the glenoid bony defect, and calculate its surface area (B) 3. Bone loss is calculated by dividing the surface area of bone loss (B) by the surface area of the best-fit circle (A)	$\frac{(B)}{A} \times 100\%$
Linear	1. Draw a best-fit circle on the inferior glenoid surface 2. Measure a distance from the center of the circle to the posterior edge of the glenoid (A) 3. Measure a distance from the center of the circle to the anterior edge of the glenoid (B) 4. Bone loss is calculated by dividing the defect distance (A–B) by the glenoid diameter	$\frac{(A-B)}{2 \times A} \times 100\%$
Superimposed	1. Requires bilateral shoulder CT scans 2. Draw a best-fit circle on the inferior two-thirds of the normal glenoid (A) 3. Superimpose the best-fit circle on the injured glenoid (B) 4. Bone loss is calculated by dividing the defect's surface area (A–B) by the surface area of the best-fit circle of the normal glenoid (A)	$\frac{(A-B)}{A} \times 100\%$

CT computed tomography

Imaging

Plain radiographs are the initial diagnostic imaging modality to evaluate for anterior glenoid bone loss. A standard series should include an anteroposterior (AP), a true AP (Grashey view), axillary, and modified scapular Y views. The axillary view helps visualize the anteroinferior glenoid. A specialty view called the West Point view is a modification of the axillary view and has demonstrated significantly higher specificity of anteroinferior glenoid bone loss. It is also essential to evaluate for any humeral-sided bone loss, such as a Hill-Sachs lesion, which can be seen as blunting of the superolateral aspect of the proximal humerus on an AP view. However, the Stryker notch view is the best radiographic view to evaluate for a Hill-Sachs lesion.

MRI with or without arthrography is the gold standard for evaluating soft-tissue pathologies, including capsulolabral complex tears, which are essential lesions in shoulder instability cases. While MRI is useful in assessing osseous pathology, a CT scan is more effective. A 3D reconstruction CT scan with an en face view of the glenoid is optimal for quantifying bone loss. Multiple methods exist to measure anterior glenoid bone loss, including the surface area, linear, and superimposed circle methods (Table 20.1). The most precise technique is the surface area method as the others can underestimate or overestimate the amount of bone loss [26]. However, the linear method is likely the most convenient in an office-based setting.

Bone Augmentation with a Distal Tibia Allograft

A bone augmentation procedure is typically required for significant anterior glenoid bone loss as this is associated with high failure rates with soft-tissue stabilization alone [9, 11, 27]. There is a controversy regarding the cutoff point for critical bone loss, and in the literature, the bone loss cutoff ranges between 13.5% and 25% [9, 11, 12]. However, a multitude of factors can influence the decision to opt for a bony augmentation procedure, such as soft-tissue pathologies (e.g., anterior labral periosteal sleeve avulsion), concurrent large and medial Hill-Sachs lesions, failed prior soft-tissue stabilization, and specific demographics such as young male contact sport athletes [28].

Although open Latarjet coracoid transfer remains the gold standard bone augmentation procedure, multiple other graft options offer a valid and alternative approach, each with advantages and disadvantages. Compared with the Latarjet procedure, DTA negates the risk for donor-site morbidity, preserves subscapularis integrity, and reduces graft-related complications, iatrogenic neurovascular injury, and osteolysis [29, 30]. DTA also provides an osteochondral surface and graft curvature similar to the native glenoid that can be fashioned depending on the amount of bone loss. The anatomic reconstruction of the glenoid allows for improved humeral head articulation, restoring stability and normal shoulder biomechanics and enabling a return to high-demand physical activity [2, 14, 22, 23]. Potential disadvantages include graft availability, cost, risk of disease transmission, and slower integration compared to autogenous grafts [31, 32].

Step 1: Distal Tibia Allograft Preparation.

There are multiple DTA types. We prefer a fresh DTA over a fresh-frozen allograft as it has a higher potential for osteointegration and less bone resorption. However, fresh allografts carry a higher risk of disease transmission, and patients should be counseled about the risk of such adverse events.

We typically use a commercially available graft workstation that facilitates graft preparation (Fig. 20.5). The graft size should be approximately fashioned to the following dimensions: 1 cm wide, 1 cm deep, and 2 cm in length (Figs. 20.6 and 20.7). However, one must tailor the size depending on the size of the defect. Thereafter, further graft preparation depends on the preferred fixation method, such as screws, suture-buttons, or suture anchors. Our preferred approach is to use 4.5 mm fully threaded cortical screws.

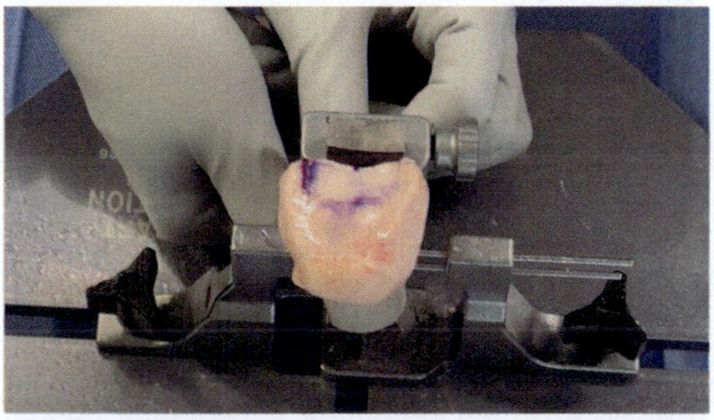

Fig. 20.5 The distal tibia allograft preparation using a commercially available workstation

Step 2: The Deltopectoral Approach.

The surgery is performed in the beach chair with the head of the table inclined to 60 degrees. A bump is placed under the ipsilateral scapular medial border, facilitating glenoid exposure. The affected upper extremity and hemithorax are draped, and the affected arm is placed in an arm holder.

The incision utilized is more medial and vertical in orientation when compared to the conventional deltopectoral approach to enhance exposure to the anterior glenoid. An incision is

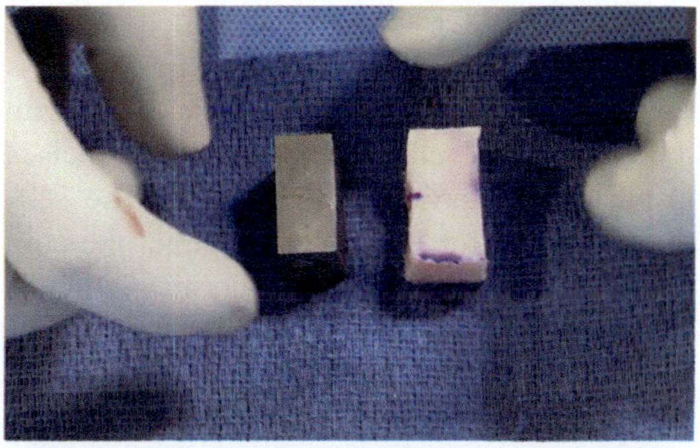

Fig. 20.6 The distal tibia allograft is fashioned with a length of 20 mm and a width of 10 mm

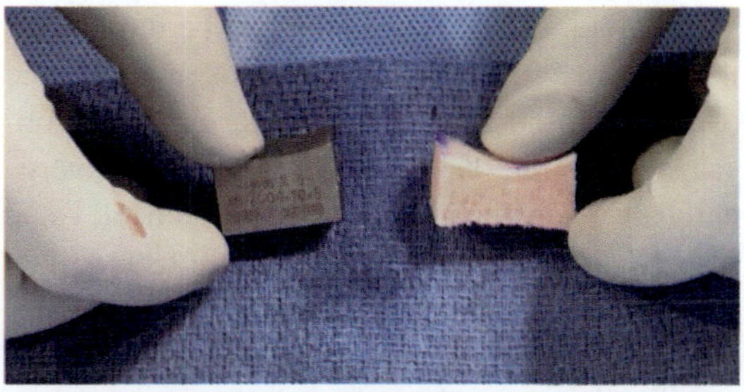

Fig. 20.7 The distal tibia allograft is fashioned with a depth of 10 mm

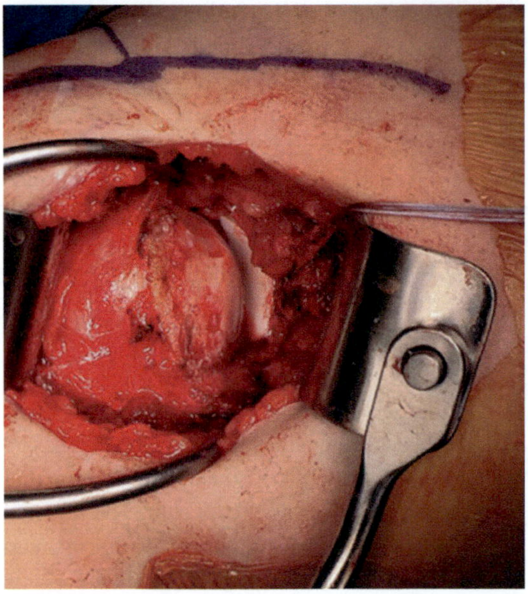

Fig. 20.8 Exposure of the glenoid in a patient with a prior failed anterior stabilization procedure. (Frank et al. [22])

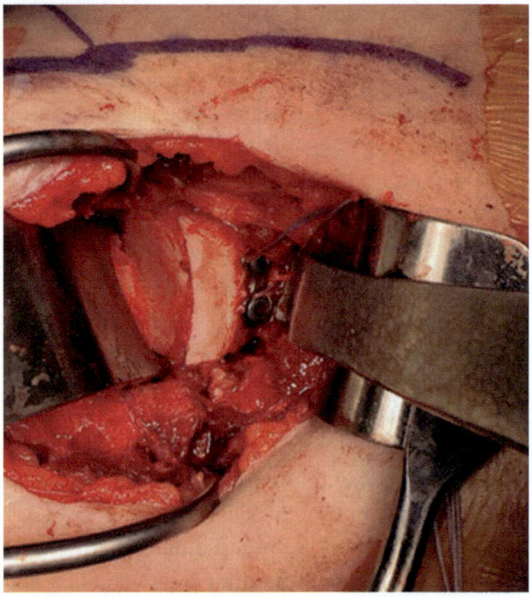

Fig. 20.9 An intraoperative photograph demonstrating the completed open anterior distal tibial allograft augmentation using screw fixation. (Frank et al. [22])

made from the coracoid and taken inferiorly toward the axillary crease. The deltopectoral approach is developed, and the cephalic vein is dissected carefully and retracted laterally with the deltoid. The clavipectoral fascia is incised just lateral to the conjoined tendon. The self-retaining retractor is utilized to retract the conjoined tendon and pectoralis major medially and the deltoid laterally.

Step 3: Glenoid Preparation and Graft Fixation.

The subscapularis tendon and muscle are then visualized, and the subscapularis tendon is split horizontally at its middle third. The subscapularis tendon split is carried medially through the subscapularis muscle. Gauze can then be introduced through the subscapularis split to enhance the exposure of the capsule just posterior to the subscapularis split. The capsule is then split vertically at the anterior glenoid and then elevated medially with any remaining labrum to facilitate exposure of the anterior glenoid. This exposure might be difficult in cases with a prior soft-tissue stabilization procedure due to the presence of scar tissue and the lack of a discrete capsule and labrum. In cases of a prior failed Latarjet procedure, a careful dissection for hardware removal is essential as the distance to the neurovascular structures is much shorter (Fig. 20.8) [33].

A humeral head retractor, such as the Fukuda retractor, is used to facilitate glenoid exposure. The anterior glenoid surface is freshened with an electrical burr. The prepared distal tibia graft is then applied to the anterior glenoid and is fixed provisionally with K-wires. One must ensure that the graft is flush with the glenoid articular margin. Each K-wire is sequentially drilled with a cannulated 3.2 mm drill bit, and then a 4.5 mm cannulated fully threaded screw with a washer is applied (Fig. 20.9). The capsule is then repaired, and the subscapularis split is then closed.

Postoperative Rehabilitation

Postoperative rehabilitation consists of three phases. Phase one includes an immobilization period of 6 weeks to ensure graft healing. However, passive ROM is allowed with pendulums. Phase two consists of starting active ROM and continuously improving passive ROM for

6 weeks. Phase three includes continued ROM rehabilitation, rotator cuff strengthening, and sport-specific conditioning. Patients are expected to return to sport at 4–6 months, depending on sport type and level of competition.

References

1. Provencher MT, Bhatia S, Ghodadra NS, Grumet RC, Bach BR Jr, Dewing CB, et al. Recurrent shoulder instability: current concepts for evaluation and management of glenoid bone loss. J Bone Joint Surg Am. 2010;92(Suppl 2):133–51. https://doi.org/10.2106/jbjs.J.00906.
2. Provencher MT, Ghodadra N, LeClere L, Solomon DJ, Romeo AA. Anatomic osteochondral glenoid reconstruction for recurrent glenohumeral instability with glenoid deficiency using a distal tibia allograft. Arthroscopy. 2009;25(4):446–52. https://doi.org/10.1016/j.arthro.2008.10.017.
3. Thacher RR, Retzky JS, Dekhne MS, Oquendo YA, Greditzer HG. Current concepts in the measurement of Glenohumeral bone loss. Curr Rev Musculoskelet Med. 2023;16(9):419–31. https://doi.org/10.1007/s12178-023-09852-0.
4. DeFroda SF, Donnelly JC, Mulcahey MK, Perez L, Owens BD. Shoulder instability in women compared with men: epidemiology, pathophysiology, and special considerations. JBJS Rev. 2019;7(9):e10. https://doi.org/10.2106/jbjs.Rvw.19.00007.
5. Nakagawa S, Iuchi R, Hanai H, Hirose T, Mae T. The development process of bipolar bone defects from primary to recurrent instability in shoulders with traumatic anterior instability. Am J Sports Med. 2019;47(3):695–703. https://doi.org/10.1177/0363546518819471.
6. Brophy RH, Marx RG. The treatment of traumatic anterior instability of the shoulder: nonoperative and surgical treatment. Arthroscopy. 2009;25(3):298–304. https://doi.org/10.1016/j.arthro.2008.12.007.
7. De Carli A, Vadalà AP, Lanzetti R, Lupariello D, Gaj E, Ottaviani G, et al. Early surgical treatment of first-time anterior glenohumeral dislocation in a young, active population is superior to conservative management at long-term follow-up. Int Orthop. 2019;43(12):2799–805. https://doi.org/10.1007/s00264-019-04382-2.
8. Prada C, Al-Mohrej OA, Patel A, Flood B, Leroux T, Khan M. Managing bone loss in shoulder instability-techniques and outcomes: a scoping review. Curr Rev Musculoskelet Med. 2021;14(6):447–61. https://doi.org/10.1007/s12178-021-09727-2.
9. Shaha JS, Cook JB, Song DJ, Rowles DJ, Bottoni CR, Shaha SH, et al. Redefining "critical" bone loss in shoulder instability: functional outcomes worsen with "subcritical" bone loss. Am J Sports Med. 2015;43(7):1719–25. https://doi.org/10.1177/0363546515578250.
10. Tennent DJ, Donohue MA, Posner MA. Bone loss and Glenohumeral instability. Sports Med Arthrosc Rev. 2017;25(3):131–5. https://doi.org/10.1097/jsa.0000000000000156.
11. Shin SJ, Kim RG, Jeon YS, Kwon TH. Critical value of anterior glenoid bone loss that leads to recurrent Glenohumeral instability after arthroscopic Bankart repair. Am J Sports Med. 2017;45(9):1975–81. https://doi.org/10.1177/0363546517697963.
12. Burkhart SS, De Beer JF. Traumatic glenohumeral bone defects and their relationship to failure of arthroscopic Bankart repairs: significance of the inverted-pear glenoid and the humeral engaging hill-Sachs lesion. Arthroscopy. 2000;16(7):677–94. https://doi.org/10.1053/jars.2000.17715.
13. Hurley ET, Matache BA, Wong I, Itoi E, Strauss EJ, Delaney RA, et al. Anterior shoulder instability part II-Latarjet, Remplissage, and glenoid bone-grafting-an international consensus statement. Arthroscopy. 2022;38(2):224–33.e6. https://doi.org/10.1016/j.arthro.2021.07.023.
14. Provencher MT, Peebles LA, Aman ZS, Bernhardson AS, Murphy CP, Sanchez A, et al. Management of the Failed Latarjet Procedure: outcomes of revision surgery with fresh distal Tibial allograft. Am J Sports Med. 2019;47(12):2795–802. https://doi.org/10.1177/0363546519871896.
15. Reider B. The non-Latarjet. Am J Sports Med. 2018;46(5):1027–9. https://doi.org/10.1177/0363546518764666.
16. Tokish JM, Brinkman JC, Hassebrock JD. Arthroscopic technique for distal Tibial allograft bone augmentation with suture anchor fixation for anterior shoulder instability. Arthrosc Tech. 2022;11(5):e903–e9. https://doi.org/10.1016/j.eats.2022.01.010.
17. Kwapisz A, Fitzpatrick K, Cook JB, Athwal GS, Tokish JM. Distal clavicular osteochondral autograft augmentation for glenoid bone loss: a comparison of radius of restoration versus Latarjet graft. Am J Sports Med. 2018;46(5):1046–52. https://doi.org/10.1177/0363546517749915.
18. Liles JL, Ganokroj P, Peebles AM, Mologne MS, Provencher CMT. Fresh distal Tibial allograft: an updated graft preparation technique for anterior shoulder instability. Arthrosc Tech. 2022;11(6):e1027–e31. https://doi.org/10.1016/j.eats.2022.02.005.
19. Gilat R, Wong SE, Lavoie-Gagne O, Haunschild ED, Knapik DM, Fu MC, et al. Outcomes are comparable using free bone block autografts versus allografts for the management of anterior shoulder instability with glenoid bone loss: a systematic review and meta-analysis of "the non-Latarjet". Knee Surg Sports Traumatol Arthrosc. 2021;29(7):2159–74. https://doi.org/10.1007/s00167-020-06194-z.
20. Provencher MT, Frank RM, Golijanin P, Gross D, Cole BJ, Verma NN, et al. Distal tibia allograft glenoid reconstruction in recurrent anterior shoulder instabil-

ity: clinical and radiographic outcomes. Arthroscopy. 2017;33(5):891–7. https://doi.org/10.1016/j.arthro.2016.09.029.
21. Wong I, John R, Ma J, Coady CM. Arthroscopic anatomic glenoid reconstruction using distal Tibial allograft for recurrent anterior shoulder instability: clinical and radiographic outcomes. Am J Sports Med. 2020;48(13):3316–21. https://doi.org/10.1177/0363546520960119.
22. Frank RM, Romeo AA, Richardson C, Sumner S, Verma NN, Cole BJ, et al. Outcomes of Latarjet versus distal tibia allograft for anterior shoulder instability repair: a matched cohort analysis. Am J Sports Med. 2018;46(5):1030–8. https://doi.org/10.1177/0363546517744203.
23. Waterman BR, Chandler PJ, Teague E, Provencher MT, Tokish JM, Pallis MP. Short-term outcomes of glenoid bone block augmentation for complex anterior shoulder instability in a high-risk population. Arthroscopy. 2016;32(9):1784–90. https://doi.org/10.1016/j.arthro.2016.01.051.
24. Dickens JF, Slaven SE, Cameron KL, Pickett AM, Posner M, Campbell SE, et al. Prospective evaluation of glenoid bone loss after first-time and recurrent anterior Glenohumeral instability events. Am J Sports Med. 2019;47(5):1082–9. https://doi.org/10.1177/0363546519831286.
25. Hettrich CM, Magnuson JA, Baumgarten KM, Brophy RH, Kattan M, Bishop JY, et al. Predictors of bone loss in anterior Glenohumeral instability. Am J Sports Med. 2023;51(5):1286–94. https://doi.org/10.1177/03635465231160286.
26. Bakshi NK, Cibulas GA, Sekiya JK, Bedi A. A clinical comparison of linear- and surface area-based methods of measuring glenoid bone loss. Am J Sports Med. 2018;46(10):2472–7. https://doi.org/10.1177/0363546518783724.
27. Frank RM, Romeo AA, Provencher MT. Glenoid reconstruction with distal tibia allograft for recurrent anterior shoulder instability. Orthopedics. 2017;40(1):e199–205. https://doi.org/10.3928/01477447-20161006-06.
28. Ozbaydar M, Elhassan B, Diller D, Massimini D, Higgins LD, Warner JJ. Results of arthroscopic capsulolabral repair: Bankart lesion versus anterior labroligamentous periosteal sleeve avulsion lesion. Arthroscopy. 2008;24(11):1277–83. https://doi.org/10.1016/j.arthro.2008.01.017.
29. Gupta A, Delaney R, Petkin K, Lafosse L. Complications of the Latarjet procedure. Curr Rev Musculoskelet Med. 2015;8(1):59–66. https://doi.org/10.1007/s12178-015-9258-y.
30. van der Linde JA, Wessel RN, Trantalis JN, van den Bekerom MPJ. Review of Latarjet (1954) on the treatment of recurrent shoulder dislocations. Journal of ISAKOS. 2018;3(4):242–8. https://doi.org/10.1136/jisakos-2017-000153.
31. Tokish JM, Fitzpatrick K, Cook JB, Mallon WJ. Arthroscopic distal clavicular autograft for treating shoulder instability with glenoid bone loss. Arthrosc Tech. 2014;3(4):e475–81. https://doi.org/10.1016/j.eats.2014.05.006.
32. Willemot LB, Elhassan BT, Verborgt O. Bony reconstruction of the anterior glenoid rim. J Am Acad Orthop Surg. 2018;26(10):e207–e18. https://doi.org/10.5435/jaaos-d-16-00649.
33. LaPrade CM, Bernhardson AS, Aman ZS, Moatshe G, Chahla J, Dornan GJ, et al. Changes in the neurovascular anatomy of the shoulder after an open Latarjet procedure: defining a surgical safe zone. Am J Sports Med. 2018;46(9):2185–91. https://doi.org/10.1177/0363546518773309.

21 The Frozen Distal Tibial Allograft: Justification and an All-Arthroscopic Approach

Fares Hamdan Al-Jahdali and Ivan Wong

Case Example

History:

This is a 24-year-old healthy woman who had a dislocation of her right shoulder while playing rugby. She underwent a Bankart repair and did well for a year. However, she dislocated her shoulder again after doing some overhead lifting and has been experiencing shoulder instability with multiple dislocations (Fig. 21.1).

Examination:

She had full range of motion (passively and actively).

She had 5/5 strength of her deltoid and rotator cuff muscle.

She had positive apprehension, relocation, and rebound test.

She was neurovascularly intact.

Imaging:

Her CT scan shows glenoid bone loss (15%) and addition to Hill-Sachs lesion (Fig. 21.2).

Plan:

Arthroscopic Bankart and remplissage procedure.

Arthroscopic anatomic glenoid reconstruction using distal tibia allograft (DTA) (Fig. 21.3).

F. H. Al-Jahdali
Orthopaedic Surgery, Department of Surgery, Faculty of Medicine, Dalhousie University, Halifax, NS, Canada

Department of Orthopedics, Prince Mohammed Bin Abdulaziz Hospital, Ministry of National Guard-Health Affairs, Madinah, Saudi Arabia
e-mail: fr756992@dal.ca

I. Wong (✉)
Orthopaedic Surgery, Department of Surgery, Faculty of Medicine, Dalhousie University, Halifax, NS, Canada
e-mail: research@drivanwong.com

© The Author(s), under exclusive license to Springer Nature Switzerland AG 2026
R. M. Frank, J. M. Tokish (eds.), *Management of Shoulder Instability*,
https://doi.org/10.1007/978-3-032-18089-6_21

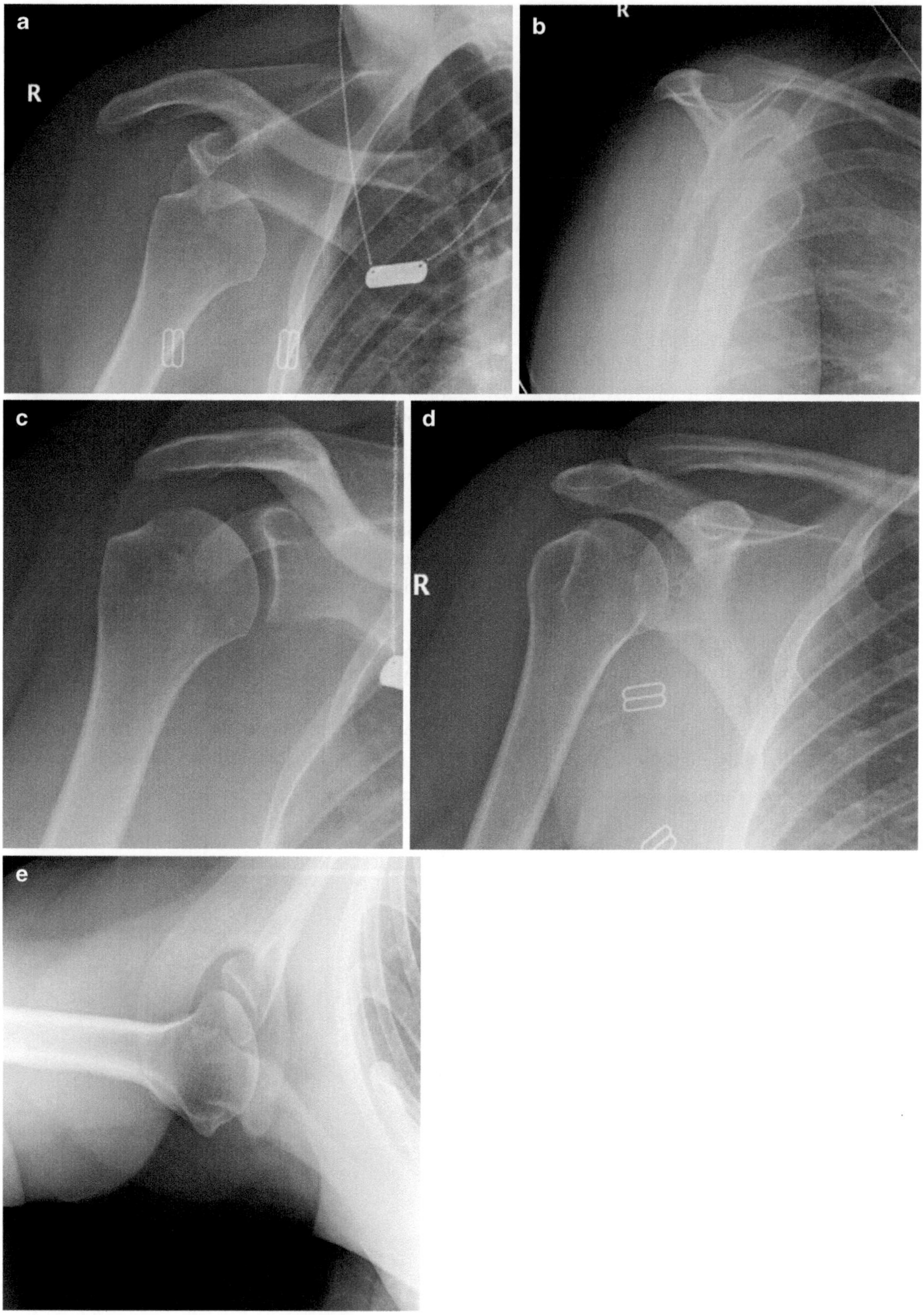

Fig. 21.1 (**a**–**e**) AP and scapular Y view showing right shoulder dislocation with AP and oblique view of her right shoulder post reduction

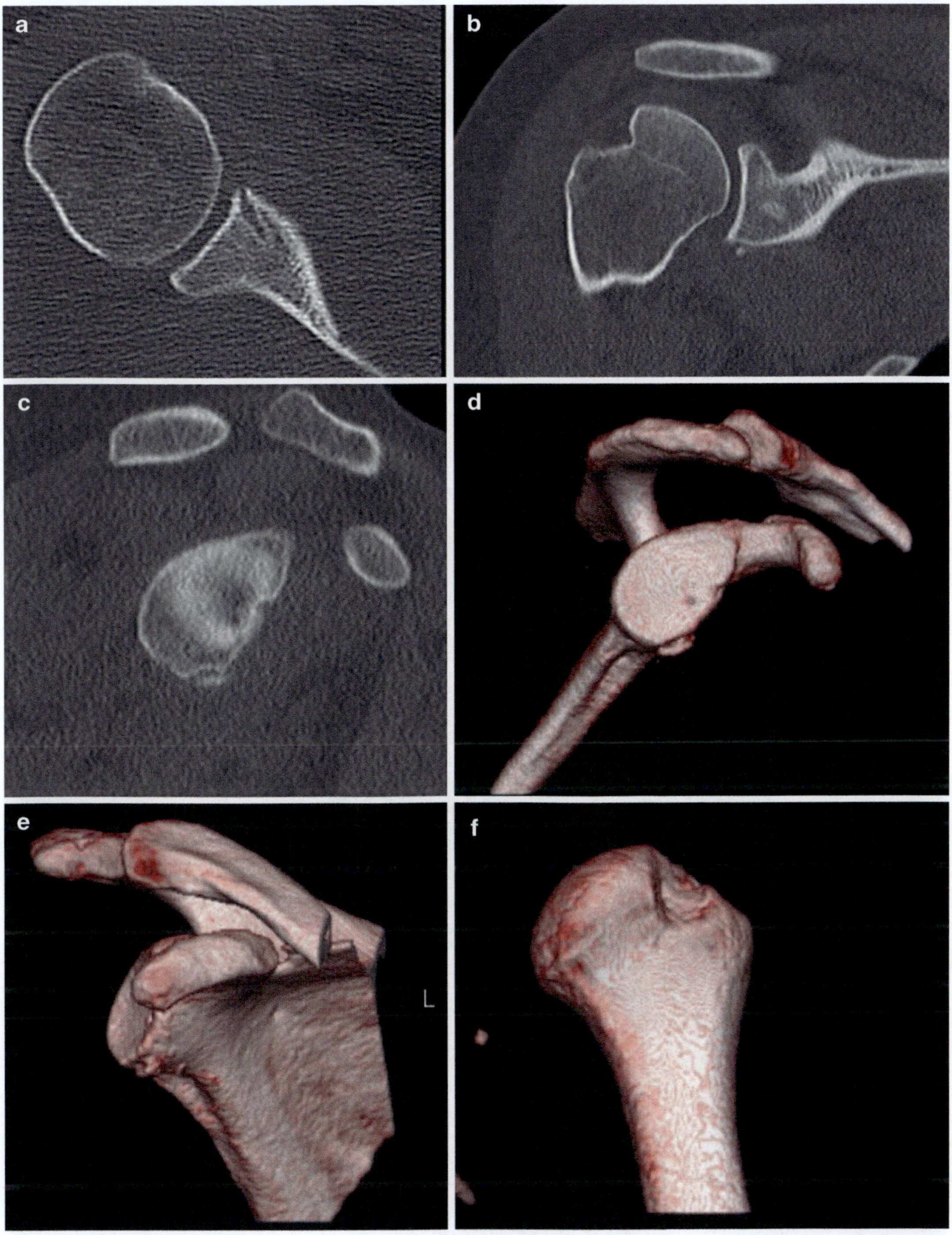

Fig. 21.2 (**a**–**f**) Preoperative CT scan with glenoid showing bony Bankart and Hill-Sachs lesion

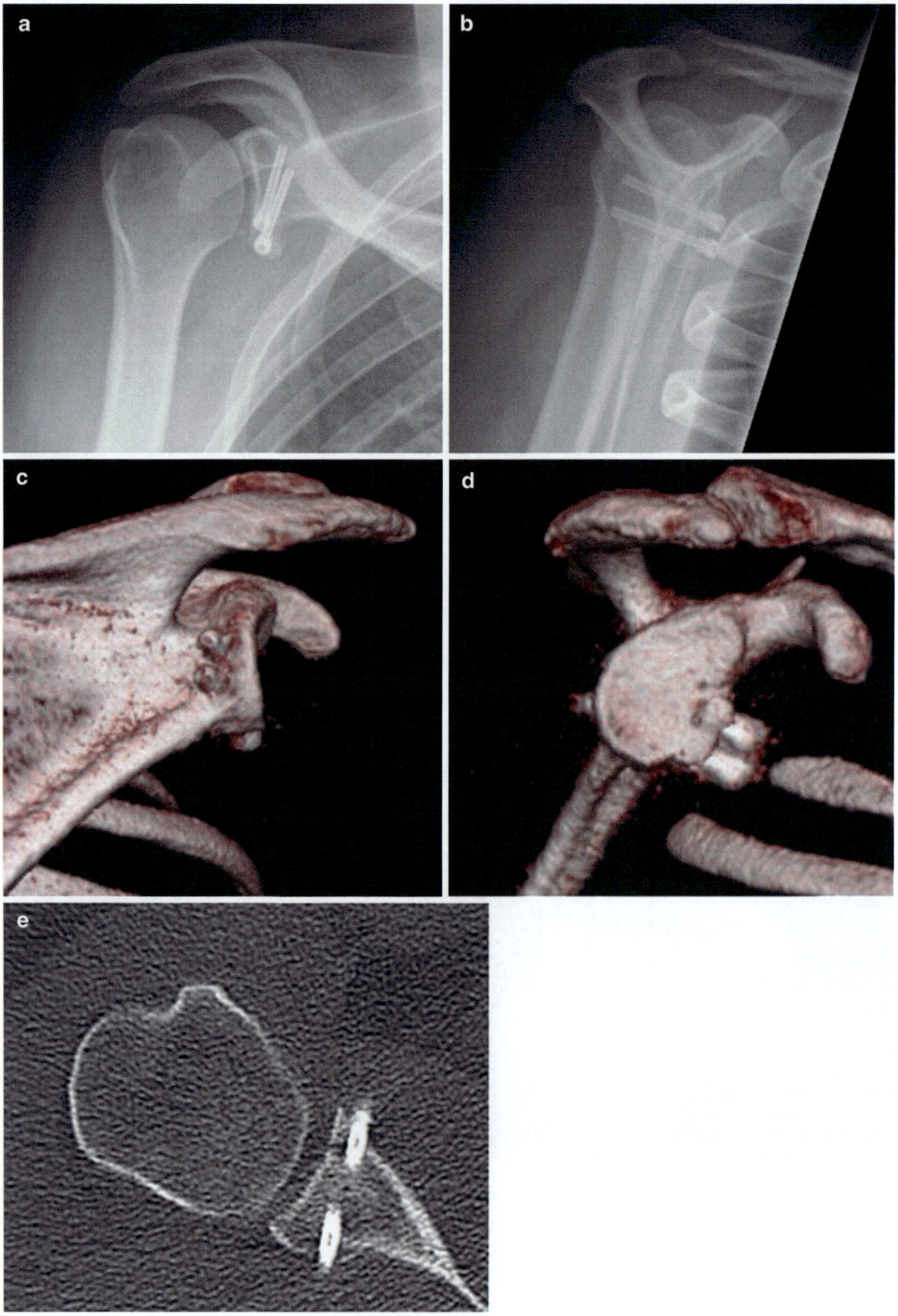

Fig. 21.3 (**a**–**e**) Postoperative CT scan showing the bone graft healing and position

Distal Tibia Allograft in Anterior Shoulder Instability

The glenohumeral joint has the greatest range of motion, and due to the complexity and its delicate balance between stability and mobility, it is at a higher risk of dislocation making up 50% of all dislocations [1, 2]. Most of the traumatic shoulder dislocations are anterior (96%) leading to bony and soft tissue injury. Glenohumeral instability has been associated with a recurrence rate ranging from 30% to 90% [3–5]. Failing to address glenoid bone loss (GBL) and only addressing soft tissue is a risk factor for failure, making the risk of recurrence as high as 67% [4]. The anteroinferior rim of the glenoid is important for anteroinferior glenohumeral stability, with biomechanical studies showing that 20% anterior GBL reduces the force required to anteriorly translate glenohumeral joint [6, 7].

There are multiple options to address GBL including the Latarjet procedure and bony augmentation using autograft and allografts. The Latarjet procedure is considered the gold standard surgical treatment [8]. The combination of coracoid bone grafting and the sling effect of the conjoined tendon has shown to be successful static restraint against anterior dislocation; however, more recently, it has been shown that it is a nonanatomic reconstruction due to the non-cartilaginous surface of the coracoid and shifting this to the anterior rim of glenoid through a subscapularis split makes future surgery more difficult. Moreover, the Latarjet has a potential of graft osteolysis and resorption [9–11]. Fresh distal tibia allograft (DTA) for glenoid reconstruction in anterior shoulder instability was recently described and has gained popularity recently [12, 13]. DTA is a strong weight-bearing bone and can consequently accommodate more drilling and instrumentation. It also has excellent conformity with the native glenoid and has less contamination risk due to being a peripheral portion of the body [12]. In addition, Moroder et al. has shown in his level 1 Neer Award paper comparing Latarjet to free bone block that the conjoined sling is not necessary to maintain shoulder stability in patients with glenoid bone loss if the glenoid bone is reconstructed [14]. Wong et al. (2018) has shown that arthroscopic anatomic glenoid reconstruction (AAGR) with frozen DTA has shown comparable healing rate, final graft size, and the anteroposterior dimensions of the reconstructed glenoid as compared to the Latarjet [15]. This procedure has also shown promising radiographic and clinical outcomes at 1 year and 2 years postoperatively while minimizing complication rates [16, 17]. These positive outcomes of the AAGR with screw fixation have lasted at a minimum of 5-year follow-up with a low recurrence rate and an excellent safety profile, which demonstrates that AAGR with DTA is a great surgical option for patients with anterior shoulder instability with GBL [18].

Surgical Technique

Patient Position

The patient is positioned in the lateral decubitus position using a vacuum bean bag positioner, allowing the patient to rotate back approximately 30 degrees so that the glenoid surface is parallel to the floor (Fig. 21.4). A bolster is placed to support the scapula and the arm is placed in a pneumatic limb positioner (Spider 2; Smith & Nephew, Memphis, TN) and abducted 60 degrees in balanced suspension. Anesthesia should be consulted with lateral decubitus positioning to keep blood pressure at 100 mmHg systolic so that pump pressure can be kept as low as possible. An inflow/outflow pump with pressure settings of 35 mmHg can allow the entire procedure to have adequate viewing while minimizing any fluid extravasation, thus making the procedure safer and less painful.

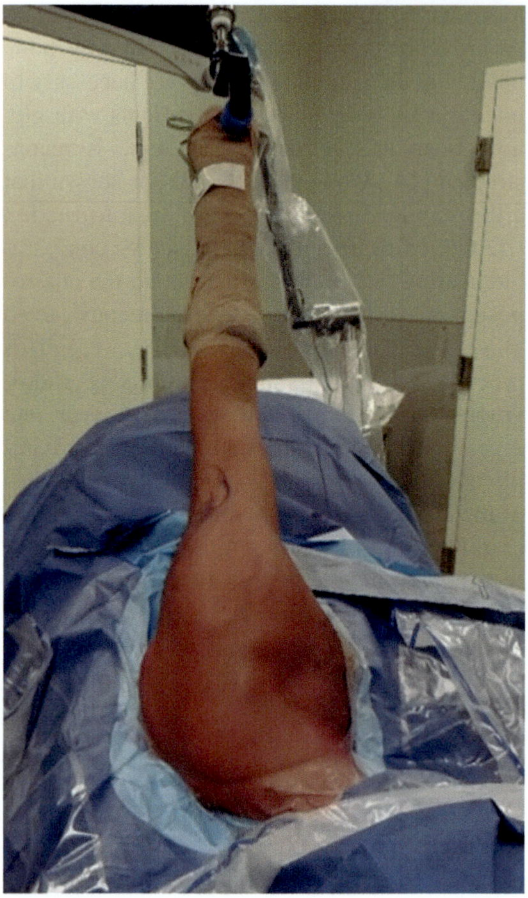

Fig. 21.4 The picture shows the patient is positioned in the lateral decubitus position using a vacuum bean bag positioner and the arm is placed in a pneumatic limb positioner and abducted 60 degrees in balanced suspension

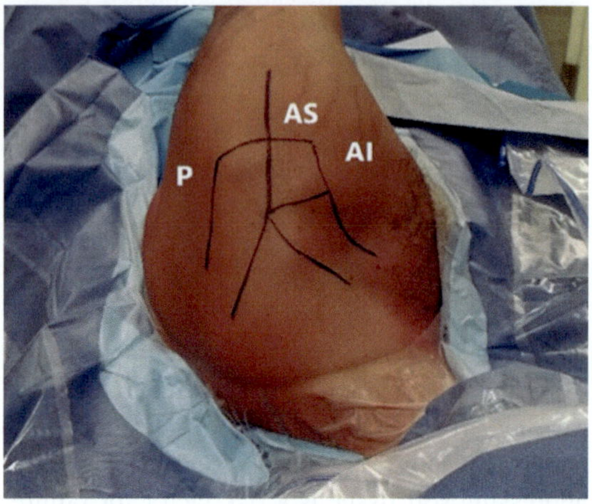

Fig. 21.5 This picture shows skin landmarks being drawn, acromion, clavicle, acromioclavicular joint, and scapular spine. Posterior, anterosuperior (AS), and anteroinferior (AI) portals

Portal Placement and Diagnostic Arthroscopy

After positioning, skin landmarks are drawn, including the coracoid, acromion, clavicle, acromioclavicular joint, and scapular spine. Posterior, anterosuperior (AS), and anteroinferior (AI) portals are also located and marked (Fig. 21.5). A standard 15-point diagnostic arthroscopy is performed starting at the posterior portal according to Snyder's technique [19]. To create the AI portal, an outside-in technique is used. Using a shaver and thermal probe, the rotator interval is released to visualize the acromioclavicular ligament, the tip of the coracoid, and the conjoined tendon. The arthroscope is switched to the AS portal for the viewing portal. A traction suture is placed around the anterosuperior labrum at 3 o'clock through the AI portal using a suture passer (Spectrum II; ConMed, Utica, NY). This traction suture assists in manipulation of the labrum and visualization of the bone bed, is used to secure the Bankart repair at the end of the case, and is used to measure the inferior to superior shift translating the tissue from 3 o'clock to 12 o'clock at the end of the procedure. An episiotomy of the labrum between the traction suture and the biceps anchor is made to maximize view and allow for a real inferior to superior capsular shift. Elevation of the anterior capsule labral complex is best done with a chisel ablator tip (Arthrocare 90 Smith and Nephew), starting the release medially and extending it laterally toward the articular surface. This improves the quality of tissue so that even ALPSA/GLAD-type lesions have good soft tissue to recreate the bankart shift. In addition, this allows for better visualization than using an elevator knife to release the tissue from the labrum/articular surface. An elevator knife can be used below the 6 o'clock location to free any labral adhesions to the glenoid rim and neck (Fig. 21.6), with a shaver being used to debride any further soft tissue residue (Fig. 21.7) [20]. A switching stick can be introduced through the posterior portal to retract the subscapularis.

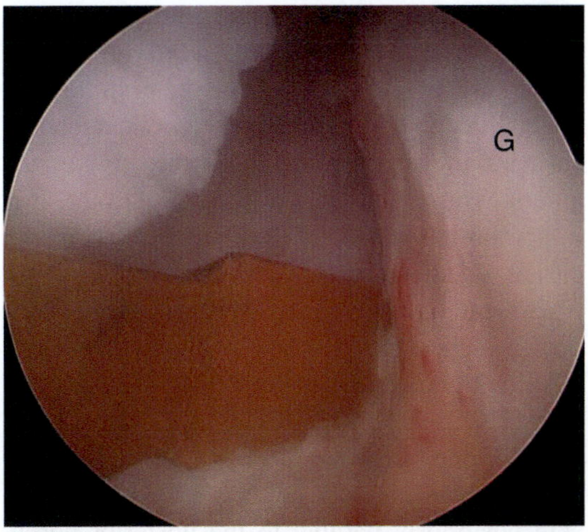

Fig. 21.6 Arthroscopic picture showing an elevator knife being used to free labral adhesions to the glenoid rim and neck

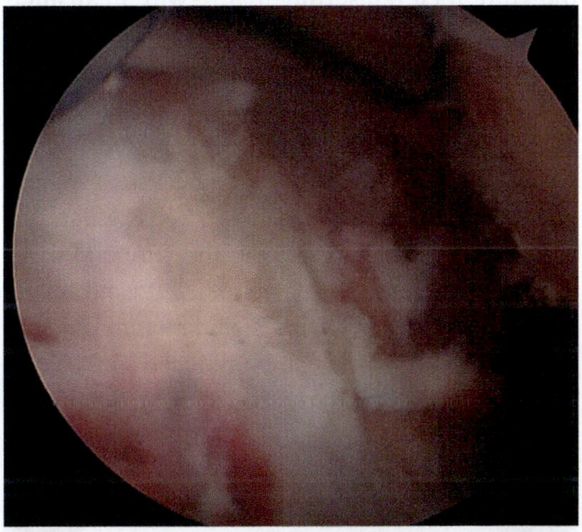

Fig. 21.7 Arthroscopic picture showing a shaver being used to debride any further soft tissue residue

The anteroinferior rim of the glenoid is decorticated using a burr (Stonecutter; Smith & Nephew) to provide a healthy, bleeding surface for graft union. Using a calibrated probe, the bare spot on the glenoid is used as a reference point for a calculation of glenoid dimension [20], which is then used to size the bone graft.

Hill-Sachs

The Hill-Sachs lesions should be addressed if calculating the on-track off-track to be in the peripheral track lesion as described by Itoi [21–23]. The anatomic glenoid reconstruction technique described here will produce a normal-sized glenoid no matter what size of graft is inserted after the bone has fully remodeled. Thus, a large Hill-Sachs lesion may result in an off-track lesion after final remodeling of bone. If this is the case, remplissage will be performed at the beginning of surgery using two q-fix anchors (Smith & Nephew) and a mattress suture configuration technique [24].

Graft Preparation and Placement

A frozen nonirradiated DTA is prepared based on intraoperative glenoid measurements. Utilizing the posterolateral corner of the DTA is better as it replicates the native contour of the glenoid, but the anterolateral corner works as well (Fig. 21.8a, b). The graft is then cut in typically dimension of 10 mm (anterior to posterior) × 15 mm (medial to

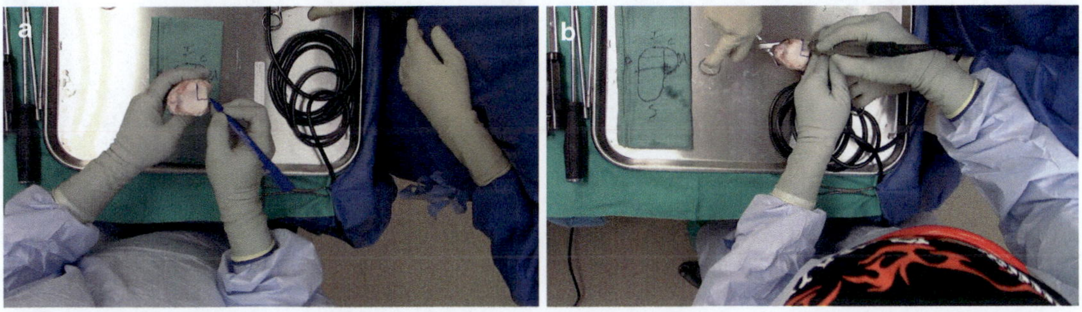

Fig. 21.8 (**a**, **b**) Graft being prepared based on the preoperative glenoid measurements utilizing the posterolateral corner of the DTA

lateral) × 20 mm (superior to inferior). A trapezoidal edge should be included so that the base of the graft will be in full contact with the medial edge of the native glenoid away from the articular cartilage (Fig. 21.8a, b). The alpha/beta guide (Depuy Mitek) with the positioning wire is used to drill two holes (10 mm apart) using a 2.8 mm drill [20]. The graft is then tapped and top-hat washers are placed to prevent hoop stress during screw compression. A clear double-barrel cannula is used and attached to the graft with the use of threaded cannulated screws [20] (Fig. 21.9).

The subscapularis is retracted inferiorly using a switching stick from the posterior portal and tension is released by internally rotating the humerus. The Halifax portal is created using an inside-out technique, instead of performing a subscapularis split [25] (Fig. 21.10). The thick switching stick is then advanced from the posterior portal, parallel to the glenoid, going above subscapularis and lateral to conjoined tendon before going through the skin [25]. If the conjoined tendon is tight preventing a parallel portal to the glenoid surface, the arm can be adducted and elbow flexed to 90 degrees.

Using the two slotted cannulas over the switching stick allows dilation of the Halifax portal with a channel dilator (Depuy Mitek). The portal is further dilated using a finger to make sure the clavipectoral fascia is well released lateral to the conjoin so that the graft can pass without entrapment into the glenohumeral joint. Two slotted cannulas are then replaced to prevent soft tissue entrapment while passing the graft through the Halifax portal lateral to the conjoined tendon, superior to subscapularis, and directly on the anterior rim of the glenoid (Fig. 21.11a, b). It is important to look at the graft from all portals to ensure adequate reduction and accurate graft placement. The switching stick in the posterior portal can be utilized to help manipulate the graft position to make sure that it is level with the glenoid [25].

Two long wires are used to drill through the double-barrel cannula going all the way to the skin posteriorly parallel to the posterior portal. Micro-adjustment of the graft to angulate or translate to recreate the glenoid surface can be done by removing one K-wire, rotating or tilting the graft, then reinserting that K-wire in an alternating fashion. The barrel is removed and a 2.8 mm calibrated cannulated drill is used to drill until posterior glenoid cortex is perforated. Screw length measurements can be made most accurately with the calibrations read near the top-hats. Cannulated titanium screws (max diameter: 4.5 mm) are then passed over the wire and tightened in an alternating fashion. The usual length of the screws are between 34 and 36 mm [20, 25].

The subscapularis can be reduced in the front of the graft by pulling on the traction stitch and/

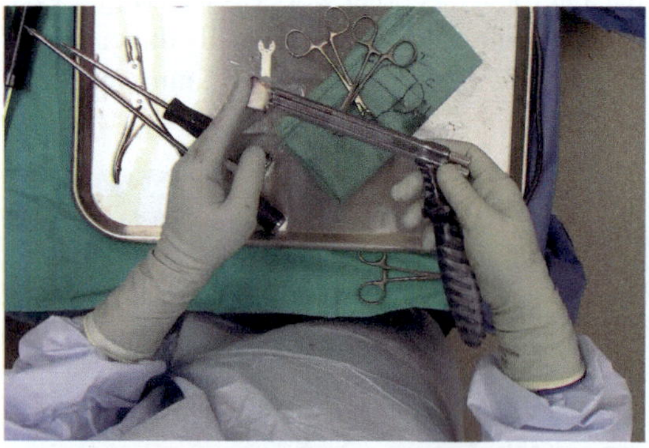

Fig. 21.9 Graft being held with the graft prep tool (Smith & Nephew) after the two holes being drilled and a clear double-barrel cannula is used and attached to the graft with the use of threaded cannulated screws for graft placement through the Halifax portal

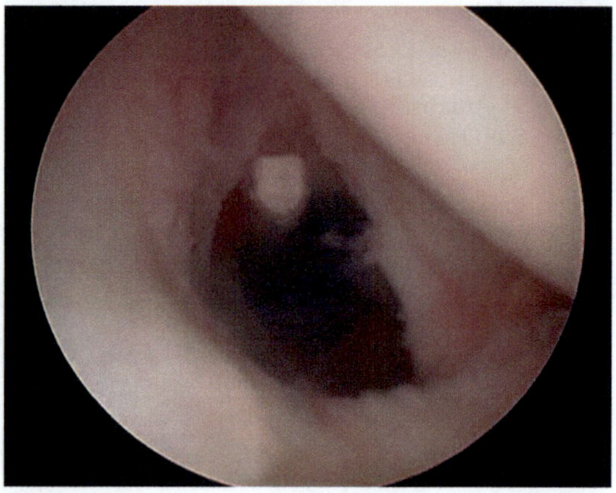

Fig. 21.10 Arthroscopic picture showing subscapularis being retracted inferiorly using a switching stick from the posterior portal to create the Halifax portal through an inside-out technique

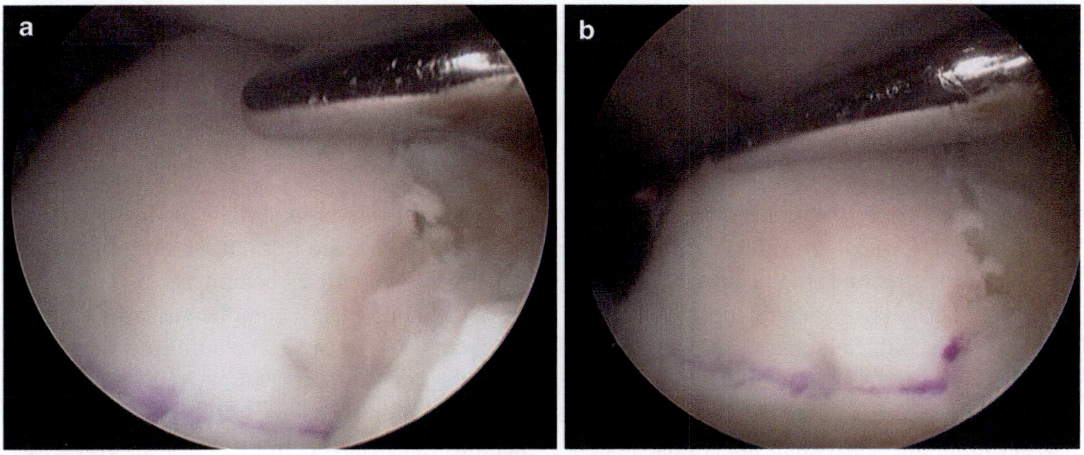

Fig. 21.11 (**a**, **b**) Arthroscopic picture showing the graft through the medial portal lateral to the conjoined tendon, superior to subscapularis, and directly on the anterior rim of the glenoid confirming that it is parallel to the glenoid using the switching stick

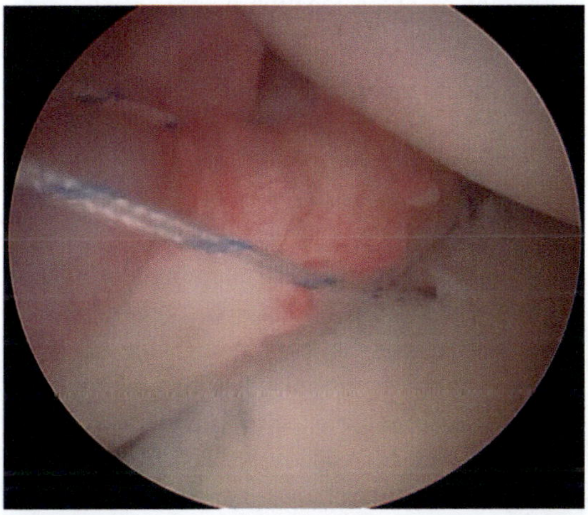

Fig. 21.12 Arthroscopic picture showing standard Bankart repair being performed at the end for added soft tissue support

or using a switching stick from the AI portal. Once the graft is placed, the arm should be abducted to 60 degrees and arm rotated back to neutral to allow a well-tensioned Bankart repair above the graft. Single-loaded all suture anchors are used (Q-fix, 1.8 mm single-loaded Smith and Nephew) at the 5 o'clock position on the native glenoid and then a standard Bankart repair is performed to add additional soft tissue support and to make the allograft extraarticular (Fig. 21.12). The traction suture is used to shift the tissue from 3'oclock where the traction suture was placed to 12 o'clock for an approximate 2 cm inferior to superior capsular shift. A second Q-fix anchor at the 3 o'clock position is used, and finally, the traction suture is fixed to the 12 o'clock position using a knotless 2.8 mm bioraptor (Smith and Nephew) to refix the labrum. A viewing from all portals should be done focusing on the AS portal to confirm that the humerus is stable and no longer dislocatable anteriorly [20]. All instruments then should be removed, and a shoulder examina tion should be performed to check for stability.

Postoperative Rehabilitation

An abduction shoulder brace (Slingshot 3.0 Breg Inc., Carlsbad, CA, USA) is used postoperatively. For the first 48–72 h, it is recommended to use ice compression to decrease swelling and pain. The brace is used for the first 2 weeks after surgery with passive range of motion exercises (shoulder, elbow, wrist, and hand). Active range of motion is not recommended before 6 weeks postoperatively; however, the introduction of isometric passive rotator cuff and deltoid exercises are allowed. The brace is discontinued after 6 weeks, and patients can work toward full active range of motion (ROM) and begin active-assisted exercises. Strengthening begins after patients have regained their full ROM.

Discussion

Lateral decubitus is the preferred position for AAGR with DTA [20] since it provides a better viewing of the structures in the anterior shoulder, including the anterior glenoid neck, subscapularis, and coracoid. In addition, the lateral position gives easier access to the posterior shoulder for the guidewires to exit the shoulder without the risk of hitting the beach-chair apparatus.

AAGR provides more anatomic stability than Latarjet because DTA has a better anatomic match and a smoother cartilaginous surface than the coracoid. The distal tibia is less abrasive to the humeral head and has the advantage of being fully customizable in terms of size and shape. In addition, the Latarjet gets stability from the conjoined tendon along with the bone block; however, AAGR with DTA allows a soft tissue repair (i.e., Bankart) over top of the bone graft imparting additional stability to the construct.

One of the main advantages of AAGR is that most of the arthroscopic portals it uses are those that shoulder surgeons are already familiar with (i.e., anteroinferior, anterosuperior, and posterior portals). The only new portal required for this procedure is the far medial portal, also known as the Halifax portal. It is created using an inside-out technique which provides a safe passage of the DTA and enables screws to be placed parallel to the glenoid. It has been shown in a cadaveric study that the portal is far away from neurovascular structures, which demonstrates the safety of the portal [26, 27] Moreover, it has been shown that surgeons only need around nine cases for surgical proficiency with this technique to obtain good graft positioning [27].

Both AAGR and Latarjet have showed comparable clinical outcomes. In a systematic review, McNeil et al. (2020) reported that AAGR results in satisfactory patient-reported outcomes (90% satisfaction) with a minimum follow-up of 15 months and also demonstrated significant improvements postoperatively. Wong et al. (2020) also showed promising clinical and radiographic outcomes at the minimum 2-year follow-up [17]. Similarly, Hurley et al. (2021) showed excellent midterm patient-reported outcomes of both open Latarjet and arthroscopic Latarjet postoperatively [28].

Even though both AAGR and the Latarjet have low recurrence rates, the Latarjet generally has more reported complications than the AAGR. Latarjet has a complication rate that varies from 15% to 30%, including nerve injuries that are not present with AAGR [29–31] In patients who underwent AAGR with DTA, graft healing rates ranged from 96.6% to 100% [29, 30], in comparison to a 9% nonunion rate for the Latarjet as reported by Griesser et al. (2013) in a systematic review [30]. Reoperation due to hardware complications and graft nonunion is still a concern for both treatment options (Latarjet and DTA) [31]; however, the revision for Latarjet is more challenging than the revision for AAGR due to the nonanatomic nature of the procedure [32].

The main limitation of DTA is access to bone graft in some institutions. Physicians at institutions without access to tissue banks may have limitations associated with obtaining frozen DTA for this procedure. There may be higher costs for these institutions as compared with hospitals with access to tissue banks. Lacking a bone bank may cause limitations with preoperative planning; however, DTA is rarely used for other purposes and is still relatively easier to obtain as compared to other types of grafts. In addition, iliac crest can be used as the graft for the same technique of AAGR as we have demonstrated it to be effective as our experience with DTA with a significant improvement in patient-reported outcome scores and high rates of graft union [33].

Conclusion

AAGR with DTA shows promising short- to mid-term outcomes with low complication rates and a low recurrence rate. This technique has a fast-learning curve and has demonstrated an excellent safety profile. In addition, due to the anatomic nature of the procedure, it is easier to revise than a Latarjet. AAGR with DTA is considered as a reliable treatment option for anterior shoulder instability with glenoid bone loss.

References

1. Dugas JR, Crozier MW. Traumatic anterior instability: treatment options for initial instability. Sports Med Arthrosc [Internet]. 2018;26(3):95–101.
2. Cutts S, Prempeh M, Drew S. Anterior shoulder dislocation. Ann R Coll Surg Engl. 2009;91(1):2–7.
3. Hovelius L, Olofsson A, Sandström B, Augustini B-G, Krantz L, Fredin H, et al. Nonoperative treatment of primary anterior shoulder dislocation in patients forty years of age and younger: a prospective twenty-five-year follow-up. JBJS. 90:945.
4. McLaughlin HL, Cavallaro WU. Primary anterior dislocation of the shoulder. Am J Surg. 1950;80(6):615–21.
5. Simonet WT, Cofield RH. Prognosis in anterior shoulder dislocation. Am J Sports Med. 1984;12(1):19–24.
6. Barchilon VS, Kotz E, Barchilon Ben-Av M, Glazer E, Nyska M. A simple method for quantitative evaluation of the missing area of the anterior glenoid in anterior instability of the glenohumeral joint. Skeletal Radiol. 2008;37(8):731–6.
7. Yamamoto N, Muraki T, Sperling JW, Steinmann SP, Cofield RH, Itoi E, et al. Stabilizing mechanism in bone-grafting of a large glenoid defect. JBJS. 2010;92(11)
8. Burkhart SS, De Beer JF. Traumatic glenohumeral bone defects and their relationship to failure of arthroscopic Bankart repairs: Significance of the inverted-pear glenoid and the humeral engaging Hill-Sachs lesion. Arthroscopy. 2000;16(7):677–94.
9. Kralinger FS, Golser K, Wischatta R, Wambacher M, Sperner G. Predicting recurrence after primary anterior shoulder dislocation. Am J Sports Med. 2002;30(1):116–20.
10. Lo IKY, Parten PM, Burkhart SS. The inverted pear glenoid: an indicator of significant glenoid bone loss. Arthroscopy. 2004;20(2):169–74.
11. Voos JE, Livermore RW, Feeley BT, Altchek DW, Williams RJ, Warren RF, et al. Prospective evaluation of arthroscopic bankart repairs for anterior instability. Am J Sports Med. 2010;38(2):302–7.
12. Provencher MT, Ghodadra N, LeClere L, Solomon DJ, Romeo AA. Anatomic osteochondral glenoid reconstruction for recurrent glenohumeral instability with glenoid deficiency using a distal tibia allograft. Arthroscopy. 2009;25(4):446–52.
13. Provencher MT, Frank RM, Golijanin P, et al. Distal tibia allograft glenoid reconstruction in recurrent anterior shoulder instability: clinical and radiographic outcomes. Arthroscopy. 2017;33(5):891–7.
14. Moroder P, Schulz E, Wierer G, Auffarth A, Habermeyer P, Resch H, Tauber M. Neer Award 2019: Latarjet procedure vs. iliac crest bone graft transfer for treatment of anterior shoulder instability with glenoid bone loss: a prospective randomized trial. J Shoulder Elbow Surg. 2019;28(7):1298–307. https://doi.org/10.1016/j.jse.2019.03.035. Epub 2019 May 23. PMID: 31129017
15. Wong IH, King JP, Boyd G, Mitchell M, Coady C. Radiographic analysis of glenoid size and shape after arthroscopic coracoid autograft versus distal tibial allograft in the treatment of anterior shoulder instability. Am J Sports Med. 2018;46(11):2717–24. https://doi.org/10.1177/0363546518789348. Epub 2018 Aug 10. PMID: 30095986
16. Amar E, Konstantinidis G, Coady C, Wong IH. Arthroscopic treatment of shoulder instability with glenoid bone loss using distal tibial allograft augmentation: safety profile and short-term radiological outcomes. Orthop J Sports Med. 2018;6(5):2325967118774507. https://doi.org/10.1177/2325967118774507. PMID: 29854863; PMCID: PMC5971393
17. Wong I, John R, Ma J, Coady CM. Arthroscopic anatomic glenoid reconstruction using distal tibial allograft for recurrent anterior shoulder instability: clinical and radiographic outcomes. Am J Sports Med. 2020;48(13):3316–21.
18. Wong IH, Sparavalo S, Ma J, Remedios S. Arthroscopic anatomic glenoid reconstruction has excellent outcomes at medium-term follow up for treating anterior shoulder instability with bone loss. 2022 AAOS Conference Proceedings. Available from: https://index.mirasmart.com/AAOS2022/PDFfiles/AAOS2022-001863.PDF.
19. Snyder SJ. Shoulder arthroscopy. 2nd ed. Philadelphia: Lip- pincott Williams & Wilkins; 2002.
20. McNeil D, Coady C, Wong IH. Arthroscopic anatomic glenoid reconstruction in lateral decubitus position using allograft with nonrigid fixation. Arthrosc Tech. 2018;7(11):e1115–21.
21. Burkhart SS, DeBeer JF, Tehrany AM, Parten PM. Quantifying glenoid bone loss arthroscopically in shoulder instability. Arthroscopy. 2002;18(5):488–91.
22. Itoi E. Opinion editorial—first-time shoulder dislocation: my approach. In: Matsen FAIII, Cordasco FA, Sperling JW, et al., editors. Rockwood and Matsen's the shoulder. 6th ed. Philadelphia: Elsevier; 2021. ISBN: 9780323698368.
23. Yamamoto N, Shinagawa K, Hatta T, et al. Peripheral-Track and Central-Track Hill-Sachs lesions: a new concept of assessing an On-Track lesion. Am J Sports Med. 2020;48:33–8.
24. Callegari JJ, Phillips CJ, Denard PJ. All-inside Knotless Remplissage technique. Arthrosc Tech. 2021;10(6):e1479–84. Published 2021 May 7. https://doi.org/10.1016/j.eats.2021.02.014.
25. Wong IH, Urquhart N. Arthroscopic anatomic glenoid reconstruction without subscapularis split. Arthrosc Tech. 2015;4(5):e449–56.

26. Moga I, Konstantinidis G, Wong IH-B. The safety of a far medial arthroscopic portal for anatomic glenoid reconstruction: a cadaveric study. Orthop J Sports Med September. 2018; https://doi.org/10.1177/2325967118795404.
27. Moga I, Konstantinidis G, Coady C, Ghosh S, Wong IH. Arthroscopic anatomic glenoid reconstruction: analysis of the learning curve. Orthop J Sports Med. 2018;6(11):2325967118807906. https://doi.org/10.1177/2325967118807906. PMID: 30480021; PMCID: PMC6240977
28. Hurley ET, Ben Ari E, Lorentz NA, Mojica ES, Colasanti CA, Matache BA, et al. Both open and arthroscopic latarjet result in excellent outcomes and low recurrence rates for anterior shoulder instability. Arthrosc Sport Med Rehabil. 2021;3(6):e1955–60.
29. Gupta A, Delaney R, Petkin K, Lafosse L. Complications of the Latarjet procedure. Curr Rev Musculoskelet Med. 2015;8(1):59–66.
30. Griesser MJ, Harris JD, BW MC, Hussain WM, Jones MH, Bishop JY, et al. Complications and reoperations after Bristow-Latarjet shoulder stabilization: a systematic review. J Shoulder Elb Surg. 2013;22(2):286–92.
31. Banas MP, Dalldorf PG, Sebastianelli WJ, DeHaven KE. Long-term followup of the modified Bristow procedure. Am J Sports Med. 1993;21(5):666–71.
32. Giannakos A, Vezeridis PS, Schwartz DG, Jany R, Lafosse L. All-arthroscopic revision Eden-Hybinette procedure for failed instability surgery: technique and preliminary results. Arthroscopy. 2017;33(1):39–48.
33. Oldfield M, Burns J, Wong I. Arthroscopic anatomic bone augmentation using iliac crest autograft is safe and effective for anterior shoulder instability with bone loss. Arthrosc Sports Med Rehabli. 2021;3(6):e1671–7.

22 The Iliac Crest J-Bone Graft: Justification and Technical Pearls

Giovanni Spagna and Philipp Moroder

Introduction

Intact articular glenohumeral surfaces are the first static stabilization for the shoulder due to a concavity compression mechanism.

Significant bone defect at the anterior glenoid rim is associated with recurrent anterior shoulder instability [1]. The most typical lesion in recurrent anterior shoulder dislocation is an anterior labrum lesion [2]. A Bankart repair in patients with glenoid osseous defect is not recommended because of the high recurrence rate [3]. Several surgical techniques open and arthroscopic have been developed for the restoration of the anterior glenoid. Historically, the first autograft concept was developed more than hundred years ago from Eden and Hybinette [4]. Using an iliac crest bone grafting ensure an anatomic joint restoration in contrast to the widely used Latarjet operation where the coracoid is transferred with attached conjoined tendon as an anterior mechanical barrier. The advantage of the J-bone graft procedure is not only the anatomical glenoid restoration but the press-fit insertion of a bicortical J-shaped iliac crest graft at the glenoid defect site without any foreign material such as screws for the graft fixation [5]. The J-bone graft technique demonstrates a comparable clinical outcome with the Latarjet procedure [6].

Illustrative Clinical Case (Figs. 22.1, 22.2, and 22.3)

A 34-year-old male presented to the clinic with several years of recurrent anteroinferior glenohumeral instability. The patient reported frequent rest pain and at night was unable to sleep on the affected shoulder.

In the physical exam, the patient had a normal axillary innervation. The range of motion reported no limitation, and rotator cuff tests were negative with good symmetrical force. Gagey test was negative. Apprehension and relocation tests were positive.

X-rays showed no degenerative changes.

An MRI was performed demonstrating an anterior labral lesion as well as a Hill-Sachs defect. A CT scan with 3D reconstruction showed an anterior glenoid bone loss.

After an insufficient conservative treatment, the patient decided to proceed with surgery given his inability to be active and work overhead.

G. Spagna (✉) · P. Moroder
Department of Shoulder and Elbow Surgery, Schulthess Klinik, Zurich, Switzerland

© The Author(s), under exclusive license to Springer Nature Switzerland AG 2026
R. M. Frank, J. M. Tokish (eds.), *Management of Shoulder Instability*,
https://doi.org/10.1007/978-3-032-18089-6_22

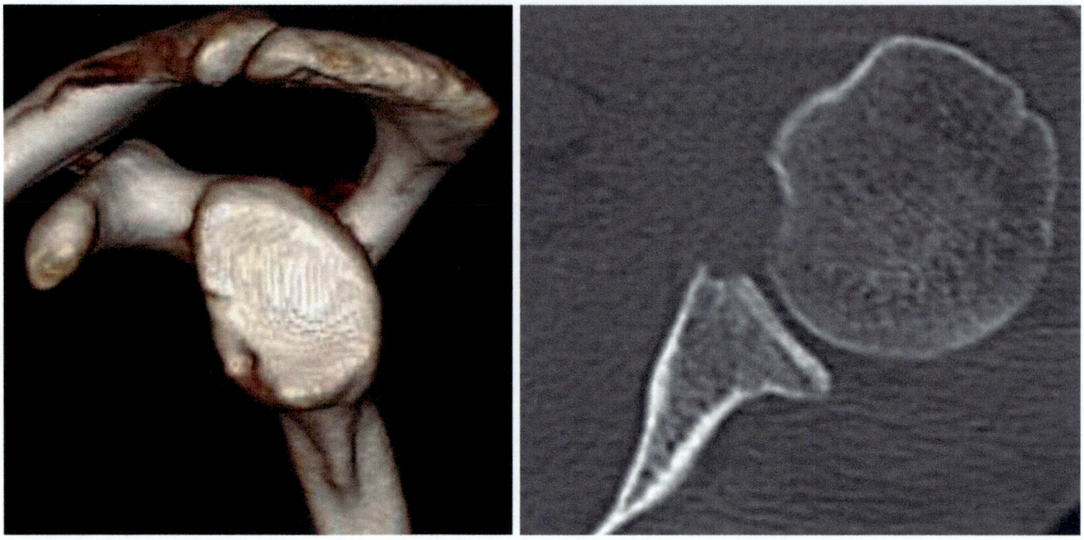

Fig. 22.1 Preoperative CT scan with 3D reconstruction showed an anterior glenoid bone loss of 15%

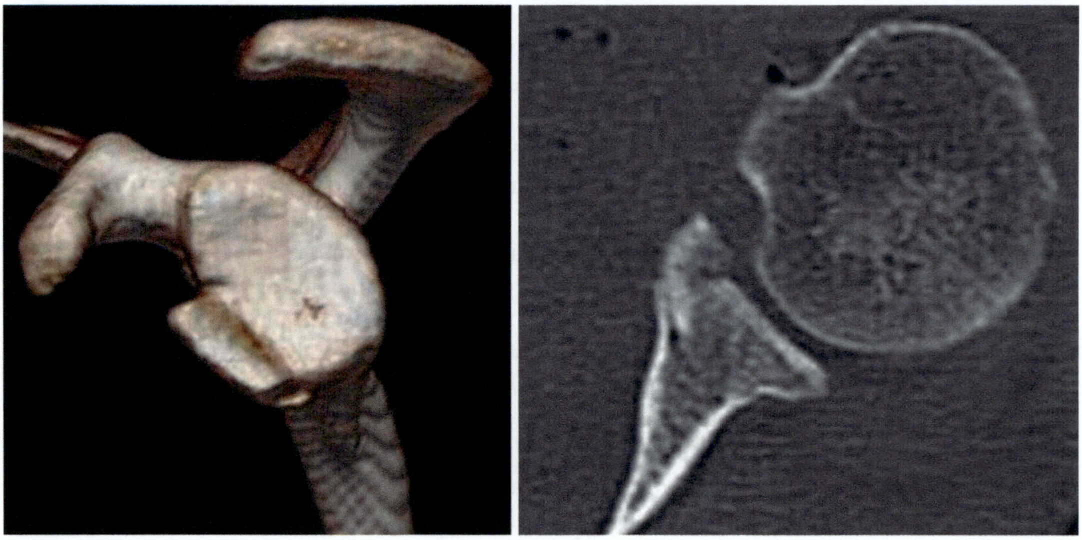

Fig. 22.2 Postoperative CT scan with 3D reconstruction showing the position of the J-bone graft

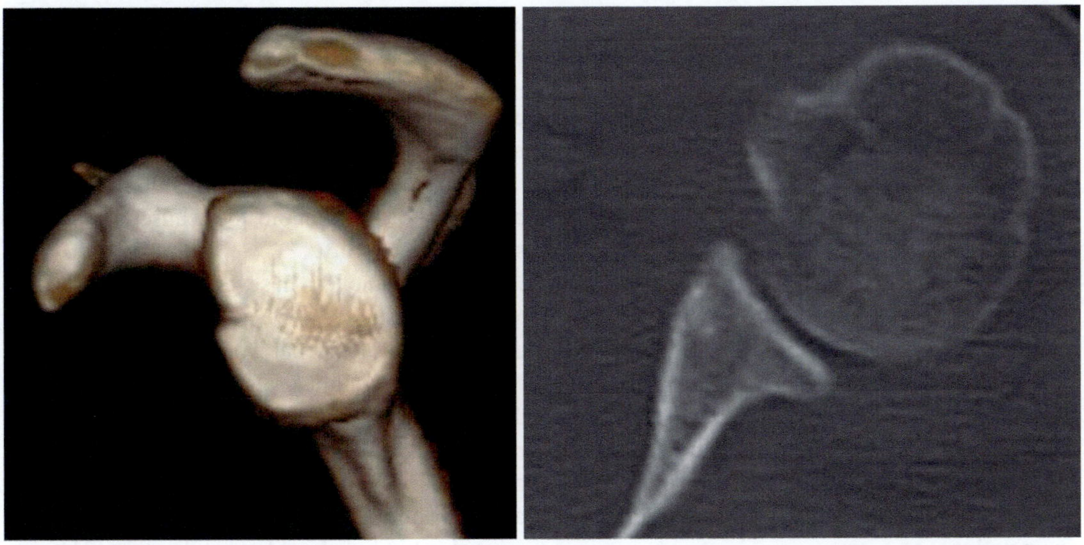

Fig. 22.3 CT scan with 3D reconstruction 1 year postoperative showing integration of the graft and remodeling

Preoperative Considerations

History

A thorough patient medical history of the recurrent anterior dislocation is necessary before the operation. The age of the patient is very important because male under the age of 30 have an increased risk of recurrent instability [7]. Sport, job, and activity level as well as patient's ambitions should be evaluated to understand if it is a risk patient such as an overhead athlete.

The questions should include the time and the mechanism of the first dislocation, the necessity of a closed reduction under sedation in a hospital, as well as an overview of following instability episodes, possibly recording the number of dislocations. It is important to understand the uncomfortable movements leading to apprehension, instability, and pain.

Signs and Symptoms

The typical feeling of instability in patients with anterior shoulder instability is a movement with the arm in abduction and external rotation. In this "apprehension" position, the humeral head is anteriorly translated and by structural damages of the glenoid or the labrum and ligament complex results in a discomfort feeling or a dislocation. Patients could experience pain in this uncomfortable position. The presence of chronic pain is referrable to early degenerative changes or structural lesions. It is important to exclude a lesion of the axillary nerve by hypesthesia and weakness in the lateral shoulder and deltoid region.

Physical Examination

A detailed physical examination should be performed bilaterally, initially with inspection to compare asymmetry or muscle atrophy and identify local inflammation signs like redness, swelling, or scars from previous surgical procedures and then palpation, active and passive range of motion, and sensory and motor testing. Specific provocative tests based on humeral displacement on the glenoid should be performed such as the apprehension test [8], the relocation test [9], and the surprise or anterior-release test [10]. These tests are helpful to confirm the diagnoses and to exclude a possibly overlooked glenohumeral posterior instability. A structural defect should be differentiated from a functional shoulder instability where a pathological muscle activation pattern causes shoulder instability even in the absence of structural damage [11].

Risk factors for glenohumeral joint instability should be assessed, such as hyperlaxity or hypermobility with the Beighton score [12], sulcus sign [13], Walch test [14], Gagey test [15], and the load-and-shift test [16] to exclude an excessive anterior translation of the humeral head. Evaluation of the integrity of the rotator cuff muscles should complete the physical examination.

Imaging

Radiographies are the first-line diagnostic investigation for anterior shoulder instability. A true anteroposterior and axillary view are important to evaluate a correct centering of the humeral head, to identify a possible bone lesion, or to assess the presence of developmental changes or instability arthropathy.

Computer tomography is essential to rule out fractures not visible in conventional radiographs or to quantify the extent and severity of fractures already diagnosed in previous radiographs. A 3D computed tomography with digital subtraction of the humeral head allows to quantify the glenoid bone loss of a Bankart fragment as well as the glenohumeral track and Hill-Sachs lesion size. CT is also useful to assess humeral and glenoid version [17].

MRI arthrography is the most accurate method for diagnosing labral tears, anterior capsule or ligament lesions, rotator cuff tendon tears, cartilage defects, or SLAP lesions.

Indications and Contraindications

Bone graft stabilization techniques such as the J-bone graft procedure are generally favored over a Bankart repair in anterior shoulder instability with a significative anterior glenoid osseous defect. A soft tissue repair in this case would be considered insufficient due to the higher risk of recurrence [18].

A large glenoid bone loss results in a loss of concavity of the glenoid that causes an anterior shoulder instability.

Glenoid bone loss in several study was defined as a value usually between 20 and 25% [1]. The definition of a critical value even for smaller defects with a clinical significance is still under debate [20]. For patients with critical anterior glenoid defect, a bone grafting technique or a Latarjet operation is indicated. Patient's functional demand and sport activities are relevant in considering this kind of shoulder stabilization [21].

The surgical indication of the J-bone graft procedure is very similar to the Latarjet procedure; however, it might be better suited for patients requiring full range of rotation and less suited for patients with smaller glenoid bone loss [21].

Contraindications to the J-bone graft procedure are significant degenerative changes, untreated neuromuscular pathologies including seizure, and a history of chronic glenohumeral joint infection.

Surgical Technique

Patient Positioning.

The open J-bone graft anterior shoulder stabilization using the implant-free technique is performed with the patient laying in a beach chair position under general anesthesia and usually an interscalene block. The shoulder, arm, and ipsilateral iliac crest are prepped and draped. Free draping of the arm allows for unrestricted shoulder motion and better visualization during the procedure.

Surgical Landmarks/Incisions

The operative access is through a deltopectoral approach. Landmarks for the approach such as the clavicle, the acromion, and the coracoid process are marked. A skin incision is performed starting from the coracoid tip aiming toward the axilla. In most patients, a skin incision of about 5–6 cm is sufficient (Fig. 22.4). After preparation through the subcutaneous layer, the clavipectoral fascia is exposed and opened vertically. The cephalic vein is identified in the interval between the pectoralis major and the deltoid muscle. The deltopectoral interval is then opened and the cephalic vein is retracted laterally together with the deltoid muscle. The conjoined tendon becomes visible medially and the curvature of the humeral head laterally. The bursa is excised and the conjoined tendon is retracted in order to expose the subscapularis which is then horizontally split between the middle and inferior third, paying attention not to harm the capsule laying beneath.

A Gelpi retractor is used to separate the two parts of the subscapularis and a periosteal elevator is used to detach the underlying capsule. Then a Hohmann retractor is positioned at the anterior scapula neck to better expose the anterior capsule (Fig. 22.5). After horizontal capsulotomy, the Gelpi retractor is repositioned to additionally split the capsule, and a Fukuda retractor is inserted to expose the anterior glenoid rim, visible in case of significant bone defect as a straight line. The bony surface is freed from scar tissue, and at this point in case of a previous Bankart repair, the previous anchor sutures are removed.

Using a 15 mm osteotome, a vertical osteotomy is created at the scapula neck medial to the anterior glenoid rim. It is important to perform the osteotomy in an angle of 20 degrees to the glenoid surface in the transosseus plane while keeping a 5 mm distance to the apex of the anterior glenoid rim (Fig. 22.6). The correct placement of the osteotomy is crucial for subsequent graft positioning. The osteotomy should have a vertical extent of about 2 cm and should bridge a depth of 10 to 12 mm. At this point, a pitfall could be an articular glenoid fracture while performing the osteotomy if the angulation and distance from the articular surface are not respected.

In order to facilitate graft insertion, the entry of the slot is widened slightly toward the glenoid surface. The retractors are loosened and the surgical site is covered.

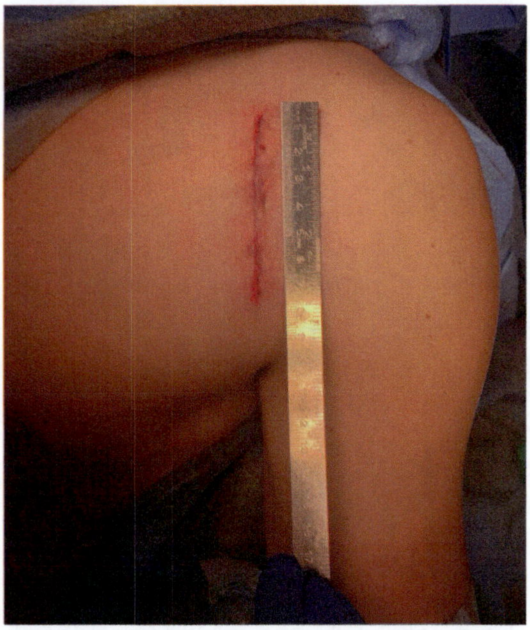

Fig. 22.4 A skin incision is performed starting from the coracoid tip aiming towards the axilla. In most patients a skin incision of about 5-6 cm is sufficient

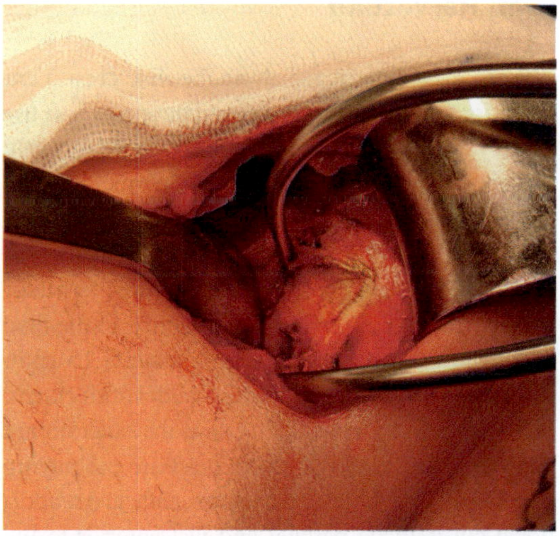

Fig. 22.5 A Gelpi retractor is used to separate the 2 parts of the subscapularis and a periosteal elevator is used to detach the underlying capsule. Then a Hohmann retractor is positioned at the anterior scapula neck to better expose the anterior capsule

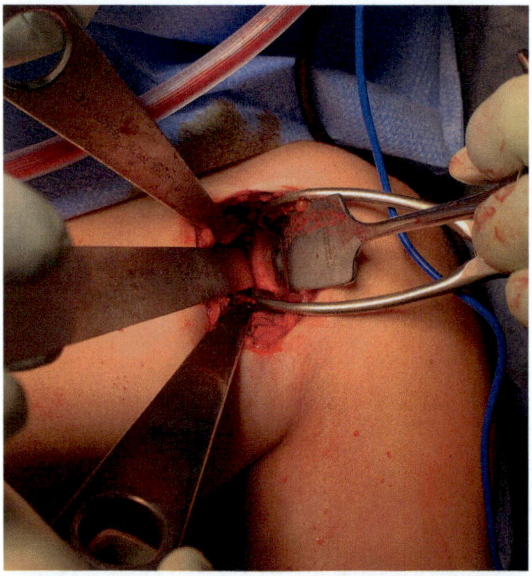

Fig. 22.6 A vertical osteotomy is performed at the scapula neck medially to the anterior glenoid rim with an angle of 20 degrees to the glenoid surface in the transosseus transverse plane, keeping a 5 mm distance to the apex of the anterior glenoid rim

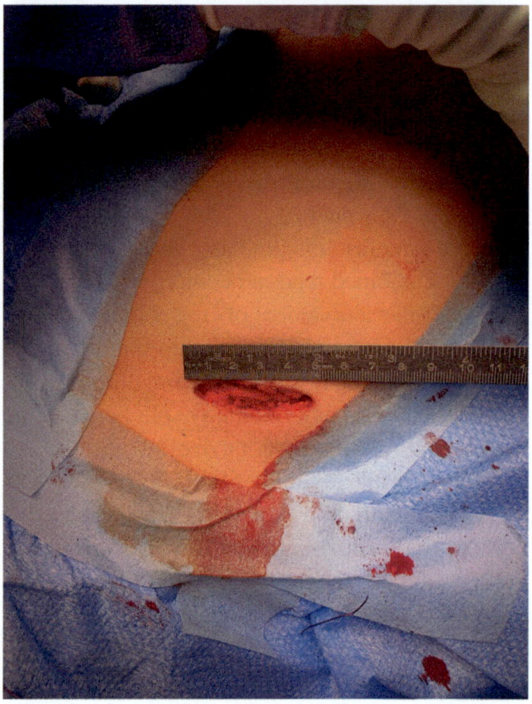

Fig. 22.7 Graft harvesting: a 3 cm incision is made along the iliac crest 5 cm posteriorly to the anterior superior iliac spine. Soft tissue layers are split and the musculature is detached from the iliac crest

Graft Harvesting

A 3 cm incision is made along the iliac crest 5 cm posterior to the anterior superior iliac spine. Soft tissue layers are split, and the musculature is fairly detached from the iliac crest. After further detachment, using a periosteal elevator, superior and inferior Hohmann retractors are inserted in order to expose the iliac crest (Fig. 22.7). With the osteotome, two clefts are made perpendicular to the iliac crest with a distance of approximately 15 mm, which relate to define the cranio-caudal graft extent. With the use of an oscillating saw, the outer cortex and the superior aspect of the crest are cut paying attention to leave the inner cortex intact. An additional cut is made parallel and just anterior to the inner cortex trying to exploit as much as the width of the iliac crest as possible. Then a final osteotomy is made on the outer cortex with about 15 mm distance to the apex of the crest. Finally, the osteotome is used to lose and harvest the graft (Fig. 22.8). At this point, the internal cortex is visible and the local defect is then filled with a hemostatic bone sponge and local anesthetic in order to reduce the postoperative pain. The soft tissue layers are than readapted. An intracutaneous suture is performed.

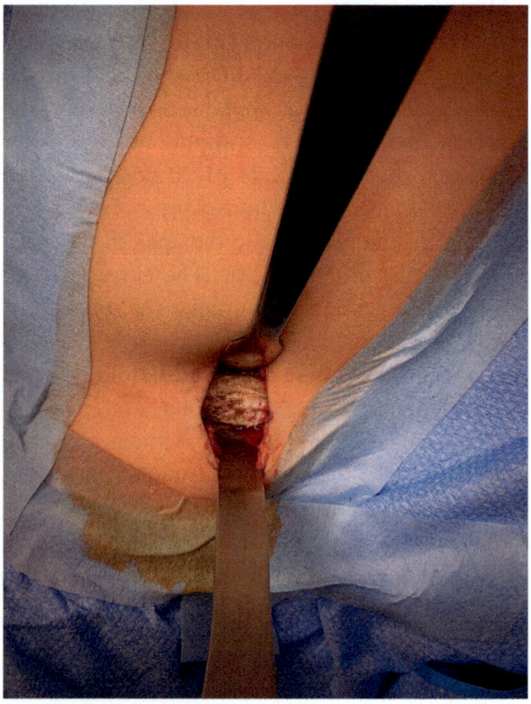

Fig. 22.8 After further detachment using a periosteal elevator a superior and inferior Hohmann retractor are inserted in order to expose the iliac crest

Shaping of the Graft

The harvested cortical cancellous bone block is then fixated with a special clamp to stabilize the harvest during the shaping process. As a first step, a vertical cut will be performed parallel to the former superior cortex. Then a horizontal cut is made parallel to the former outer cortex which will become the keel of the graft. These two steps are repeated until the whole cancellous bone is removed from the keel (Fig. 22.9). To facilitate the graft insertion, the tip of the keel is sharpened and the edges of the keel are trimmed, giving the graft the shape of a letter "J" which is why this technique is called the J-bone graft (Figs. 22.10, 22.11, and 22.12).

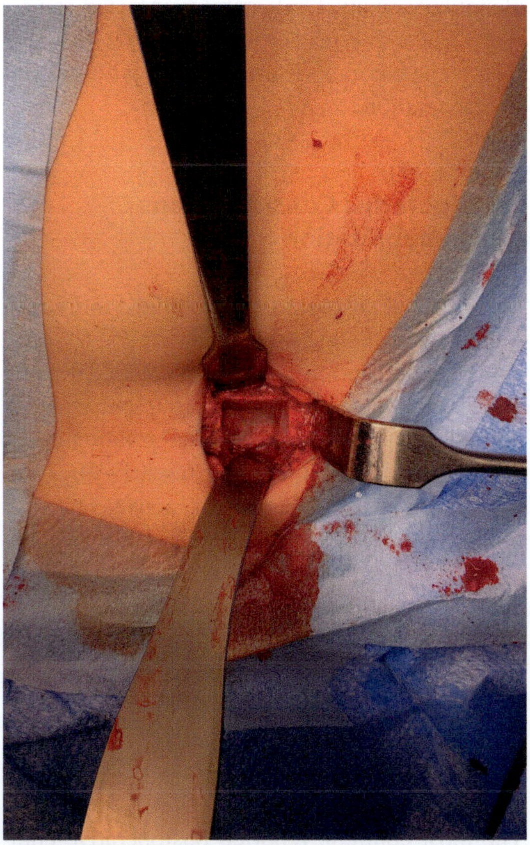

Fig. 22.9 Iliac crest showing the direction of the osteotomy

Graft Insertion

The keel of the J-bone graft is then inserted with the special clamp used for the stabilization during the shaping process directly into the osteotomy at the glenoid neck (Fig. 22.13). Then a spike impactor is used for further advancement of the keel by placing it on different levels of the graft always close to the medial border because lateral forces might break the graft in two pieces

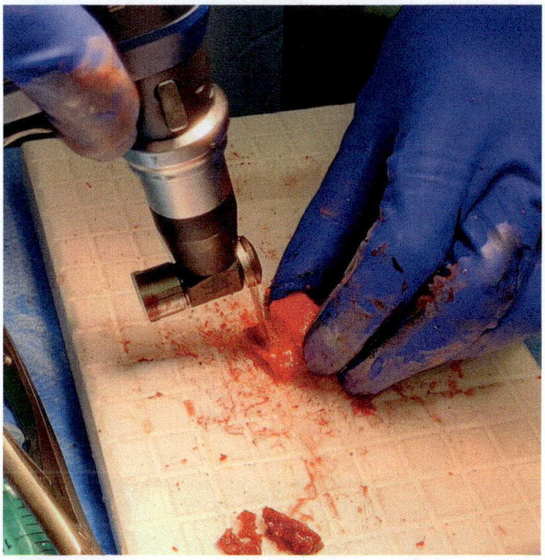

Fig. 22.10 Shaping of the graft

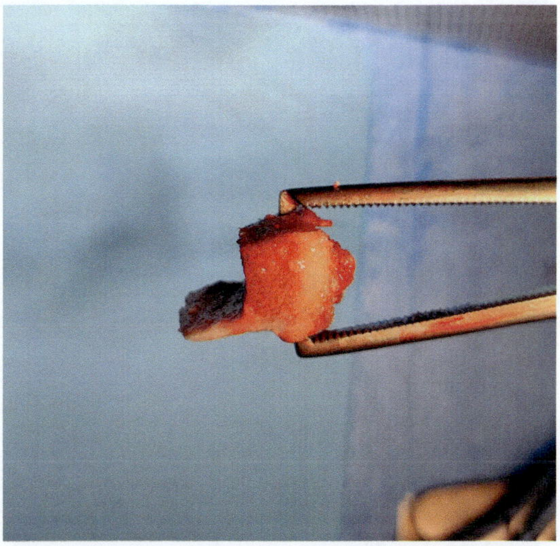

Fig. 22.11 Graft shape

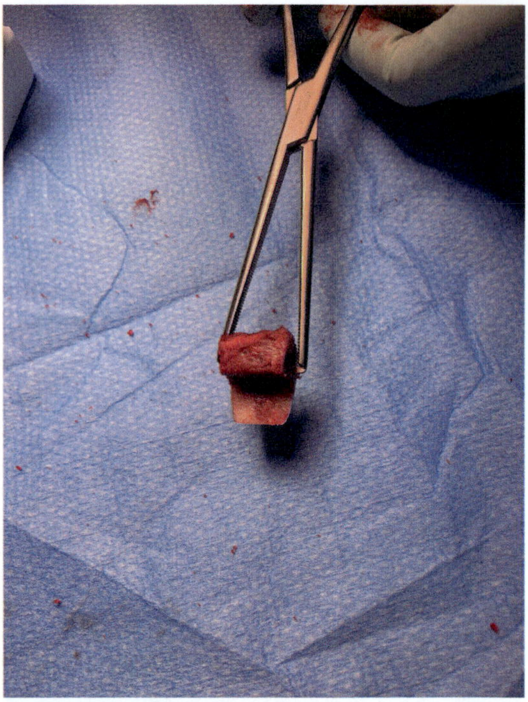

Fig. 22.12 Graft shape

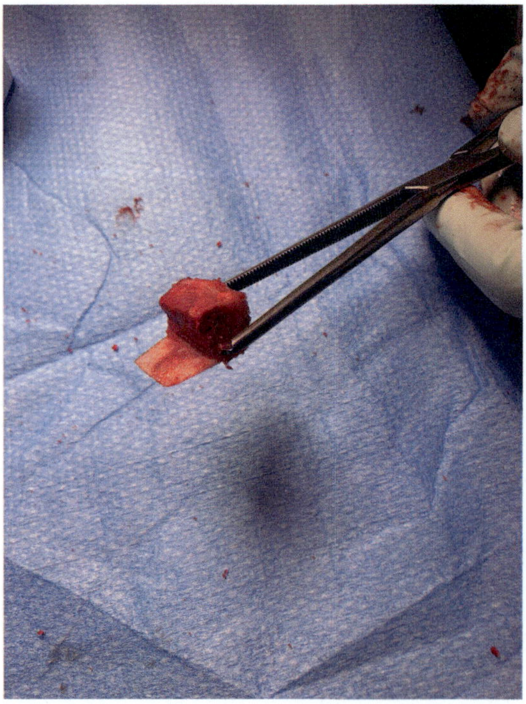

Fig. 22.13 Graft shape

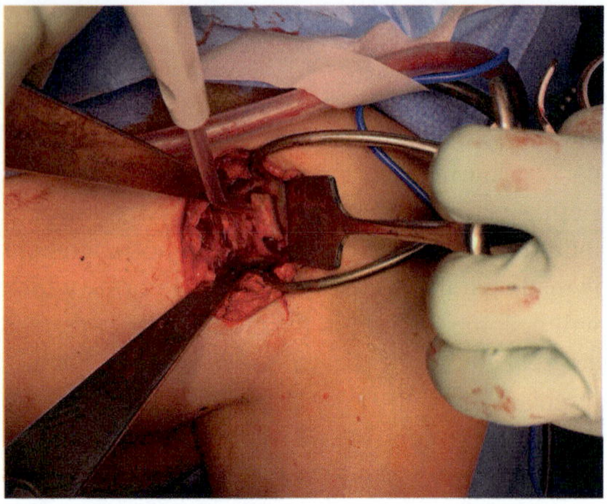

Fig. 22.14 Graft Insertion

(Fig. 22.14). The graft lateral surface, which is most formed of cancellous bone, is leveled down using a high-speed burr in order to reshape the glenoid concavity. Graft stability is tested using a periosteal elevator. The capsular split first and then the subscapularis are repaired with side-to-side adaptation.

Postoperative Considerations and Rehabilitation

Postoperative, the arm is immobilized in internal rotation using a sling for the following 3–6 weeks. Passive mobilization exercises are started directly at the first day after surgery but only with a limited range of motion. External rotation of the shoulder is strictly limited for 6 weeks after surgery. Progressive increase of active range of motion and strengthening exercises of the rotator cuff and the scapulothoracic muscles are initiated after 6 weeks to regain free range of motion of the glenohumeral joint. Return to sport is usually possible 6 months after the operation.

Complications

The most common reported postoperative complication is a hypoesthesia at the donor site as well as postoperative hematomas. For this reason, it is important to seal the bony harvesting site with wax in order to control the bleeding.

A bone graft fracture is a very rare complication after a postoperative fall [22].

A potential complication of the procedure is graft osteolysis in case the technique is used in patients with intact glenoid and without glenoid bone loss, as well as the general risks of a surgical intervention [23].

Results

A randomized trial showed similar clinical and radiological results of the J-bone graft procedure compared to the Latarjet procedure at short-term follow-up with an advantage in terms of postoperative range of motion especially in the internal rotation [6]. The bone graft undergoes a remodeling process based on Wolff's law within 1 year after surgery, with subsequent anatomic glenoid reconstruction [24].

Clinical follow-up after 8 years [5] and 18 years [22] investigating the long-term outcome of the J-bone graft procedure showed how glenohumeral stability and shoulder function are maintained over time with excellent results in the range of motion and strength compared to the contralateral uninjured site.

After this procedure, recurrence of instability can be observed with low rates [6]. The progression of instability arthropathy cannot be stopped like with any other technique, especially in patients with preoperative signs of arthropathy [22].

References

1. Yamamoto N, Itoi E, Abe H, et al. Effect of an anterior glenoid defect on anterior shoulder stability: a cadaveric study. Am J Sports Med. 2009;37(5):949–54.
2. Yiannakopoulos CK, Mataragas E, Antonogiannakis E. A comparison of the spectrum of intra-articular lesions in acute and chronic anterior shoulder instability. Arthroscopy. 2007;23(9):985–90.
3. Tauber M, Resch H, Forstner R, Raffl M, Schauer J. Reasons for failure after surgical repair of anterior shoulder instability. J Shoulder Elb Surg. 2004;13(3):279–85.
4. Villatte G, Spurr S, Broden C, et al. The Eden-Hybbinette procedure is one hundred years old! A historical view of the concept and its evolutions. Int Orthop. 2018;42(10):2491–5.
5. Auffarth A, Schauer J, Matis N, Kofler B, Hitzl W, Resch H. The J-bone graft for anatomical glenoid reconstruction in recurrent post-traumatic anterior shoulder dislocation. Am J Sports Med. 2008;36(4):638–47.
6. Moroder P, Schulz E, Wierer G, et al. Neer Award 2019: Latarjet procedure vs. iliac crest bone graft transfer for treatment of anterior shoulder instability with glenoid bone loss: a prospective randomized trial. J Shoulder Elbow Surg. 2019;28(7):1298–307.
7. Zacchilli MA, Owens BD. Epidemiology of shoulder dislocations presenting to emergency departments in the United States. J Bone Joint Surg Am. 2010;92:542–9.
8. Rowe CR, Zarins B. Recurrent transient subluxation of the shoulder. J Bone Joint Surg Am. 1981;63(6):863–72. https://doi.org/10.2106/00004623-198163060-00001.
9. Jobe FW, Kvitne RS, Giangarra CE. Shoulder pain in the overhand or throwing athlete. The relationship of anterior instability and rotator cuff impingement. Orthop Rev. 1989;18(9):963–75.
10. Lo IK, Nonweiler B, Woolfrey M, Litchfield R, Kirkley A. An evaluation of the apprehension, relocation, and surprise tests for anterior shoulder instability. Am J Sports Med. 2004;32(2):301–7. https://doi.org/10.1177/0095399703258690
11. Moroder P, Danzinger V, Maziak N, et al. Characteristics of functional shoulder instability. J Shoulder Elbow Surg. 2020;29(1):68–78.
12. Baum J, Larsson LG. Hypermobility syndrome—new diagnostic criteria. J Rheumatol. 2000;27(7):1585–6.
13. Jia X, Ji JH, Petersen SA, Freehill MT, McFarland EG. An analysis of shoulder laxity in patients undergoing shoulder surgery. J Bone Joint Surg Am. 2009;91(9):2144–50.
14. Coudane H, Walch G, Sebesta A. Chronic anterior instability of the shoulder in adults. Methodology. Rev Chir Orthop Reparatrice Appar Mot. 2000;86(Suppl 1):94–5.
15. Gagey OJ, Gagey N. The hyperabduction test. J Bone Joint Surg. 2001;83(1):69–74.
16. Hawkins R, Bokor DJ. Clinical evaluation of shoulder problems. Philadelphia: Saunders; 1990.
17. Moroder P, Resch H, Schnaitmann S, Hoffelner T, Tauber M. The importance of CT for the preoperative surgical planning in recurrent anterior shoulder instability. Arch Orthop Trauma Surg. 2013;133(2):219–26.
18. Burkhart SS, De Beer JF. Traumatic glenohumeral bone defects and their relationship to failure of arthroscopic Bankart repairs: significance of the inverted-pear glenoid and the humeral engaging hill-Sachs lesion. Arthroscopy. 2000;16(7):677–94.

19. Yamamoto N, Muraki T, Sperling JW, et al. Stabilizing mechanism in bone-grafting of a large glenoid defect. J Bone Joint Surg Am. 2010;92(11):2059–66.
20. Shaha JS, Cook JB, Song DJ, et al. Redefining "critical" bone loss in shoulder instability: functional outcomes worsen with "subcritical" bone loss. Am J Sports Med. 2015;43(7):1719–25.
21. Kim SJ, Kim SH, Park BK, Chun YM. Arthroscopic stabilization for recurrent shoulder instability with moderate glenoid bone defect in patients with moderate to low functional demand. Arthroscopy. 2014;30(8):921–7.
22. Moroder P, Plachel F, Becker J, et al. Clinical and radiological long-term results after implant-free, autologous, iliac crest bone graft procedure for the treatment of anterior shoulder instability. Am J Sports Med. 2018;46(12):2975–80.
23. Moroder P, Blocher M, Auffarth A, et al. Clinical and computed tomography-radiologic outcome after bony glenoid augmentation in recurrent anterior shoulder instability without significant glenoid bone loss. J Shoulder Elbow Surg. 2014;23(3):420–6.
24. Moroder P, Hirzinger C, Lederer S, et al. Restoration of anterior glenoid bone defects in posttraumatic recurrent anterior shoulder instability using the J-bone graft shows anatomic graft remodeling. Am J Sports Med. 2012;40(7):1544–50.

Glenoid Fracture: Tips for Reduction and Fixation

23

Douglas W. Bartels and Michael T. Freehill

Introduction

Glenohumeral dislocation is the most common adult joint dislocation with epidemiologic studies reporting an incidence as high as 23.1 per 100,000 person-years [1, 2]. Labral injury is an expected byproduct of glenohumeral dislocation, but glenoid fracture (also known as bony Bankart injury) is a potentially devastating pathology with variable prevalence reported as high as 41% for first-time dislocators [3, 4]. In the setting of recurrent dislocation, bone loss is found to be even more common with an average 22.8% loss of native glenoid width compared to 6.8% loss in first-time dislocators [5]. When interpreting these numbers, it is important to distinguish between acute fractures with the bone fragment still present and chronic injury with resultant bony absorption as this has drastic implication on treatment strategy and outcomes. Numerous studies have outlined the detrimental effect of glenoid bone loss on recurrent instability rates following Bankart repair [6–8]. Additionally, the literature suggests that 51.9% of fragment absorption occurs within the first year following injury with further absorption occurring in a time-dependent fashion [9]. Given this, it is the authors' belief that bony Bankart lesions should be treated acutely when possible. This position is supported by literature that suggests worse clinical outcomes when bony Bankart fractures are managed in the chronic setting versus the acute setting [10]. When treated operatively, bony Bankart lesions have been shown to demonstrate healing of the osseous fragment as well as excellent clinical outcomes at medium- and long-term follow-up [11, 12]. Therefore, it is important to have a solid grasp on the various techniques used to fix glenoid fractures before bony absorption occurs. Our goal is to present two approaches for surgical management of anterior glenoid fracture in a case-based fashion followed by a discussion of treatment considerations in patients presenting with glenoid fractures.

D. W. Bartels
Mayo Clinic Health Systems – Eau Claire, Department of Orthopaedic Surgery, Eau Claire, WI, USA

Stanford University School of Medicine, Department of Orthopaedic Surgery, Redwood City, CA, USA
e-mail: Bartels.douglas@mayo.edu

M. T. Freehill (✉)
Stanford University School of Medicine, Department of Orthopaedic Surgery, Redwood City, CA, USA
e-mail: freehill@stanford.edu

© The Author(s), under exclusive license to Springer Nature Switzerland AG 2026
R. M. Frank, J. M. Tokish (eds.), *Management of Shoulder Instability*,
https://doi.org/10.1007/978-3-032-18089-6_23

Case 1

Case Presentation

A 79-year-old right-hand dominant male presented to the clinic with right-sided shoulder pain in the setting of a mechanical fall onto his shoulder 3 days prior to presentation. He endorsed the immediate onset of deep right shoulder pain as well as the subjective sensation of instability. He did not have a true dislocation event. Prior to this injury, the patient did not note any issues with the shoulder and has no surgical history with regard to the right upper extremity. He remained active until the injury, working as a physician and continuing to live an independent life.

Pertinent physical exam findings included a prominent sulcus with inferior subluxation of the humerus when the arm was brought past 110° of forward flexion or abduction. Strength was near symmetric compared to the contralateral extremity with negative belly press and lift-off tests. Additionally, he had a positive apprehension and relocation test and negative Mayo-Shear and jerk tests. Sensation was symmetric to light touch in all nerve distributions bilaterally and radial pulse was palpable.

Imaging

Radiographs of the shoulder were obtained including Grashey and axillary x-rays. On the Grashey view (Fig. 23.1a), there was some suggestion of bony abnormality near the inferior aspect of the glenoid. When looking at the axillary (Fig. 23.1b), again there was some evidence of compression or bony injury at the anteroinferior aspect of the glenoid. Magnetic resonance imaging (MRI) (Fig. 23.2a and b) was also obtained which demonstrated a 10x25 mm bony Bankart lesion to the anteroinferior aspect of the glenoid. This fragment was measured to be about 21% of the native glenoid surface. Based on the Kim classification [13], this would be described as a medium lesion (12.5–25%). There was adjacent depression of a glenoid fragment without significant displacement of the fracture. Notably, while there was evidence of rotator cuff tendinosis, no full-thickness tearing was appreciated.

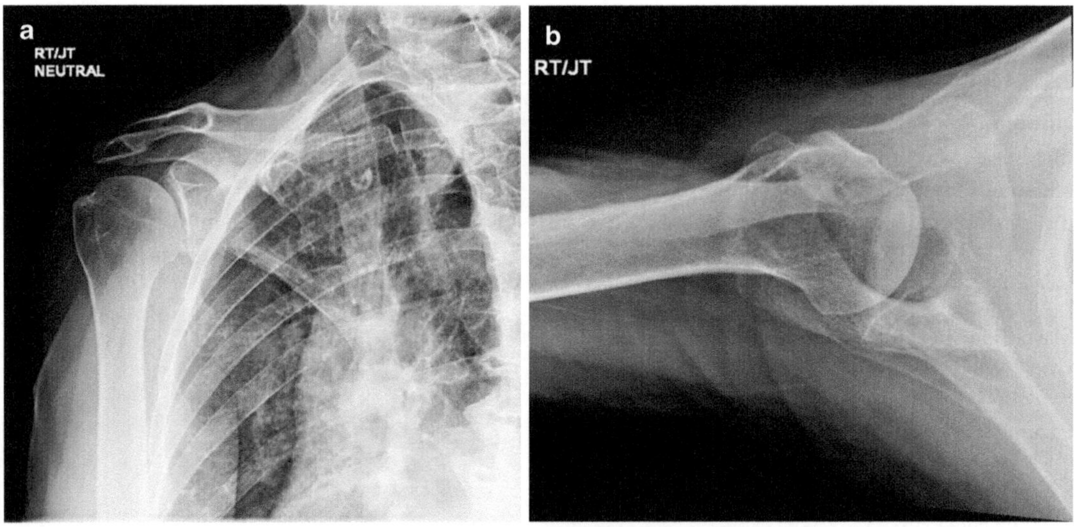

Fig. 23.1 (**a**) Grashey view of the right shoulder with some suggestion of bony abnormality at the inferior aspect of the glenoid. (**b**) Axillary view of the right shoulder demonstrating bony injury at the anterior glenoid

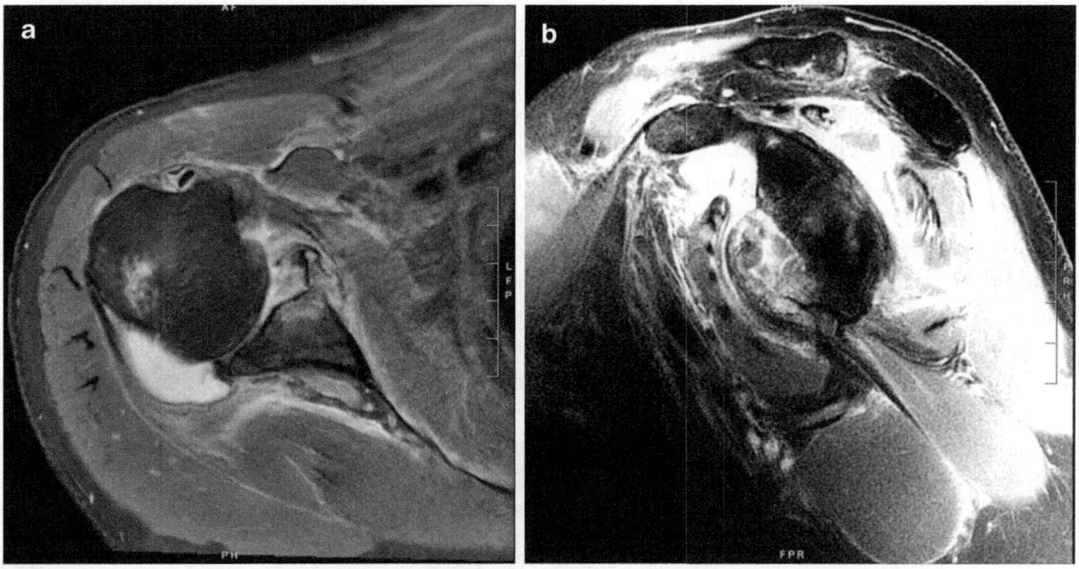

Fig. 23.2 (**a**) Axial MRI cut demonstrating anteroinferior glenoid fracture with associated glenoid compression injury. (**b**) Sagittal MRI demonstrating 10x25 mm glenoid fracture over the anteroinferior aspect of the glenoid

Treatment Options

A discussion was had with the patient regarding treatment options available in the setting of his known bony Bankart injury. Given the patient's age, one could certainly consider nonoperative management; however, given his reproducible instability on physical exam as well as his desire to continue high level activity including riding bikes, nonoperative management seemed a less reliable treatment plan.

From a surgical standpoint, a number of options exist. Given that this was an acute injury, our preference was for attempted repair of the bony Bankart lesion to the glenoid. This has traditionally been accomplished either arthroscopically or open with suture anchors or with metal screws. Given the size of the lesion, we believed this would best be managed arthroscopically with suture anchor fixation.

Surgical Technique

Our surgical approach for this case is based off the bony Bankart bridge technique by Millett and Braun [14]. In the preoperative area, anesthesia placed in an indwelling interscalene catheter. The patient was placed on a standard operative table in the supine position where general endotracheal anesthesia was administered. Exam under anesthesia demonstrated grade 2 anterior-based translation confirming glenohumeral instability. He was transitioned to the lateral decubitus position and prepped and draped in sterile fashion. A 60 mL of lactated ringers was injected into the glenohumeral joint space through the posterior viewing portal for insufflation. An anterior working portal was made just above the upper border of the subscapularis. Diagnostic arthroscopy revealed the bony Bankart lesion resulting in an inverted pear appearance of the glenoid. Additionally, the long head of the biceps tendon was found to have considerable synovitis.

Given the appearance of the long head of the biceps, the decision was made to perform a biceps tenodesis. The arthroscope was removed and a 3 cm incision was made in the axillary crease. The plane between the conjoined tendon and the inferior border of the pectoralis major tendon was developed. The long head of the biceps was identified and removed from the bicipital groove. An all-suture double-loaded anchor was placed in the bicipital groove and an onlay tenodesis was performed.

The arthroscope was reintroduced, and an accessory high anterolateral portal was created. This was made in such a way that the portal was just anterior to the leading edge of the supraspinatus tendon and more lateral than the standard anterior working portal. All visualization occurred through the high anterolateral portal. Work was completed through the standard anterior and posterior portals as well as a percutaneous 7 o'clock portal located just above the posterior-inferior glenohumeral ligament. A tissue liberator and motorized shaver were utilized to develop the plane between native glenoid and the bony Bankart fragment (Fig. 23.3). Gross debris and hematoma were removed from the fracture bed. A medial neck-based double-loaded all-suture anchor was placed at the medial most aspect of the fracture bed through the anterior portal (Fig. 23.4). Using a rigid bone penetrator device, the sutures were then placed around the bony Bankart fracture. These sutures were then docked for later fixation. Another all-suture double-loaded anchor was then placed at the inferior aspect of the bed of the glenoid lesion. This was done percutaneously through a 7 o'clock portal. These sutures were passed through capsulolabral tissue in a horizontal and vertical fashion, which we call a modified Mason-Allen configuration. The horizontal component restores the labral bumper, while the vertical component includes a nip-and-tuck technique which provides capsular volume reduction via a capsulorrhaphy. The horizontal component was tied first, followed by the vertical component. This was repeated at the superior aspect of the lesion with a second double-loaded all-suture anchor again in modified Mason-Allen configuration which reapproximated the entire lesion (Fig. 23.5). The four sutures that were previously placed around the bony Bankart fragment were then fixed on the

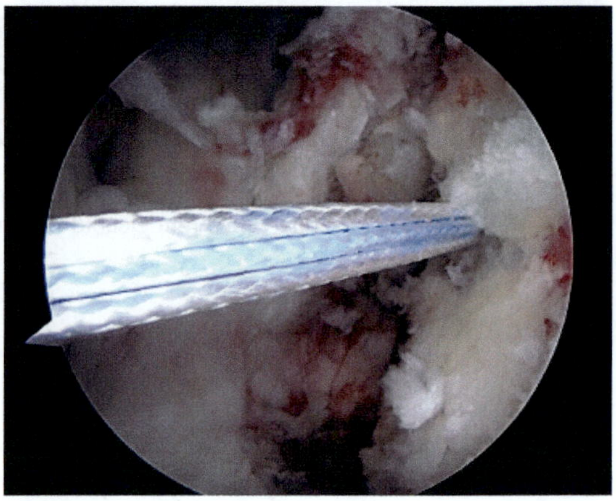

Fig. 23.4 Arthroscopic image depicting placement of an all-suture anchor on the most medial aspect of the glenoid fracture, before passage of suture around the bony Bankart lesion. Viewing from high anterior portal

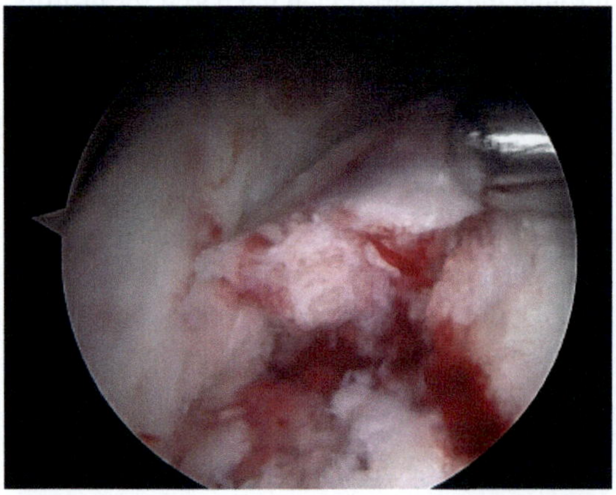

Fig. 23.3 Arthroscopic image depicting motorized shaver used to debride the glenoid fracture bed. Viewing from the high anterior portal. The shaver at the 5:00 position of anteroinferior glenoid

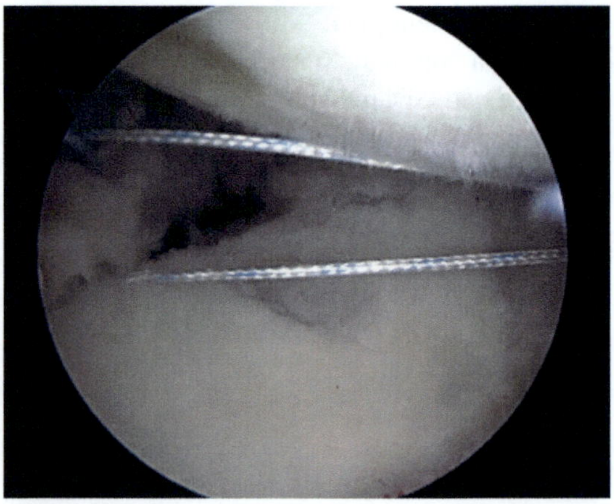

Fig. 23.5 Arthroscopic image showing vertical limb of modified Mason-Allen stitch prior to knot tying directly superior to the bony Bankart lesion. Viewing from high anterior portal

face of the glenoid using a 2.9 mm knotless BioComposite anchor (Arthrex, Naples, FL) to complete the double-row construct (Fig. 23.6). This brought the bony Bankart fragment back to its appropriately seated position, maximizing the bony apposition of the fragment and the glenoid (Fig. 23.7). Wounds were closed in a standard fashion and dressing applied. An abduction pillow and sling was placed.

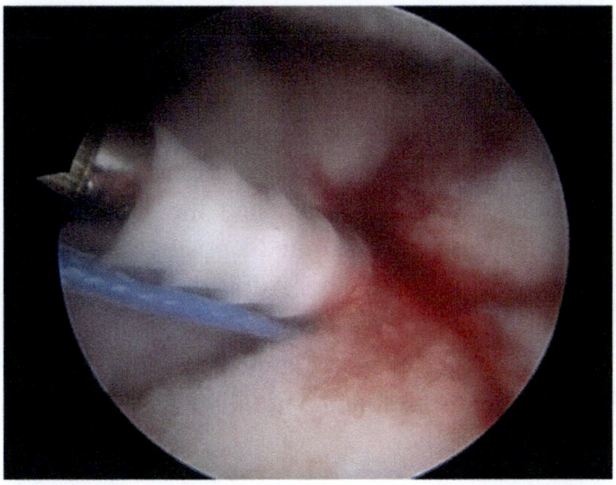

Fig. 23.6 Arthroscopic image showing insertion of the lateral fixation knotless suture anchor on the glenoid face to complete the double-row repair of the bony Bankart bridge construct. Viewing from the high anterior portal

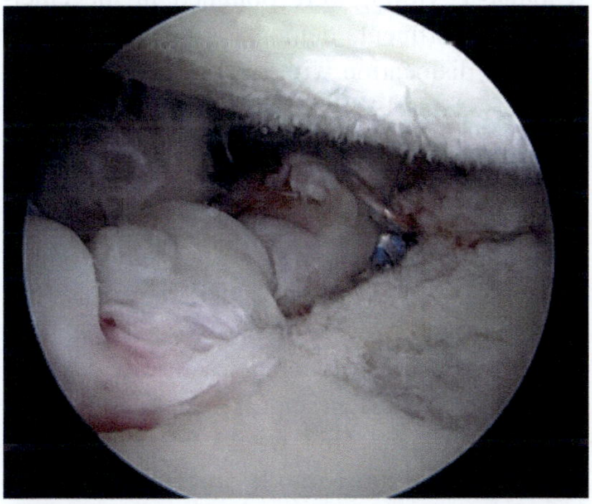

Fig. 23.7 Arthroscopic image depicting final construct of the bony Bankart bridge repair with fracture in an appropriately seated position. View from high anterior portal

Postoperative Management

The patient was started on the author's Bankart capsulorrhaphy physical therapy protocol. This entails use of a sling for 6 weeks postoperatively. Passive range of motion at the elbow began at the first postoperative visit. Shoulder pendulums and scapular motions began at the 2-week mark. Formal physical therapy began at the 3-week mark per our standard Bankart/capsulorrhaphy protocol, secondary to robust fixation, beginning with passive range of motion, followed by active-assist range of motion, and finally active range of motion. Active range of motion would be initiated sometime between 6 and 8 weeks postoperatively. Strengthening was initiated following return of range of motion generally around the 10-week mark. Around the 4-month mark, patient was given clearance for activity including cycling and swimming.

Technical Pearls

1. Patient position in the lateral decubitus position is critical for proper visualization of the glenoid. While technically possible to perform in the beach chair position, our belief is that the lateral position offers significant ease in terms of visualization for shoulder stabilization procedures.
2. We utilized a high anterolateral portal for visualization, and work was completed through standard low anterior and posterior portals. We believe visualization from this portal allows for a bird's-eye view of the glenoid and in turn the bony lesion. This ultimately allows for precise passage of sutures for both the capsulorrhaphy and fixation of the bony Bankart fragment.
3. The 7 o'clock portal is extremely useful for anchor placement at the true inferior aspect of the glenoid [15]. In the authors' experience, utilizing the standard low anterior portal for the 6 or 6:30 o'clock glenoid anchor place-

ment is technically challenging and can result in inappropriate positioning of the anchor. This portal is typically located more lateral and inferior than the posterior viewing portal. A spinal needle can be used to localize the appropriate position of the portal before making skin incision. The anchor can then be placed percutaneously while still completing all suture passage between the anterior and posterior portals. It is critical to stay above the posterior-inferior glenohumeral ligament to avoid potential injury to the axillary nerve.

4. Capsulorrhaphy superior and inferior to the bony Bankart lesion utilizing a double-loaded suture anchor in a modified Mason-Allen configuration was performed. We believe the use of a modified Mason-Allen configuration offers a number of advantages over the more traditional simple stitch configuration. Namely, the horizontal component acts as a ripstop to prevent the vertical component from cutting through tissue. This maintains the integrity of the repair. Additionally, this allows creation of a labral bumper and the benefit of compression from the vertical component.
5. A double row repair of the bony Bankart fragment was performed in this case. This is preferred by the authors over a single-row repair as we believe this more anatomically reduces the fragment, preventing the fragment from everting or toggling, and ultimately pulling away from the fracture bed. Additionally, we believe this provides greater fragment stability at time-zero compared to traditional single-row techniques.

Case 2

Case Presentation

A 32-year-old right-hand dominant male presented to the clinic with left shoulder pain and instability in the setting of a known prior dislocation 3 weeks prior. He reports that he was playing baseball when he jammed his left arm into a base, resulting in immediate pain. He presented to the local emergency department where he was found to have an anterior shoulder dislocation requiring reduction under sedation. Since the injury, he has had recurrent subluxation episodes with normal activities of daily living. Prior to this injury, he noted that he had experienced a number of subluxation episodes with higher-intensity activity such as swinging a bat, but no true dislocation events. Ultimately, he would like to get back to sports including baseball.

Pertinent physical exam findings include limited active motion in all planes secondary to extreme discomfort. Passive motion was also limited secondary to pain and the sensation of instability. He demonstrated a positive apprehension and relocation test. Additional provocative testing was deferred due to gross instability and pain. Sensation was symmetric to light touch in all nerve distributions bilaterally and radial pulse was palpable.

Imaging

Radiographs, including anteroposterior (AP) and scapular-Y views, were obtained in the emergency department demonstrating an anterior shoulder dislocation with likely glenoid fracture (Fig. 23.8a and b). Postreduction AP x-ray demonstrated apparent concentric reduction of the glenohumeral joint with an anterior inferomedial displaced bony fragment (Fig. 23.9). A computed tomography (CT) scan with 3-dimensional reconstructions was obtained to better characterize the glenoid fracture (Fig. 23.10a and b). This redemonstrated the glenoid fracture which was measured to represent approximately 30% of the articular surface. This would be classified as large based on the Kim classification [13]. The inferior portion of the fragment was thought to be an intact piece of bone, whereas the superior portion was believed to have some fragmentation.

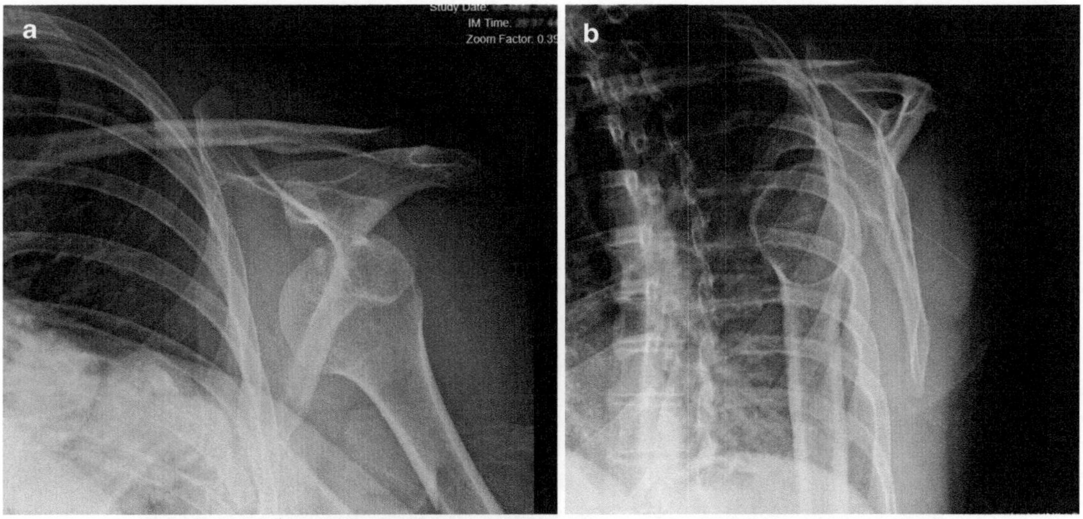

Fig. 23.8 (**a**) AP radiograph demonstrating glenohumeral dislocation with bony abnormality near the anterior face of the glenoid suggestive of glenoid fracture. (**b**) Scapular-Y radiograph demonstrating anterior glenohumeral dislocation

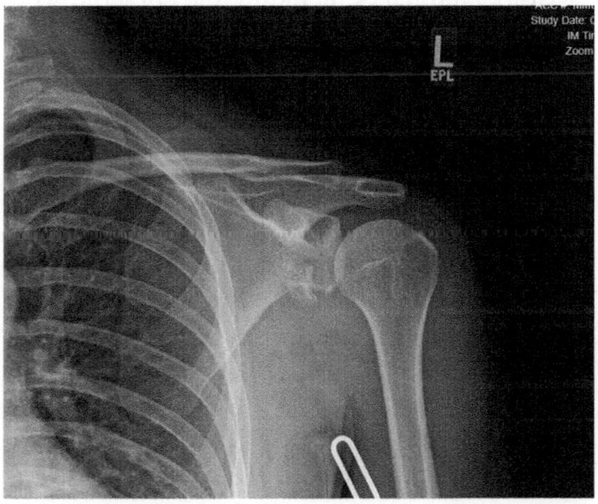

Fig. 23.9 Postreduction AP radiograph demonstrating apparent concentric reduction of glenohumeral joint with displaced glenoid fracture

Treatment Options

A thorough discussion regarding treatment options in the setting of the patient's known large glenoid fracture took place. Nonoperative management and likelihood of success were discussed. Given the large nature of the fracture fragment and the fact the patient was having subluxation episodes with normal daily activity, this was deferred. Additionally, he wanted to get back to high-level sporting activities which would likely only be feasible with operative intervention.

From a surgical standpoint, a number of options exist. One could consider attempted arthroscopic management of the fracture; however, given the size of the bony fragment, we

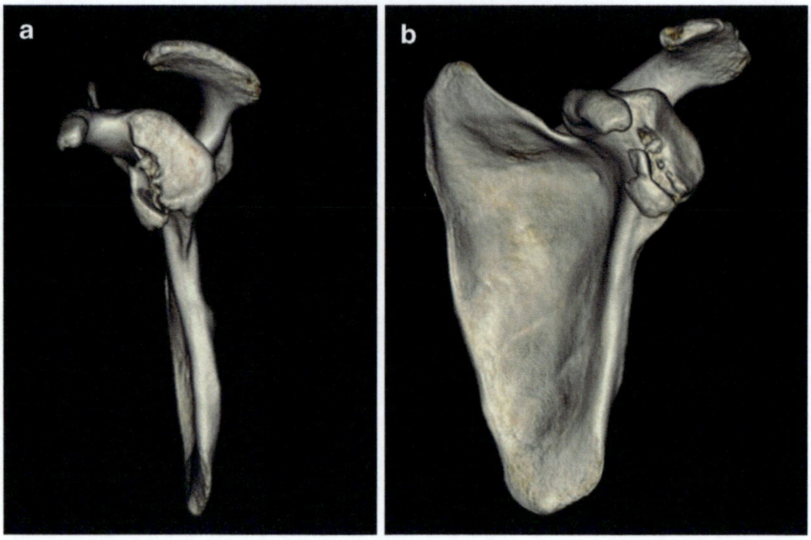

Fig. 23.10 (**a**) CT with 3-dimensional reconstructions demonstrating a large anterior glenoid fracture measured to be approximately 30% of the native glenoid width. (**b**) CT with 3-dimensional reconstructions demonstrating the large glenoid fracture with some fragmentation of the superior aspect of the fracture

believed fracture fixation would be more predictable with an open approach. Based on available imaging, we believed the inferior portion of the glenoid fracture could be reduced and fixed with screws. Given the fragmentation of the superior aspect of the fracture, we would attempt screw fixation but be prepared for fixation augmentation with suture anchors. If the fragment itself was not found to be amenable to open reduction internal fixation, then a Latarjet coracoid bone block transfer stabilization procedure would be performed.

Surgical Technique

The patient was brought to the operating room and placed supine on the operative table. The decision was made to forgo a preoperative block given the proximity of the axillary nerve to the operative field and the desire for a postoperative exam. General endotracheal anesthesia was administered and exam under anesthesia demonstrated grade 3 translation with frank instability anteriorly at baseline. He was transitioned to the beach chair position with a towel bump placed under the scapula on the operative side.

Bony landmarks including the coracoid were marked on the patient. A 6 cm incision was made from the coracoid toward the axillary crease. The deltopectoral interval was developed with the cephalic vein safely retracted. The interval between the conjoined tendon and subscapularis was gently developed until the subscapularis could be seen in its entirety. The subscapularis was then split just under the midway point with curved Mayo scissors. The capsule was identified and a sharp Hohmann was placed inferiorly to retract the lower subscapularis. A vertical capsulotomy was performed with a long blade 15 knife facing superiorly so as to avoid potential iatrogenic injury to the axillary nerve. A humeral head retractor was placed lateral and a Bankart retractor medially which brought the glenoid fracture into view. Additionally, a sharp Hohmann retractor was placed inferiorly which allowed for excellent visualization of the glenoid and fracture fragment. An absorbent sponge can be placed along the scapular spine anteriorly to aid with achieving hemostasis. The bony fragment was gently elevated and gross debris and hematoma were evacuated from the fracture bed. As suspected from preoperative imaging, the inferior fragment was robust and amenable to screw fixation, whereas the superior fragment was small and would require suture anchor fixation. The inferior fragment was then reduced and held in anatomic position with use of a K-wire (Fig. 23.11). A cannulated drill was used to overdrill the K-wire and a 4.5 mm fully-threaded screw was placed with good purchase. An all-suture anchor was placed in the superior fracture bed cheating a bit anterior at the mid-glenoid. Suture ends were then brought around the superior fracture fragment and associated labrum and tied in place providing excellent fixation. The capsule was closed in a pants-over-vest fashion, and the subscapularis was reapproximated with interrupted figure-of-eight #2 Ethibond (J&J MedTech, New Brunswick, NJ) sutures with the arm in 30 degrees of external rotation. The wound was closed in layers and the patient was placed in an abduction pillow sling.

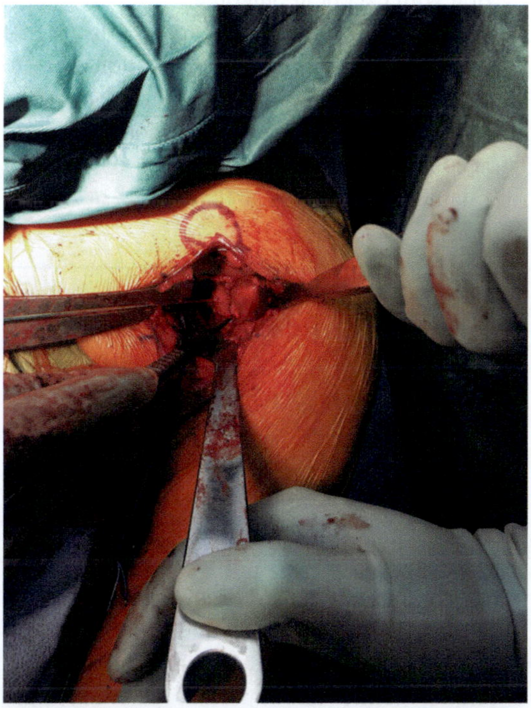

Fig. 23.11 Intraoperative photograph showing provisional reduction of inferior glenoid fracture fragment with a K-wire

Postoperative Management

The patient was placed on the author's Bankart physical therapy program; however, this was to be delayed until the 6-week postoperative mark to avoid loading forces across the anterior glenoid. Note the start times of PT are different in the two cases. Although subjective, it was decided to delay the initiation of PT secondary to the size of the bony fragment. In this particular case, allowing bony healing was deemed most important and more at risk than the smaller bony fragment from case 1. Passive range of motion at the elbow began at the first postoperative visit. Shoulder pendulums and scapular motions began at the 2-week mark. Postoperative radiographs were obtained at the 6-week mark demonstrating appropriate reduction of the fracture (Fig. 23.12a and b), and he was weaned out of the sling to begin his formal physical therapy regimen.

Technical Pearls

1. Utilize a utilitarian approach that allows for management of the fracture through multiple techniques as needed depending on the appearance and characteristics of the fracture at direct visualization. In this case, a deltopectoral approach with a subscapularis split was performed which allowed direct visualization of the fracture and ultimately open reduction and internal fixation with suture anchor augmentation. Employing a subscapularis split rather than taking down the subscapularis eliminates the concern over subscapularis healing back to the lesser tuberosity. If the fracture was found not to be amenable to primary repair, this approach would allow for a bone block stabilization procedure to be performed such as a Latarjet.
2. Use K-wires with eventual cannulated screws. This allows for maintenance of fracture reduction while obtaining final fixation. This is cru-

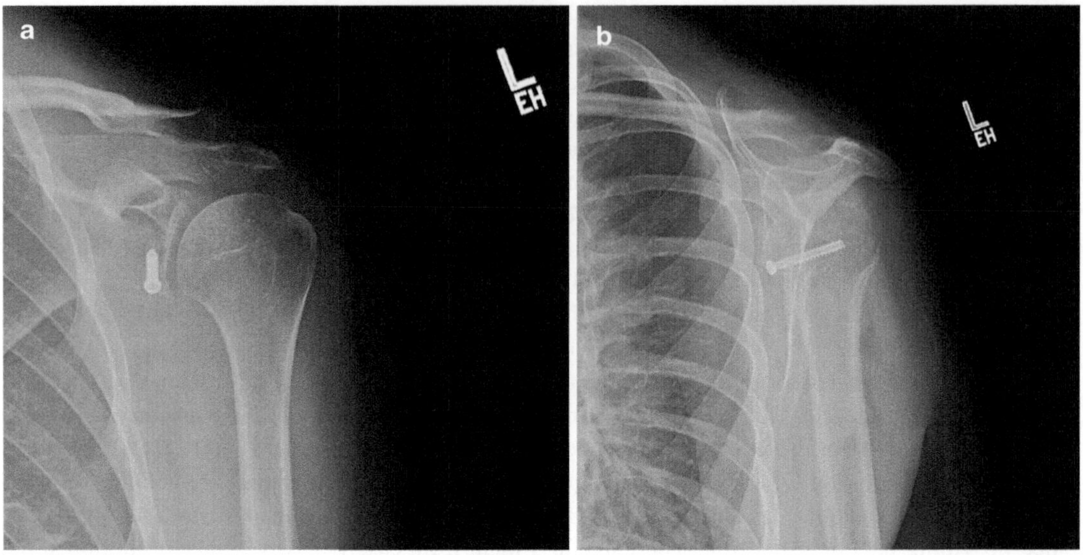

Fig. 23.12 (**a**) Postoperative Grashey view radiograph demonstrating screw fixation of glenoid fracture. (**b**) Postoperative scapular-Y radiograph demonstrating screw fixation of the inferior glenoid fragment

cial when attempting to place screws in small bone fragments that may not be amenable to fixation with traditional fracture reduction techniques. Cannulated screws are acceptable if minimum diameter is 4 mm or greater. Smaller caliber is at risk for breakage. Additionally, titanium possesses a Modulus of Elasticity closer to bone and thus may allow healing of the fracture with potential avoidance of stress shielding the bone.

3. In larger fractures, use a two-screw construct if the bony anatomy permits. This reduces the likelihood of rotational instability and improves the overall stability of the fixation construct.
4. Recognize typical screw length when fixing glenoid fractures. In situ fixation of glenoid fractures will generally be done with screws around 24–36 mm in length. While anatomy can be variable, avoiding placement of excessively long screws can reduce soft tissue irritation.
5. Be willing to combine fracture fixation techniques depending on the nature of the glenoid fracture. In this case, the inferior portion of the fracture was robust and amenable to screw fixation. The superior fragment was smaller and likely would have split with attempted screw fixation. Thus, suture anchor fixation was utilized for fracture fixation augmentation with excellent outcome.
6. When performing capsular repair, ensure that the arm is in an appropriate position so as to avoid postoperative stiffness and restrictions in range of motion. The author prefers to accomplish this in 30 degrees of external rotation.

Anterior Glenoid Fracture Treatment Considerations

A thorough understanding of the characteristics of a glenoid fracture is critical in planning the best approach for reduction and fixation of glenoid fractures. Knowing this, patients with glenoid fractures will often require a combination of imaging modalities prior to presenting to the operating room. Standard in any workup of suspected glenoid fracture should be a series of radiographs including AP, axillary, and scapular-Y views. While an important part of injury workup, radiographs alone are often insufficient in quantifying glenoid involvement compared to advanced imaging [16].

A CT scan is effective in terms of assessing extent of injury in the setting of glenoid fracture [16–18]. A CT allows for precise characterization of the size and shape of the bony Bankart lesion. Additionally, it allows for assessment of glenoid bone loss in the setting of resorption or recurrent subluxation. A CT with 3-dimensional reconstructions has become increasingly popular as it allows for en face view of the glenoid surface in its entirety rather than assessing individual slices of a standard CT scan [19]. Quantifying the size of the bony fragment and how large it is as a percentage of native glenoid is critical as it helps guide treatment. In the setting of acute fracture, percentage of involvement of the bony fragment can be calculated using an en face sagittal CT with 3-dimensional reconstruction. With this, a best-fit circle over the inferior two-thirds of the glenoid using the inferior glenoid cortex as reference is created. The greatest width of the bony Bankart fragment is then divided by the greatest width of the best-fit circle and multiplied by 100 to create a percentage of native glenoid involvement [13].

MRI has long been considered gold standard for assessing soft tissue injury in the setting of glenohumeral instability. Recent advancements in MRI technology have brought into question the need for CT in evaluating bone involvement and loss in glenoid fracture, with the potential advantage of diminishing radiation exposure. While data exists to support MRI in quantifying bone loss [16, 20, 21], further validation is needed as comparative studies show mixed results [22].

A number of classification systems have been proposed to describe glenoid fractures with the goal of guiding treatment [23, 24]. The classification system used by the authors in the previously discussed cases was proposed by Kim et al. [13]. With this system, advanced imaging is used to describe the bony lesions as small (<12.5%), medium (12.5–25%), or large (>25%) based on the percent of fragment present as a percentage of native glenoid bone. Sugaya et al. [12] and Kitayama et al. [11] showed that excellent bony healing and clinical outcomes can be achieved with surgical repair of bony Bankart lesions.

Small Lesions (<12.5%)

Surgical management of small lesions with arthroscopic single-row Bankart repair has been shown to have favorable outcomes [13, 25]. Kim et al. [13] report that lesions <12.5% of native glenoid width respond well to arthroscopic single-row fixation with incorporation of the glenoid fracture fragment in the repair. Their patient cohort saw improvement in clinical outcomes with a recurrence rate of 6.3%, a number similar to the recurrence rate reported for standard soft tissue Bankart repairs [26]. A technique similar to that proposed by Maziak et al. [27] can be implemented for surgical management of these small fractures. With this technique, a single-row repair is performed by placing anchors superior and inferior to the fragment as well as an anchor in the fracture bed to capture the bony fragment. A number of technical pearls should be considered when performing these arthroscopic repairs. First, the authors preferred technique involves use of at least three anchors when performing soft tissue or small bony Bankart repair. A recent review cited instability recurrence of 11.4% when three anchors or more were used versus 15% when less than three anchors were used [28]. While the numbers presented in this study did not reach statistical significance, literature support for three of more suture anchors exists [8]. Second, the authors highly suggest anchor placement low on the glenoid, near the 6 o'clock position. A number of options exist for successful anchor placement in this position including curved guides, low anterior trans-subscapularis portals, or with the 7 o'clock portal. As previously described in case 1, we prefer the use of the 7 o'clock percutaneous portal for inferior anchor placement. Literature suggests anchor placement in this position is important in terms of reducing instability recurrence rates and optimizing outcomes [29].

Medium Lesions (12.5–25%)

Kim et al. [13] described medium lesions as those involving between 12.5% and 25% of native glenoid bone width. They reported on their outcomes of single-row arthroscopic repair in this patient group, citing good outcomes and a low recurrence rate of 5.6%. The authors' preferred technique for medium lesions is based off the technique first described by Millet and Braun [14] known as the bony Bankart bridge. With this technique, a double-row repair is performed with suture from a medial row anchor wrapping around the fracture and incorporating into a knotless lateral row anchor on the face of the glenoid. Using this technique, Millett et al. [30] and his colleagues [31] report low revision surgery rates, low complication rates, and good clinical outcomes at both short-term and midterm follow-up. We prefer the bony Bankart bridge technique for a number of reasons including improved fracture reduction and stability compared to single-row techniques [32, 33]. As discussed previously, a number of technical pearls exist to facilitate reduction and fixation with this technique including positioning in the lateral decubitus position, viewing from a high anterolateral portal, use of a rigid passing device to facilitate passage of suture around the bony fragment, and modified Mason-Allen stitch configuration above and below the fracture fragment.

Large Lesions (>25%)

While a number of techniques exist for fixation of large glenoid fractures including arthroscopic endobutton fixation [34], arthroscopic fixation with bioabsorbable screws [35], and open fixation with bioabsorbable pins [36], our preferred technique is open reduction internal fixation with titanium cannulated screws. While results for the aforementioned techniques are good, open screw fixation of large glenoid fractures has excellent long-term patient satisfaction rates, clinical outcomes, and low recurrence rates [24, 37–39] Additionally, a biomechanical study has shown that addition of screw fixation significantly improves construct stiffness and load to failure when compared to suture anchor fixation alone [40]. The open approach is favored by the authors for many reasons including the facile nature of the deltopectoral approach and fracture fixation compared to arthroscopic techniques as well as the ability to transition to bone block stabilization techniques should bony anatomy not be amenable to repair.

Posterior Glenoid Fracture Treatment Considerations

Posterior shoulder instability is much less common than anterior shoulder instability, occurring in only about 10% of patients experiencing shoulder instability [41]. These injuries are more common among football players, weightlifters, patients with seizure disorders, and in the setting of electrical shock [42]. In severe cases of posterior instability, glenoid fracture can accompany soft tissue injury. Nacca et al. [43] report posterior glenoid bone defects of greater than 20% that are treated with soft tissue repair alone remain unstable. This highlights the importance of bony repair when dealing with medium to large posterior glenoid fractures. For this reason, the treatment algorithm for dealing with posterior glenoid fractures is largely similar to that of anterior glenoid fractures. For small lesions, arthroscopic single-row repair incorporating the fracture fragment has been described with good outcomes [44]. In medium to large lesions, a modification of the anterior bony Bankart bridge has been described in which the fracture fragment is repaired through a double-row suture anchor technique [45]. In their series of seven patients, there were no patients with persistent instability and all had returned to sport and activity at preinjury levels.

Summary

Glenoid fracture in the setting of shoulder instability is a relatively common occurrence and potentially devastating to patient outcomes if not properly treated in the acute setting. The preferred approach to surgical management can be guided by size of the fracture fragment with different techniques indicated for small, medium, and large fractures. An understanding of technical pearls for both arthroscopic and open management of glenoid fractures is critically important for surgeons treating patients with these injuries.

References

1. Shields DW, Jefferies JG, Brooksbank AJ, Millar N, Jenkins PJ. Epidemiology of glenohumeral dislocation and subsequent instability in an urban population. J Shoulder Elb Surg. 2018;27(2):189–95.
2. Leroux T, Wasserstein D, Veillette C, Khoshbin A, Henry P, Chahal J, et al. Epidemiology of primary anterior shoulder dislocation requiring closed reduction in Ontario, Canada. Am J Sports Med. 2014;42(2):442–50.
3. Griffith JF, Antonio GE, Tong CW, Ming CK. Anterior shoulder dislocation: quantification of glenoid bone loss with CT. AJR Am J Roentgenol. 2003;180(5):1423–30.
4. Griffith JF. Measuring glenoid and humeral bone loss in shoulder dislocation. Quant Imaging Med Surg. 2019;9(2):134–43.
5. Dickens JF, Slaven SE, Cameron KL, Pickett AM, Posner M, Campbell SE, et al. Prospective evaluation of glenoid bone loss after first-time and recurrent anterior glenohumeral instability events. Am J Sports Med. 2019;47(5):1082–9.
6. Zhang M, Liu J, Jia Y, Zhang G, Zhou J, Wu D, et al. Risk factors for recurrence after Bankart repair: a systematic review and meta-analysis. J Orthop Surg Res. 2022;17(1):113.
7. Dekker TJ, Peebles LA, Bernhardson AS, Rosenberg SI, Murphy CP, Golijanin P, et al. Risk factors for recurrence after arthroscopic instability repair-the importance of glenoid bone loss >15%, patient age, and duration of symptoms: a matched cohort analysis. Am J Sports Med. 2020;48(12):3036–41.
8. Boileau P, Villalba M, Héry JY, Balg F, Ahrens P, Neyton L. Risk factors for recurrence of shoulder instability after arthroscopic Bankart repair. J Bone Joint Surg Am. 2006;88(8):1755–63.
9. Nakagawa S, Mizuno N, Hiramatsu K, Tachibana Y, Mae T. Absorption of the bone fragment in shoulders with bony Bankart lesions caused by recurrent anterior dislocations or subluxations: when does it occur? Am J Sports Med. 2013;41(6):1380–6.
10. Porcellini G, Paladini P, Campi F, Paganelli M. Long-term outcome of acute versus chronic bony Bankart lesions managed arthroscopically. Am J Sports Med. 2007;35(12):2067–72.
11. Kitayama S, Sugaya H, Takahashi N, Matsuki K, Kawai N, Tokai M, et al. Clinical outcome and glenoid morphology after arthroscopic repair of chronic osseous Bankart lesions: a five to eight-year follow-up study. J Bone Joint Surg Am. 2015;97(22):1833–43.
12. Sugaya H, Moriishi J, Kanisawa I, Tsuchiya A. Arthroscopic osseous Bankart repair for chronic recurrent traumatic anterior glenohumeral instability. J Bone Joint Surg Am. 2005;87(8):1752–60.
13. Kim YK, Cho SH, Son WS, Moon SH. Arthroscopic repair of small and medium-sized bony Bankart lesions. Am J Sports Med. 2014;42(1):86–94.
14. Millett PJ, Braun S. The "bony Bankart bridge" procedure: a new arthroscopic technique for reduction and internal fixation of a bony Bankart lesion. Arthroscopy. 2009;25(1):102–5.
15. Davidson PA, Rivenburgh DW. The 7-o'clock postero-inferior portal for shoulder arthroscopy. Am J Sports Med. 2002;30(5):693–6.
16. Walter WR, Samim M, LaPolla FWZ, Gyftopoulos S. Imaging quantification of glenoid bone loss in patients with glenohumeral instability: a systematic review. AJR Am J Roentgenol. 2019:1–10.
17. Itoi E, Lee SB, Amrami KK, Wenger DE, An KN. Quantitative assessment of classic anteroinferior bony Bankart lesions by radiography and computed tomography. Am J Sports Med. 2003;31(1):112–8.
18. Sugaya H. Techniques to evaluate glenoid bone loss. Curr Rev Musculoskelet Med. 2014;7(1):1–5.
19. Chuang TY, Adams CR, Burkhart SS. Use of preoperative three-dimensional computed tomography to quantify glenoid bone loss in shoulder instability. Arthroscopy. 2008;24(4):376–82.
20. Gyftopoulos S, Beltran LS, Yemin A, Strauss E, Meislin R, Jazrawi L, et al. Use of 3D MR reconstructions in the evaluation of glenoid bone loss: a clinical study. Skeletal Radiol. 2014;43(2):213–8.
21. Stecco A, Guenzi E, Cascone T, Fabbiano F, Fornara P, Oronzo P, et al. MRI can assess glenoid bone loss after shoulder luxation: inter- and intra-individual comparison with CT. Radiol Med. 2013;118(8):1335–43.
22. Bishop JY, Jones GL, Rerko MA, Donaldson C. 3-D CT is the most reliable imaging modality when quantifying glenoid bone loss. Clin Orthop Relat Res. 2013;471(4):1251–6.
23. Bigliani LU, Newton PM, Steinmann SP, Connor PM, McLlveen SJ. Glenoid rim lesions associated with recurrent anterior dislocation of the shoulder. Am J Sports Med. 1998;26(1):41–5.
24. Scheibel M, Magosch P, Lichtenberg S, Habermeyer P. Open reconstruction of anterior glenoid rim fractures. Knee Surg Sports Traumatol Arthrosc. 2004;12(6):568–73.
25. Nakagawa S, Mae T, Yoneda K, Kinugasa K, Nakamura H. Influence of glenoid defect size and bone fragment size on the clinical outcome after arthroscopic Bankart repair in male collision/contact athletes. Am J Sports Med. 2017;45(9):1967–74.
26. Hurley ET, Manjunath AK, Bloom DA, Pauzenberger L, Mullett H, Alaia MJ, et al. Arthroscopic Bankart repair versus conservative management for first-

time traumatic anterior shoulder instability: a systematic review and meta-analysis. Arthroscopy. 2020;36(9):2526–32.
27. Maziak N, Minkus M, Krüger D, Scheibel M. Arthroscopic reconstruction of multifragmented anteroinferior glenoid rim fractures. JBJS Essent Surg Tech. 2019;9(4)
28. Brown L, Rothermel S, Joshi R, Dhawan A. Recurrent instability after arthroscopic Bankart reconstruction: a systematic review of surgical technical factors. Arthroscopy. 2017;33(11):2081–92.
29. Frank RM, Mall NA, Gupta D, Shewman E, Wang VM, Romeo AA, et al. Inferior suture anchor placement during arthroscopic Bankart repair: influence of portal placement and curved drill guide. Am J Sports Med. 2014;42(5):1182–9.
30. Millett PJ, Horan MP, Martetschläger F. The "bony Bankart bridge" technique for restoration of anterior shoulder stability. Am J Sports Med. 2013;41(3):608–14.
31. Godin JA, Altintas B, Horan MP, Hussain ZB, Pogorzelski J, Fritz EM, et al. Midterm results of the bony Bankart bridge technique for the treatment of bony Bankart lesions. Am J Sports Med. 2019;47(1):158–64.
32. Spiegl UJ, Smith SD, Todd JN, Coatney GA, Wijdicks CA, Millett PJ. Biomechanical comparison of arthroscopic single- and double-row repair techniques for acute bony Bankart lesions. Am J Sports Med. 2014;42(8):1939–46.
33. Greenstein AS, Chen RE, Knapp E, Brown AM, Roberts A, Awad HA, et al. A biomechanical, cadaveric evaluation of single- versus double-row repair techniques on stability of bony Bankart lesions. Am J Sports Med. 2021;49(3):773–9.
34. Taverna E, Guarrella V, Freehill MT, Garavaglia G. Arthroscopic reduction with endobutton fixation for glenoid fracture. Joints. 2017;5(2):127–30.
35. Scheibel M, Hug K, Gerhardt C, Krueger D. Arthroscopic reduction and fixation of large solitary and multifragmented anterior glenoid rim fractures. J Shoulder Elb Surg. 2016;25(5):781–90.
36. Maier D, Izadpanah K, Ogon P, Mützel M, Bayer J, Südkamp NP, et al. Open fixation of acute anterior glenoid rim fractures with bioresorbable pins: analysis of clinical and radiological outcome. Arch Orthop Trauma Surg. 2015;135(7):953–61.
37. Raiss P, Baumann F, Akbar M, Rickert M, Loew M. Open screw fixation of large anterior glenoid rim fractures: mid- and long-term results in 29 patients. Knee Surg Sports Traumatol Arthrosc. 2009;17(2):195–203.
38. Osti M, Gohm A, Benedetto KP. Results of open reconstruction of anterior glenoid rim fractures following shoulder dislocation. Arch Orthop Trauma Surg. 2009;129(9):1245–9.
39. Pfister G, Murison JC, Sabate-Ferris A, Danis J, De l'Escalopier N, Mathieu L. Open screw fixation of large anterior glenoid rim fractures using a deltopectoral approach with subscapularis splitting. Tech Hand Up Extrem Surg. 2022;
40. Clavert P, Aim F, Bonnevialle N, Arboucalot M, Ehlinger M, Bauer T. Biomechanical properties of transosseous bony Bankart repair in a cadaver model. Orthop Traumatol Surg Res. 2019;105(2):271–4.
41. Brelin A, Dickens JF. Posterior shoulder instability. Sports Med Arthrosc Rev. 2017;25(3):136–43.
42. Robinson CM, Seah M, Akhtar MA. The epidemiology, risk of recurrence, and functional outcome after an acute traumatic posterior dislocation of the shoulder. JBJS. 2011;93(17):1605–13.
43. Nacca C, Gil JA, Badida R, Crisco JJ, Owens BD. Critical glenoid bone loss in posterior shoulder instability. Am J Sports Med. 2018;46(5):1058–63.
44. Poehling-Monaghan KL, Krych AJ, Dahm DL. Arthroscopic repair of a posterior bony Bankart lesion. Arthrosc Tech. 2015;4(6):e669–73.
45. Lacheta L, Goldenberg BT, Horan MP, Millett PJ. Posterior bony Bankart bridge technique results in reliable clinical 2-year outcomes and high return to sports rate for the treatment of posterior bony Bankart lesions. Knee Surg Sports Traumatol Arthrosc. 2021;29(1):120–6.

24 The Deep Hill-Sachs Lesion: Open Bone Grafting with Allograft

Jason Khoury and George S. Athwal

Introduction

Hill-Sachs (HS) lesions and reverse Hill-Sachs (rHS) lesions are humeral head impression fractures that occur after either anterior or posterior shoulder dislocation, respectively. During contact of the glenoid rim with the humeral head at the time of dislocation, the denser bone of the glenoid rim compresses the softer cancellous bone of the humeral head to create the defect [1]. This reduces the humeral articular surface available for the glenoid track, producing an articular arc mismatch that may lead to recurrent or persistent instability [2]. Currently, there are no well-accepted criteria for when to address humeral head bone loss, particularly when there is concomitant glenoid bone loss. The Latarjet procedure and other glenoid bone block augmentation procedures have become the workhorse for addressing shoulder instability with substantial bone loss. Some may even consider humeral head reconstruction redundant to anterior inferior glenoid bone grafting [1]. However, not all off-track HS lesions can be converted to on-track lesions with a glenoid bony augmentation [3]. The decision to surgically treat humeral bone loss in shoulder instability is a complex one, particularly in the primary setting and when there is concomitant glenoid bone loss. The treatment goal should be to restore the native sphericity of the humeral head and thus reestablish stability without sacrificing range of motion [4]. Methods for addressing humeral bone loss depend largely on the degree of bone loss present as well as patient factors and surgeon comfort. The larger lesions tend to have greater effect on stability and thus are more likely to require operative fixation [5, 6]. In this chapter, we will focus on the use of osteoarticular allograft for the reconstruction of large humeral head defects both in the context of anterior and posterior instability.

Case Example

A 33-year-old left-hand dominant male presented with recurrent right anterior shoulder instability. He had a previous open anterior stabilization that failed, followed by an arthroscopic Bankart repair and soft tissue remplissage 2 years prior. He presented due to a recurrent instability event. He was known to have a seizure disorder that was well controlled on medication with no recent seizure. On examination, he had full range of motion and no hyperlaxity but grossly positive anterior apprehension and relocation tests. There were no infectious signs, and his neurovascular examination was normal. Radiographs and CT scan demonstrated anterior glenoid bone loss measuring 25% of the glenoid surface area and a substantial

J. Khoury · G. S. Athwal (✉)
McFarlane Hand & Upper Limb Centre, St. Joseph's Health Care, London, ON, Canada
e-mail: jason.khoury@mcgill.ca

© The Author(s), under exclusive license to Springer Nature Switzerland AG 2026
R. M. Frank, J. M. Tokish (eds.), *Management of Shoulder Instability*,
https://doi.org/10.1007/978-3-032-18089-6_24

HS defect involving 20% of the humeral head articular surface. Given the bipolar nature of bone loss with <30% humeral head involvement, the surgeon decided to proceed with a glenoid augmentation procedure by performing an arthroscopic Latarjet fixed with two partially threaded titanium cortical screws. The shoulder was tested at the end of the glenoid-based procedure, and the HS lesion was found to be non-engaging in all functional positions, so the humerus was not addressed. The patient was placed into a sling and started active and active-assisted range of motion at 6 weeks. At 3 months, a CT scan was performed and showed stable fixation with interval healing of the bone block, so the patient was started on a progressive strengthening program.

Four years after glenoid bony augmentation, the patient had a traumatic fall from standing height and re-dislocated the affected shoulder, with three subsequent instability episodes and symptomatic instability on examination. Repeat radiographs and CT scan demonstrate a non-united bone block with broken hardware and an enlarging HS defect measuring 40% of the humeral articular arc (Fig. 24.1). Given multiple failed instability surgeries with substantial bipolar bone loss, the decision was taken to proceed with bony reconstruction of the humerus and glenoid using side- and size-matched humeral osteochondral allograft and distal clavicle autograft, respectively.

After interscalene regional block and general anesthetic, the patient was administered weight-appropriate antibiotics and placed into the beach-chair position at 20 degrees (T-Max, Smith & Nephew, London). The medial border of the scapula may be supported by the backrest to provide some resistance when reconstructing the glenoid. The arm was placed into a pneumatic arm positioner (Spyder, Smith & Nephew, London). An anterior deltopectoral approach was utilized with extension proximally for distal clavicle harvest. The deltopectoral interval was entered and dissection was erred laterally in order to avoid the brachial plexus given the absence of the coracoid from the previous failed Latarjet procedure. A biceps tenodesis was performed to the proximal portion of the pectoralis major. The acromioclavicular (AC) joint was opened longitudinally and a 15 mm osteoarticular bone block was harvested from the distal clavicle. The AC joint ligaments were closed primarily. A subscapularis peel approach was used, taking the subscapularis and capsule in one layer. The anterior portion of the glenoid vault was exposed and the previous non-united bone block and hardware were removed. A surgical dislocation of the humerus was done by bringing the arm into externally rotated and extension to expose the humeral bone defect posteriorly. Tension was removed from the brachial plexus by bringing the humeral head superiorly and maintaining the arm in adduction. It is helpful to place straight blunt retractors (such as Darrach retractors) posterior to the humeral head to use as a skid and lever the head out. Using a burr, the defect was fashioned into a wedge shape with orthogonal edges to the remaining articular surface in order to accommodate the new graft. The bone defect was then measured using a sterile ruler, noting its depth, width, length, and approximate circumference, as described by Miniaci et al. [7]. A fresh-frozen side- and size-matched humeral head osteochondral allograft was prepared on the back table and marked according to the defect measurements. It is best to err on making the graft slightly larger and then refining its shape as needed. The wedge shape was cut using an oscillating saw, and then small adjustments were made in one plane at a time using a burr in order to mirror the defect. It is important for the articular edges to match the native articular cartilage. Once the graft was fashioned appropriately, it was provisionally fixed with K-wires and then fixed with four 3.5 mm cortical screws from anterior to posterior (Fig. 24.2). Anteriorly based screws achieve adequate fixation, avoid penetration of the allograft cartilaginous surface, mitigate the risk of impingement of the screw head, and simplify

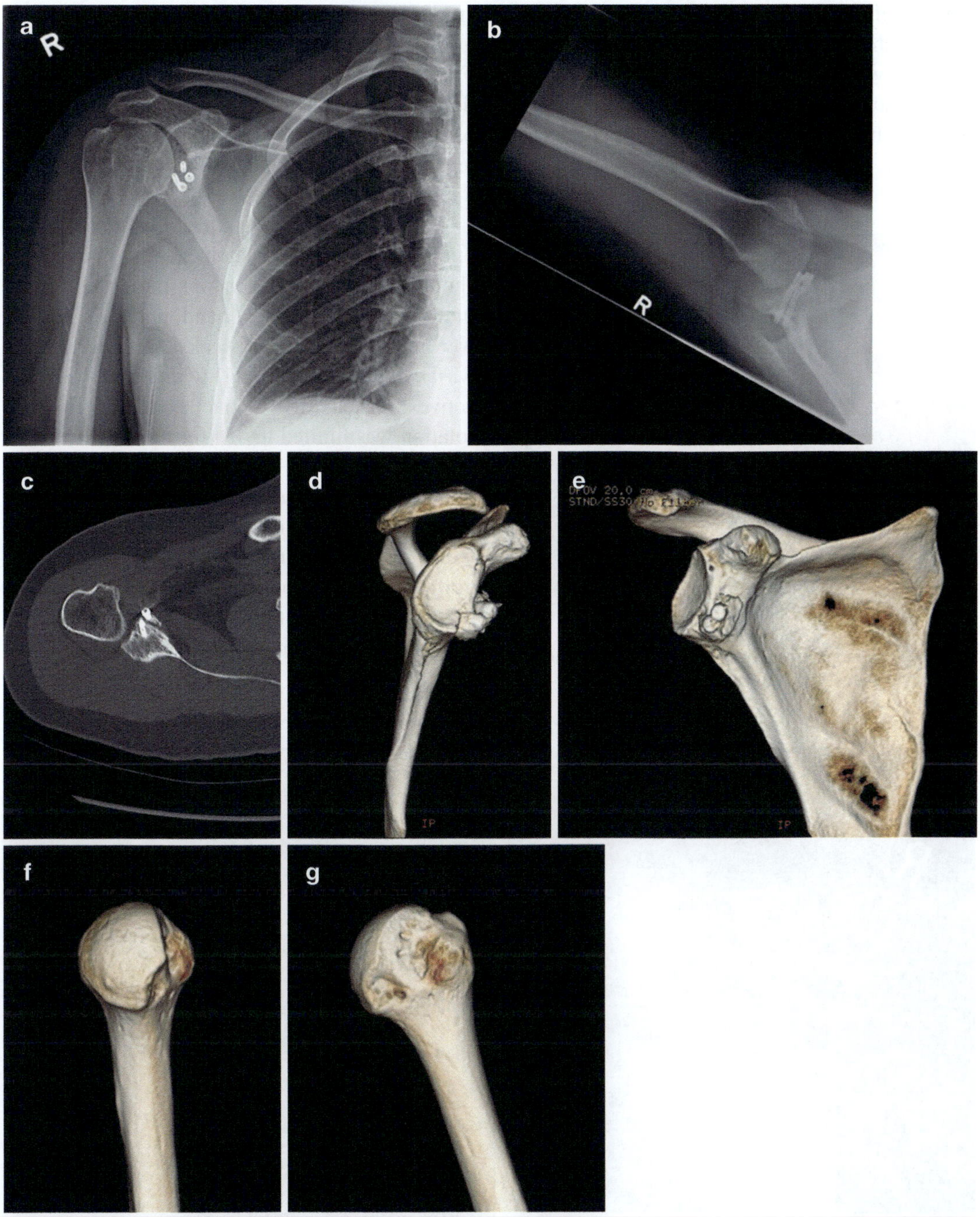

Fig. 24.1 Preoperative imaging after failure of an arthroscopic Latarjet procedure. (**a**) AP view of the shoulder demonstrating broken hardware; (**b**) axillary view demonstrating broken hardware, displaced and non-united bone block, and large HS lesion; (**c**) CT scan axillary cut redemonstrating broken hardware and displaced and non-united bone block; (**d** and **e**) 3D CT showing degree of anterior glenoid bone loss; (**f** and **g**) lateral and posterior view of the humeral head on 3D CT reconstruction demonstrating large HS lesion

removal if the screw heads become prominent [8]. The shoulder was reduced, the distal clavicle autograft was pinned and fixed with three 3.5 mm cortical screws to recreate the anterior glenoid rim, and the labrum was repaired. It is important to check stability of the reconstruction and smooth range of motion by assessing joint congruity in functional shoulder positions. Fluoroscopy was used to confirm hardware position. The subscapularis repair was performed based on the technique by Lapner et al. using a tension-band technique, transosseus tunnels, and a mini-fragment plate [9].

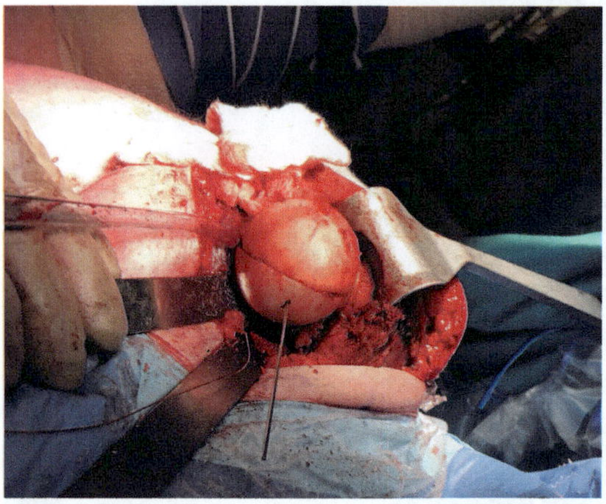

Fig. 24.2 Intraoperative photo of the osteoarticular graft fitted to the defect and provisionally fixed with a K-wire

Postoperatively, the patient was given antibiotics and placed into a shoulder immobilizer. No shoulder range of motion was permitted for the first 6 weeks, but elbow, hand, and wrist motion were encouraged. At 6 weeks, shoulder motion was initiated, beginning with pendular, then active assisted, then active exercises. External rotation was limited to 45° for the first 3 months given the nature of recurring instability. Control radiographs were taken at each visit to ensure appropriate graft and hardware positioning, as well as to confirm graft healing (Fig. 24.3). Some graft resorption should be expected. There were no recurrent dislocations at 5-year follow-up, and the graft has remained stable with minimal resorption.

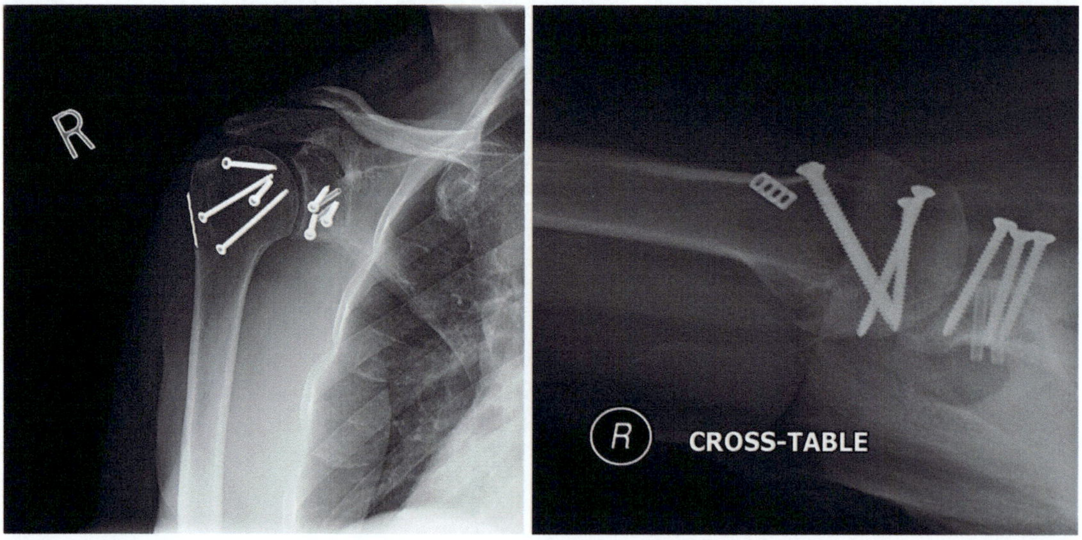

Fig. 24.3 Postoperative radiographs (AP and axillary) demonstrating intact hardware and healing of the osteoarticular allograft and distal clavicle autograft with reconstitution of the humeral head articular arc

Imaging

Standard radiographs should be obtained, including an AP view, true AP (or Grashey) view, scapular-Y, and an axillary view. The internal rotation view is best to evaluate HS lesions. Other views specific for evaluation of a HS defect include the Stryker notch view and apical oblique view of Garth [1, 10].

Computer tomography (CT) scans with 3D reconstructions have become the mainstay in the preoperative evaluation of bone loss and are better at determining the width, depth, orientation, and location of HS lesions [11]. The on-track/off-track concept has gained widespread use for determination of a functionally important lesion, and this can be calculated on 3D-reconstructed CT scans [12]. A CT scan with 3D reconstructions with and without humeral subtraction is the author's preferred imaging modality in the preoperative evaluation of patients with shoulder instability as it best delineates the bony architecture of the humerus and glenoid and thus identify what must be addressed surgically.

Ultrasound has been shown to have similar sensitivity in the detection of HS lesions compared to CT arthrography although clinical application is limited by dependence on operator experience and limited evaluation of other structures and the orientation of the lesion [1, 10].

Magnetic resonance imaging (MRI) has also shown to have high accuracy for detection of HS lesions and allows for the detection of other intra-articular pathology [10]. This modality is especially important in older patients after shoulder dislocation as there is a high incidence of associated rotator cuff pathology [13]. If MRI is selected, evaluation of bone loss and determination of on-track or off-track lesions can still be performed [11]. In a recent review article by Khan et al., magnetic resonance arthrography (MRA) was shown to have the greatest sensitivity, specificity, intra-rater, and inter-rater agreement among all modalities [11]. However, studies are limited in their size with significant technical variability and reproducibility was only moderate [11]. Further limitations of MR imaging include its higher cost, presence of metal artifact, and the need for intra-articular injection of contrast medium if an arthrogram is performed [11].

Classification of Hill-Sachs Defects

Humeral bone defects can be quantified anatomically by measuring their size. This can be done on axillary or Stryker notch radiographs, 2D or 3D CT scans, CT arthrogram, 2D or 3D MRI, MRA, or arthroscopically [11]. Typically, width, length, and depth are noted. A more practical method is to note the size of the lesion as a percentage of the entire articular arc or humeral head diameter after application of a best-fit circle on axial CT slices [14, 15]. Gerber et al. developed a variation of this by comparing the articular arc angle to the defect angle on a best-fit circle applied to the proximal humerus on axial CT slices taken at or immediately below the level of the coracoid tip [16].

The definition of a functionally significant HS lesion was reintroduced by Burkhart and DeBeer to explain failure of arthroscopic Bankart repairs [17]. They defined an engaging lesion as one in which the long axis of the humeral head defect aligns with the rim of the anterior glenoid in a functional position of abduction and external rotation. Yamamoto et al. studied this further by observing the imprint of the glenoid on the humeral head, known as the glenoid track. With the arm in 60° of abduction relative to the scapula, or 90° relative to the trunk, the glenoid track measured 84% of the glenoid width, extending medially from the cuff insertion [18]. Further work by Di Giacomo et al. elaborated on this to calculate whether a lesion was considered engaging or "off-track" [12]. HS defects that extend medial to the glenoid track have a sufficiently large articular arc mismatch such that the glenoid rim may "fall into" the humeral head defect and allow for dislocation—just as a car tire may fall into a pothole rather than roll over it if the hole is large enough and suitably orientated [12]. Thus, the determination of a functionally important HS lesion is given by its size, location, orientation, and the presence or absence of glenoid bone loss.

When to Address Humeral Bone Loss

When a surgeon is faced with a HS lesion in the context of anterior shoulder instability, how should they determine whether it needs to be addressed surgically? Size assessed on CT or MRI is the most widely studied method, but there is no well-defined critical threshold for guiding surgical management [11]. One of the most used classifications is one proposed by Warner and Flatow. Lesions with <20% articular arc involvement are clinically insignificant, lesions between 20% and 40% have variable clinical significance, and lesions >40% of the humeral head are clinically significant and warrant surgical consideration [6, 13, 19]. Chen et al. developed an algorithm that stratifies lesions based on the percentage of articular arc involvement on axillary radiographs or axial CT scan. In patients with <20% articular arc involvement, the glenoid was addressed alone. With 20–30% articular arc involvement, the glenoid was addressed first and then a soft tissue filling procedure with either infraspinatus or latissimus dorsi was performed if there was residual instability. Allograft reconstruction was only addressed in cases of severe (30–45%) humeral bone defect and was performed in conjunction with anterior glenoid stabilization. Arthroplasty was reserved for >45% defects [13]. With the increasing use of glenoid bony augmentation, the decision to address the HS lesion is even further complicated as an engaging lesion may become non-engaging once the glenoid width is reestablished or widened to supraphysiologic size [1, 3].

The reason that there is no established consensus on specific decision-making strategies and threshold values for critical HS size is likely twofold. First, there exists a wide variability of measurement techniques in the literature which has made it difficult to compare bone loss between studies [11]. Second, the clinical significance of a HS lesion is not solely based on its size. Rather, it depends on a multitude of factors such as location, orientation, concomitant glenoid bone loss, patient-specific factors, and risk factors for recurrent instability [1]. With this in mind, the search for a single critical defect size may be elusive as the relative contribution from all these elements will alter the threshold for surgical intervention. In this case, the surgeon should choose a technique that will fully address the instability all while minimizing operative time, cost, and surgical trauma. If instability can be managed by addressing either the glenoid or the humerus, then an attempt should be made to do so. In the case of smaller HS lesions, it is generally easier to address the glenoid bone loss only, regardless of the degree of glenoid bone loss present. In the case of large HS lesions with minimal glenoid bone loss, it may be easier to address the humeral bone loss only and supplement with a glenoid soft tissue procedure. However, some surgeons would still elect to conduct glenoid-sided procedures, with soft tissue interposition for the HS defect. In the case where there is moderate to severe glenoid and/or humeral bone loss present, the surgeon must try to determine which is more clinically relevant, or whether both need to be addressed, and work within their comfort level and with available local resources.

Reverse HS lesions, or the so-called McLaughlin lesion, are equally challenging to manage. The surgeon should consider that in general, humeral bone loss after a posterior shoulder dislocation is comparatively greater and more functionally significant than humeral bone loss after anterior dislocation [19, 20]. This is because posterior dislocations tend to occur from higher-energy mechanisms such as seizures and high-energy trauma and thus result in humeral bone loss that is larger with greater involvement of the articular arc [19, 21–23]. It is also important to distinguish between posterior shoulder dislocation and posterior instability. Contrary to the association between anterior dislocation and anterior instability, posterior dislocation is not a common feature of posterior instability [24]. Rather, posterior instability more commonly presents due to episodes of posterior subluxation from repetitive microtrauma from loading of the shoulder in the provocative position of flexion and internal rotation or secondary to ligamentous laxity [24, 25]. So although rHS lesions have been reported in up to 86% of patients after first-time posterior dislocation, they are not nearly as common in cases of posterior instability without frank dislocation [20, 24]. Other risk factors for recurrent posterior instability are age < 40, seizure disorder, posterior glenoid bone loss, glenoid dysplasia, and increased glenoid retroversion [24]. Glenoid bone loss and retroversion have garnered increasing attention in patients with recurrent posterior instability [24, 25]. Posterior glenoid bone loss after an initial instability event has been measured at 5.4% of the glenoid width or 4.2% of the glenoid surface, considerably smaller than glenoid bone loss associated with anterior instability [24, 25]. In a biomechanical study by Nacca et al., a critical posterior defect size of 20% led to persistent instability after posterior labral repair [26]. Similarly, shoulders with >13.5% surface area of glenoid bone loss were found to have an increased risk of reoperation after labral repair alone [26]. Increased glenoid retroversion is also a risk factor for posterior instability and is associated with increased posterior glenoid bone loss and failure of soft tissue only capsulolabral repair [24, 25, 27]. Further research is thus needed to evaluate the functional significance of a rHS lesion in the presence of altered glenoid morphology and progressive posterior bone loss [24].

Surgical decision-making in the context of a reverse HS lesion and posterior shoulder dislocation thus suffers from similar limitations as those discussed for anterior instability. Robinson et al. recommended disimpaction and bone grafting for lesions with <25% articular involvement detected <2 weeks after injury, subscapularis transfer if the lesion is detected >2 weeks after injury, and structural allograft for any lesion with >40–50% articular involvement [23]. Other authors have advocated for surgical intervention with as little as 10% humeral head involvement [19, 28]. Paul et al. suggested osteochondral allograft in defects >40% with good bone quality and absence of osteoarthritis [29]. Gerber et al. recommended osteochondral allograft reconstruction for defects 30–55% of the articular arc [16]. On the other hand, arthroplasty has been advocated for defects involving >40–45% [21, 29]. The threshold of humeral head involvement that warrants allograft reconstruction thus varies across the literature, and there is no consensus on a single algorithmic approach. In general, due to the more extensive articular involvement of a rHS, restorative or reconstructive options are more commonly required in order to reestablish a more physiologic arc of motion. As such, there is considerably more literature on allograft reconstruction in the context of rHS lesions compared to HS lesions.

A special consideration for posterior dislocation is that they are commonly missed and so the surgeon must also consider the chronicity of the injury [23]. Greater chronicity predisposes to greater osteopenia, progressively larger lesions, more difficult reduction, and greater incidence of OA and thus may limit available surgical techniques [16]. Gerber et al. treated 13 patients with chronic posterior dislocations (>4 weeks) with osteoarticular grafts at a mean delay of 6.3 months (range 1–15 months) [16]. They recommend treating these as early as possible to optimize outcomes [16].

In general, humeral bone loss involving more than 20% of the articular arc warrants further consideration for surgical intervention since they have a higher propensity to cause recurrent instability and should thus have a lower threshold for addressing surgically [13]. Anatomic reconstruction with osteochondral graft should be considered for lesions involving more than 30–40% of the articular arc. Irrespective of the individual contribution of humeral or glenoid bone loss, surgical decision-making should be based on an appreciation of their shared impact on shoulder instability and the continuous spectrum of instability that exists with varying degrees of bipolar bone loss.

The author's indications for performing osteoarticular allograft reconstruction of a humeral bone defects are:

- >30% humeral articular arc involvement
- Younger patient
- Failed prior instability surgery with a substantial HS defect

In anterior instability, the author prefers addressing bone loss on the glenoid side prior to addressing the humerus as addressing the humerus open adds considerable surgical invasiveness. In posterior dislocation, the larger rHS lesion is typically the predominant bone defect so it is addressed first. When there is posterior instability without frank dislocation or no large rHS lesion, the decision should consider the previously mentioned factors. In any case, there is a lower threshold for addressing humeral bone loss with progressively larger lesions, in cases where previous instability surgery has failed, and in patients with high risk of dislocation such as contact athletes or those with a seizure disorder [1, 7].

Contraindications include active infection, advanced age, and diffuse osteoarthritis. Relative contraindications include patients who will be unable to follow postoperative instructions, osteoporosis, infections of distant sites, and comorbidities that could alter bone healing potential [21].

Preoperative Considerations

A careful history and physical examination must be performed. In our experience, patients with voluntary dislocation or with an uncontrolled seizure disorder will perform poorly after surgical reconstruction and are at high risk of recurrence. In patients with acute posterior dislocations without high-energy trauma, the surgeon must maintain a high index of suspicion for an underlying seizure disorder. In the absence of an epileptic disorder, it may be appropriate to investigate for other causes such as metabolic abnormality, alcoholism, hypoglycemic convulsion, or an intracranial mass and treat them prior to addressing the shoulder [23]. In the setting of revision surgery, previous operative reports and imaging should be obtained.

When treating a patient with humeral bone loss, the decision to proceed with osteochondral allograft will ultimately depend on:

- Clinical history—number and ease of dislocation, chronicity of instability or dislocation, etiology of instability (e.g., seizure disorder, alcoholism), and voluntary or involuntary instability
- Humeral defect size, orientation, and location
- Presence and size of associated glenoid bone loss
- Patient-specific factors such as age, comorbidities, ligamentous laxity, handedness, activity level, occupation, ability to comply with postoperative restrictions, and patient expectations
- Presence of concomitant glenohumeral wear
- Bone quality
- Presence of other intra-articular pathology such as chondral defects, capsulolabral tears, rotator cuff tears, humeral avulsion of the glenohumeral ligament (HAGL), or capsular laxity
- Revision for previous failed instability procedure
- Surgeon comfort level and experience
- Local availability of implants, equipment, and osteoarticular allograft

Treatment

Once the decision has been made to address humeral bone loss surgically, the surgeon must select the appropriate technique. Soft tissue procedures used for HS lesions such as remplissage are nonanatomic and may limit external rotation [30, 31]. They are thus reserved for small to moderate lesions only. Similarly, reconstruction of rHS lesions were traditionally managed by the technique described by McLaughlin and then modified by Neer, where the lesser tuberosity and subscapularis tendon were transferred into the defect site to prevent engagement. Although this technique has good success in moderately sizes lesions, it is nonanatomic, de-tensions the subscapularis, and may limit future arthroplasty options by altering the anatomy of the proximal humerus [10].

The treatment of larger lesions thus focuses on anatomic techniques. Options generally include humeroplasty, humeral head bony augmentation, and arthroplasty. Humeroplasty is reserved for acute lesions <3 weeks old, whereby the depressed fragments are elevated and the void is filled with bone graft [19]. This technique is more difficult if there is comminution of the articular surface (as is often seen in rHS lesions) or if there is poor bone quality and is thus better suited for small to moderate lesions [22]. Arthroplasty or partial resurfacing should be reserved for older or lower-demand patients, presence of concomitant glenohumeral cartilage wear, or salvage scenarios [19]. Humeral derotational osteotomy has largely fallen out of favor due to a higher complication rate [19].

Humeral head bony augmentation—the focus of this chapter—has the advantage of reconstituting the articular arc of the humeral head, thus preventing the defect from engaging the glenoid rim, offering a cartilaginous surface for joint contact and maintaining normal range of motion without compromising the structural anatomy of the humeral head and thus allowing for revision to arthroplasty if needed. Overall, techniques are similar whether attempting to reconstruct a HS or rHS lesion.

The goals of surgery in the treatment of large HS lesions are to:

1. Fill the defect
2. Restore the articular congruity of the humeral head
3. Maintain a normal arc of motion
4. Eliminate instability

Surgical Techniques

There is limited evidence on the use of osteoarticular allografts in the treatment of a HS lesion with anterior instability. The surgeon may choose to have the patient in a beach-chair position or in the lateral decubitus position. The procedure has been described with both open and arthroscopic techniques [7, 31–40]. The open procedure can be done anteriorly through a deltopectoral incision or posteriorly between the infraspinatus and teres minor or through a bipennate split of the infraspinatus [7, 31, 33–38]. If the shoulder is approached anteriorly, anterior glenoid stabilization can be done with either a soft tissue repair or with supplementary bone block augmentation, usually done after humeral reconstruction [7, 35–37]. If the shoulder is approached posteriorly, soft tissue anterior stabilization is usually done arthroscopically prior to the humeral reconstruction [31, 34, 38].

The treatment of rHS defects is usually done through an open anterior deltopectoral approach [4, 16, 21, 41–49]. However, it has also been described arthroscopically in two cases [50, 51]. The posterior shoulder should be accessible within the surgical field and can be used to facilitate reduction of the humeral head in chronic cases or address posterior glenoid-sided pathology if needed. The surgeon may opt to begin with an arthroscopy to confirm the diagnosis or address other intra-articular pathology such as an HAGL or posterior labral injury [20, 45, 47, 49].

When addressing bone loss, the subscapularis can be managed to the surgeon's preference with either a complete or limited subscapularis peel or tenotomy. Ker and colleagues suggest a pedicled lesser tuberosity osteotomy to preserve the integrity of the anterior humeral circumflex artery (AHCA) and its ascending arcuate branch [52]. This preserves the subscapularis tendinous origin and can theoretically maintain blood flow to the humeral head, potentially limit osteonecrosis, and decrease graft resorption [52]. Other authors have described a subscapularis peel or tenotomy with preservation of the AHCA and arcuate artery [16, 21, 42].

Graft options to reconstruct humeral head bone loss include fresh, fresh-frozen, or cryopreserved humeral or femoral head osteochondral allograft or iliac crest autograft [2, 4, 16, 21, 38, 40–48, 50, 52]. If femoral head is used, it is preferred to obtain a smaller graft to better match the native radius of curvature of the humeral head [46]. Fresh talus allograft has also been described in the reconstruction of rHS lesions with the purported benefit of dense subchondral supporting bone, a similar radius of curvature to the humeral head and greater availability due to not requiring size matching [5, 20, 53, 54]. Non-irradiated grafts are preferred to avoid graft resorption and prominent hardware [7]. Fresh allograft can maintain chondrocyte viability but are much more limited in their availability and must be implanted within 2 weeks after a series of microbiological and serological testing [5]. Side- and size-matched humeral head allograft is preferred in larger lesions in order to best match the patient's native articular arc [7]. However, given limitations in availability of osteoarticular grafts, the use of non-matched grafts is also acceptable.

Osteochondral graft can be harvested as a wedge-shaped segment or an osteochondral plug [7, 32, 34, 45]. Multiple small plugs can be stacked to form a mosaicplasty [39]. Alternatively, a large circular to elliptical plug can be fashioned using the multiple osteochondral autograft transport systems (OATS) available on the market. 3D-printed guides have also been used [41]. Fixation can be press-fit or fixed with fully or partially threaded screws, headless compression screws, or suture anchors.

Miniaci et al. addressed large HS defects with fresh-frozen size- and side-matched osteoarticular allograft in 18 patients who all had >25% humeral head involvement [7]. All patients in their cohort had a previous failed instability surgery. At the time of surgery, nine were found to have recurrent anterior Bankart lesions and three had <20% glenoid bone erosion. Seizure disorder was identified as a common mechanism of injury [7]. Tjoumakaris et al. addressed bipolar bone loss in a marine with recurrent anterior shoulder instability using a fresh-frozen size-matched humeral head allograft to reconstruct the humeral defect. The authors harvested a bicortical bone block from the same humeral allograft to reconstruct the glenoid bone defect [35]. Liow et al. treated 10 patients with anterior instability and bipolar bone loss (25% humeral articular surface and 15% glenoid surface area) using a combined humeral head allograft and Latarjet procedure [37]. Snir et al. used osteochondral plugs harvested from a side- and size-matched fresh-frozen humeral head allograft and press-fit them arthroscopically in the humeral defect [39]. Soft tissue Bankart lesions were addressed arthroscopically and glenoid bony augmentation, if necessary, was staged [39].

When addressing rHS lesions, Diklic et al. had successful outcomes after allograft reconstruction in 13 patients with chronic posterior dislocation with 25–50% articular surface involvement [4]. Gerber et al. treated 22 shoulders with locked posterior dislocations and rHS between 30 and 55% of the articular arc using segmental fresh-frozen humeral or femoral head as well as structural iliac crest bone graft. Two patients required conversion to arthroplasty more than 15 years after surgery, and one patient was revised early to arthroplasty due to persistent posterior subluxation and collapse of the allograft [16]. Martinez et al. followed six patients with fresh-frozen humeral head allograft after posterior shoulder dislocation and 40–50% articular arc involvement. All returned to work at 4 months, and there were no nonunions, infections, or recurrent instability events. At 10 years, three patients had no pain or mechanical symptoms, and three patients were converted to arthroplasty more than 8 years after surgery [55]. In a more recent study, Marcheggiani Mucciolo et al. treated 12 patients with chronic locked posterior dislocations with 30–50% articular arc involvement with osteochondral humeral head allografts. They reported significant functional improvement with minimal osteoarthritis and no reoperations at a mean of 66 months [42].

Postoperative Considerations

Typical postoperative instructions after osteoarticular allograft reconstruction include a standard abduction shoulder sling and restriction on shoulder range of motion for a period of 6 weeks. Elbow, hand, and wrist range of motion are encouraged. From 6 weeks to 3 months, active assisted and active range of motion of the shoulder are initiated. At 3 months, a gentle progressive strengthening program is started under supervision with a physiotherapist. Radiographs are repeated at 2, 6, and 12 weeks to ensure graft integration. Known graft-related complications include graft resorption leading to hardware prominence, graft collapse, avascular necrosis, and nonunion. Other complications to be aware of include progressive osteoarthritis, stiffness, persistent subluxation, or recurrent instability episodes [7, 16].

References

1. Armitage MS, Faber KJ, Drosdowech DS, Litchfield RB, Athwal GS. Humeral head bone defects: remplissage, allograft, and arthroplasty. Orthop Clin North Am. 2010;41:417–25.
2. Saltzman BM, Riboh JC, Cole BJ, Yanke AB. Humeral head reconstruction with osteochondral allograft transplantation. Arthroscopy. W.B. Saunders. 2015;31:1827–34.
3. Calvo C, Calvo J, Rojas D, Valencia M, Calvo E. Clinical relevance of persistent off-track hill-sachs lesion after arthroscopic Latarjet procedure. Am J Sports Med. 2021;49(8):2006–12.
4. Diklic ID, Ganic ZD, Blagojevic ZD, Nho SJ, Romeo AA. Treatment of locked chronic posterior dislocation of the shoulder by reconstruction of the defect in the humeral head with an allograft. J Bone Jt Surg [Br]. 2010;92(1):92–71.
5. Capito NM, Owens BD, Sherman SL, Smith MJ. Osteochondral allografts in shoulder surgical procedures. JBJS Rev. Journal of Bone and Joint Surgery Inc. 2016;4:e3.
6. Flatow EL, Miniaci A, Evans PJ, Simonian PT, Warren RF. Instability of the shoulder: complex problems and failed repairs: part I. Relevant biomechanics, multidirectional instability, and severe loss of glenoid and humeral bone. Instr Course Lect. 1998;47:113–25.
7. Miniaci A, Gish MW. Management of anterior glenohumeral instability associated with large Hill-Sachs defects. Tech Shoulder Elb Surg. 2004;5(3):170–5.
8. Puskas GJ, Giles JW, Degen RM, Johnson JA, Athwal GS. Humeral head reconstruction for Hill-Sachs defects: a biomechanical comparison of 2 fixation techniques for bone grafting. Arthrosc J Arthrosc Relat Surg. 2014;30(1):22–8.
9. Lapner P, Pollock JW, Zhang T, Ruggiero S, Momoli F, Sheikh A, et al. A randomized controlled trial comparing subscapularis tenotomy with peel in anatomic shoulder arthroplasty. J Shoulder Elb Surg. 2020;29(2):225–34.
10. Skendzel JG, Sekiya JK. Diagnosis and management of humeral head bone loss in shoulder instability. Am J Sports Med. 2012;40:2633–44.
11. Khan S, Shanmugaraj A, Faisal H, Prada C, Munir S, Leroux T, et al. Variability in quantifying the Hill-Sachs lesion: a scoping review. Shoulder Elbow. SAGE Publications Inc. 2022;15:465.
12. Di Giacomo G, Itoi E, Burkhart SS. Evolving concept of bipolar bone loss and the hill-sachs lesion: from "engaging/non-engaging" lesion to "on-track/off-track" lesion. Arthroscopy [Internet]. 2014;30(1):90–8. https://doi.org/10.1016/j.arthro.2013.10.004.
13. Chen AL, Hunt SA, Hawkins RJ, Zuckerman JD. Management of bone loss associated with recurrent anterior glenohumeral instability. Am J Sports Med. 2005;33(6):912–25.
14. Sahajpal DT, Zuckerman JD. Chronic glenohumeral dislocation. J Am Acad Orthop Surg. 2008;16(7):385–98.
15. Cho SH, Cho NS, Rhee YG. Preoperative analysis of the Hill-Sachs lesion in anterior shoulder instability: how to predict engagement of the lesion. Am J Sports Med. 2011;39(11):2389–95.
16. Gerber C, Catanzaro S, Jundt-Ecker M, Farshad M. Long-term outcome of segmental reconstruction of the humeral head for the treatment of locked posterior dislocation of the shoulder. J Shoulder Elb Surg. 2014;23(11):1682–90.
17. Burkhart SS, De Beer JF. Traumatic glenohumeral bone defects and their relationship to failure of arthroscopic Bankart repairs: significance of the inverted-pear glenoid and the humeral engaging Hill-Sachs lesion. Arthrosc J Arthrosc Relat Surg. 2000;16(7):677–94.
18. Yamamoto N, Itoi E, Abe H, Minagawa H, Seki N, Shimada Y, et al. Contact between the glenoid and the humeral head in abduction, external rotation, and horizontal extension: a new concept of glenoid track. J Shoulder Elb Surg. 2007;16(5):649–56.
19. Provencher MT, Frank RM, LeClere LE, Metzger PD, Ryu JJ, Bernhardson LTA, et al. The Hill-Sachs lesion: diagnosis, classification, and management. J Am Acad Orthop Surg. 2012;20:242–52.
20. Aman ZS, Peebles LA, Johnson DW, Hanson JA, Provencher MT. Multidirectional shoulder instability with circumferential labral tear and bony reverse hill Sachs: treatment with 270° labral repair and fresh talus osteochondral allograft to the humeral head. Arthrosc Tech. 2021;10(3):e781–7.
21. Alkaduhimi H, Van Den Bekerom MPJ, Van Deurzen DFP. Step-by-step technique for segmental reconstruction of reverse Hill-Sachs lesions using homologous osteochondral allograft. Tech Hand Up Extrem Surg [Internet]. 2017;21(2):60–6. Available from: www.techhandsurg.com
22. Moroder P, Resch H, Tauber M. Failed arthroscopic repair of a large reverse Hill-Sachs lesion using bone allograft and cannulated screws: a case report. Arthrosc J Arthrosc Relat Surg. 2012;28(1):138–44.
23. Robinson CM, Aderinto J. Current concepts review posterior shoulder dislocations and fracture-dislocations. J Bone Jt Surg. 2005;87-A(3)
24. Bedrin MD, Owens BD, Slaven SE, LeClere LE, Donohue MA, Tennent DJ, et al. Prospective evaluation of posterior glenoid bone loss after first-time and recurrent posterior glenohumeral instability events. Am J Sports Med. 2022;50(11):3028–35.
25. Ernat JJ, Golijanin P, Peebles AM, Eble SK, Midtgaard KS, Provencher MT. Anterior and posterior glenoid bone loss in patients receiving surgery

for glenohumeral instability is not the same: a comparative 3-dimensional imaging analysis. JSES Int. 2022;6(4):581–6.
26. Nacca C, Gil JA, Badida R, Crisco JJ, Owens BD. Critical glenoid bone loss in posterior shoulder instability. Am J Sports Med. 2018;46(5):1058–63.
27. Wolfe JA, Elsenbeck M, Nappo K, Christensen D, Waltz R, LeClere L, et al. Effect of posterior glenoid bone loss and retroversion on arthroscopic posterior glenohumeral stabilization. Am J Sports Med. 2020;48(11):2621–7.
28. Duey RE, Burkhart SS. Arthroscopic treatment of a reverse hill-sachs lesion. Arthrosc Tech. 2013;2(2):e155.
29. Paul J, Buchmann S, Beitzel K, Solovyova O, Imhoff AB. Posterior shoulder dislocation: systematic review and treatment algorithm. Arthrosc J Arthrosc Relat Surg. 2011;27(11):1562–72.
30. Boileau P, O'Shea K, Vargas P, Pinedo M, Old J, Zumstein M. Anatomical and functional results after arthroscopic Hill-Sachs remplissage. J Bone Jt Surg. 2012;94(7):618–26.
31. Sochacki KR, Dillingham MF, Abrams GD, Sherman SL, Donahue J. Humeral head osteochondral allograft reconstruction with arthroscopic anterior shoulder stabilization at a long-term follow-up: a case report. JBJS Case Connect. 2020;10(2):e0555.
32. Chapovsky F, Kelly JD IV. Osteochondral allograft transplantation for treatment of glenohumeral instability. Arthrosc J Arthrosc Relat Surg. 2005;21(8):1007.e1.
33. Yagishita K, Thomas BJ. Use of allograft for large Hill-Sachs lesion associated with anterior glenohumeral dislocation A case report. Injury. 2002;33:791.
34. Kropf EJ, Sekiya JK. Osteoarticular allograft transplantation for large humeral head defects in glenohumeral instability. Arthrosc J Arthrosc Relat Surg. 2007;23(3):322.e1–5.
35. Tjoumakaris FP, Humble B, Sekiya JK. Combined glenoid and humeral head allograft reconstruction for recurrent anterior glenohumeral instability. Orthopedics. 2008;31(5):1.
36. Nathan ST, Parikh SN. Osteoarticular allograft reconstruction for Hill-Sachs lesion in an adolescent. Orthopedics. 2012;35(5)
37. Liow RYL, Adam J, Holland P, Bhatti A. Bulk osteochondral allograft for massive Hill–Sachs defect combined with Latarjet procedure for bipolar bone loss in anterior instability. Shoulder Elbow. 2022;
38. Zhuo H, Xu Y, Zhu F, Pan L, Li J. Osteochondral allograft transplantation for large Hill-Sachs lesions: a retrospective case series with a minimum 2-year follow-up. J Orthop Surg Res. 2019;14(1)
39. Snir N, Wolfson TS, Hamula MJ, Gyftopoulos S, Meislin RJ. Arthroscopic anatomic humeral head reconstruction with osteochondral allograft transplantation for large Hill-Sachs lesions. Arthrosc Tech. 2013;2(3):e289.
40. Tang J, Xu C, Zhao J. Arthroscopic bone grafting of the humeral head for treatment of a deep Hill-Sachs lesion. Arthrosc Tech. 2017;6(5):e1653–9.
41. Di Felice AP, Fusaro FM, Abad MP, Soldado F, Coll JQ. The utilization of computer planning and 3D-printed guide in the surgical management of a reverse Hill-Sachs lesion. JSES Int. 2020;4(3):569–73.
42. Marcheggiani Muccioli GM, Rinaldi VG, Lullini G, Ritali A, Mosca M, Romagnoli M, et al. Mid-term outcomes following fresh-frozen humeral head osteochondral allograft reconstruction for reverse Hill Sachs lesion: a case series. BMC Musculoskelet Disord. 2021;22(1)
43. Martinez AA, Calvo A, Domingo J, Cuenca J, Herrera A, Malillos M. Allograft reconstruction of segmental defects of the humeral head associated with posterior dislocations of the shoulder. Injury. 2008;39(3):319–22.
44. Patrizio L, Sabetta E. Acute posterior shoulder dislocation with reverse Hill-Sachs lesion of the epiphyseal humeral head. ISRN Surg. 2011;2011:1–4.
45. Black LO, Ko JWK, Quilici SM, Crawford DC. Fresh osteochondral allograft to the humeral head for treatment of an engaging reverse Hill-Sachs lesion: technical case report and literature review. Orthop J Sports Med. 2016;4(11)
46. Murphy LE, Tucker A, Charlwood AP. Fresh frozen femoral head osteochondral allograft reconstruction of the humeral head reverse Hill Sachs lesion. J Orthop. 2018;15(3):772–5.
47. Guehring M, Lambert S, Stoeckle U, Ziegler P. Posterior shoulder dislocation with associated reverse Hill-Sachs lesion: treatment options and functional outcome after a 5-year follow up. BMC Musculoskelet Disord. 2017;18(1)
48. Mastrokalos DS, Panagopoulos GN, Galanopoulos IP, Papagelopoulos PJ. Posterior shoulder dislocation with a reverse Hill–Sachs lesion treated with frozen femoral head bone allograft combined with osteochondral autograft transfer. Knee Surg Sport Traumatol Arthrosc. 2017;25(10):3285–8.
49. Mitchell JJ, Vap AR, Sanchez G, Liechti DJ, Chahla J, Moatshe G, et al. Concomitant reverse Hill-Sachs lesion and posterior humeral avulsion of the glenohumeral ligament: treatment with fresh talus osteochondral allograft and arthroscopic posterior humeral avulsion of the glenohumeral ligament and labrum repair. Arthrosc Tech. 2017;6(4):e987–95.
50. Qi W, Zhan J, Yan Z, Lin J, Xue X, Pan X. Arthroscopic treatment of posterior instability of the shoulder with an associated reverse Hill–Sachs lesion using an iliac bone-block autograft. Orthop Traumatol Surg Res. 2019;105(5):819–23.
51. Riff AJ, Yanke AB, Shin JJ, Romeo AA, Cole BJ. Midterm results of osteochondral allograft transplantation to the humeral head. J Shoulder Elb Surg. 2017;26(7):e207–15.

52. Ker AM, Veen EJD, Maharaj JC, Launay MM, Cutbush K, Gupta A. Pedicled-lesser tuberosity osteotomy for glenohumeral joint exposure: a technical note and case report highlighting its use in allograft reconstruction of a large engaging reverse Hill-Sachs lesion after posterior shoulder dislocation. JSES Rev Rep Tech. 2021;1(3):224–8.
53. Liles JL, Peebles AM, Saker CC, Ganokroj P, Mologne MS, Provencher MT. Talar allograft preparation for treatment of reverse Hill-Sachs defect in recurrent posterior shoulder instability. Arthrosc Tech. 2022;11(9):e1625–31.
54. Griswold BG, Paré DW, Herzwurm ZP, Murphy CS, Morpeth BG, Provencher MT, et al. Utility of allograft talus as a source for grafting of concurrent humeral and glenoid defects associated with anterior glenohumeral instability: an anthropometric analysis. Arthrosc J Arthrosc Relat Surg. 2021;37(3):845–51.
55. Martinez AA, Navarro E, Iglesias D, Domingo J, Calvo A, Carbonel I. Long-term follow-up of allograft reconstruction of segmental defects of the humeral head associated with posterior dislocation of the shoulder. Injury. 2013;44(4):488–91.

The Massive Hill-Sachs Lesion: Metal Replacement

25

Anthony Miniaci and Michael J. Scarcella

Introduction

Traumatic shoulder instability impacts approximately 2% of the population, with up to 95–98% of dislocations occurring in the anterior direction [1, 2]. The traumatic injury in conjunction with the complexity of the shoulder joint creates a spectrum of injury with varying degrees of soft tissue and bony involvement. Osseous injuries represent a particularly difficult pattern of injury, altering joint-contact area, congruency, and function of the static restraints [3–7]. Bony impaction injuries of the posterior humeral head were described by two radiologists, Hill and Sachs in 1940 [8]. While the true incidence of these lesions is unknown, they are associated with 40%–90% of initial anterior dislocations [9–13]. The incidence in recurrent instability can be up to 100%, with arthroscopy identifying lesions not appreciated on MRI [8, 11]. A majority of the lesions are clinically irrelevant and may be indirectly managed, with treatment guided by location, size, engagement, and track status ("on" versus "off") [14–16]. These large focal defects are particularly challenging and metallic implants represent a potential solution, even in young and active patients.

Clinical Case

A 15-year-old high school athlete presented to the emergency department following an acute contact left shoulder injury during a Friday night high school football. Shoulder deformity and limited range of motion was noted, and radiographs confirmed an anterior shoulder dislocation, which was successfully reduced under sedation (Fig. 25.1). He was seen by a local orthopedic surgeon 4 days after the injury and MRI as well as physical therapy were ordered.

Upon completion of the MRI, the student-athlete returned to his primary orthopedic surgeon. They reported five subluxation events with activities of daily living and one atraumatic dislocation with spontaneous reduction. The MRI revealed a large Hill-Sachs lesion with anterior-inferior labrum tear. No glenoid bony involvement was noted (Fig. 25.2).

The student-athlete was ultimately referred to a shoulder reconstruction specialist for further treatment options. At the time of evaluation, physical revealed left shoulder range of motion of 180 degrees forward elevation, external rotation with arm adducted to 45 degrees, and internal rotation to T6 (contralateral extremity

A. Miniaci (✉)
Florida Atlantic University, Boca Raton, FL, USA

Baptist Health Orthopedic Care,
Boca Raton, FL, USA
e-mail: Anthony.Miniaci@baptisthealth.net

M. J. Scarcella
Cleveland Clinic Sports Medicine, Department of Orthopaedic Surgery, Cleveland, OH, USA

© The Author(s), under exclusive license to Springer Nature Switzerland AG 2026
R. M. Frank, J. M. Tokish (eds.), *Management of Shoulder Instability*,
https://doi.org/10.1007/978-3-032-18089-6_25

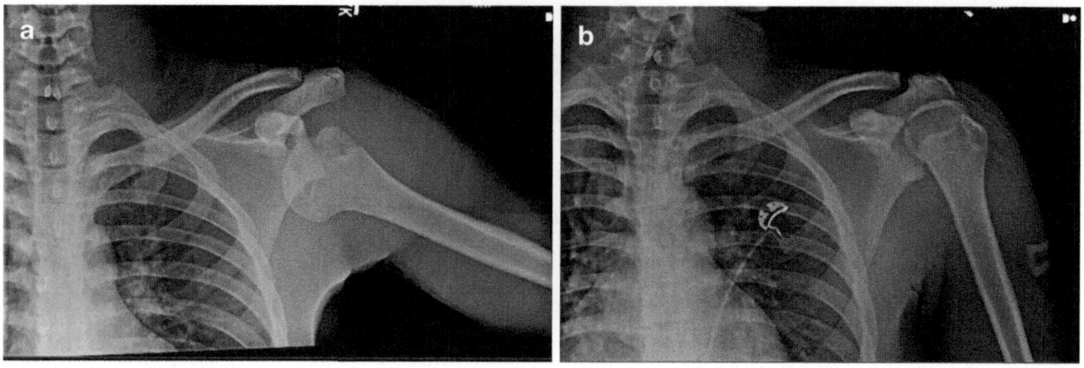

Fig. 25.1 (**a**) Initial injury radiograph demonstrating anterior shoulder dislocation. (**b**) Postreduction radiographs in the emergency department

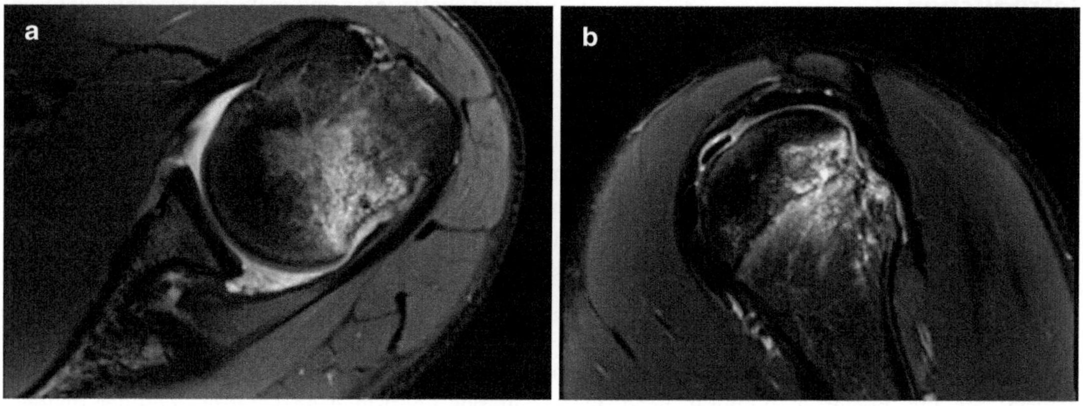

Fig. 25.2 (**a**) Axial fat saturation MRI demonstrating deep and medial Hill-Sachs lesion with associated anterior labrum involvement. (**b**) Sagittal fat saturation MRI demonstrating deep Hill-Sachs lesion

measured 180 degrees of forward elevation, external rotation with arm adducted to 70 degrees, and internal rotation to T6 level). They had a positive apprehension and relocation at 80 degrees of external rotation and a grade 3 load shift. Further provocative maneuvers revealed intact rotator cuff and upper extremity strength. Humeral head bone loss was estimated at 20–30% on MRI and a CT scan was obtained to critically evaluate bone loss (Fig. 25.3).

Humeral head bone loss was measured at 30% on CT scan and the lesion was deemed off-track without any glenoid bone loss. Based on these findings, options were discussed, and given this level of bone loss, reconstructive procedures were discussed. The options consisted of humeral allograft versus metallic replacement. The patient elected for metallic replacement with open labrum repair. Arthroscopic and soft tissue filling procedures were considered less reliable due to excessive bone loss.

The procedure is performed through a standard deltopectoral approach. In order to access the Hill-Sachs lesion, a subscapularis tenotomy is performed and the tendon tagged for later repair. The subscapularis is elevated from

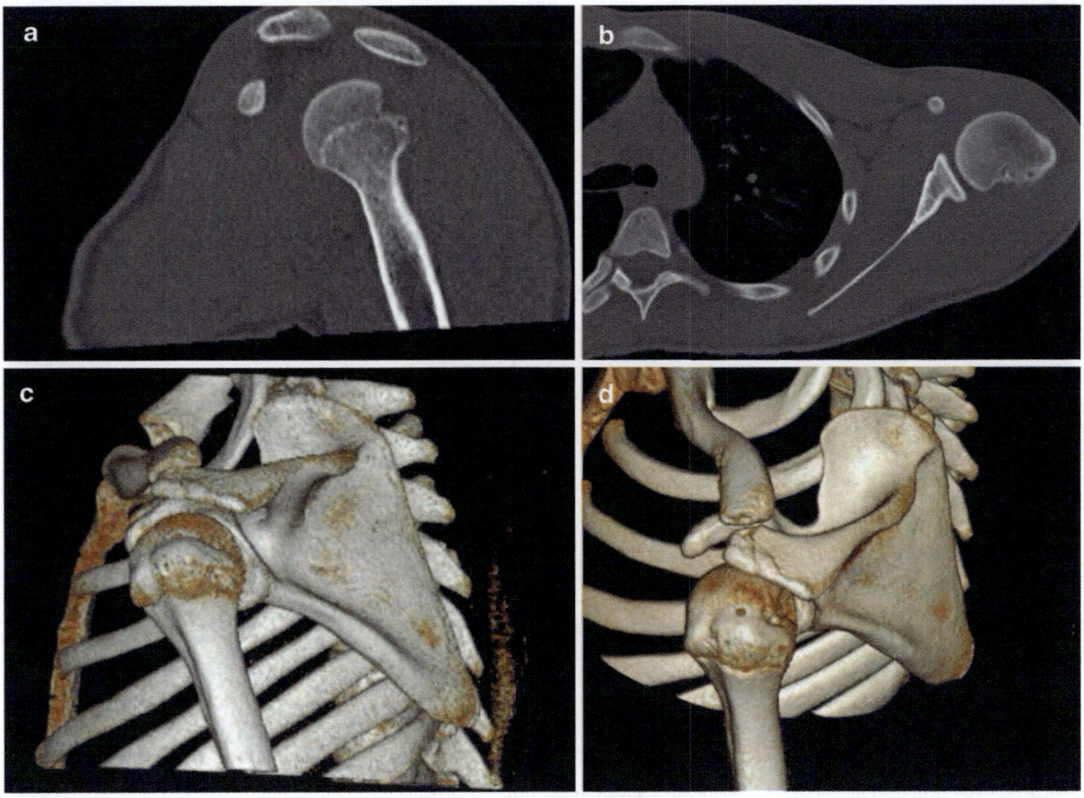

Fig. 25.3 (**a**) Axial CT scan demonstrating significant depth and medial extent of humeral head bone loss. (**b**) Sagittal CT scan further demonstrating the depth of humeral head bone loss. (**c** and **d**) 3D CT reconstruction demonstrating depth and width of humeral head involvement

the underlying capsule. The capsule is elevated off the humeral head in a hockey-stick fashion, tagged, and retracted medially for later repair. At this point, the arm can be externally rotated to deliver the humeral defect into the wound. The defect was sized 25 mm by 25 mm, and a 25 mm implant trial was overlaid demonstrating excellent coverage of the defect. A commercially available pin guide and reamer system was utilized to circumferentially prepare the defect to the appropriate depth in order to accept the metallic replacement without offset. The implant is placed and shoulder taken through a range of motion (Fig. 25.4). No impingement or catching was noted. At this time, the anterior labrum was repaired, and the capsule was advanced and repaired. No further instability was noted. Finally, the subscapularis tenotomy was repaired side to side.

The patient is initially treated in a sling for 4 weeks postoperatively. External rotation is limited until 6 weeks postoperatively, and range of motion is progressed as tolerated in all planes. Once range of motion is restored, the patient can progress with strengthening and may return to recreational events between 4 and 6 months postoperatively. At final follow-up, the patient's left shoulder demonstrated 180 degrees of forward elevation, 60 degrees of external rotation, T6 level internal rotation, no apprehension, and full strength including subscapularis. Radiographs demonstrated intact component with good alignment (Fig. 25.5).

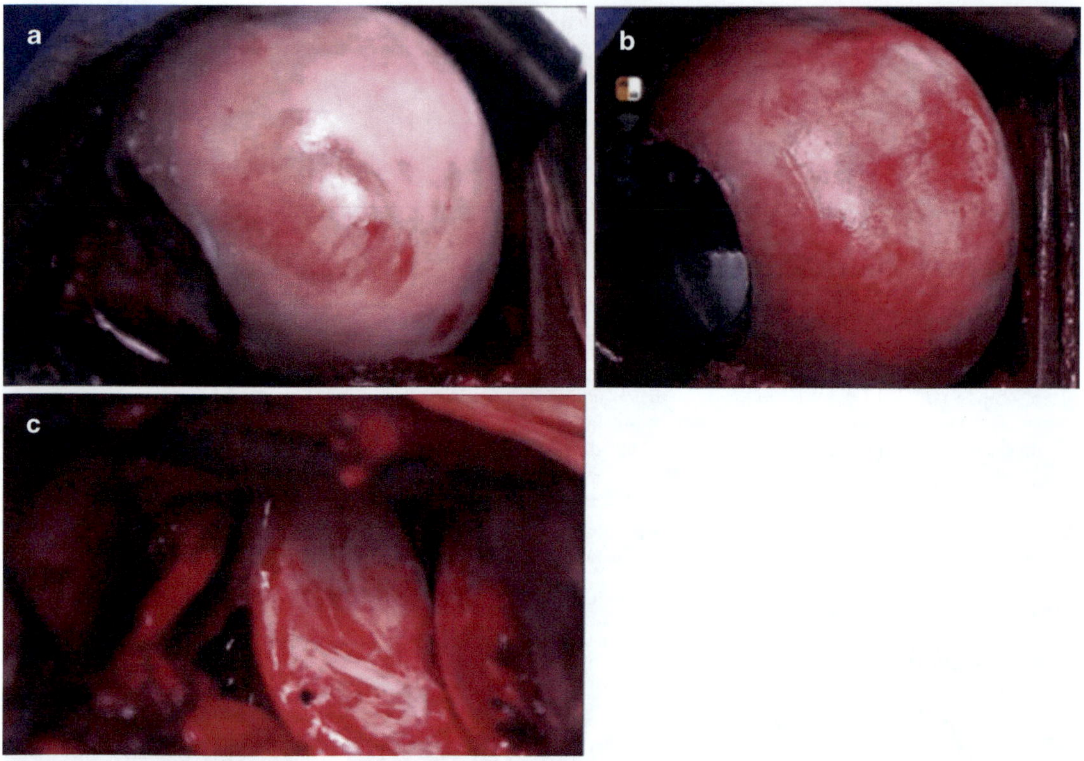

Fig. 25.4 (**a**) Humeral head defect measuring 25 mm by 25 mm. (**b**) Resurfacing replacement. (**c**) Resurfacing replacement with excellent articulation

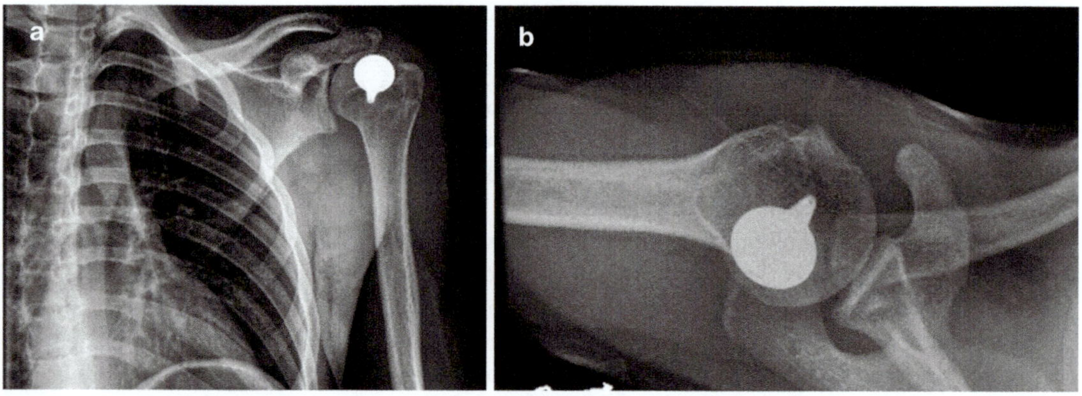

Fig. 25.5 (**a** and **b**) Postoperative radiographs demonstrating good component position and alignment

Etiology

The most common mechanism of injury is a traumatic anterior shoulder dislocation from an indirect force on the abducted and externally rotated arm. The humeral head externally rotates relative to the glenoid while translating anteriorly. Following the dislocation, the posterosuperolateral aspect of the humeral head then impacts on the anterior aspect of the glenoid rim and can create a Hill-Sachs lesion [17]. Richards et al. identified the typical location of the Hill-Sachs. On an axial view with 0 degrees representing direct anterior, the typical Hill-Sachs lesion lies between 170 degrees and 260 degrees, with a midpoint at 209 degrees [18].

The volume of bone loss associated with a Hill-Sachs lesion depends on dislocation frequency, chronicity, and force. Cetik et al. found an increasing percentage of articular surface involvement with increasing frequency of dislocations [19]. The size of the humeral head defect is also correlated to dislocations of longer duration, for example, neglected or locked dislocations [20, 21].

Biomechanics are an important consideration when addressing humeral head lesions. There is considerable variation in the normal shoulder anatomy. Specifically, the humeral head retroversion may range from 0° to 55° and inclination from 30° to 55°. Additionally, the radius of curvature ranges from 20 to 30 mm [22]. A change of 5 mm in the radius of curvature can affect shoulder range of motion by as much as 20–30° [23, 24]. Furthermore, alterations in humeral head geometry can greatly influence the contact pressure and stress distribution on the glenoid [5]. HemiCAP (Arthrosurface, Franklin MA) offers a variety of implant options which allows the surgeon to use intraoperative mapping to fit the patient's radius of curvature. The design of partial resurfacing avoids changes in humeral head angulation. The defect filling design does not change offset, fundamentally maintaining joint kinematics [25].

Giles et al. performed a biomechanical comparison of intact shoulders to remplissage, allograft reconstruction, and partial resurfacing in large engaging HSL. They created a 30–40% HSL in cadaveric shoulders and assessed range of motion and stability. Partial resurfacing resulted in no significant difference in joint stiffness or ROM compared to the intact state. The key to restoring articular geometry is selecting an implant that will completely fill the defect. Overlap into areas of native cartilage may be necessary to avoid residual defects that can engage on the glenoid [26].

Restoring the geometric center of the humeral head is important in maintaining joint kinematics and contact pressures. Hammond et al. found that partial resurfacing was better able to replicate geometric center of the intact shoulder compared to HA in cadaveric modeling. They concluded that partial resurfacing may better limit eccentric glenoid wear because the glenohumeral joint biomechanics and the moment arms of the rotator cuff and deltoid muscle are restored more closely to those of the intact shoulder [27].

Diagnosis/Imaging

As with any orthopedic injury, a thorough history must be obtained. Specific to shoulder instability, the surgeon should understand the mechanism of injury including arm position, force applied, need for reduction, number of instability events, as well as any underlying instability. Past medical history, including but not limited to collagen disorders and epilepsy, should be documented as these specifically relate to shoulder instability. A general shoulder examination should be performed with observation, paying particular attention to asymmetry, scars, and shoulder positioning. A focused instability exam of the shoulder should be performed in anterior, posterior, and inferior directions in multiple positions (sitting, standing, supine) as patients with large Hill-Sachs lesions usually exhibit apprehension that often occurs with the arm in significantly less than 90 degrees of abduction and 90 degrees of external rotation [28].

Standard shoulder radiographs should be obtained at the time of evaluation and consist of AP, Grashey, and axillary views. Injury films with a documented dislocation should be reviewed if available. Additionally, a Stryker notch view can be obtained and has been found to be the most sensitive in identifying a Hill-Sachs lesion on radiographs [29, 30]. Advanced imaging is recommended in the majority of traumatic shoulder instability cases. MRI is useful for identifying soft tissue pathology, as well as areas of potentially bony involvement. However, whenever bone loss is considered, the authors prefer CT scan with 3D rendering. Bois et al. reported that CT scan with 1-mm slices and 3D recon-

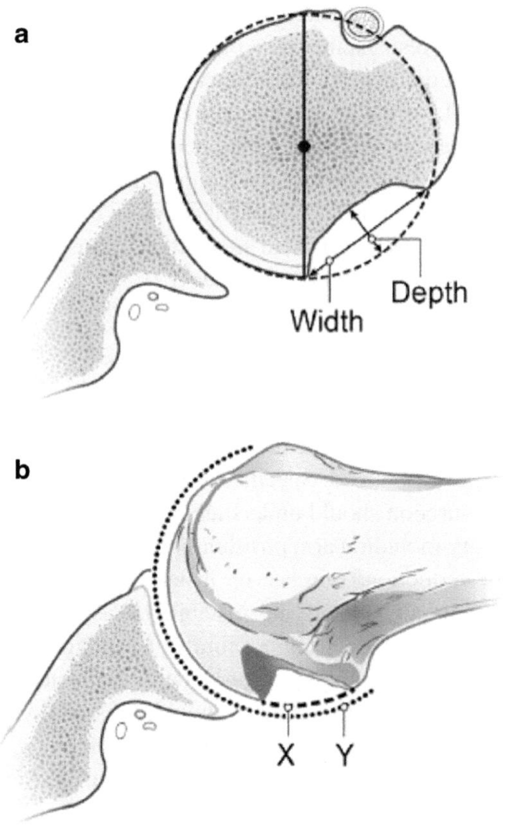

Fig. 25.6 (**a**) Lesion depth and width measurement using perfect circle. (**b**) Percentage of humeral head involvement measure [(X/Y)×100]

structions improve the accuracy of determining the size and location of the defects, with axial and sagittal being the most accurate and reproducible views for measuring the Hill-Sachs lesion [31]. Multiple measurements for quantification have been proposed, with the authors preferring methods that quantify depth, width, or percentage (Fig. 25.6) [17].

Surgical Management

Multiple algorithms exist for the management of traumatic anterior shoulder instability; however, none are universally accepted. These algorithms are based on varying assessments of clinical variables, as well as radiographic assessments or measurements [32, 33]. Furthermore, there is no consensus regarding the surgical management of large Hill-Sachs lesions (>20–25% humeral head percentage). The authors consider metallic resurfacing in cases of (1) displaced humeral head fracture dislocation with irreparable bony segment, (2) lesions greater than 30% of the humeral head in cases of chronic instability, and (3) engaging lesions greater than 20–25% humeral head without glenoid bone loss.

The surgical technique is outlined in the case presentation and is performed through a standard deltopectoral approach utilizing a subscapularis tenotomy. The authors' preferred implant is the HemiCAP (Arthrosurface, Franklin, MA, USA). Multiple diameter options and trials exist within the set. The defect is sized using a trial component making sure to obtain adequate coverage of the defect. In most cases, it is recommended to overlap a millimeter into healthy bone and cartilage to ensure full coverage. This prevents gapping or step-off. A guide pin is drilled perpendicular to the humeral head in the center of the defect. The defect is reamed with the appropriately sized reamer. A depth limiter prevents over- or underreaming so that the final component sits flush with the remaining articular cartilage. Deeper defects may be packed with bone graft from the reamers or off-shelf graft alternatives. The tapered post is seated over the center pin and seated to the appropriate depth. The tapered post is a headless titanium alloy cannulated screw that seats in cancellous bone. The articular component is a cobalt-chromium alloy, which mounts on the Morse taper of the post. Finally, the shoulder is taken through a range of motion to confirm there is congruency and no further instability or mechanical blockage to motion. The wound is irrigated, and a capsular plication is performed at closure. The subscapularis tenotomy is closed end to end.

Postoperative/Additional Considerations

Postoperatively, the patient is placed into a sling for focus and the subscapularis repair is protected. Gentle progressive range of motion can begin in forward elevation immediately after the surgery. External rotation beyond neutral is avoided until postoperative week 6, after which the patient may progress to range of motion without restrictions. Strengthening begins once the patient has obtained full range of motion. Patients may return to recreational activities between 4 and 6 months postoperatively.

Large Hill-Sachs defects present a particular challenge. The more common surgical techniques to manage off-track or "engaging" lesions consist of remplissage, allograft reconstruction, or partial resurfacing. Remplissage is a soft tissue procedure that transforms an intra-articular defect into an extra-articular defect. Therefore, normal articular geometry is not restored. There is a concern that this technique can restrict motion, and results in the literature have been mixed. [34–37] Furthermore, Park et al. demonstrated a failure rate of 15% in their series of 20 patients with large defects (>25%). Humeral head allograft is capable of restoring articular congruency and restoring stability with low rates of recurrent instability [28, 38]. However, it is technically demanding and requires a waiting period while a fresh-frozen allograft is obtained. In addition, risks associated with allograft such as disease transmission, graft resorption, collapse, or non-union are also present and not insignificant if they occur. Most of these patients are functionally compromised and are not willing to delay treatment. As an alternative, a partial humeral head implant has been described to treat these large Hill-Sachs defects associated with recurrent instability. Bessette et al. retrospectively reviewed the results of 16 patients undergoing HemiCAP partial resurfacing (Arthrosurface, Franklin MA) for Hill-Sachs defects. The mean age was 32.3 years (range, 17–49) and mean follow-up was 36.9 months. Implant diameter ranged from 25 to 40 mm. There was no patient-reported recurrent dislocation. Thirteen (81.25%) returned to activity at preinjury levels. Penn shoulder scores improved by a mean 36.4 points. All patients regained full range of motion, with the exception of two. One patient had postoperative stiffness attributed to a delay in postoperative physical therapy. The patient underwent manipulation under anesthesia 3 months after the index surgery. The other patient had a sensation of instability but no dislocation resulting in self-restricted motion. Two patients required reoperation, the previously mentioned patient and a second patient who had a seizure resulting in subscapularis rupture but no dislocation. There were no revisions or failure due to instability [39].

There are few reports on partial resurfacing, but there have been no implant-related complications reported. Radiographs have not demonstrated loosening or osteolysis. In cases of dislocations, recurrence has not been documented. [40, 41] The 2012 annual report of the Australian National Joint Replacement Registry reported survivorship data on 86 primary shoulder inlay arthroplasty procedures. No HemiCAP (Arthrosurface, Franklin MA) had been revised to the date of the report (195 implant years). In the 2013 report, stemmed hemi-resurfacing implants had a 246% higher revision rate compared to HemiCAP (Arthrosurface, Franklin MA). HA and TSA had a 207% higher revision rate. This report included partial resurfacing for all pathologies (avascular necrosis, focal defects, and Hill-Sachs lesions) [42].

References

1. Hovelius L. Incidence of shoulder dislocation in Sweden. Clin Orthop Relat Res. 1982;166:127–31.
2. Mazzocca AD, Cote MP, Solovyova O, Rizvi SH, Mostofi A, Arciero RA. Traumatic shoulder instability involving anterior, inferior, and posterior labral injury: a prospective clinical evaluation of arthroscopic repair of 270° labral tears. Am J Sports Med. 2011;39(8):1687–96. https://doi.org/10.1177/0363546511405449.
3. Bollier MJ, Arciero R. Management of glenoid and humeral bone loss. Sports Med Arthrosc Rev. 2010;18(3):140–8. https://doi.org/10.1097/JSA.0b013e3181e88ef9.
4. Bhatia S, Van Thiel GS, Gupta D, et al. Comparison of glenohumeral contact pressures and contact areas after glenoid reconstruction with latarjet or distal tibial osteochondral allografts. Am J Sports Med. 2013;41(8):1900–8. https://doi.org/10.1177/0363546513490646.
5. Greis PE, Scuderi MG, Mohr A, Bachus KN, Burks RT. Glenohumeral articular contact areas and pressures following labral and osseous injury to the antero-

inferior quadrant of the glenoid. J Shoulder Elbow Surg. 2002;11(5):442–51. https://doi.org/10.1067/mse.2002.124526.
6. Matsen FA 3rd, Chebli CM, Lippitt SB. Principles for the evaluation and management of shoulder instability. Instr Course Lect. 2007;56:23–34.
7. Montgomery WH Jr, Wahl M, Hettrich C, Itoi E, Lippitt SB, Matsen FA 3rd. Anteroinferior bone-grafting can restore stability in osseous glenoid defects. J Bone Joint Surg Am. 2005;87(9):1972–7. https://doi.org/10.2106/jbjs.D.02573.
8. Hill HA, Sachs MD. The grooved defect of the humeral head: a frequently unrecognized complication of dislocations of the shoulder joint. Radiology. 1940;35(6):690–700.
9. Calandra JJ, Baker CL, Uribe J. The incidence of Hill-Sachs lesions in initial anterior shoulder dislocations. Arthroscopy. 1989;5(4):254–7. https://doi.org/10.1016/0749-8063(89)90138-2.
10. Charalambous CP, Eastwood S. The bankart procedure: a long-term end-result study. In: Classic papers in orthopaedics; 2014. p. 313–5.
11. Saupe N, White LM, Bleakney R, et al. Acute traumatic posterior shoulder dislocation: MR findings. Radiology. 2008;248(1):185–93. https://doi.org/10.1148/radiol.2481071003.
12. Taylor DC, Arciero RA. Pathologic changes associated with shoulder dislocations. Arthroscopic and physical examination findings in first-time, traumatic anterior dislocations. Am J Sports Med. 1997;25(3):306–11. https://doi.org/10.1177/036354659702500306.
13. Yiannakopoulos CK, Mataragas E, Antonogiannakis E. A comparison of the spectrum of intra-articular lesions in acute and chronic anterior shoulder instability. Arthroscopy. 2007;23(9):985–90. https://doi.org/10.1016/j.arthro.2007.05.009.
14. Burkhart SS, Danaceau SM. Articular arc length mismatch as a cause of failed bankart repair. Arthroscopy. 2000;16(7):740–4. https://doi.org/10.1053/jars.2000.7794.
15. Saito H, Itoi E, Minagawa H, Yamamoto N, Tuoheti Y, Seki N. Location of the Hill-Sachs lesion in shoulders with recurrent anterior dislocation. Arch Orthop Trauma Surg. 2009;129(10):1327–34. https://doi.org/10.1007/s00402-009-0854-4.
16. Yamamoto N, Itoi E, Abe H, et al. Contact between the glenoid and the humeral head in abduction, external rotation, and horizontal extension: a new concept of glenoid track. J Shoulder Elbow Surg. 2007;16(5):649–56. https://doi.org/10.1016/j.jse.2006.12.012.
17. Patel RM, Amin NH, Lynch TS, Miniaci A. Management of bone loss in glenohumeral instability. Orthop Clin North Am. 2014;45(4):523–39. https://doi.org/10.1016/j.ocl.2014.06.005.
18. Richards RD, Sartoris DJ, Pathria MN, Resnick D. Hill-Sachs lesion and normal humeral groove: MR imaging features allowing their differentiation. Radiology. 1994;190(3):665–8. https://doi.org/10.1148/radiology.190.3.8115607.
19. Cetik O, Uslu M, Ozsar BK. The relationship between Hill-Sachs lesion and recurrent anterior shoulder dislocation. Acta Orthop Belg. 2007;73(2):175–8.
20. Loebenberg MI, Cuomo F. The treatment of chronic anterior and posterior dislocations of the glenohumeral joint and associated articular surface defects. Orthop Clin North Am. 2000;31(1):23–34. https://doi.org/10.1016/s0030-5898(05)70125-5.
21. Kirtland S, Resnick D, Sartoris DJ, Pate D, Greenway G. Chronic unreduced dislocations of the glenohumeral joint: imaging strategy and pathologic correlation. J Trauma. 1988;28(12):1622–31. https://doi.org/10.1097/00005373-198812000-00002.
22. Phillips J, Runciman R, Miniaci A. Mathematical modeling of humeral head geometry. Rosemont, IL: American Academy of Orthopaedic Surgeon; 2004. p. 213–8.
23. Harryman DT, Sidles JA, Harris SL, Lippitt SB, Matsen FA 3rd. The effect of articular conformity and the size of the humeral head component on laxity and motion after glenohumeral arthroplasty. A study in cadavera. J Bone Joint Surg Am. 1995;77(4):555–63. https://doi.org/10.2106/00004623-199504000-00008.
24. Jobe CM, Iannotti JP. Limits imposed on glenohumeral motion by joint geometry. J Shoulder Elbow Surg. 1995;4(4):281–5. https://doi.org/10.1016/s1058-2746(05)80021-7.
25. Scalise JJ, Miniaci A, Iannotti JP. Resurfacing arthroplasty of the humerus: indications, surgical technique, and clinical results. Tech Should Elbow Surg. 2007;8(3):152–60.
26. Giles JW, Elkinson I, Ferreira LM, et al. Moderate to large engaging Hill-Sachs defects: an in vitro biomechanical comparison of the remplissage procedure, allograft humeral head reconstruction, and partial resurfacing arthroplasty. J Shoulder Elb Surg. 2012;21(9):1142–51. https://doi.org/10.1016/j.jse.2011.07.017.
27. Hammond G, Tibone JE, McGarry MH, Jun BJ, Lee TQ. Biomechanical comparison of anatomic humeral head resurfacing and hemiarthroplasty in functional glenohumeral positions. J Bone Joint Surg Am. 2012;94(1):68–76. https://doi.org/10.2106/jbjs.I.00171.
28. Miniaci A, Gish MW. Management of anterior glenohumeral instability associated with large Hill–Sachs defects. Tech Shoulder Elbow Surg. 2004;5(3):170–5.
29. Edwards TB, Boulahia A, Walch G. Radiographic analysis of bone defects in chronic anterior shoulder instability. Arthroscopy. 2003;19(7):732–9. https://doi.org/10.1016/s0749-8063(03)00684-4.
30. Pavlov H, Warren RF, Weiss CB Jr, Dines DM. The roentgenographic evaluation of anterior shoulder instability. Clin Orthop Relat Res. 1985;194:153–8.
31. Bois AJ, Walker RE, Kodali P, Miniaci A. Imaging instability in the athlete: the right modality for the right diagnosis. Clin Sports Med. 2013;32(4):653–84. https://doi.org/10.1016/j.csm.2013.07.004.
32. Balg F, Boileau P. The instability severity index score (ISIS score): a rational approach for patient selection

in arthroscopic Bankart repair. The British Editorial Society of Bone & Joint Surgery; 2009. p. 242.
33. Di Giacomo G, Peebles LA, Pugliese M, et al. Glenoid track instability management score: radiographic modification of the instability severity index score. Arthroscopy. 2020;36(1):56–67. https://doi.org/10.1016/j.arthro.2019.07.020.
34. Boileau P, O'Shea K, Vargas P, Pinedo M, Old J, Zumstein M. Anatomical and functional results after arthroscopic Hill-Sachs remplissage. J Bone Joint Surg Am. 2012;94(7):618–26. https://doi.org/10.2106/jbjs.K.00101.
35. Franceschi F, Longo UG, Ruzzini L, Rizzello G, Maffulli N, Denaro V. Arthroscopic salvage of failed arthroscopic Bankart repair: a prospective study with a minimum follow-up of 4 years. Am J Sports Med. 2008;36(7):1330–6. https://doi.org/10.1177/0363546508314403.
36. Merolla G, Paladini P, Di Napoli G, Campi F, Porcellini G. Outcomes of arthroscopic Hill-Sachs remplissage and anterior Bankart repair: a retrospective controlled study including ultrasound evaluation of posterior capsulotenodesis and infraspinatus strength assessment. Am J Sports Med. 2015;43(2):407–14. https://doi.org/10.1177/0363546514559706.
37. Park MJ, Tjoumakaris FP, Garcia G, Patel A, Kelly JD. Arthroscopic remplissage with Bankart repair for the treatment of glenohumeral instability with Hill-Sachs defects. Arthroscopy. 2011;27(9):1187–94. https://doi.org/10.1016/j.arthro.2011.05.010.
38. Sekiya JK, Wickwire AC, Stehle JH, Debski RE. Hill-Sachs defects and repair using osteoarticular allograft transplantation: biomechanical analysis using a joint compression model. Am J Sports Med. 2009;37(12):2459–66. https://doi.org/10.1177/0363546509341576.
39. Bessette MC, Frisch NC, Kodali P, Jones MH, Miniaci A. Partial resurfacing for humeral head defects associated with recurrent shoulder instability. Orthopedics. 2017;40(6):e996–e1003. https://doi.org/10.3928/01477447-20171012-01.
40. Sweet SJ, Takara T, Ho L, Tibone JE. Primary partial humeral head resurfacing: outcomes with the HemiCAP implant. Am J Sports Med. 2015;43(3):579–87. https://doi.org/10.1177/0363546514562547.
41. Uribe JW, Botto-van Bemden A. Partial humeral head resurfacing for osteonecrosis. J Shoulder Elbow Surg. 2009;18(5):711–6. https://doi.org/10.1016/j.jse.2008.10.016.
42. National Joint Replacement Registry TAOA. Demographics and outcomes of shoulder arthroplasty: supplementary report 2012; 2014. Accessed February 4, 2023, https://aoanjrr.sahmri.com/annual-reports-2014

Part III

Posterior Shoulder Instability

Arthroscopic Posterior Bankart Repair in the Lateral Position

26

Stephanie A. Boden, Justin W. Arner, and James P. Bradley

Introduction

Posterior shoulder instability has become increasingly recognized as a distinct and important subcategory of shoulder instability with a higher incidence than historically reported. It has been reported to account for up to 10% of shoulder instability events, with the highest incidence noted in young active males [3, 17, 49]. Studies have shown that in operative shoulder instability cases, posterior labral tears occur in isolation in approximately 25% of cases and in combination with anterior labral tears in approximately 18 to 44% of cases [65, 67]. Diagnosis can be challenging due to often vague and variable complaints and a generally insidious onset of symptoms, including generalized shoulder fatigue and pain without a specific injury [12, 17]. Instability most commonly presents as recurrent posterior subluxations (RPSs), less commonly as a traumatic dislocation event, and, in rare instances, a chronic locked posterior dislocation.

S. A. Boden
Department of Orthopedic Surgery, University of Louisville, Louisville, KY, USA
e-mail: Stephanie.Boden@louisville.edu

J. W. Arner (✉) · J. P. Bradley
Department of Orthopedic Surgery, University of Pittsburgh Medical Center, Pittsburgh, PA, USA
e-mail: Justin.Arner@upmc.edu; bradleyjp@upmc.edu

Unlike anterior instability, which is generally associated with a traumatic event, posterior glenohumeral instability in the young active patient population is more often caused by repetitive microtrauma to the posteroinferior capsulolabral complex, although the etiology may be multifactorial [3, 17, 46]. Management of patients with posterior shoulder instability can be challenging due to difficulty with diagnosis, the variety of surgical techniques available, and the lack of consensus regarding management when posterior bone loss is present. Posterior glenohumeral stabilization has evolved from open to arthroscopic and anatomic techniques, which have demonstrated reliable and good clinical outcomes, high patient satisfaction, high rate of return to sport, and low complication rates [3, 31, 47, 49].

Clinical Case

Patient is a 15-year-old male right-handed baseball pitcher and football lineman who presents with a complaint of right shoulder pain for 6 months. The pain started insidiously, and he denies a specific injury or acute dislocation event. He reports pain with throwing and blocking motions. He was initially seen by an outside provider and underwent 3 months of focused physical therapy as well as a regimented throwing program without significant improvement in his pain prior to presentation in our clinic. On exami-

© The Author(s), under exclusive license to Springer Nature Switzerland AG 2026
R. M. Frank, J. M. Tokish (eds.), *Management of Shoulder Instability*,
https://doi.org/10.1007/978-3-032-18089-6_26

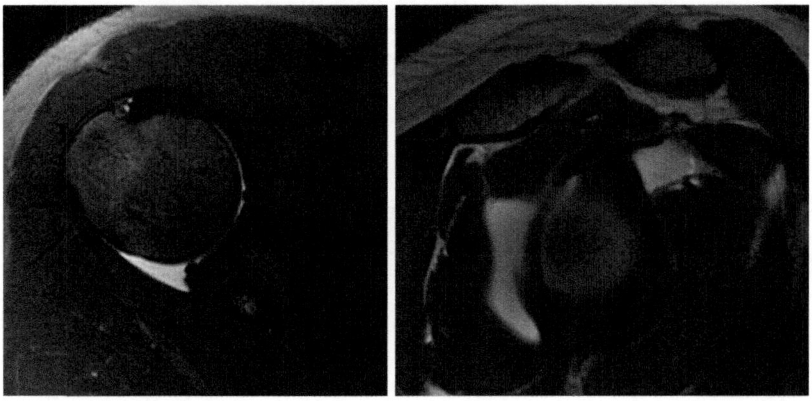

Fig. 26.1 Axial and sagittal magnetic resonance imaging demonstrating a posterior labral tear

nation, the patient is noted to have full ROM and 5/5 strength throughout. He has a positive O'Brien's test, positive D-PITT and modified D-PITT tests, positive posterior apprehension, 2+ posterior load and shift, negative impingement tests, normal scapula motion, and no GIRD. Radiographs, including an AP, axillary, and scapular Y lateral, demonstrate no abnormalities. Given concern for posterior instability, an MRI was obtained, which demonstrated a posterior labral tear (Fig. 26.1). Risks/benefits of continued conservative versus operative management were discussed with the patient and his parents at length, and given his failure to improve after focused physical therapy, as well as significant labral tear on MRI, the decision was made to proceed with arthroscopic stabilization.

Etiology/Pathogenesis

The etiology of posterior instability is generally broken down into three different categories based on primary injury mechanism including (1) repetitive microtrauma causing cumulative attenuation to the posterior capsule and labral injury, (2) acute trauma (generally a posteriorly directed force to the anterior shoulder with the arm in flexion, internal rotation, and horizontal adduction, causing an acute shear injury at the capsulolabral junction), and (3) generalized capsulolabral laxity with stretching of the posterior capsule and the dynamic posterior stabilizers. To understand these various injury mechanisms and therefore the pathogenesis of posterior shoulder instability, it is crucial to understand the anatomy and normal function of the posterior shoulder stabilizers.

Anatomy/Biomechanical Considerations

The posterior capsulolabral complex consists of the posterior labrum, posterior capsule, and the posterior band of the inferior glenohumeral ligament (IGHL). These static structures serve as the primary stabilizers to posterior humeral head translation between 45 and 90 degrees of shoulder abduction by providing a compressive force across the glenohumeral joint. The labrum adds depth and width to the glenoid fossa and acts as a mobile organ of tension superiorly and a fixed organ of compression inferiorly [37, 64]. Anatomic studies have demonstrated some variability in the insertion of the posterior labrum, and medialization of the insertion is found in a subset of the population, which can be mistaken for a labral tear [44, 57]. Cadaveric studies have shown that in 96% of cases, the posterior band of the IGHL (PIGHL) inserts between 7 and 9 o'clock, and the posterior labrum attaches to the articular cartilage and bone in up to 98% of patients [44]. The PIGHL has been shown to be consistently thinner than its anterior counterpart, potentially increasing susceptibility to injury and attenuation from repetitive stress [64].

In addition to the primary stabilizers of the glenohumeral joint, the rotator cuff musculature also plays an important role in the stabilization of the posterior glenohumeral joint by providing dynamic cavity compression of the humeral head in the glenoid. The subscapularis is the most important dynamic stabilizer to resist posterior translation of the humeral head, thereby supporting the static action of the PIGHL [13]. Patients with rotator cuff weakness or fatigue may therefore be more susceptible to injury to the posterior capsulolabral complex.

Pathogenesis

Stresses on the posterior capsulolabral complex occur with repetitive activity-specific motions that load the posterior shoulder stabilizers. Such activities include push-ups, bench press, blocking in football, tennis backhand, backswing of golf, lead shoulder for baseball batters, follow-through in overhead throwing, anterior-posterior axial loading in gymnastics, and the pull-through phase of swimming [21]. These activities can lead to excessive stress on the posterior structures and lead to posterior capsulolabral tearing.

In overhead athletes and swimmers, the mechanism is thought to be different. RPS may occur due to progressive attenuation and laxity of the posterior capsule in combination with fatigue of both static and dynamic shoulder stabilizers [3, 17, 64]. Over time, deformation of the posterior capsule leads to a patulous posterior capsular pouch. Conversely, posteroinferior capsular thickening and tightness associated with glenohumeral internal rotation deficit (GIRD) is a common adaptation among overhead pitchers with increased external rotation, and studies have shown that greater than 25–30 degrees of GIRD is associated with pathologic shearing forces on the posterosuperior labrum and rotator cuff [7, 19].

With excessive external rotation of the shoulder in the abduction external rotation (ABER) position, as seen in overhead throwing, the posterosuperior labrum, long head of biceps tendon (LHBT), and undersurface of the rotator cuff experience significant rotatory forces that can result in the peel-back phenomenon of the posterosuperior labrum at the biceps anchor (Fig. 26.2) [1, 64]. This peel-back phenomenon has been observed arthroscopically in the overhead throwing athlete but may not always be a pathologic process and has been postulated to be a purposeful adaptation to allow increased external rotation and horizontal adduction without compromising stability in the throwing motion [64]. When the posterior and superior labrum decouples, as seen with a superior labral anterior posterior (SLAP) tear that propagates inferiorly, the tension band function of the superior biceps-labrum complex is lost, thereby compromising stability and resulting in the pathologic "snap back" phenomenon of the posterosuperior labrum at the biceps anchor [1, 64]. In some instances, these tears propagate posteroinferiorly around the glenoid to the PIGHL,

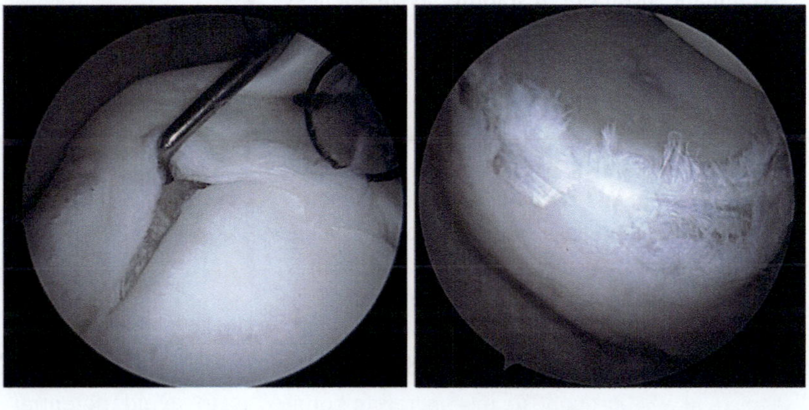

Fig. 26.2 Arthroscopic image of the "peel-back" phenomenon of the posterosuperior labrum at the biceps anchor with the arm in the abduction external rotation (ABER) position

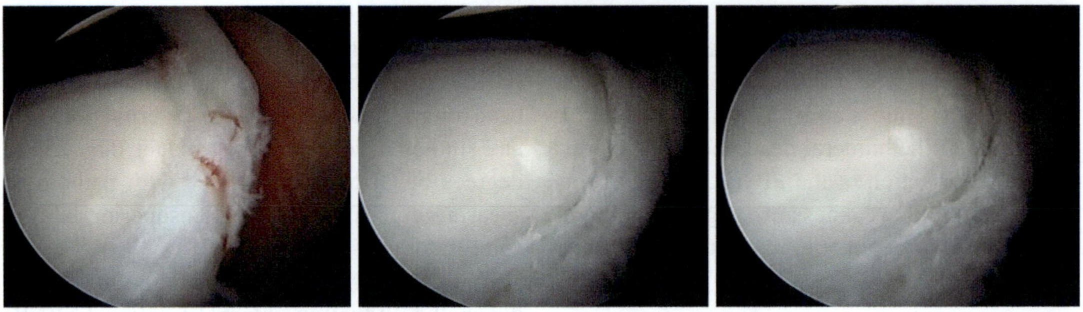

Fig. 26.3 Arthroscopic image of a thrower with a tear beginning at the posterior superior labrum with propagation posteroinferiorly to the posterior inferior glenohumeral ligament (PIGHL)

creating a type VIII SLAP tear and symptomatic RPS (Fig. 26.3) [29, 64].

RPS has also been associated with the lead arm in batters ("batter's shoulder") and the lead shoulder in golfers [35, 59]. During a forceful swing motion, the posterior shoulder stabilizers experience significant rotational and torsional stresses, with rotational velocity often exceeding 900 degrees per second [59]. These stresses to the posterior shoulder are further amplified if the bat or club does not contact the ball, as the lack of counterforce to the dynamic posterior pulling forces of the lead shoulder causes increased shear force across the glenohumeral joint during the follow-through phase of the swing [59, 74]. Over time, the repetitive stresses on the posterior stabilizers can lead to RPS, which often presents as vague posterior shoulder pain during the provocative position of shoulder adduction and flexion at the top of the back-swing in golf, pain during batting, or diminished power during the baseball/softball swing [59, 74].

Traumatic posterior instability is much less common and differs in etiology, as it results from an acute capsulolabral detachment known as a reverse Bankart tear (Fig. 26.4) [3]. This generally occurs from a posteriorly directed force to the anterior shoulder with the arm in flexion, internal rotation, and adduction, causing an acute shear injury at the capsulolabral junction. Acute traumatic instability may be associated with a reverse Hill-Sachs lesion of the humeral head, which can lead to recurrent posterior instability and posterior glenoid bone loss [3, 28].

While abnormalities in the primary posterior stabilizers can all contribute to posterior instability, studies have shown a wide variety of damaged structures with no single structure reliably injured across all patients with posterior instability [17, 21]. In a review of 200 shoulders with unidirectional posterior shoulder instability, 21% had a patulous posterior capsule with no labral detachment, 15% had an incomplete posterior labral tear, 64% had a full-thickness detachment of the posterior labrum, and 61% of shoulders with labral tears were also noted to have excessive

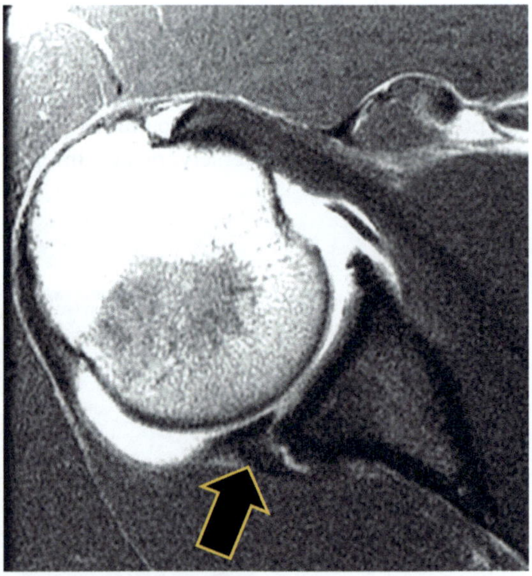

Fig. 26.4 Axial magnetic resonance imaging arthrogram demonstrating an acute posterior capsulolabral detachment

capsular laxity, with a patulous posterior capsule noted in 69% of all shoulders [17]. In a review of 48 adolescent patients with unidirectional posterior shoulder instability, 6.25% had anterior labral fraying, 10% had posterior glenoid labrum articular defect (GLAD) lesions, 43.8% had posterior labral tears, 45.8% had a patulous posterior capsule, and 35% had partial rotator cuff tears [9]. Associated intra-articular pathology is common in patients with posterior instability, necessitating a thorough and complete examination to ensure appropriate management.

Diagnosis/Imaging

History

Patients with posterior glenohumeral instability tend to present with vague and often nonspecific complaints, making initial diagnosis clinically challenging. Presenting symptoms are heterogenous and can include vague poste\ior shoulder pain, which can be associated with clicking/popping, crepitus, perceived weakness and/or loss of power, and, rarely, feelings of instability or subluxation. Overhead throwers may report pain with throwing, classically from mid-late acceleration to ball release, difficulty warming up, progressive difficulty with pitch control, diminished velocity, and need for increased recovery time between pitching outings. These players also tend to lose their launch window and commonly miss high and outside. Batters may report pain in the lead shoulder with loading and follow-through. Golfers may also report pain in the lead shoulder at the height of the backswing or follow-through. Given the wide range of vague presenting complaints, a high index of suspicion is necessary, especially in at-risk patients with repetitive loading and stress to the posterior shoulder stabilizers.

Physical Examination

Given the wide range of presenting complaints and pathology associated with posterior instability, a thorough physical examination is crucial. As with other shoulder-related pathologies, examination should proceed in an organized stepwise fashion, starting with a global assessment of the patient's kinetic chain, including proximal and distal kinetic chain segments. An assessment of scapulothoracic motion is important, as scapular winging can function as a compensatory mechanism to prevent posterior subluxation of the humeral head in patients with posterior instability by anteverting the glenoid [75].

A thorough shoulder examination is imperative for the detection of posterior shoulder instability and should include inspection, palpation, range of motion (ROM), strength testing, and provocative testing with comparison to the contralateral side. On inspection, it is important to assess for muscular atrophy, shoulder asymmetry, and scapular dysrhythmia. One should also look for the presence of a posterior subacromial "dimple" or skin tether, as this sign has been shown to be 62% sensitive and 92% specific for association with posterior positional shoulder instability [72]. Palpation may elicit crepitus and/or tenderness over the posterior joint line in patients with synovitis or posterior rotator cuff tendonitis from recurrent episodes of posterior instability [60].

Shoulder ROM should be assessed bilaterally, including forward flexion, abduction in the scapular plane, external rotation with the arm at the side, and internal rotation with the arm behind the back. Supine shoulder ROM is also important to assess. In the supine position, the shoulder is abducted 90 degrees, the scapula is stabilized by the examination table, and glenohumeral internal and external rotation are measured. Total arc of motion is the summation of total internal and external rotation measurements and has been found to be the most important evaluation in overhead athletes. A 25-degree difference in internal rotation between sides is suggestive of GIRD, and objective parameters of GIRD have been described as greater than an 8-degree deficit in total arc of motion, greater than a 20-degree deficit in glenohumeral rotation, and/or more than a 5-degree increase in external rotation compared to the contralateral side [64]. It is important to assess for the total arc of motion and GIRD in throwing athletes, as contraction of the posteroinferior capsule alters the center of rotation of the humeral head to a more posterosuperior location in the position of abduction and external rotation, therefore increasing the risk of posterosuperior pathology. Pathologic GIRD has been associated with micro-instability from rotator-interval laxity, which can lead to posterosuperior labral tears and progression of SLAP tears to type VIII SLAP tears with resultant posterior shoulder instability [63].

Strength testing should also be performed in both shoulders, focusing on the rotator cuff musculature. In patients with RPS, subtle rotator cuff weakness is not uncommon, as the rotator cuff provides dynamic stability to the posterior shoulder. Supraspinatus strength is assessed with the arm in a 90-degree abduction in the scapular plane with downward force applied to the arm. The strength of the posterior rotator cuff muscles (infraspinatus and teres minor) is assessed with resisted external rotation, while the arm is adducted and in 90 degrees of elbow flexion. Subscapularis strength is assessed via the lift-off, belly press, and bear hug tests.

Specific tests for evaluation of posterior glenohumeral instability include the load-and shift, sulcus sign, Kim, jerk, and posterior stress tests (Table 26.1). A combination of positive tests that

Table 26.1 Provocative tests for posterior instability

Test	How to perform	Interpretation of results	Sensitivity	Specificity
Load and shift test [54, 69]	Patient in supine position Arm in 90° abduction, neutral rotation Axial load applied with anterior and then posterior force to the shoulder Translation of the humeral head over the glenoid rim is graded from 0 to 3+	Posterior load and shift over the glenoid rim indicative of a component of posterior instability Inferior translation often associated with posterior subluxation and can be indicative of MDI	37.5%	89.2%
Sulcus sign [70]	Patient in seated position Arm adducted at the side, neutral position Downward traction applied	The sulcus sign represents excessive inferior translation of the humeral head Suggests inferior instability, possible involvement of IGHL	28%[a]	97%[a]
Jerk test [43]	Patient standing or seated position Examiner stands on the affected side with the elbow in one hand and the distal clavicle and scapular spine in the other Arm in flexion and internal rotation The flexed elbow is pushed posteriorly, while the shoulder girdle is pushed anteriorly	Pain and a sudden jerk indicate a positive test as the subluxated humeral head relocates into the glenoid fossa	73% 97%[b]	98%
Kim test [43]	Patient in seated position Arm in 90° abduction in the scapular plane The examiner holds the elbow in one hand and the lateral aspect of the proximal arm in the other hand While elevating the patient's arm to 45°, a downward and posterior force is applied to the upper arm	Sudden onset of pain indicates a positive test, signifying posteroinferior shoulder instability	94% 97%[b]	80%

(continued)

Table 26.1 (continued)

Test	How to perform	Interpretation of results	Sensitivity	Specificity
Posterior stress test	Patient in seated position Arm held in 90° forward flexion, adduction, and internal rotation Examiner stabilizes the medial border of the scapula and applies a posteriorly directed force to the arm	Apprehension, subluxation, dislocation, or reproduction of pain indicates a positive test	Not reported	Not reported
Circumduction test	Patient standing, examiner behind patient Elbow in full extension, arm in 90° forward elevation, and slight adduction The examiner applies a posteriorly directed load The arm then circumducted with a combination of abduction and extension until the head reduces into the glenoid fossa	A palpable clunk as the humeral head reduces into the glenoid fossa indicates a positive test If no pain or guarding with a positive test, it often indicates chronic posterior instability	Not reported	Not reported
Modified dynamic labral shear test [11, 38]	Patient standing The arm was placed in 110° abduction and external rotation in the scapular plane and then moved to 70° abduction in the scapular plane	Posterior joint line pain indicates a positive test as the labrum is sheared between the humeral head and the glenoid during an internal impingement motion	72%	98%

[a]Sensitivity and specificity for inferior instability; not specifically reported in the literature for posterior instability
[b]Sensitivity of the Kim test increases to 97% when combined with a positive jerk test

make up the "Pitt 3 Pack" (dynamic posterior instability test (D-PIT), Whipple, O'Brien; Figs. 26.5 and 26.6) has been found to be 94.4% sensitive and 95% specific for a posterior labral tear (Table 26.2) [38, 56]. Generalized ligamentous laxity should be assessed using the Beighton scale, as this may contribute to multidirectional instability (MDI). Positive impingement signs on exam are often associated with scapular dyskinesia or secondary impingement syndrome from repetitive stress to the posterior rotator cuff muscles.

Imaging

Initial work-up for posterior instability should consist of plain radiographs of the shoulder, including anteroposterior (AP) films in the scapular plane, as well as axillary and scapular Y lateral views. In most patients with RPS, these images will be normal. Posterior dislocation or subluxation, posterior glenoid bone loss, a posterior bony Bankart fragment, and glenoid dysplasia may be appreciated on the lateral view radiographs when present. The axillary radiograph is particularly helpful in assessing glenoid retroversion, which is an established risk factor for RPS [18]. Sagittal plane acromial morphology can be assessed on the scapular Y radiographs, and a posterior acromial height (PAH) >23 mm has been associated with a significantly increased risk of posterior instability [50].

Advanced cross-sectional imaging should be obtained in cases of suspected posterior instability with either magnetic resonance imaging (MRI), magnetic resonance arthrography (MRA), or computed tomography (CT). It is important to keep in mind that advanced imaging should be used as a method to confirm a suspected clinical diagnosis, and diagnosis should not rely solely on abnormal MRI findings, as some lesions that

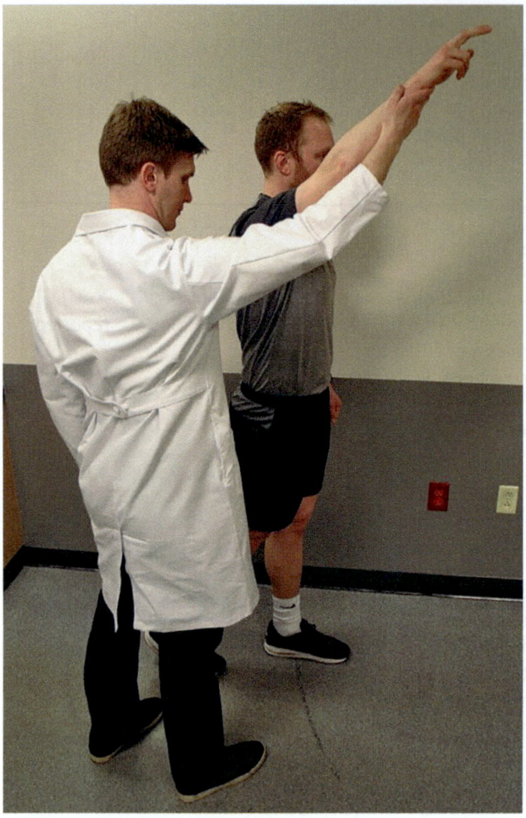

Fig. 26.5 The D-PIT (dynamic posterior instability) test should be performed when assessing for posterior shoulder instability. The patient places their shoulder in approximately 135° of forward flexion with the elbow in extension and pushes to the floor in a throwing motion as the examiner provides resistance. Posterior shoulder pain indicates a positive test. The modified D-PIT (mDPIT) involves the examiner stabilizing the posterior humeral head by applying pressure, often improving the patient's pain

appear on MRI may be asymptomatic or adaptive in nature. MRA has been shown to be the most sensitive diagnostic imaging test for the detection of posterior labral and capsular lesions [2, 4]. The authors typically do not perform MRAs and believe MRI provides the necessary detail. The Kim classification may be used to describe posterior labral tear morphology (Table 26.3) [40].

Dynamic MRI ABER sequences may improve the diagnostic accuracy of posterior labral tears, SLAP tears, and bony glenoid lesions and may be of particular use in predicting the presence of dynamic labral peel back at the time of arthroscopy [15, 51]. The addition of an axial sequence in internal rotation has also been suggested in the setting of posterior instability, as this position tensions the posterior capsulolabral structures and may prove helpful in identifying otherwise hidden lesions [2, 27]. CT scans can be helpful in patients with posterior glenoid bone loss and/or reverse Hill-Sachs lesions, as well as those with significant glenoid retroversion, glenoid dysplasia, or abnormal bony morphology. When evaluating osseous morphology and bony defects, it is helpful to obtain a non-contrast CT scan with thin slices, three-dimensional reconstructions, and humeral head subtraction views.

Findings suggestive of posterior instability on MRI include flattening of the glenoid articular surface, glenoid dysplasia (lazy J or delta type), increased glenoid retroversion, posteroinferior glenoid deficiency, reverse bony Bankart lesion, posterior translation of the humeral head relative

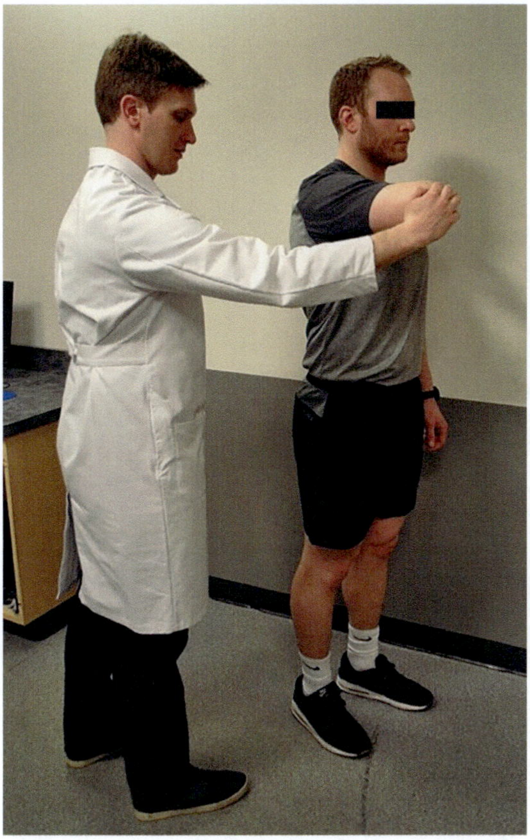

Fig. 26.6 The Whipple test is performed by having the patient put their hand on the contralateral shoulder and lift their elbow toward the ceiling. Posterior shoulder pain indicates a positive test. The modified Whipple test involves the examiner stabilizing the posterior humeral head by pushing on it with his or her thumb. Improvement in pain is expected

to the glenoid, reverse Hill-Sachs lesion (McLaughlin lesion), flattening of the posterior labrum, posterior labral tear or splitting, type VIII SLAP tear, Kim lesion (incomplete postero-inferior labral tears), posterior labrocapsular periosteal sleeve avulsion (POLPSA), PIGHL tear, reverse humeral avulsion of the glenohumeral ligament (rHAGL), Bennett lesion (mineralization of the PIGHL), a posterior capsular tear or rent, increased posterior capsular area, and subscapularis tendon avulsion [2–4, 32, 45]. Compared with age-matched controls, patients with posterior labral tears and symptomatic posterior shoulder instability have increased glenoid retroversion, increased incidence of glenoid dysplasia, and increased posterior capsular area on MRA [32].

Table 26.2 "Pitt 3 Pack" tests for posterior instability

Test	How to perform	Interpretation of results	Sensitivity	Specificity
O'Brien's active compression test [11]	Patient standing or in a seated position Arm in 90° forward flexion, 10° adduction, and internal rotation (thumb pointed down) with the elbow in extension Downward force applied to the arm The arm was then externally rotated, and the same downward force was applied	Deep pain with the arm in internal rotation position that improves with the arm in external rotation indicates a positive test, which suggests superior labral pathology	94.4%[a]	95%[a]
Dynamic posterior instability test (D-PIT) [38, 56]	Patient standing Shoulder placed in approximately 135° forward flexion with the elbow in extension (ball-release position) The examiner provides resistance against the arm while the patient continues the throwing motion	Posterior shoulder pain indicates a positive test For the modified DPIT (mDPIT), the examiner applied pressure to the posterior aspect of the humeral head to prevent posteroinferior subluxation, thus improving the patient's pain		
Whipple test	Patient standing or in a seated position Arm in 90° forward flexion and adduction with the hand opposite the contralateral shoulder The examiner applies downward force while the patient resists	Pain indicates a positive test, suggestive of a partial supraspinatus tear or superior labrum tear		

[a]A combination of three positive tests is 94.4% sensitive and 95% specific for a posterior labral tear

Table 26.3 Kim's classification of posterior labral tear morphology

Type	Description	MRA example	Arthroscopic image
I	Incomplete detachment	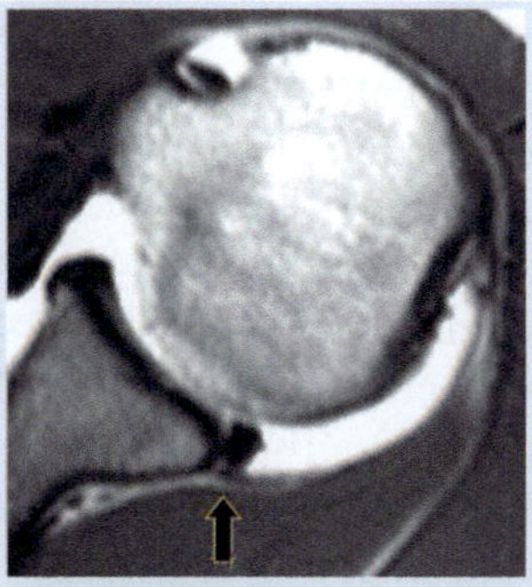	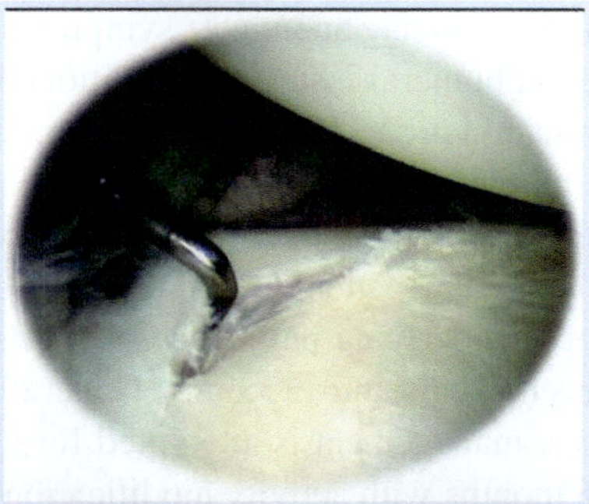
II	Concealed complete detachment ("Kim lesion") *Appears as a crack at the posteroinferior junction between the glenoid articular cartilage and the labrum, which requires probing to identify deeper complete detachment of the labrum from the glenoid rim* [41]	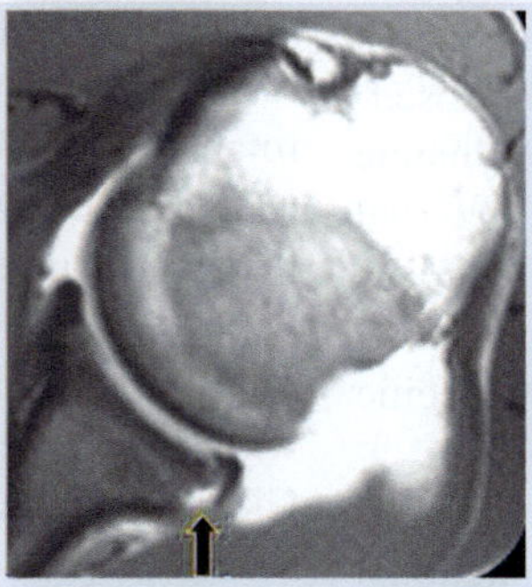	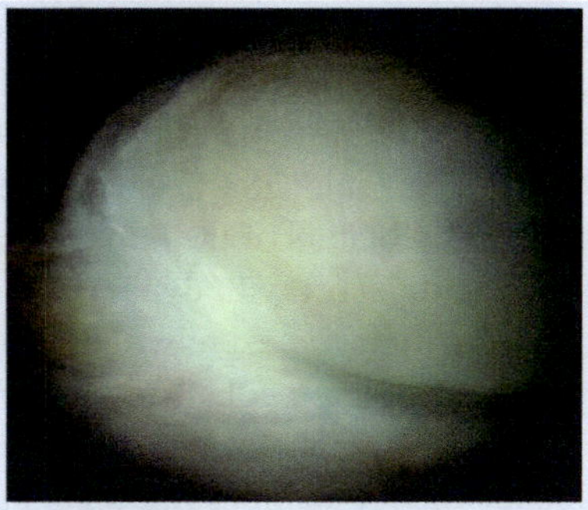
III	Chondrolabral erosion	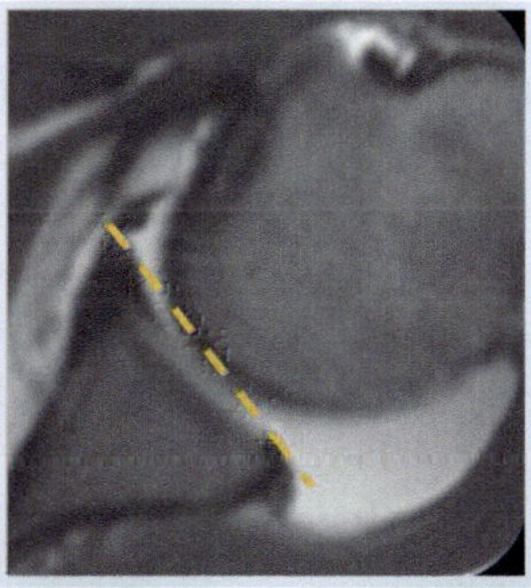	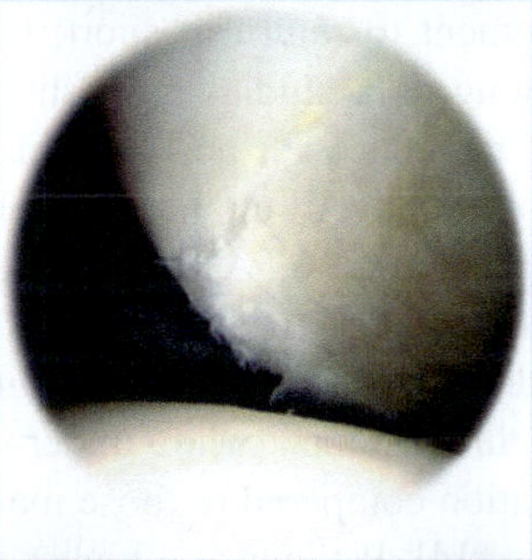
IV	Posteroinferior labrum flap tear	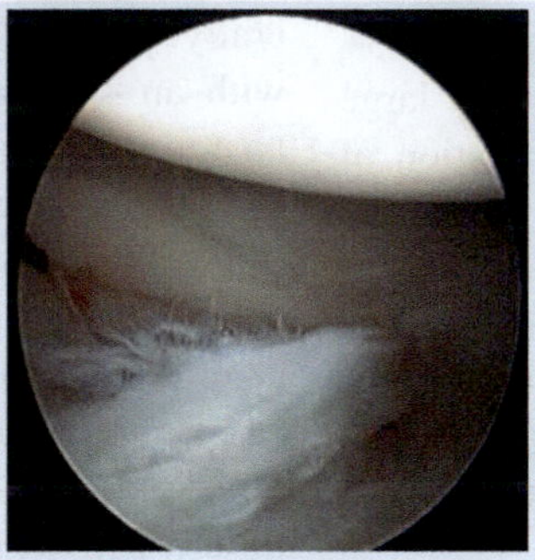	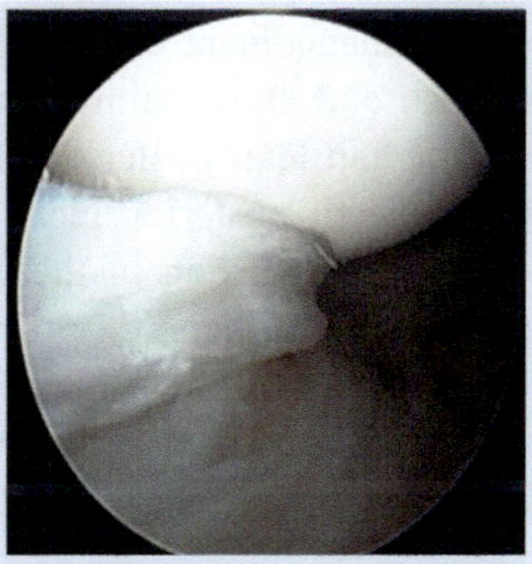

Management Options

Initial management of symptomatic posterior glenohumeral instability traditionally consists of rehabilitation focused on diminishing pain, improving function, and minimizing the risk of recurrence. Treatment should be individualized, taking the patient's symptoms, specific pathology, underlying pathogenesis, and sport-specific needs/goals into account. Generally, nonoperative management is attempted for a minimum of 6 months with activity modification and physical therapy consisting of three phases: (1) regain static proprioceptive control using simple closed-chain kinetic movements, (2) improve dynamic stability via isokinetic balancing of the internal and lateral rotators of the humerus, and (3) focus on return-to-sport with dynamic, proprioceptive, open-chain kinetic exercises and a sport-specific return to play protocol [14, 24].

Historically, up to 70% of athletes managed nonoperatively demonstrated enough functional improvement to return to sport; however, more recent long-term studies have shown that up to 70% of patients with posterior instability managed conservatively ultimately undergo surgical stabilization [14, 76]. A prospective comparative study of 51 patients with posterior shoulder instability demonstrated improved functional outcomes in patients who underwent surgical stabilization compared to those managed nonoperatively [14]. Patients at a higher risk of failing conservative management include those with 3+ posterior load and shift, painful jerk test, large labral tear or flap tear, posterior subluxation of the humeral head, posterior glenoid bone loss >11%, a humeral avulsion of the glenohumeral ligament, excessive glenoid retroversion, and greater PAH [8, 22, 42, 76]. It is important to recognize that failed nonoperative management can increase the risk of progression of posterior glenoid bone loss.

Operative Management

Surgical stabilization is recommended in patients with persistent symptoms or functional limitations after a trial of conservative management, as well as those at a higher risk of failing nonoperative management. Since the recognition of posterior instability as a unique diagnosis, a variety of techniques for posterior stabilization have been described, including extracapsular bone block procedures, the McLaughlin and modified McLaughlin technique (transfer of subscapularis and lesser tuberosity to reverse Hill-Sachs lesion), reverse Putti-Platt procedure (no longer performed given high rates of recurrent instability and loss of internal rotation), staple capsulorrhaphy (no longer performed due to high failure rates), glenoid osteotomy, capsular shift, humeral rotational osteotomy, thermal capsulorrhaphy (fallen out of favor given higher long-term failure rates and concern for thermal-related complications), labral repair, intra-articular bone block procedures, and capsulolabral reconstruction with capsular shift, among others [3, 23, 26, 30]. Glenoid osteotomy is not recommended by the authors, as retroversion has not been shown to be a risk factor for failure of posterior instability repair, only for the development of posterior instability. Patients with significant glenoid retroversion can do very well after posterior capsulolabral repair, and a small series by Waltenspül et al. demonstrated poor long-term outcomes following glenoid osteomy for posterior instability in the setting of significant glenoid retroversion [73].

Management preferences over time have generally shifted from open to arthroscopic repair with an emphasis on restoring and conserving anatomy. Open bony augmentation procedures are generally reserved for patients with significant posterior bone loss or dysplasia. While critical and subcritical bone loss is well defined in anterior instability, it remains controversial in cases of posterior instability. Arner et al. found a threshold of 11% posterior glenoid bone loss to be critical, with a 10 times higher failure rate when treated with arthroscopic repair and a 25 times higher failure rate in patients with 15% bone loss [8]. While many of the surgical procedures listed above have been shown to have acceptable outcomes for the treatment of recurrent posterior glenohumeral instability, arthroscopic posterior capsulolabral repair with a minimum of three to four suture anchors has become the mainstay of contemporary operative management for recurrent posterior glenohumeral instability [3, 30, 49]. With advances in arthroscopic techniques, the all-arthroscopic capsulolabral repair has been found to more reliably address a wide array of pathologies associated with posterior instability while minimizing surgical morbidity and time needed for recovery [7]. The arthroscopic approach has the advantage of clear visualization of the entire glenoid, labrum, capsule, rotator cuff, and other intra-articular pain generators, which facilitates patient-specific repair for a variety of pathologies. Recent studies have demonstrated excellent clinical outcomes after arthroscopic capsulolabral repair for RPS with low recurrence rates, high patient satisfaction, and high rates of return to play in both collision and overhead throwing athletes, making this approach the current standard of care for the majority of patients indicated for operative management of posterior instability [7, 17, 29, 49]. Goals of surgical management are to restore anatomy to improve glenohumeral mechanics and stability, prevent further instability and subluxation, and allow for functional return to desired activities and sports.

Indications

Indications for arthroscopic stabilization continue to evolve as more long-term and prospective studies provide additional insight into specific risk factors for failure of conservative management. After diagnosis of RPS, primary indications for arthroscopic posterior capsulolabral stabilization include persistent symptoms of instability or pain after 12 or more weeks of physical therapy focused on stretching and rotator cuff strengthening, a large labral tear or flap tear on MRA, chondrolabral retroversion of greater than 10°, reverse HAGL or discrete posterior capsular tear, reverse osseous Bankart lesion, or an inability to return to desired sport or activity level after conservative management.

Contraindications

Contraindications to isolated arthroscopic posterior capsulolabral stabilization also continue to evolve, as studies further elucidate which patient populations are at increased risk of failure of arthroscopic repair. Current contraindications to all-arthroscopic repair include significant glenoid bone loss (traditionally classified as >25%, however, more recent studies have suggested that a bone loss of 11% may be a better threshold for critical bone loss in the setting of posterior instability), large reverse Hill-Sachs lesions (>30%), capsular tissue loss from prior surgery, excessive glenoid retroversion (type C glenoid), significant osteoarthritis, or patients who have failed prior arthroscopic stabilization (relative contraindication). Patients with neuromuscular abnormalities and habitual dislocators should be approached with caution. Additionally, patients unable to comply with postoperative restrictions, including a brief period of immobilization and a subsequent structured rehabilitation program, may not be suitable surgical candidates.

Author's Preferred Surgical Technique: A Case-Based Approach

Based on experience as well as the best available clinical and biomechanical evidence to date, our preferred index technique for management of recurrent posterior instability that has failed or has a high chance of failing conservative management is arthroscopic posterior capsulolabral repair in the lateral decubitus position with knotless constructs. Repair should be tailored to the patient's specific injury pattern, intra-articular pathology, and sport-specific needs.

Preoperative Preparation

Before surgery, MRI should be reviewed meticulously with specific attention paid to the degree of glenoid retroversion and associated intra-articular pathology, including the extent of labral injury, capsular injury, and glenoid bone loss. It is imperative to understand the individual patient's specific injury pattern, pathology, and functional needs to ensure proper surgical management. For example, capsular plication should be avoided or minimal in overhead throwing athletes to avoid over-constraining the glenohumeral joint, whereas high-risk collision athletes with significant capsulolabral pathology will likely require capsular plication for improved outcomes. Patients should be adequately counseled on the surgical risks, including stiffness, infection, neurovascular injury, and recurrent instability.

Patient Positioning

Arthroscopic capsulolabral repair can be performed in the lateral decubitus or beach chair positions with comparable long-term outcomes [52]. Our preference is the lateral decubitus position, as it facilitates complete visualization with excellent access to the posterior joint and capsule. After induction of general anesthesia and before moving to the lateral position, examination under anesthesia is performed on both the injured and contralateral shoulders. In our clinical case, the patient was found to have a 2+ posterior load and shift on the operative shoulder compared with a 1+ on the contralateral side. The sulcus sign was negative bilaterally.

The patient is then placed in the lateral decubitus position on a beanbag with an axillary roll. Adequate padding of the legs, bony prominences, and peroneal nerve is ensured, and the patient is secured to the table. The operative arm is placed in 10 pounds of balanced longitudinal traction with 45 degrees of shoulder abduction and 20 degrees of forward elevation to displace the humeral head anteriorly and inferiorly, bringing the posterior labrum into unobstructed view (Fig. 26.7). The operative extremity is then prepped to maintain a wide operative field. A sterile bump or manual lateral traction can be applied during arthroscopy to create more distraction between the humeral head and glenoid if desired, thereby improving circumferential visualization and access to the labrum and capsule, particularly inferiorly.

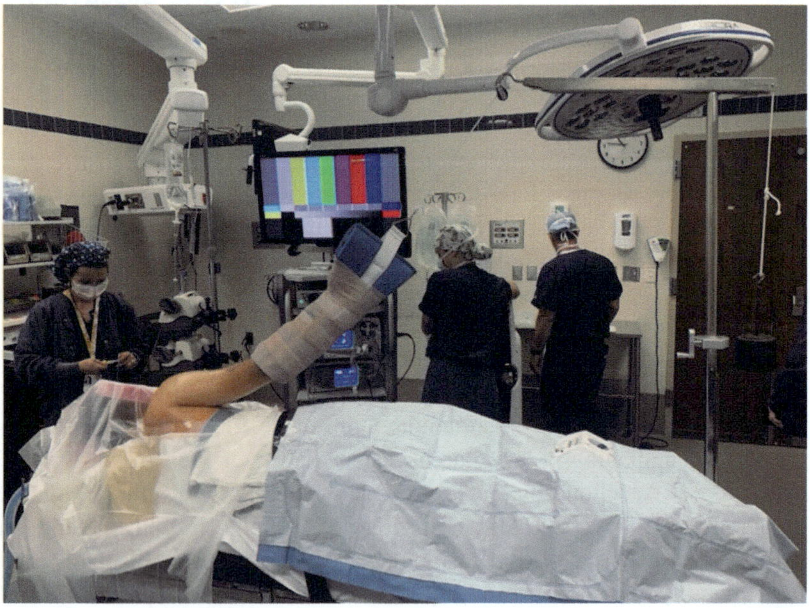

Fig. 26.7 The operative arm is placed in 10–15 pounds of balanced longitudinal traction with 45 degrees of shoulder abduction and 20 degrees forward elevation. This brings the posterior labrum into unobstructed view by displacing the humeral head anteriorly and inferiorly

Portal Placement

Prior to portal placement, the glenohumeral joint is insufflated with 30 cc of sterile saline to facilitate safe insertion of the arthroscope cannula and blunt trocar, thereby minimizing potential articular cartilage damage. Following insufflation, the posterior portal is established first, in a modified position approximately 1 cm distal and 1 cm lateral to the standard posterior portal. This modified posterior portal allows a tangential trajectory of instruments toward the posterior glenoid rim, facilitating proper anchor placement. Posterior portals that are placed too far superior or medial in the posterior capsule may cause difficulty with the correct angle for placement of suture anchors. After the posterior portal is established, the anterior portal can be made high in the rotator interval using either an "inside out" technique with a switching stick (author's preferred method) or an "outside in" technique with a spinal needle. A 5.75 × 7 mm clear cannula is placed in the anterior portal. The arthroscope can be switched to the anterior portal for additional viewing of the posterior capsule and labrum. When needed, a 7 o'clock portal can be made percutaneously to facilitate placement of inferior anchors near the 6 o'clock position.

Diagnostic Arthroscopy

Following appropriate portal placement, diagnostic arthroscopy should be performed using a 30-degree arthroscope through the posterior viewing portal to evaluate for pathology. A 70-degree scope is commonly utilized for visualization, particularly inferiorly. It is important to visualize the humeral head articular surface, glenoid articular surface, posterior labrum, posterior capsule, inferior glenohumeral ligament, superior labrum and attachment, biceps tendon, anterior capsule, anterior and inferior labrum, axillary pouch, subscapularis tendon, rotator interval, subcoracoid recess, and undersurface of the superior and posterior rotator cuff tendons. For the passage of an arthroscopic probe and other instruments for repair, a switching stick is used to place a posterior 8.25-mm distally threaded clear cannula, as smaller cannulas are unable to accommodate the 45-degree suture hook.

In our clinical case, diagnostic arthroscopy revealed no chondrosis of the humeral head or glenoid. A posterior labral tear was noted from the 10-o'clock to 6-o'clock position on the glenoid (Fig. 26.8). Aberrant anatomy of the middle glenohumeral ligament was noted with thickening and attachment to the anterosuperior labrum. The rotator cuff and anterior labrum were intact. No pathology was noted about the LHBT. Dynamic evaluation of the shoulder was performed by taking the shoulder out of longitudinal traction and placing it in abduction and external rotation, revealing a pathologic snapback of the superior labrum (Fig. 26.9). At this point, the decision was made to proceed with superior and posterior labral repair.

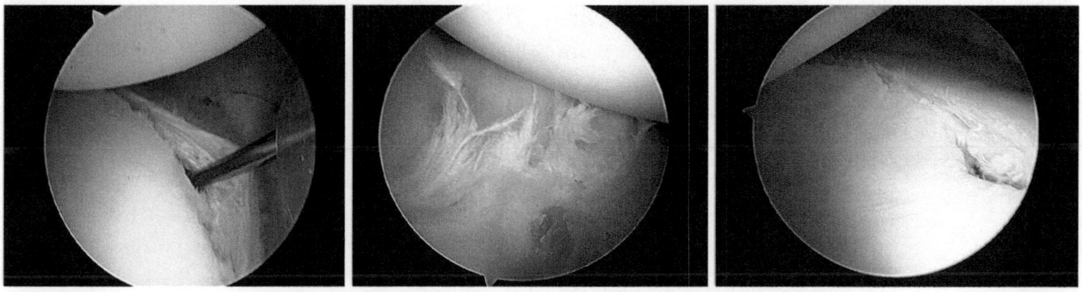

Fig. 26.8 Arthroscopic view of a posterior labral tear extending from the 10 o'clock to 6 o'clock position on the posterior glenoid

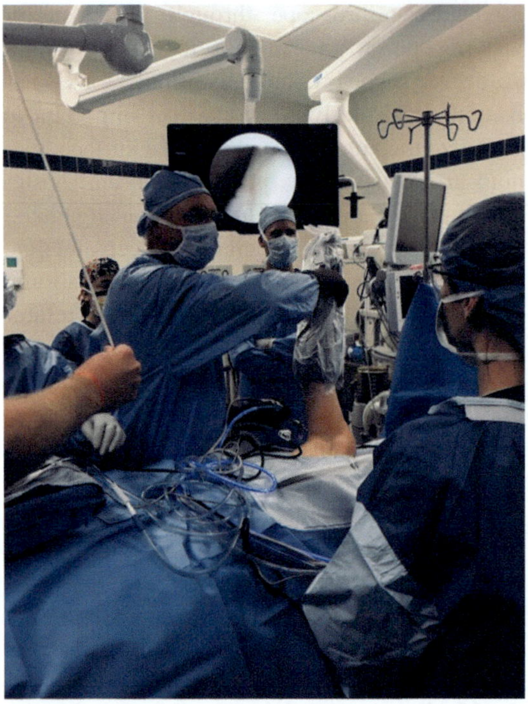

Fig. 26.9 Dynamic evaluation of the posterior labrum is performed by taking the shoulder out of longitudinal traction and placing it in the abduction external rotation position. This position allows evaluation for the pathologic snap-back phenomenon of the posterosuperior labrum at the biceps anchor

Glenoid Labrum Preparation

After complete visualization of the extent of the labral tear and associated pathology using both the anterior and posterior portals, while viewing from the posterior portal, an arthroscopic chisel and rasp are used from the anterior superior portal to elevate and mobilize the torn and often scarred labrum from the glenoid rim across the entire extent of the tear (Fig. 26.10). This is done until the labrum is free floating without tension. The arthroscopic shaver is used to gently decorticate the glenoid rim to achieve a healthy bleeding surface for improved healing. A shaver can be used to debride the labrum, although this should be limited to the labrum with large flaps or extensive fraying to preserve as much labrum as possible for incorporation into the repair. In cases where a capsular plication is desired, a meniscal rasp is used to abrade the capsule adjacent to the labral tear. In our clinical case, capsular plication was not desired to avoid over-constraint, as the patient is an overhead baseball pitcher. In contact athletes, greater capsular plication is recommended.

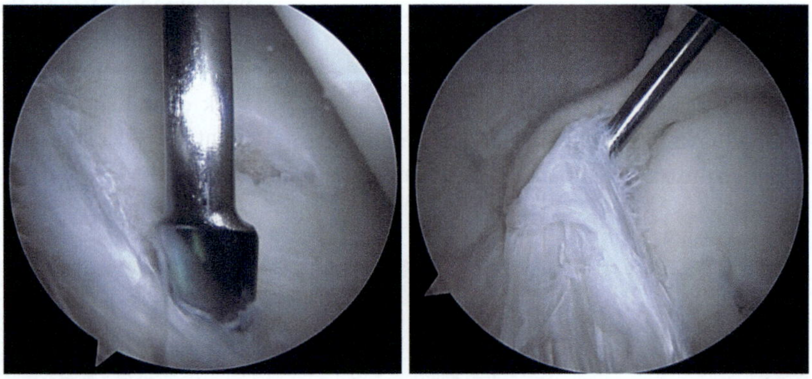

Fig. 26.10 An arthroscopic chisel is used to elevate and mobilize the posterior labrum from the glenoid rim across the entire extent of the labral tear. A rasp and shaver are used to decorticate and prepare the glenoid rim for improved healing prior to suture anchor placement

Anchor Placement and Labral Repair

Following glenoid labrum preparation, knotless suture anchors are placed at the articular margin of the glenoid rim from an inferior to superior direction (Fig. 26.11). Inferiorly, the labrum attaches to the face of the glenoid, while superiorly, it is off the face. It is essential to maintain this anatomical relationship. We generally use four to five anchors, but depending on the tear extent and size of the glenoid, a minimum of three knotless suture anchors should be utilized. Based on the patient's glenoid size, we prefer 2.4 mm or 2.9 mm BioComposite PushLock suture anchors with SutureTape (Arthrex Naples, FL). SutureTape increases the surface area of fixation, strengthening the repair construct, and has a higher pullout strength. A drill guide is placed on the glenoid rim, and the drill is directed onto the chondral surface to ensure anatomic repair of the labrum on the glenoid face. Care should be taken to avoid prominent anchors during placement, which may occur with a low, tangential drilling angle <30 degrees.

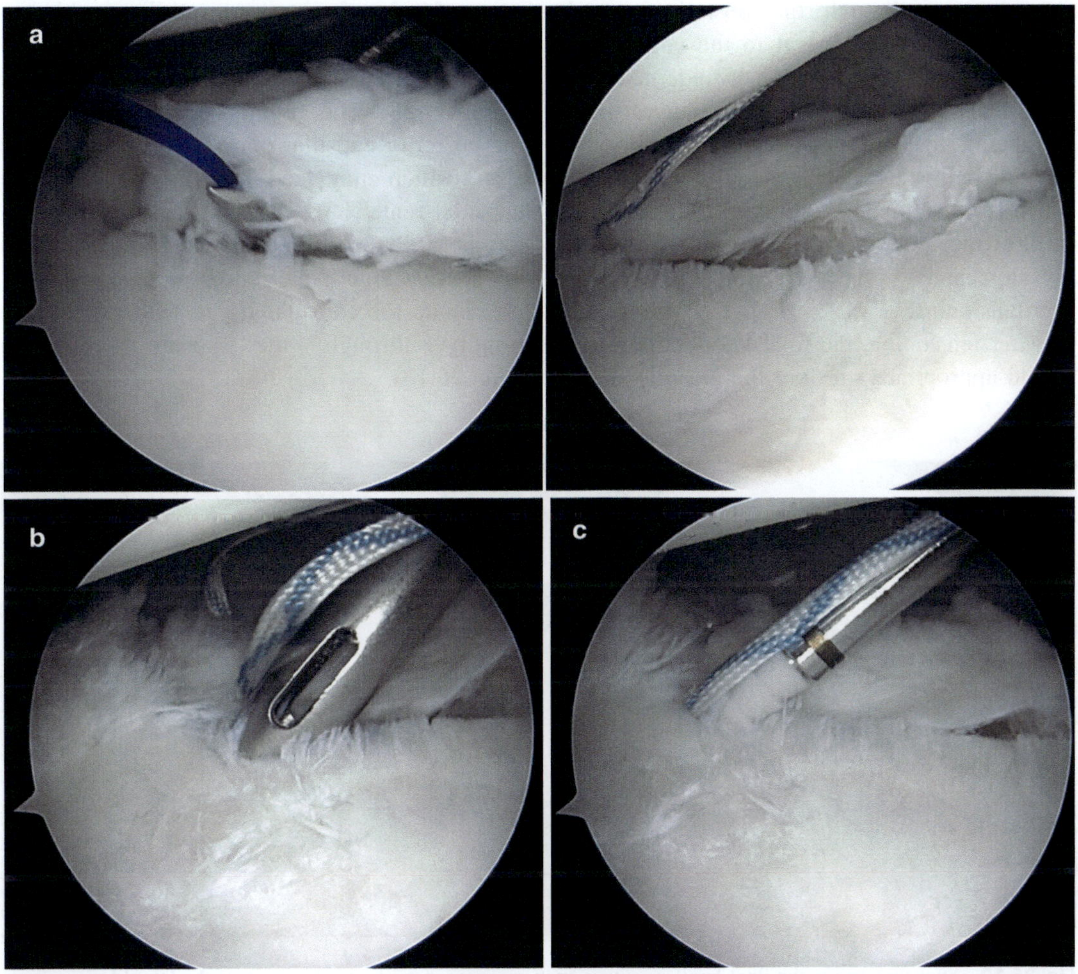

Fig. 26.11 (**a**) A curved suture hook loaded with a PDS suture is passed through the capsule based on the desired amount of capsulorrhaphy and then under the labrum against the glenoid articular margin. The PDS passing suture is tied to a Suture Tape, which is shuttled through the posterior working cannula. (**b**) The anchor is drilled, and the tape is delivered through the anchor islet. (**c**) The tape is then appropriately tensioned, and the anchor is inserted

Suture anchors are placed appropriately from inferior to superior. For our clinical case, the tear was from the 6:00 to 10:00 o'clock position on the glenoid, so anchors were placed at 7:00, 8:00, 9:00, and 10:00 o'clock positions. Commonly, a separate 7 o'clock portal is necessary to obtain the appropriate trajectory for the most inferior anchor. Care was taken to only incorporate the labrum into the repair and not the capsule, again because the patient is primarily an overhead throwing athlete. In non-throwing athletes, and especially patients with a patulous posterior capsule, capsular tissue should be appropriately incorporated into the repair by advancing the suture passer through the posterior capsule approximately 1 cm lateral to the edge of the labral tear and then directing it underneath the labral tear to the edge of the articular cartilage. Advancing the suture passer from inferior to superior helps to restore tension to the PIGHL, which is imperative to restore posterior stability. In throwing athletes, care is taken to limit the capsulorrhaphy in order to avoid over-tensioning.

After tensioning, the final knotless construct should appropriately restore the posterior labral bumper anatomically on the glenoid face (Fig. 26.12). If further capsular tensioning is needed after anchor placement, suture capsulorrhaphies can be performed by suturing capsule directly to the repaired labrum in the intervals between the suture anchors; however, appropriate capsular plication should be accomplished with the suture anchors, so further tensioning is not needed. Posterior labral tearing also commonly occurs in concert with anterior and superior labral tearing. All pathologies that appear to be pathologic based on history and physical examination should be appropriately addressed.

Rotator interval closure is not necessary in cases of isolated posterior instability, as biomechanical studies have demonstrated no additional benefit to closure with regard to posterior stability [53]. The authors recommend closing the posterior capsular portal to prevent a stress riser, which may lead to enlargement of the capsular rent. The authors prefer closure with a number 0 PDS suture using a suture passer and an arthroscopic penetrating grasper to reapproximate the capsular tissue with a knot tied blindly through the posterior cannula (Fig. 26.13).

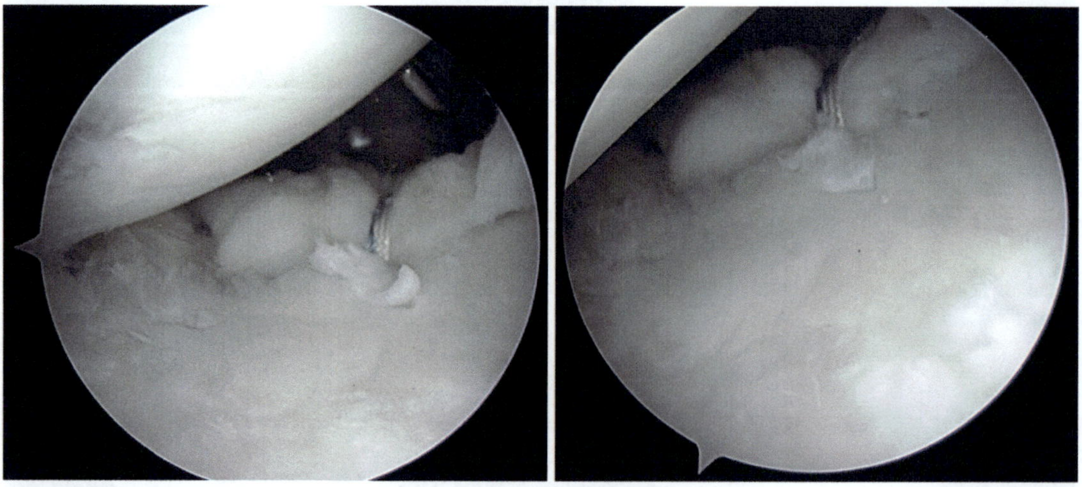

Fig. 26.12 After tensioning, the final knotless suture anchor constructs appropriately restore the labral bumper anatomically on the glenoid face

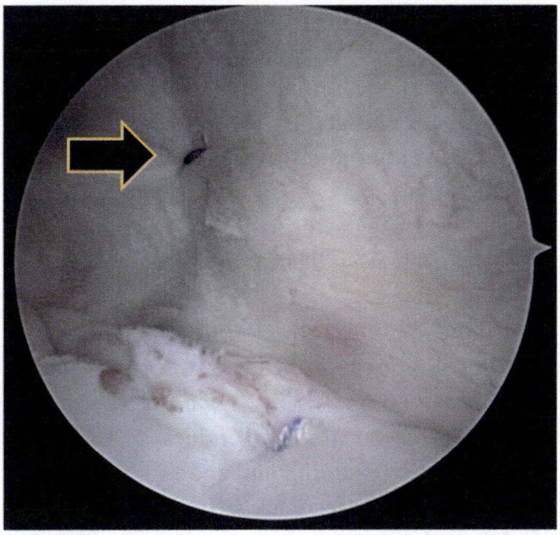

Fig. 26.13 An arthroscopic penetrator with a PDS suture is used to close the posterior capsular portal

Pearls

- The authors prefer the lateral decubitus position rather than the beach chair position to facilitate arthroscopic access to both the anterior and posterior labrum.
- Positioning the arm in balanced traction of 10–15 pounds with 45 degrees of shoulder abduction and 20 degrees of forward flexion provides the best access to the posterior labrum, as it displaces the humeral head anteroinferiorly.
- The authors utilize a modified posterior portal that is 1 cm lower and 1 cm more lateral than the standard posterior viewing portal to allow a tangential trajectory of instruments toward the posterior glenoid rim, facilitating proper anchor placement.
- Capsular plication should be individualized to the patient's specific activity needs, with more plication in collision athletes with a patulous posterior capsule, and minimal to no plication in overhead throwing athletes to avoid over-constraint.
- In patients with a patulous posterior capsule, the capsular tissue should be abraded, and a concomitant capsular plication should be performed using sutures from the suture anchors.
- Knotless anchor constructs are preferred, as they have improved pullout strength, allow a more anatomic repair to the glenoid face, allow faster repair, and minimize the risk of cartilage wear from friction with knots.
- In patients who require anchor placement at the 6 o'clock position, a small percutaneous 7 o'clock portal can help facilitate placement without further compromising posterior capsular stability.
- The use of a spinal needle will help ensure proper placement of the 7 o'clock portal (4 cm lateral to the posterolateral acromion), with the ideal capsular entry located 1 cm lateral to the glenoid rim and at a 45-degree angle.
- The authors recommend routine closure of the posterior capsular portal in all cases of posterior instability.

Pitfalls

- Patients with generalized ligamentous laxity (Beighton score 5 or greater) and posterior shoulder instability should fully exhaust a rehabilitation program before consideration of surgical management.
- Proper suture anchor placement can be difficult if the posterior portal is created too high or medial in the capsule.
- When abrading the posterior capsule, overly aggressive use of the motorized shaver may inadvertently penetrate the thin capsular tissue; we therefore favor the use of a rasp for this purpose.
- Placement of anchors too close to one another can lead to glenoid bone fragmentation.
- Posterior capsular plication in overhead throwers can lead to over-constraint, which should be avoided if return to throwing activities is desired.
- Failure to close the posterior capsule can lead to capsular insufficiency, as widening of the portal rent can occur over time.

Postoperative Management

Postoperative management and rehabilitation consist of a series of phases: (1) initial immobilization; (2) passive range of motion; (3) active range of motion; (4) rotator cuff, deltoid, and periscapular strengthening; and (5) sport-specific rehabilitation. Initially, after surgery, the patient is placed in a sling with an abduction pillow for 6 weeks. The abduction pillow places the shoulder in 30 degrees of abduction and prevents internal rotation in order to protect the posterior capsulolabral repair. A cryotherapy device is used for the first 3 days after surgery to diminish swelling and pain. Starting the day after surgery, active ROM of the elbow, wrist, and fingers is encouraged. A formal physical therapy program is initiated after 3 weeks, with a focus on graduated, gentle, pain-free passive ROM up to 90 degrees of forward flexion and abduction in the scapular plane, as well as external rotation to 0 degrees.

Active-assistive ROM exercises are initiated, and isometric internal and external rotation with the arm at the side and elbow flexed to 90 degrees are added according to the patient's tolerance. Motion should be pain-free, and the shoulder position can be adjusted to allow painless muscle contraction. During the 3- to 6-week phase, active external rotation can be initiated if it remains pain-free. Active horizontal abduction can be added with the patient lying prone; however, movement should be restricted from 45 degrees of horizontal adduction to full horizontal abduction to avoid excessive stress to the posterior capsule.

The sling is discontinued at 6 weeks postoperatively, and therapy should progress with continued ROM exercises and pain-free, gentle internal rotation. Full passive and active ROM should be achieved by 2–3 months postoperatively. After achieving full, painless active and passive ROM, the focus shifts to rotator cuff strengthening. After 3 months, push-ups are added to the strengthening exercises, starting with wall push-ups and progressing to floor push-ups as tolerated without raising the body beyond the scapular plane. Shoulders should be positioned in 80–90 degrees of abduction, and caution is applied during the ascent phase of the push-up to avoid excessive stress to the posterior capsule. Isotonic strengthening with an emphasis on the rotator cuff and posterior deltoid is continued. Active internal rotation using surgical or rubber tubing may be added, and horizontal abduction can be performed through an increased range, starting at 90 degrees of horizontal adduction as tolerated.

Around 4 months postoperatively, weights can be progressed as tolerated, and eccentric rotator cuff strengthening should be initiated. An arm ergometer can be used for endurance exercises. Isokinetic strengthening and endurance exercises (high speeds—200+ degrees/second) for shoulder internal/external rotation (arm at side) and horizontal abduction may be added. Prerequisite strength requirements of the rotator cuff are 5–10 pounds for external rotation and 15–20 pounds for internal rotation. The shoulder should be pain-free and have no significant amount of swelling.

Patients who demonstrate at least 80% strength and endurance compared with the contralateral side, as measured by isokinetic testing, can begin a sport-specific rehabilitation protocol. This should include a total body conditioning program with emphasis on the shoulder (rotator cuff, posterior deltoid), as well as sport-specific skill mastery, and is usually initiated between 4 and 6 months after surgery. For overhead throwing athletes, this begins with an interval throwing program. Between 7 and 8 months after surgery, endurance activities are progressed, stretching and strengthening of the upper extremity continue, and swimming may be added as part of the exercise program (the butterfly stroke is not recommended). Non-throwing athletes can generally return to full sport between 6 and 9 months postoperatively, after they demonstrate full ROM and strength, along with restoration of glenohumeral stability. Throwing athletes should be approached more cautiously but typically are able to complete their interval throwing program around 9 months postoperatively. Clearance to return to sports is needed by the operating surgeon. The author's preferred interval throwing protocol is outlined in Table 26.4.

Table 26.4 Interval throwing protocol after arthroscopic posterior stabilization

Phase	Description	
45’	Step 1: A. Warm-up throwing B. 45′ (25 throws) C. Rest 15 minutes D. Warm-up throwing E. 45′ (25 throws)	Step 2: A. Warm-up throwing B. 45′ (25 throws) C. Rest 10 minutes D. Warm-up throwing E. 45′ (25 throws) F. Rest 10 minutes G. Warm-up throwing H. 45′ (25 throws)
60’	Step 3: A. Warm-up throwing B. 60′ (25 throws) C. Rest 15 minutes D. Warm-up throwing E. 60′ (25 throws)	Step 4: A. Warm-up throwing B. 60′ (25 throws) C. Rest 10 minutes D. Warm-up throws E. 60′ (25 throws) F. Rest 10 minutes G. Warm-up throwing H. 60′ (25 throws)
90’	Step 5: A. Warm-up throwing B. 90′ (25 throws) C. Rest 15 minutes D. Warm-up throwing E. 90′ (25 throws)	Step 6: A. Warm-up throwing B. 90′ (25 throws) C. Rest 10 minutes D. Warm-up throwing E. 90′ (25 throws) F. Rest 10 minutes G. Warm-up throwing H. 90′ (25 throws)
120’	Step 7: A. Warm-up throwing B. 120′ (25 throws) C. Rest 15 minutes D. Warm-up throwing E. 120′ (25 throws)	Step 8: A. Warm-up throwing B. 120′ (25 throws) C. Rest 10 minutes D. Warm-up throwing E. 120′ (25 throws) F. Rest 10 minutes G. Warm-up throwing H. 120′ (25 throws)
150’	Step 9: A. Warm-up throwing B. 150′ (25 throws) C. Rest 15 minutes D. Warm-up throwing E. 150′ (25 throws)	Step 10: A. Warm-up throwing B. 150′ (25 throws) C. Rest 10 minutes D. Warm-up throwing E. 150′ (25 throws) F. Rest 10 minutes G. Warm-up throwing H. 150′ (25 throws)

(continued)

Table 26.4 (continued)

Phase	Description	
180'	Step 11: A. Warm-up throwing B. 180′ (25 throws) C. Rest 15 minutes D. Warm-up throwing E. 180′ (25 throws) Step 12: A. Warm-up throwing B. 180′ (25 throws) C. Rest 10 minutes D. Warm-up throws E. 180′ (25 throws) F. Rest 10 minutes G. Warm-up throwing H. 180′ (25 throws)	Step 13: A. Warm-up throwing B. 180′ (25 throws) C. Rest 15 minutes D. Warm-up throwing E. 180′ (25 throws) Step 14: Begin throwing off the mound or return to the respective position

The throwing program should be performed every other day, unless otherwise specified by your physician or rehabilitation specialist. Throws should use the crow-hop method and emphasize proper mechanics with each throw

Outcomes

Arthroscopic posterior capsulolabral repair with suture anchors for stabilization of symptomatic unidirectional posterior glenohumeral instability has demonstrated high patient satisfaction rates, significant improvements in pain and function, and high rates of return to sport at mid-term follow-up (Table 26.5) [17, 31, 47, 49, 64]. Contact athletes and those with a traumatic etiology generally have the best outcomes postoperatively [5, 36, 48]. Throwers have similar RTS rates as non-throwers but are less reliably able to return to pre-injury level, especially when their main position is pitcher [29, 31, 48]. Throwers with concomitant partial-thickness rotator cuff tears who undergo debridement at the time of posterior capsulolabral repair have demonstrated noninferior outcomes compared to those without rotator cuff injury [6]. Active-duty military patients with posterior instability have demonstrated reliable outcomes after arthroscopic capsulolabral repair with or without bicep tenodesis, with 90–94% able to return to active-duty service at pre-injury activity level [33, 34]. Modern arthroscopic capsulolabral repair with knotless suture anchors and patient-specific capsular plication has become the gold standard for surgical management of symptomatic posterior instability, with reliable improvement in pain, function, patient satisfaction, and return to activities (although less reliable return to pre-injury level of activities).

Table 26.5 Results of contemporary primary arthroscopic capsulolabral repair for posterior instability

Study	Shoulders	Follow-up (mo)	Outcomes
Bradley et al. [17]	200	36	90% RTS, 64% RTS at pre-injury level Greater improvements in ASES scores and higher RTS in patients with bone suture anchors
Arner et al. [5]	56	44.7	93% RTS, 79% RTS at pre-injury level Excellent or good results (ASES >60; stability <6) were found in 96.5% of athletes and a 96% satisfaction rate
McClincy et al. [48]	96	37	94% throwers RTS, 60% RTS at pre-injury level Throwers with a discrete labral tear were ten times more likely to return to throwing. Throwers with suture anchor repair were also ten times more likely to RTS. Equivocal outcomes between throwers and pitchers, but lower RTS rates in pitchers
Katthagen et al. [36]	41	49.2	78.6% RTS, 78.6% RTS at pre-injury level Greater improvements in mean ASES and SANE scores for patients with traumatic instability
Fourman et al. [29]	46	79	Non-throwers: 94.7% RTS, 73.7% RTS at pre-injury level Throwers: 70.4% RTS, 37% RTS at pre-injury level No significant difference in stability, satisfaction rate, or RTS rates between throwers and non-throwers
McClincy et al. [49]	82	36	89% adolescents RTS, 71% RTS at pre-injury level 8.5% failure rate (continued pain or instability requiring revision surgery)
Asturias et al. [9]	48	45	RTS not reported 12.5% failure rate in adolescents (recurrent pain or instability requiring revision surgery) Higher risk of complications among younger patients
Vaswani et al. [71]	105	99.6	83.6% RTS, 37.2% RTS in throwing athletes that did not require revision surgery 8.6% revision rate at a mean of 2.8 years
Green et al. [34]	30	96.6	90% return to active-duty military at pre-injury level 10% failure rate (persistent instability or activity-limiting pain)
Green et al. [33]	32	73.5	93.8% return to active-duty military at pre-injury level

RTS return to sport, *ASES* American shoulder and elbow surgeons shoulder score, *SANE* single assessment numeric evaluation

Complications

The most common complication after arthroscopic posterior capsulolabral repair is recurrent instability, which has been reported to occur at a rate between 8 and 13% [9, 34, 49, 71]. Patients at higher risk for failure requiring revision surgery include those with ≤3 anchors at the time of primary repair, glenoid bone loss >11%, female sex, concomitant rotator cuff injury, dominant arm involvement, and smaller glenoid bone width [8, 16]. Postoperative stiffness is a rare complication that has been shown to occur in patients who undergo capsular plication. The risk of postoperative stiffness can be minimized with early posterior capsular stretching.

Several intraoperative complications can occur during arthroscopic posterior stabilization. Neurovascular structures at risk if the 7 o'clock posterior portal is placed too inferiorly include the posterior humeral circumflex artery as well as the suprascapular nerve and artery, which are on average 39 ± 4 mm and 28 ± 2 mm from the proper portal placement [25]. The axillary nerve is also at risk during arthroscopy, particularly during placement of inferior suture anchors at the 6 o'clock position on the glenoid rim, as it lies 12.4 mm away from this position, and plication of the inferior capsule, as the nerve is located on average 2.5 mm from the IGHL [61]. Given the close proximity of the axillary nerve to the IGHL, thermal devices should be avoided in this area.

Complications related to anchors have also been reported. These include articular surface damage from migration of anchors, as well as premature absorption, osteolysis, synovitis, cyst formation, and dissemination of implant fragments into the joint space with some earlier-generation bioabsorbable anchors composed of polylactic acid (PLA) [58, 66, 68]. More recent improvements in mechanical and resorptive properties of bioabsorbable suture anchor materials, including biocomposites and polyetheretherketone (PEEK) anchors, have led to a decrease in these biocompatibility issues, although there is still a paucity of long-term clinical and radiographic outcome studies [39, 55].

Anchor placement can also be associated with complications, including iatrogenic chondral damage. As previously discussed, there is a higher risk of chondral damage during anchor placement with a tangential drilling angle <30 degrees. This risk can be minimized with a properly placed posterior portal to allow a higher angle of approach to the glenoid rim. Additionally, malposition of anchors has been associated with pain, stiffness, and even failure of the repair [55].

Infection is also a rare but important complication after shoulder arthroscopy, with a reported rate of between 0.2% and 0.3% and a higher risk found in patients with chronic anemia, malnutrition, male sex, morbid obesity, and patients with diagnosed depression [10, 20]. The usual causal organism is *Cutibacterium acnes (C. acnes; formerly known as Propionibacterium acnes, or P. acnes)*, which is a gram-positive anaerobic bacterium [10]. Topical benzoyl peroxide application preoperatively, in addition to preoperative antibiotic prophylaxis, has been shown to significantly reduce the prevalence of *C. acnes* infections after shoulder arthroscopy [10].

Venous thromboembolism (VTE) is a rare but documented risk after shoulder arthroscopy, with a reported rate of 0.01–0.2% in large database reviews [62]. Risk factors include prior VTE, older age, medical comorbidities (increased Charlson Comorbidity Index), longer operative time, prolonged hospital stays, and surgery at an altitude over 4000 feet [62]. While lateral decubitus positioning with the arm in traction has been proposed as a possible risk for increased VTE, there is no conclusive evidence that positioning affects VTE risk [62]. Given the low rates of VTE and unclear benefit of prophylaxis, routine VTE prophylaxis after shoulder arthroscopy is not currently recommended.

Summary

Posterior glenohumeral instability remains a challenging clinical entity that accounts for up to 10% of shoulder instability events. Diagnosis is often delayed due to vague and variable presenting complaints and a typically insidious onset of symptoms, including generalized shoulder fatigue and pain without a specific injury. A number of characteristic imaging findings can be found on MRI, and careful examination of images can help ensure proper diagnosis and treatment approaches. Conservative management should be attempted in most cases for a minimum of 12 weeks with a focus on rotator cuff and periscapular strengthening.

After failure of conservative management, arthroscopic capsulolabral repair with patient-specific capsular plication has become the standard of care for symptomatic unidirectional posterior glenohumeral instability to restore anatomic stability to the glenohumeral joint. Overhead throwers are a unique population in comparison to collision athletes and non-throwers and should be approached with this in mind. In overhead throwers with RPS and a posterior labral tear, we recommend repair of the posterior labrum without capsular plication and an emphasis on capsular stretching for concomitant GIRD when present. In collision athletes and non-throwers with a patulous posterior capsule, we recommend an arthroscopic superiorly directed capsular plication with incorporation of capsular tissue into the knotless suture anchor labral repair. It is imperative to have a regimented post-operative rehabilitation program with specific sport-specific return to play criteria. Further research is needed to continue to unravel the complex mechanics and pathogenesis of RPS in throwing athletes, with a goal of improving symptoms and rates of RTS at the pre-injury level.

Financial Disclosure Dr. Bradley: Receives royalties from Arthrex and DJO.

References

1. Abrams GD, Safran MR. Diagnosis and management of superior labrum anterior posterior lesions in overhead athletes. Br J Sports Med. 2010;44(5):311–8.
2. Albano D, Messina C, Sconfienza LM. Posterior shoulder instability: what to look for. Magn Reson Imaging Clin N Am. 2020;28(2):211–21.
3. Antosh IJ, Tokish JM, Owens BD. Posterior shoulder instability. Sports Health. 2016;8(6):520–6.
4. Arirachakaran A, Boonard M, Chaijenkij K, et al. A systematic review and meta-analysis of diagnostic test of MRA versus MRI for detection superior labrum anterior to posterior lesions type II-VII. Skeletal Radiol. 2017;46(2):149–60.
5. Arner JW, McClincy MP, Bradley JP. Arthroscopic stabilization of posterior shoulder instability is successful in American football players. Arthroscopy. 2015;31(8):1466–71.
6. Arner JW, McClincy MP, Bradley JP. In throwers with posterior instability, rotator cuff tears are common but do not affect surgical outcomes. Am J Orthop (Belle Mead NJ). 2018;47(1)
7. Arner JW, Peebles LA, Bradley JP, Provencher MT. Anterior shoulder instability management: indications, techniques, and outcomes. Arthroscopy. 2020;36(11):2791–3.
8. Arner JW, Ruzbarsky JJ, Midtgaard K, et al. Defining critical glenoid bone loss in posterior shoulder capsulolabral repair. Am J Sports Med. 2021;49(8):2013–9.
9. Asturias AM, Bastrom TP, Pennock AT, Edmonds EW. Posterior shoulder instability: surgical outcomes and risk of failure in adolescence. Am J Sports Med. 2020;48(5):1200–6.
10. Belk JW, Kraeutler MJ, Smith JR, et al. Prevention of Cutibacterium acnes infection in arthroscopic shoulder surgery: a systematic review. J Shoulder Elb Surg. 2020;29(5):867–73.
11. Ben Kibler W, Sciascia AD, Hester P, Dome D, Jacobs C. Clinical utility of traditional and new tests in the diagnosis of biceps tendon injuries and superior labrum anterior and posterior lesions in the shoulder. Am J Sports Med. 2009;37(9):1840–7.
12. Bernhardson AS, Murphy CP, Aman ZS, LaPrade RF, Provencher MT. A prospective analysis of patients with anterior versus posterior shoulder instability: a matched cohort examination and surgical outcome analysis of 200 patients. Am J Sports Med. 2019;47(3):682–7.
13. Blasier RB, Soslowsky LJ, Malicky DM, Palmer ML. Posterior glenohumeral subluxation: active and passive stabilization in a biomechanical model. J Bone Joint Surg Am. 1997;79(3):433–40.
14. Bodendorfer BM. CORR insights(R): recurrent instability and surgery are common after nonoperative treatment of posterior glenohumeral instability in NCAA division I FBS football players. Clin Orthop Relat Res. 2021;479(4):701–3.
15. Borrero CG, Casagranda BU, Towers JD, Bradley JP. Magnetic resonance appearance of posterosuperior labral peel back during humeral abduction and external rotation. Skeletal Radiol. 2010;39(1):19–26.
16. Bradley JP, Arner JW, Jayakumar S, Vyas D. Risk factors and outcomes of revision arthroscopic posterior shoulder capsulolabral repair. Am J Sports Med. 2018;46(10):2457–65.
17. Bradley JP, McClincy MP, Arner JW, Tejwani SG. Arthroscopic capsulolabral reconstruction for posterior instability of the shoulder: a prospective study of 200 shoulders. Am J Sports Med. 2013;41(9):2005–14.
18. Brelin A, Dickens JF. Posterior shoulder instability. Sports Med Arthrosc Rev. 2017;25(3):136–43.
19. Burkhart SS, Morgan CD, Kibler WB. The disabled throwing shoulder: spectrum of pathology part I: pathoanatomy and biomechanics. Arthroscopy. 2003;19(4):404–20.
20. Cancienne JM, Brockmeier SF, Carson EW, Werner BC. Risk factors for infection after shoulder arthroscopy in a large medicare population. Am J Sports Med. 2018;46(4):809–14.
21. Chalmers PN, Hammond J, Juhan T, Romeo AA. Revision posterior shoulder stabilization. J Shoulder Elb Surg. 2013;22(9):1209–20.
22. Christensen DL, Elsenbeck MJ, Wolfe JA, et al. Risk factors for failure of nonoperative treatment of posterior shoulder labral tears on magnetic resonance imaging. Mil Med. 2020;185(9–10):e1556–61.
23. Cognetti DJ, Hughes JD, Kay J, et al. Bone block augmentation of the posterior glenoid for recurrent posterior shoulder instability is associated with high rates of clinical failure: a systematic review. Arthroscopy. 2022;38(2):551–563 e555.
24. Cruz-Ferreira E, Abadie P, Godeneche A, et al. Posterior shoulder instability: prospective non-randomised comparison of operative and non-operative treatment in 51 patients. Orthop Traumatol Surg Res. 2017;103(8S):S185–8.
25. Davidson PA, Rivenburgh DW. The 7-o'clock postero-inferior portal for shoulder arthroscopy. Am J Sports Med. 2002;30(5):693–6.
26. DiMaria S, Bokshan SL, Nacca C, Owens B. History of surgical stabilization for posterior shoulder instability. JSES Open Access. 2019;3(4):350–6.
27. Farber JM, Buckwalter KA. Sports-related injuries of the shoulder: instability. Radiol Clin North Am. 2002;40(2):235–49.
28. Festbaum C, Minkus M, Akgun D, et al. Conservative treatment of acute traumatic posterior shoulder dislocations (Type A) is a viable option especially in patients with centred joint, low gamma angle, and

middle or old age. Knee Surg Sports Traumatol Arthrosc. 2022;30(7):2500–9.
29. Fourman MS, Arner JW, Bayer S, Vyas D, Bradley JP. Type VIII SLAP repair at midterm follow-up: throwers have greater pain, decreased function, and poorer return to play. Arthroscopy. 2018;34(12):3159–64.
30. Frank RM, Romeo AA, Provencher MT. Posterior glenohumeral instability: evidence-based treatment. J Am Acad Orthop Surg. 2017;25(9):610–23.
31. Fried JW, Hurley ET, Duenes ML, et al. Return to play after arthroscopic stabilization for posterior shoulder instability-a systematic review. Arthrosc Sports Med Rehabil. 2021;3(1):e249–56.
32. Galvin JW, Parada SA, Li X, Eichinger JK. Critical findings on magnetic resonance arthrograms in posterior shoulder instability compared with an age-matched controlled cohort. Am J Sports Med. 2016;44(12):3222–9.
33. Green CK, Scanaliato JP, Duvall O, et al. Biceps tenodesis combined with arthroscopic posterior labral repair for type VIII SLAP lesions in active-duty military patients yields excellent return to military duty. Arthroscopy. 2022;38:2620.
34. Green CK, Scanaliato JP, Fares AB, et al. Midterm outcomes after arthroscopic repair of type VIII SLAP lesions in active duty military patients younger than 35 years. Orthop J Sports Med. 2022;10(5):23259671221095908.
35. Hovis WD, Dean MT, Mallon WJ, Hawkins RJ. Posterior instability of the shoulder with secondary impingement in elite golfers. Am J Sports Med. 2002;30(6):886–90.
36. Katthagen JC, Tahal DS, Montgomery SR, Horan MP, Millett PJ. Association of traumatic and atraumatic posterior shoulder instability with glenoid retroversion and outcomes after arthroscopic capsulolabral repair. Arthroscopy. 2017;33(2):284–90.
37. Kibler WB, Grantham WJ, Pike JSM, Sciascia AD. Glenoid labral injuries are more common posteriorly than superiorly and are combined across multiple areas of the glenoid. Arthrosc Sports Med Rehabil. 2022;4(2):e535–44.
38. Kibler WB, Sciascia A, Tokish JT, et al. Disabled throwing shoulder: 2021 update: part 2-pathomechanics and treatment. Arthroscopy. 2022;38(5):1727–48.
39. Kim JH, Kim YS, Park I, et al. A comparison of open-construct PEEK suture anchor and non-vented biocomposite suture anchor in arthroscopic rotator cuff repair: a prospective randomized clinical trial. Arthroscopy. 2020;36(2):389–96.
40. Kim SH, Ha KI, Park JH, et al. Arthroscopic posterior labral repair and capsular shift for traumatic unidirectional recurrent posterior subluxation of the shoulder. J Bone Joint Surg Am. 2003;85(8):1479–87.
41. Kim SH, Ha KI, Yoo JC, Noh KC. Kim's lesion: an incomplete and concealed avulsion of the posteroinferior labrum in posterior or multidirectional posteroinferior instability of the shoulder. Arthroscopy. 2004;20(7):712–20.
42. Kim SH, Park JC, Park JS, Oh I. Painful jerk test: a predictor of success in nonoperative treatment of posteroinferior instability of the shoulder. Am J Sports Med. 2004;32(8):1849–55.
43. Kim SH, Park JS, Jeong WK, Shin SK. The Kim test: a novel test for posteroinferior labral lesion of the shoulder--a comparison to the jerk test. Am J Sports Med. 2005;33(8):1188–92.
44. Koga A, Itoigawa Y, Wada T, et al. Anatomic analysis of the attachment of the posteroinferior labrum and capsule to the glenoid: a cadaveric study. Arthroscopy. 2020;36(11):2814–9.
45. Ladd LM, Crews M, Maertz NA. Glenohumeral joint instability: a review of anatomy, clinical presentation, and imaging. Clin Sports Med. 2021;40(4):585–99.
46. Lanzi JT Jr, Chandler PJ, Cameron KL, Bader JM, Owens BD. Epidemiology of posterior glenohumeral instability in a young athletic population. Am J Sports Med. 2017;45(14):3315–21.
47. Matar RN, Shah NS, Gardner TJ, Grawe BM. Return to sport after surgical treatment for posterior shoulder instability: a systematic review. JSES Int. 2020;4(4):797–802.
48. McClincy MP, Arner JW, Bradley JP. Posterior shoulder instability in throwing athletes: a case-matched comparison of throwers and non-throwers. Arthroscopy. 2015;31(6):1041–51.
49. McClincy MP, Arner JW, Thurber L, Bradley JP. Arthroscopic capsulolabral reconstruction for posterior shoulder instability is successful in adolescent athletes. J Pediatr Orthop. 2020;40(3):135–41.
50. Meyer DC, Ernstbrunner L, Boyce G, et al. Posterior acromial morphology is significantly associated with posterior shoulder instability. J Bone Joint Surg Am. 2019;101(14):1253–60.
51. Modi CS, Karthikeyan S, Marks A, et al. Accuracy of abduction-external rotation MRA versus standard MRA in the diagnosis of intra-articular shoulder pathology. Orthopedics. 2013;36(3):e337–42.
52. Moeller EA, Houck DA, McCarty EC, et al. Outcomes of arthroscopic posterior shoulder stabilization in the beach-chair versus lateral decubitus position: a systematic review. Orthop J Sports Med. 2019;7(1):2325967118822452.
53. Mologne TS, Zhao K, Hongo M, et al. The addition of rotator interval closure after arthroscopic repair of either anterior or posterior shoulder instability: effect on glenohumeral translation and range of motion. Am J Sports Med. 2008;36(6):1123–31.
54. Morey VM, Singh H, Paladini P, et al. The Porcellini test: a novel test for accurate diagnosis of posterior labral tears of the shoulder: comparative analysis with the established tests. Musculoskelet Surg. 2016;100(3):199–205.
55. Nho SJ, Provencher MT, Seroyer ST, Romeo AA. Bioabsorbable anchors in glenohumeral shoulder surgery. Arthroscopy. 2009;25(7):788–93.

56. Nickoli MSLT, Arner JW, Conway JE, Bradley JP. The dynamic posterior instability test (D-PIT). Musculoskel J Hosp Special Surg. 2021;
57. Nourissat G, Radier C, Aim F, Lacoste S. Arthroscopic classification of posterior labrum glenoid insertion. Orthop Traumatol Surg Res. 2014;100(2):167–70.
58. Nusselt T, Freche S, Klinger HM, Baums MH. Intraosseous foreign body granuloma in rotator cuff repair with bioabsorbable suture anchor. Arch Orthop Trauma Surg. 2010;130(8):1037–40.
59. OKeefe KJ, Haupt E, Thomas WC, et al. Batter's shoulder: clinical outcomes and return to sport. Cureus. 2020;12(4):e7681.
60. Pollock RG, Bigliani LU. Recurrent posterior shoulder instability. Diagnosis and treatment. Clin Orthop Relat Res. 1993;291:85–96.
61. Price MR, Tillett ED, Acland RD, Nettleton GS. Determining the relationship of the axillary nerve to the shoulder joint capsule from an arthroscopic perspective. J Bone Joint Surg Am. 2004;86(10):2135–42.
62. Rapp CM, Shields EJ, Wiater BP, Wiater JM. Venous thromboembolism after shoulder arthroplasty and arthroscopy. J Am Acad Orthop Surg. 2019;27(8):265–74.
63. Rose MB, Noonan T. Glenohumeral internal rotation deficit in throwing athletes: current perspectives. Open Access J Sports Med. 2018;9:69–78.
64. Sheean AJ, Kibler WB, Conway J, Bradley JP. Posterior labral injury and glenohumeral instability in overhead athletes: current concepts for diagnosis and management. J Am Acad Orthop Surg. 2020;28(15):628–37.
65. Song DJ, Cook JB, Krul KP, et al. High frequency of posterior and combined shoulder instability in young active patients. J Shoulder Elb Surg. 2015;24(2):186–90.
66. Spoliti M. Glenoid osteolysis after arthroscopic labrum repair with a bioabsorbable suture anchor. Acta Orthop Belg. 2007;73(1):107–10.
67. Swan ER, Lynch TB, Sheean AJ, et al. High incidence of combined and posterior labral tears in military patients with operative shoulder instability. Am J Sports Med. 2022;50(6):1529–33.
68. Take Y, Yoneda M, Hayashida K, Nakagawa S, Mizuno N. Enlargement of drill holes after use of a biodegradable suture anchor: quantitative study on consecutive postoperative radiographs. Arthroscopy. 2008;24(3):251–7.
69. Tzannes A, Murrell GA. Clinical examination of the unstable shoulder. Sports Med. 2002;32(7):447–57.
70. Tzannes A, Paxinos A, Callanan M, Murrell GA. An assessment of the interexaminer reliability of tests for shoulder instability. J Shoulder Elb Surg. 2004;13(1):18–23.
71. Vaswani R, Arner J, Freiman H, Bradley JP. Risk factors for revision posterior shoulder stabilization in throwing athletes. Orthop J Sports Med. 2020;8(12):2325967120967652.
72. Von Raebrox A, Campbell B, Ramesh R, Bunker T. The association of subacromial dimples with recurrent posterior dislocation of the shoulder. J Shoulder Elb Surg. 2006;15(5):591–3.
73. Waltenspul M, Haller T, Ernstbrunner L, et al. Long-term results after posterior open glenoid wedge osteotomy for posterior shoulder instability associated with excessive glenoid retroversion. J Shoulder Elb Surg. 2022;31(1):81–9.
74. Wanich T, Dines J, Dines D, Gambardella RA, Yocum LA. Batter's shoulder': can athletes return to play at the same level after operative treatment? Clin Orthop Relat Res. 2012;470(6):1565–70.
75. Warner JJ, Navarro RA. Serratus anterior dysfunction. Recognition and treatment. Clin Orthop Relat Res. 1998;349:139–48.
76. Woodmass JM, Lee J, Johnson NR, et al. Nonoperative management of posterior shoulder instability: an assessment of survival and predictors for conversion to surgery at 1 to 10 years after diagnosis. Arthroscopy. 2019;35(7):1964–70.

27 Posterior Bankart Repair in the Beach Chair Position

Stephen E. Marcaccio, James Dove, Edward J. Testa, Patrick Morrissey, and Brett D. Owens

Introduction

While only representing less than 10% of shoulder instability events, posterior glenohumeral instability is becoming an increasingly appreciated clinical entity, and isolated posterior labral repairs constitute nearly a quarter of operatively managed shoulder instability events [1, 2]. Unilateral posterior shoulder instability can be attributed to a variety of potential etiologies, including seizures/electrocution, trauma, or repeated overhead activities [3]. Patient presentations vary widely, with some patients reporting vague shoulder discomfort with activities and others being notably unstable, presenting with subluxation and/or dislocation events [4]. Surgical treatment remains an appropriate approach for patients who have failed nonoperative management. However, the approach to surgical intervention falls on a broad spectrum and depends upon factors including soft tissue and bony pathology, with numerous potential open and arthroscopic surgical options [5].

The exact pathology that must be addressed operatively depends upon several factors, including the exact etiology of posterior glenohumeral instability and the anatomy involved. A thorough patient history, clinical examination, and imaging studies, such as radiographs, magnetic resonance imaging (MRI, +/− arthrography), and/or computed tomography (CT) scans, are imperative for the surgeon to create an appropriate operative plan [6]. The spectrum of pathophysiology involved in posterior glenohumeral instability includes posterior/posterior-inferior labral tears (posterior Bankart lesions) [7], avulsions of the posterior periosteum [8], reverse humeral avulsion of the glenohumeral ligament (HAGL) lesions [9], capsular laxity/capsulolabral detachments [10], humeral head defects (i.e., reverse Hill-Sachs lesions) [11], glenoid retroversion [12], posterior glenoid bone loss [13], and acromial morphology [14] (Fig. 27.1).

Surgical management remains the mainstay of treatment options for refractory symptoms caused by posterior glenohumeral instability. Numerous

S. E. Marcaccio (✉) · J. Dove · E. J. Testa
P. Morrissey · B. D. Owens
Department of Orthopaedic Surgery, Warren Alpert Medical School of Brown University, Providence, RI, USA

© The Author(s), under exclusive license to Springer Nature Switzerland AG 2026
R. M. Frank, J. M. Tokish (eds.), *Management of Shoulder Instability*,
https://doi.org/10.1007/978-3-032-18089-6_27

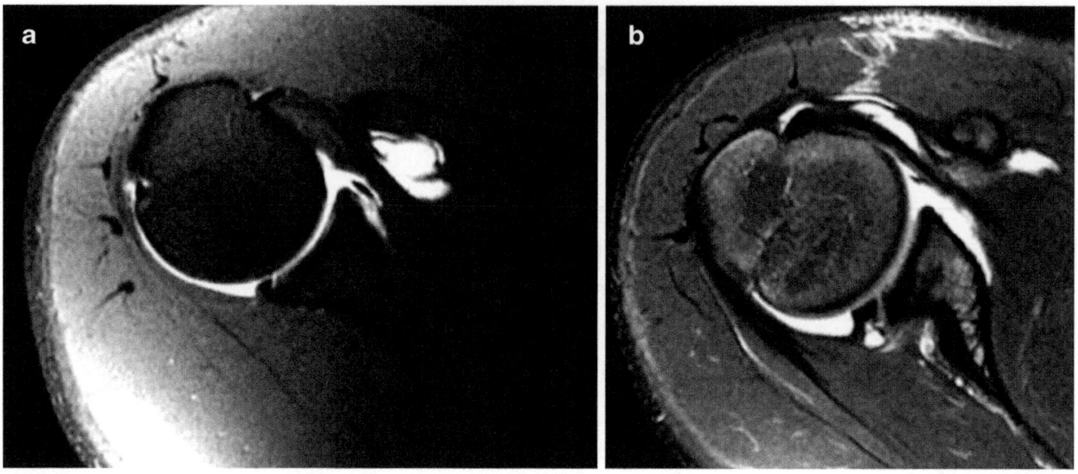

Fig. 27.1 (**a**) T2-weighted axial magnetic resonance image demonstrating a posterior labral tear. (**b**) Posterior labral tear with paralabral cyst. Antosh et al. [1]

operative treatment techniques have been described to address the specific pathology thought to be related to the cause of instability. Such procedures include arthroscopic or open posterior capsulolabral repair, filling an engaging humeral head bony defect with subscapularis tendon (i.e., reverse remplissage) [15], glenoid neck opening wedge osteotomy to treat pathologic retroversion [16], posterior glenoid bone blocks for posterior glenoid erosion [17], or even arthroplasty [18]. Concerns noted with some of these procedures include early development of arthritis, clinical failure, graft fracture, and neurologic injury [17]. While many of the aforementioned procedures involve open approaches, many patients with posterior glenohumeral instability can be treated with a less-invasive, arthroscopic approach. Moreover, recent literature suggests that arthroscopic treatment may result in superior patient-centric outcomes, lower recurrence rates, and greater return to sports (RTS) [19]. For this reason, arthroscopic posterior Bankart repair is an essential surgery for the orthopaedist's armament of techniques in the treatment of posterior shoulder instability.

Case Examples

Case 1: 17-Year-Old Male with Reverse Hill-Sachs and HAGL Lesions After Lacrosse Injury

A 17-year-old, right-hand-dominant male lacrosse player presented to the clinic 1 week after a presumed right shoulder dislocation after being hit during a lacrosse game. The patient immediately presented to an emergency department, and the shoulder was reduced. Unfortunately, no prereduction radiographs from the emergency department were available, but the notes described an anterior dislocation and reduction maneuver. Postreduction radiographs showed a humeral head incongruity consistent with a reverse Hill-Sachs lesion (Fig. 27.2). The patient's exam revealed a full range of motion, five out of five strength in the rotator cuff, and

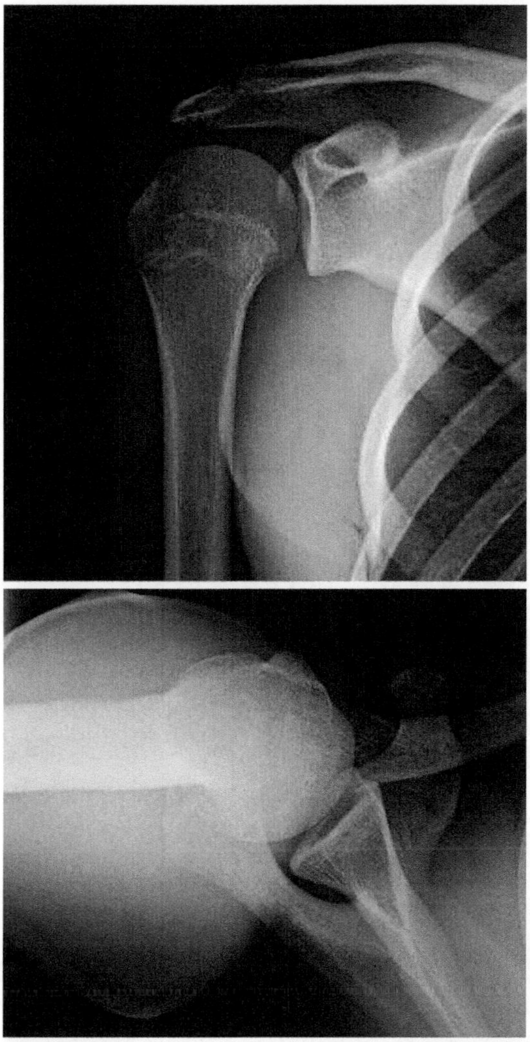

Fig. 27.2 17 yo M lacrosse player, two views of right shoulder status postreduction maneuver in the emergency department (courtesy of Dr. Brett Owens, MD)

negative Neer and Hawkins, Speeds, O'Brien's, and crossover tests but a grade 2+ posterior load shift test and a positive posterior apprehension test. His left shoulder exam was normal. An MR arthrogram confirmed the diagnosis of a reverse Hill-Sachs lesion with an associated posterior capsular tear and a reverse humeral avulsion glenohumeral (HAGL) lesion (Fig. 27.3). The patient, being a tri-sport high school varsity athlete and wishing to return to play in collision sports, elected to undergo surgical management.

The case was performed in the beach chair position with an interscalene block plus monitored anesthesia care. An initial diagnostic arthroscopy confirmed the diagnosis of a posterior labral flap tear, posterior capsular tear, and a reverse HAGL lesion. A standard anterior superior working portal was made at this point. First, the posterior inferior labral flap tear was debrided. Next, a 2.4-mm suture anchor was placed at the eight o'clock position and used for a posterior labral repair plus capsullorhaphy. To address the HAGL lesion, sutures were shuttled across the posterior inferior capsule and posterior band of the IGHL, which reduced to the humeral neck. This reduction was secured with an additional knotless 2.4-mm anchor. Finally, two interrupted stitches were placed through the horizontal posterior capsular rent. The stability of the repair was tested by confirming the elimination of posterior translation on a load shift maneuver. Examination at 3 months after operation revealed full ROM and negative load shift and apprehension tests.

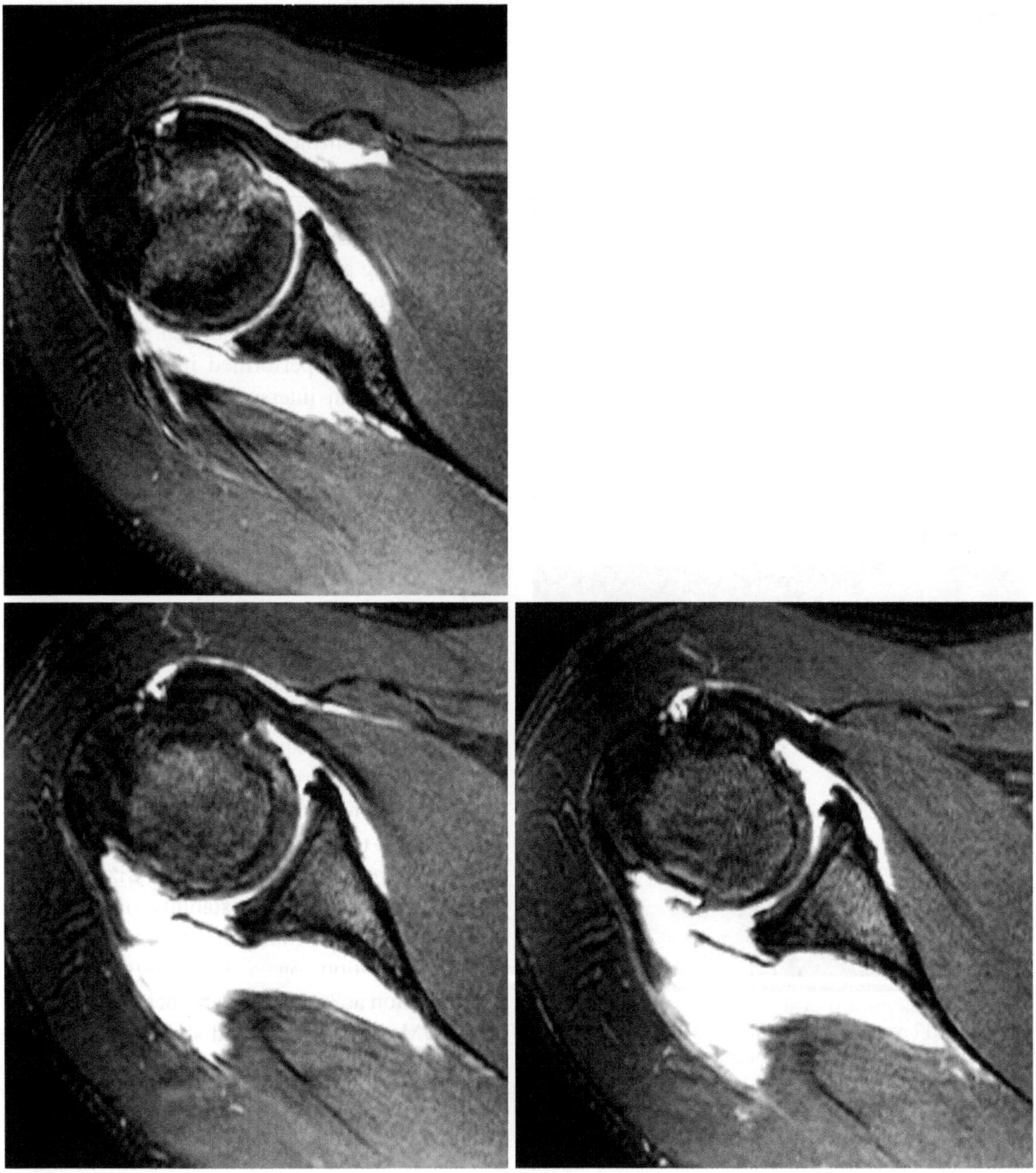

Fig. 27.3 Selected T2 axial images of MR arthroram in 17 yo M lacrosse player showing reverse Hill-Sachs lesion and reverse HAGL lesion. (Courtesy of Dr. Brett Owens, MD)

Case 2: 21-Year-Old Male with Large Reverse Hill-Sachs Lesion and Locked Posterior Glenohumeral Dislocation

A 21-year-old, right-hand-dominant male presented in clinic 5 weeks after a work-related injury with a right-sided, locked posterior glenohumeral dislocation. This patient had a history of seizures and has had multiple posterior shoulder dislocations bilaterally. After this episode, he presented to a local emergency department and received X-rays, which were read as normal. Weeks later, he underwent an MRI ordered by his primary care provider and was referred to an orthopedist. Physical examination of his right shoulder was remarkable for a clear posterior dislocation of the humeral head with very limited ROM about the shoulder. Examination of his contralateral shoulder showed full ROM, five out of five rotator cuff strength but grade 2+ anterior and posterior load shift testing, and a positive anterior and posterior apprehension test. Right shoulder radiographs revealed a posterior shoulder dislocation with a large reverse Hill-Sachs defect without significant glenoid bone loss (Fig. 27.4a–c). An MRI of the right shoulder revealed complete destruction of the posterior inferior labrum and capsule, an intact subscapularis, and mild glenoid retroversion (Fig. 27.5). The patient consented to a closed versus open reduction and arthroscopy to address posterior instability.

This case was performed in the beach chair position with general anesthesia and an interscalene block. The humeral head was first closed

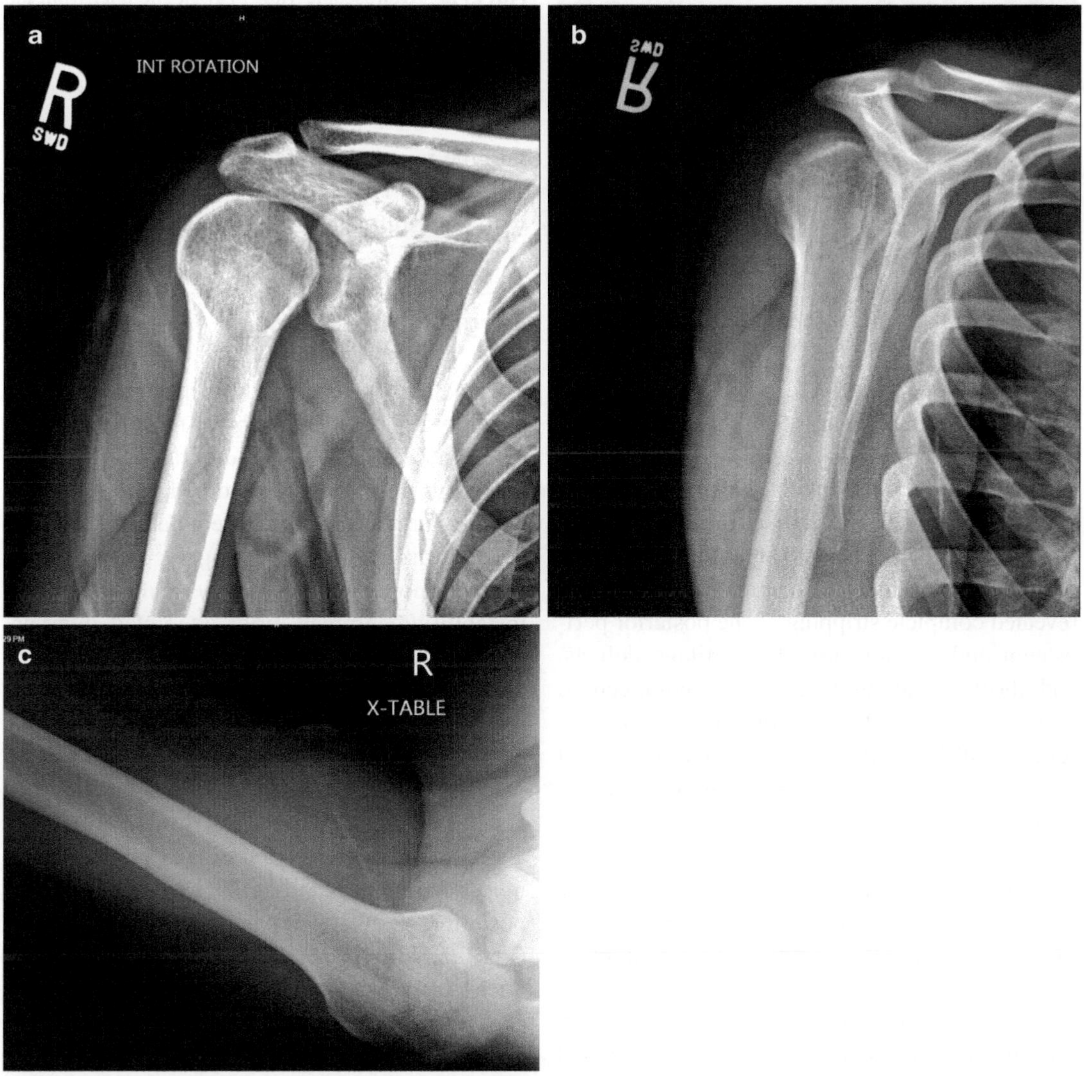

Fig. 27.4 (**a**) AP radiograph of right shoulder demonstrating locked posterior glenohumeral dislocation. (Courtesy of Dr. Brett Owens, MD). (**b**) Scapular Y radiograph demonstrating locked posterior shoulder dislocation. (Courtesy of Dr. Brett Owens, MD). (**c**) Axillary lateral view of right shoulder showing locked posterior shoulder dislocation with large anterior glenoid bone defect. (Courtesy of Dr. Brett Owens, MD)

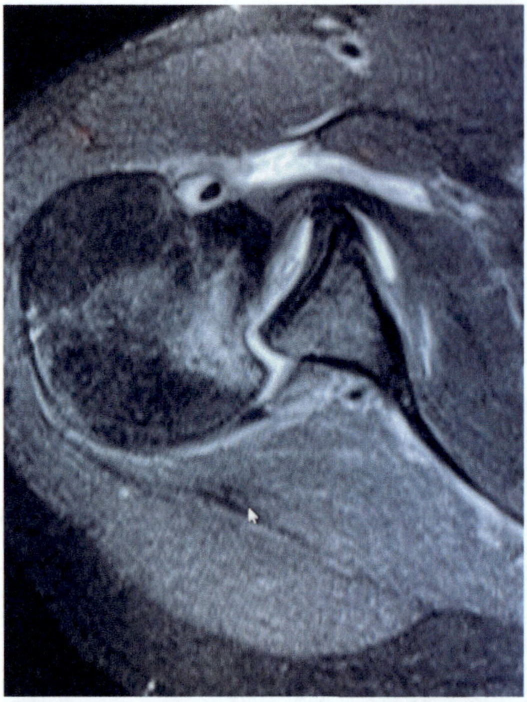

Fig. 27.5 MRI arthrogram (axial image) demonstrating locked posterior glenohumeral dislocation of the right shoulder with significant reverse Hill-Sachs defect. (Courtesy of Dr. Brett Owens, MD)

reduced with forward flexion, posterior pressure, and internal rotation to unlock the bony defect. Next, standard posterior and anterior arthroscopic portals were made. A diagnostic arthroscopy revealed complete stripping of the posterior periosteum and labrum, articular cartilage defects, and fibrillation along the central glenoid, central humeral head cartilage fibrillation, and a large reverse Hill-Sachs defect in the anterior humeral head (Fig. 27.6). After a thorough debridement, a posterior lateral portal was made at the seven o'clock position. A posterior Bankart repair was performed with three 2.9-mm knotless suture anchors starting at the six o'clock position and marching up the glenoid rim. Next, two double-loaded anchors were placed into the anterior Hill-Sachs defect through a percutaneous insertion kit, and a series of eight sutures were passed through the subscapularis tendon in a horizontal mattress fashion, completing the reverse remplissage procedure. The subscapularis was tenodesed into the reverse Hill-Sachs defect with appropriate tension. The stability of the repair was tested with load shift testing and was deemed stable.

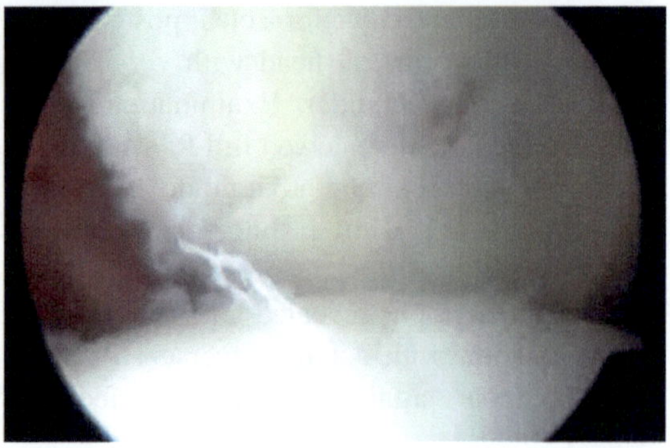

Fig. 27.6 Arthroscopic view of right shoulder from lateral portal demonstrating cartilage fibrillation and large reverse Hill-Sachs defect. (Courtesy of Dr. Brett Owens, MD)

Surgical Indications

Each patient presenting within the large spectrum of posterior shoulder instability must be carefully evaluated clinically and radiographically, as the treatment for patients should be highly individualized. Surgeons should have a detailed, patient-centric discussion regarding activity/sporting level, symptomatology, degree and direction of instability/recurrence, prior attempted interventions, and a history of ligamentous laxity. Imaging studies should be carefully reviewed for all concomitant pathology: labral tears, capsulolabral attenuation, reverse Hill-Sachs lesions, glenoid version, reverse HAGL lesions, glenoid bone loss, etc. Large and engaging reverse Hill-Sachs lesions, glenoid retroversion, and posterior glenoid bone loss exceeding 20% may fail isolated posterior Bankart repair [10, 12, 13, 20] (Fig. 27.1). In the setting of smaller reverse Hill-Sachs lesions, an arthroscopic reverse remplissage may be considered, while larger reverse Hill-Sachs lesions may necessitate management with open procedures, such as a lesser tuberosity transfer (i.e., McLaughlin procedure for patients with 20–45% head involvement), allograft reconstruction, or even arthroplasty (usually reserved for cases with greater than 45% head involvement) [21]. In the setting of a deficient posterior glenoid, open bony procedures such as the addition of bone blocks or a posterior glenoid opening wedge osteotomy may prevent recurrence [17].

Surgical Technique

When arthroscopic posterior Bankart repair is indicated, it is important to perform the procedure in a reproducible manner, utilizing a systematic approach with the following steps.

Anesthesia

The goals of anesthesia administration during the perioperative period include maximizing patient comfort intraoperatively, providing adequate muscular relaxation for ease of intraoperative exposure and facilitation of implant placement, and optimizing perioperative pain control in order to minimize both intraoperative and postoperative narcotic use [20]. These goals can be accomplished with a combination of both regional and general anesthetics. A preoperative interscalene block is performed on the operative side in the holding area under the use of ultrasound guidance. The use of the preoperative block has been shown to decrease intraoperative and postoperative narcotic requirements as well as improve subjective pain control postoperatively [22]. Often, the preoperative regional block is combined with procedural sedation in a multimodal approach to intraoperative pain control and relaxation [22]. However, there is concern about the adequacy of the preoperative block or the patient's ability to tolerate procedural sedation due to medical reasons (e.g., complex airway management due to obstructive sleep apnea, tolerance to anxiolytic medications requiring elevated and potentially dangerous doses), so general intravenous anesthesia techniques can be utilized to maximize patient safety and muscular relaxation [23].

Patient Positioning

Despite continued debate about the optimal position, there is no evidence that one position is superior for posterior instability repair, and surgeons should utilize the positioning that works best for their practice. The beach chair (BC) position is a safe, efficient, and effective method for performing a shoulder arthroscopy. In the BC position, patients are supine with the buttocks at the break of the bed and the hips flexed to 60°, a pillow or bone foam placed under the legs with the knees flexed to 30°, the back of the bed lifted to approximately 60°, the border medial of the scapula at the edge of bed, the nonoperative arm secured across the abdomen or in arm holder, the head secured in neutral position with a foam mask over the face to maximize cerebral perfusion, and the operative arm attached to an arm holder with sterile adhesive [24–26] (Fig. 27.7).

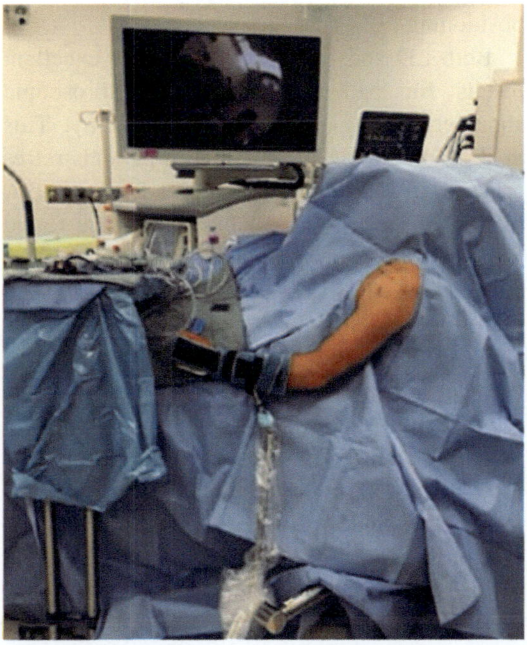

Fig. 27.7 Image of beach chair positioning for a left shoulder procedure, exposing the entire left sholder and left upper extremity, with the forearm secured into an arm holder. The arthroscopic monitor is seen in the center, beyond the sterile surgical field. [1]

The BC position was developed in the 1980s by Dr. Russell Warren, among others, to increase surgical efficiency and decrease neurologic complication rates [27]. There are several well-accepted advantages of the BC position, including reduced incidence of brachial plexus traction neuropraxia, decreased risk of neurologic injury during portal placement, the option to use regional anesthesia, and the ease of transition to open surgery [28–31]. Theoretical advantages to the BC position include increased arm mobility, improved intra-articular visualization, ease of setup, decreased surgical time, and an upright anatomic position that is ideal for instruction [29, 30].

Proponents of lateral decubitus (LD) positioning for shoulder arthroscopy note that the BC position comes with several disadvantages, including inferior visualization of the posterior and posterior-inferior aspects of the joint, neurologic injury from cerebral hypoperfusion, and concern for cranial nerve injury from the head positioning [32–36].

Both LD and BC positioning offer excellent results for patients undergoing arthroscopic shoulder surgery for posterior instability. This year, Bishop et al. examined 126 patients retrospectively (69 LD, 57 BC) who underwent a primary posterior shoulder labral repair and found no difference in postoperative patient-reported or clinical outcomes [37]. Similarly, Moeller et al. performed a systematic review that included 15 studies and 731 shoulders (626 LD, 104 BC) and found no difference in return-to-sport or recurrent instability rates [38]. Likewise, a large systematic review of 25 studies with 1085 patients (140 BC, 945 LD) who underwent surgery for posterior shoulder instability showed no significant difference in failure rates (BC 0 to 9% versus LD 0 to 29%) and revision rates (BC 8–9% versus LD 3.5 to 29%). Interestingly, the authors note a statistical trend toward lower recurrence rates and higher return to preinjury level rates in the BC position but state that inter-study variability precludes making any definitive recommendations [3].

Exam Under Anesthesia (EUA)

After anesthesia has been induced, an exam under anesthesia is performed to compare glenohumeral stability with the patient's contralateral side. A load and shift test is performed, placing one hand on the proximal forearm and the other hand on the humeral diaphysis, initiating both anteriorly and posteriorly directed force with the humerus abducted to approximately 60 degrees [4, 20] (Fig. 27.8). Further, anterior and posterior drawer tests can be performed, where the examiner uses one hand to stabilize the scapula and the other to apply anterior and posterior translation to the proximal humerus [39]. While both of these maneuvers function to assess the degree of glenohumeral instability, they differ in that the anterior and posterior drawer exam does not evaluate the glenohumeral joint with a pre-applied load [39]. It can be helpful to correlate physical examination findings in the office with the EUA; for BC surgery, we prefer our office examination to be performed in the adjacent seated position

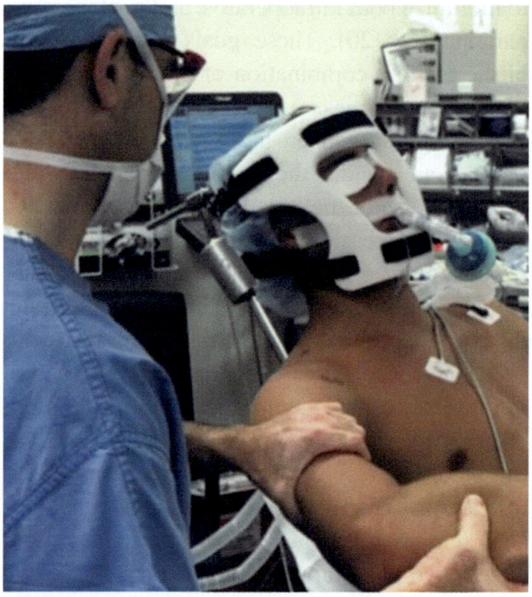

Fig. 27.8 Clinical image of patient in beach chair position, right shoulder exposed, with clinician performing examination under anesthesia of the right shoulder before prepping and draping to begin the procedure [20]

with the arm in a low abduction arc to closely mimic our EUA technique (Fig. 27.8).

Surgical Draping and Diagnostic Arthroscopy

After a thorough examination, the operative extremity is draped, and the arm is placed in a mechanical arm holder, which helps facilitate positioning throughout the surgical procedure (Fig. 27.9). Anatomic landmarks are palpated and marked on the extremity, including the distal clavicle, anterior and posterior acromial borders, scapular spine, acromio-clavicular joint, and the coracoid process. Planned locations for the portals to be utilized during the procedure are then marked, including the standard posterior-anterior working portals. Additional portals used for posterior capsulolabral repairs include the posterolateral and anterosuperior portals [1, 40]. The posterolateral portal, or the seven-o'clock portal, is essential for successful stabilization of posterior capsulolabral lesions as it facilitates access to the posteroinferior aspect of the glenohumeral joint for implant insertion [1, 40, 41]. The portal is often located about 2 cm lateral and 1 cm anterior to the original posterior portal, remaining in line with the posterior border of the distal clavicle (Fig. 27.10) [1, 41]. After the glenohumeral joint is accessed via the posterior portal, the anterior working portal (also known as the mid-glenoid portal) is established via outside-in needle localization just lateral to the coracoid process, entering the glenohumeral joint within the rotator interval, just above the subscapularis tendon [1, 40]. A diagnostic arthroscopy is performed via the original posterior portal, being careful to both characterize known pathology and identify any additional pathology that may have been missed on preoperative evaluation. This includes evaluation of the biceps tendon; rotator cuff musculature; glenohumeral articular surface; anterior, superior, and posterior labrum; and surrounding shoulder capsular and ligamentous structures [40] (Fig. 27.11). Another useful adjunctive diagnostic evaluation is the arthroscopic load shift. This is a load shift performed with the camera in the anterosuperior portal, providing direct observation of humeral translation on the glenoid. This can be especially helpful in bidirectional cases in which a balanced capsulorrhaphy may be necessary [42].

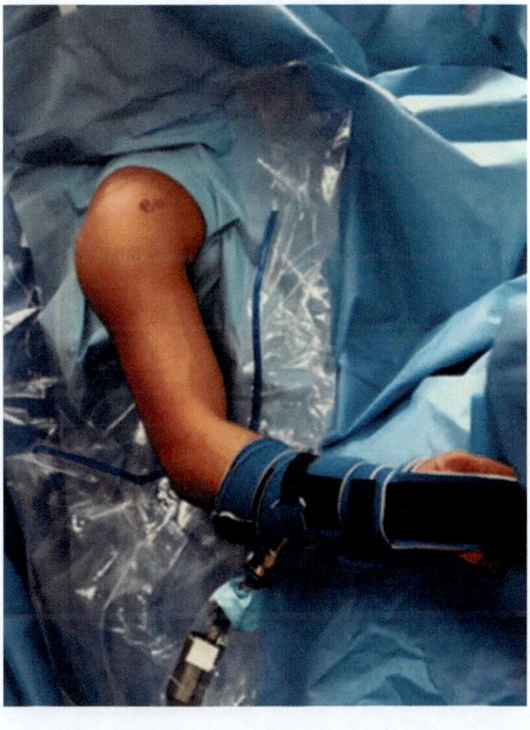

Fig. 27.9 Clinical image of patient in beach chair position, right shoulder exposed after prepping and draping. The forearm is secured in the arm holder, and the surgeon has access to the anterior and posterior shoulder. The clear drape is used to collect arthroscopic fluid that drains during the procedure [20]

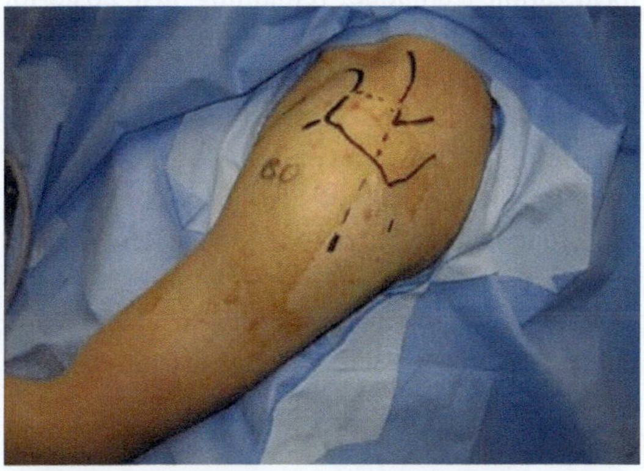

Fig. 27.10 Clinical image of left shoulder in beach chair position afte prepping and draping. The blue markings demonstrate the bone anatomy of the shoulder, including distal clavicle and acromion. The small markings represent various portal placements utilized in specific procedures [1]

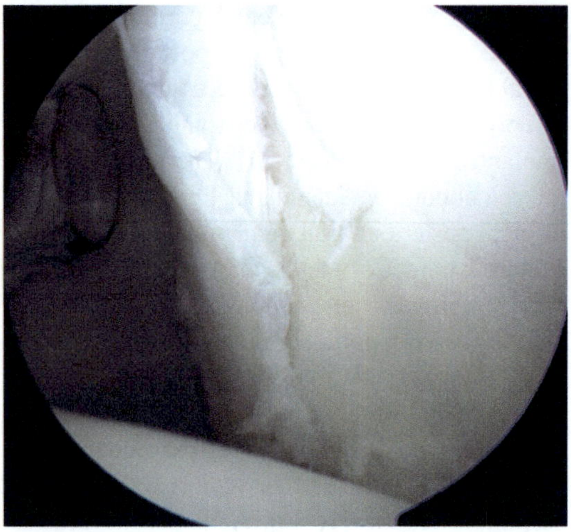

Fig. 27.11 Arthroscopic image of right shoulder from anterosuperolateral (ASL) portal, demonstrating posterior labral tear

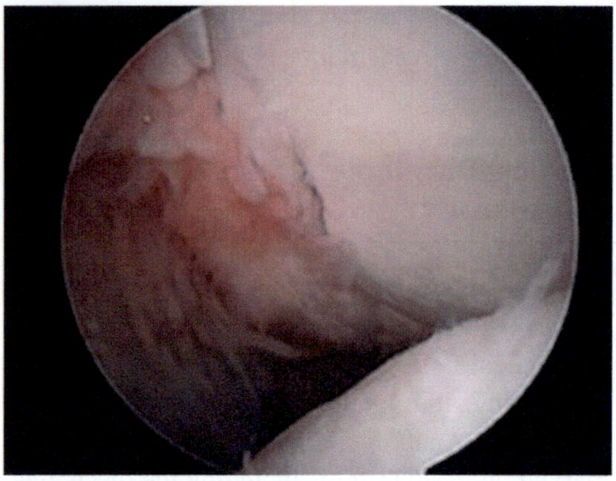

Fig. 27.12 Arthroscopic view of a right shoulder from the anterosuperolateral portal, demonstrating view of the humeral head and glenoid. This view assists with visualizing the anterior and posterior glenoid without blocking instrumentation access from anterior or posterior portals. [1]

Posterior Glenoid Labrum Preparation

Once a thorough diagnostic arthroscopy is performed, the anterosuperior portal is established via outside-in needle localization, entering the glenohumeral joint just lateral to the biceps tendon, high within the rotator interval. This portal provides excellent visualization of the inferior glenoid without interfering with the passage of instrumentation through the posterior portals (Fig. 27.12) [1, 40]. Finally, the posterolateral portal is established via an outside-in needle localization technique, remaining just posterior to the humeral head, being careful to avoid both damaging the articular cartilage and plunging into the capsule inferior to the glenoid, which risks injury to the axillary nerve (Fig. 27.13) [41]. Once this portal is established, labral preparation is initiated with the use of an elevator device introduced into the joint through either the mid-glenoid or anterosuperior portal while viewing either from the posterior portal or the anterior-based portal not occupied with instrumentation (Fig. 27.14). This serves to mobilize the injured capsulo-labral complex from any scar tissue that may have formed. Further, preparing the labrum from an anteriorly based portal allows for optimal trajectory of instrumentation while reducing the risk of glenohumeral chondral or labral damage [41]. After the capsulolabral complex is ade-

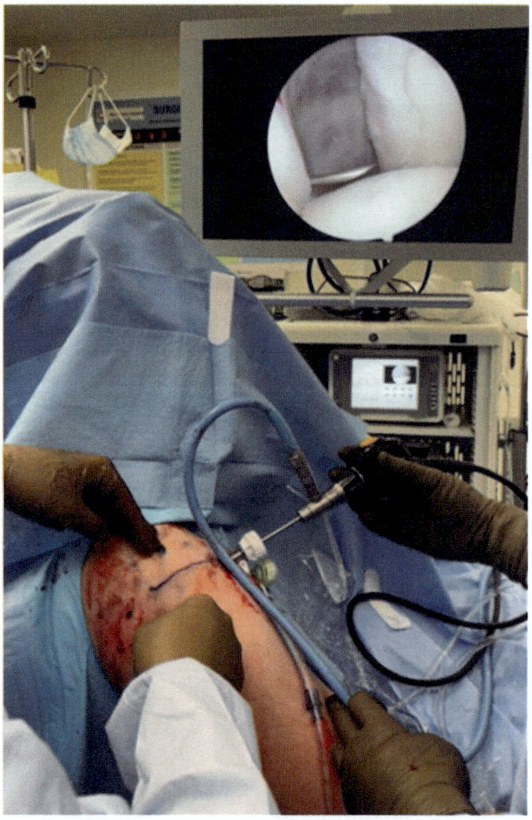

Fig. 27.13 Clinical image of the right shoulder exposed during surgery, beach chair position. The arthroscopic monitor is showing the surgeon's arthroscopic view from the anterosuperolateral (ASL) portal, which shows the posterior aspect of the glenoid, and the surgeon using a needle to pinpoint the exact location of the planned portal

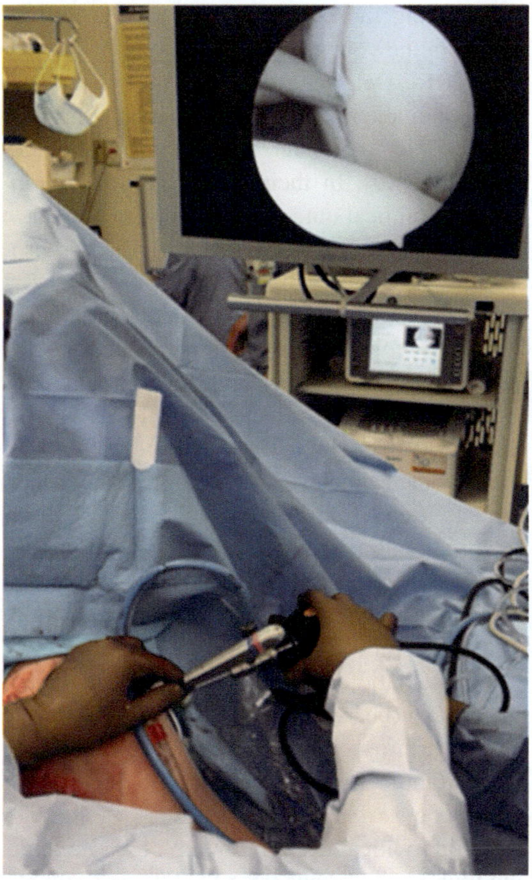

Fig. 27.14 Clinical image of the right shoulder exposed during surgery, beach chair position. The arthroscopic monitor is showing the surgeon's arthroscopic view from the anterosuperolateral (ASL) portal, which shows the posterior aspect of the glenoid, and the surgeon placing an instrument to prepare the posterior labrum for repair

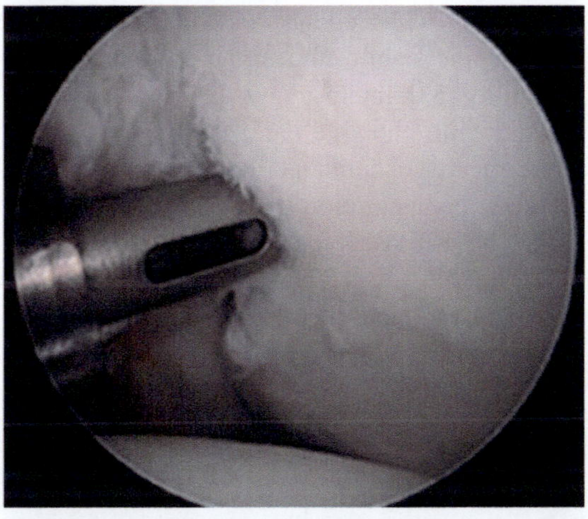

Fig. 27.15 Arthroscopic view of right shoulder from the anterosuperlateral portal, demonstrating anchor placement for posterior labrum repair. [1]

quately mobilized, an arthroscopic shaver or bur can be utilized to prepare the bony glenoid surface and promote an ideal bony bed for labral healing [1, 40] (Fig. 27.15).

Posterior Glenoid Labrum Repair

Once the capsulolabral complex is mobilized and the anatomic location for repair is prepared with an adequate bed of bleeding tissue, labral repair is initiated. The most inferior aspect of the capsulo-labral injury should be addressed first (beginning at the six o'clock position), as each capsulolabral repair stitch will progressively decrease the volume of the glenohumeral joint [41, 43]. While this concept is important for successful outcomes when treating shoulder instability, the gradual decrease in glenohumeral joint volume can make visualization difficult and interfere with accurate anchor placement, leading to suboptimal capsulolabral stabilization [40, 41]. Once shuttling is complete, the anchor is planned and placed on the rim. Both knotted and knotless suture anchors have been shown to be effective in the fixation of the labral injury [48]. This process is repeated, moving superiorly, with anchors placed approximately every 5 mm apart on the posterior glenoid edge, with the number of anchors determined by the extent of the capsulolabral injury (Fig. 27.16) [40, 41, 43]. Once completed, arthroscopic load shift can be repeated to ensure elimination of pathologic translation.

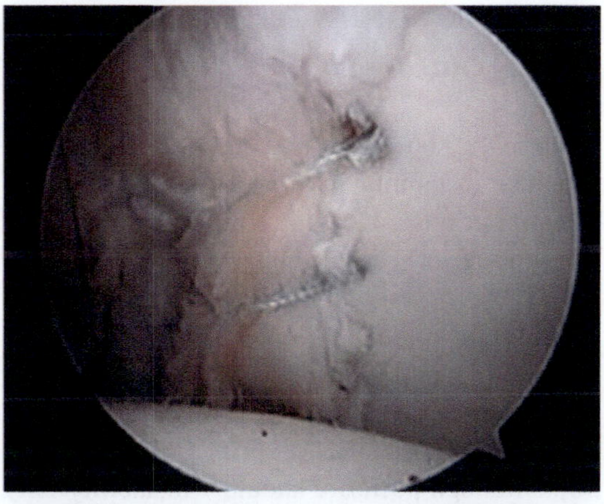

Fig. 27.16 Arthroscopic view of right shoulder from anterosuperolateral (ASL) portal, demonstrating completed posterior labral repair with sutures in place. [1]

Postoperative Rehabilitation

Postoperatively, patients are immobilized in an abduction sling for approximately four to 6 weeks. Some physicians advocate for immobilization in external rotation postoperatively to reduce the stress applied to the posterior capsulolabral repair with internal rotation of the arm [44]. It is our preferred practice to employ the use of an external rotation sling for 6 weeks. In the initial postoperative period, patients should perform active elbow and wrist range of motion (ROM), as well as pendulum exercises to prevent stiffness and shoulder shrugs to improve scapulothoracic coordination [1, 41]. Two weeks postoperatively, patients initiate active assisted ROM of the shoulder with flexion to 90 degrees, abduction to 60 degrees, and external rotation to 45–60°, continuing to avoid internal rotation [1, 45]. At about 6 weeks, the patient discontinues the sling and initiates active range of motion of the shoulder in all planes in a graduated strength and motion protocol, including light strengthening of the rotator cuff musculature [1, 45]. Patients often are allowed to return to full activity after completing a sport-specific training program, typically around four to 6 months postoperatively [41]. It should be noted that postoperative rehabilitation protocols should be tailored to the individual patient and should be adjusted based on the patient's injury pathology, surgical treatment, and long-term activity goals.

Clinical Outcomes

Historically, operative procedures for posterior shoulder instability have included a variety of options such as a glenoid or humeral osteotomy, open posterior capsulorrhaphy, posterior bone block procedures, and arthroscopic stabilization [46–48]. Over the last several years, however, there has been a significant trend to treat these injuries arthroscopically to avoid a large open procedure, especially for primary repairs [49, 50]. Although posterior shoulder instability only comprises about 10% of all shoulder instability, it is becoming more recognized and successfully treated in the young, active population [51].

In 2015, DeLong et al. performed one of the first systematic reviews to examine outcomes for arthroscopic treatment of posterior shoulder instability [19]. In their review, they also captured the clinical outcomes for open treatment to help determine superiority between the two procedures. By examining 53 studies (27 arthroscopic, 26 open), DeLong et al. concluded that arthroscopic stabilization for posterior shoulder instability was an effective and reliable treatment, but throwing athletes were less likely to return to their preinjury levels of sport compared with contact athletes. They also concluded that patients treated arthroscopically had superior outcomes compared with patients who underwent open procedures, specifically regarding recurrence of instability, patient satisfaction, RTS, and return to the previous level of play [19]. The systematic review did not specify patient positioning (beach chair versus lateral decubitus) for the arthroscopic procedures. Also in 2015, Leivadiotou et al. reviewed six studies of arthroscopic treatment of posterior shoulder instability with a mean follow-up of 44.4 months and found a recurrence rate of 5.37% and a 92.5% RTS rate [52]. Both of these early systematic reviews showed promising results from arthroscopic treatment of posterior shoulder instability.

More recently, in 2017, Jain et al. performed a systematic review to describe factors that are associated with poorer outcomes following arthroscopic stabilization for posterior shoulder instability [53]. Interestingly, they concluded that patients with chondral damage, previous shoulder surgery, concomitant shoulder surgery, and workers' compensation status led to poorer outcomes for arthroscopic repair of posterior shoulder instability. In a young military population, Galvin et al. found that the presence or absence of glenoid dysplasia did not affect the outcome following arthroscopic posterior labral repair, but a history of mental health encounters and an infantry military occupational specialty (MOS) were associated with poorer clinical outcomes [54]. Glenoid dysplasia was defined by the classification described by Weishaupt et al. [55]. Others, however, have recommended performing bony procedures, such as a glenoid osteotomy or posterior bone block, at the time of the primary repair if the glenoid dysplasia is severe (retroversion greater than 25°) [51]· [45]. These rare instances, however, are outside of the scope of this discussion for arthroscopic primary repair of posterior shoulder instability.

As posterior shoulder instability has been shown mostly to affect athletes, including weightlifters, football linemen, baseball players, and military personnel [51]· [56], RTS or return to activity is a significant outcome measure. In a systematic review from 2020, Matar et al. reported a RTS rate that ranged from 57.9% to 100% and a return to preinjury level rate that ranged from 47.4% to 100% [57]. Revision rates ranged from 0% to 36.8%. Although the majority of the studies included did not classify RTS rate based on sport, two studies found a lower RTS rate for throwing athletes compared to non-throwing athletes [58]· [59]. Ultimately, Matar et al. concluded high rates of RTS among all athletes who underwent arthroscopic stabilization for posterior shoulder instability [57]. More recently, in 2022, Gouveia et al. performed a systematic review for RTS after surgical stabilization for posterior shoulder instability and similarly found a high rate of return for all athletes, but only about two-thirds of athletes returned to their preinjury levels of sport [60]. Arthroscopic stabilization for posterior shoulder instability provides athletes with an effective and reliable option to return to play, although counseling and expectations should be discussed with the patients, as some are unable to return to their prior level of sport.

References

1. Antosh IJ, Tokish JM, Owens BD. Posterior shoulder instability: current surgical management. Sports Health. 2016;8(6):520–6.
2. Song DJ, Cook JB, Krul KP, Bottoni CR, Rowles DJ, Shaha SH, et al. High frequency of posterior and combined shoulder instability in young active patients. J Shoulder Elb Surg. 2015;24(2):186–90.
3. de Sa D, Sheean AJ, Morales-Restrepo A, Dombrowski M, Kay J, Vyas D. Patient positioning in arthroscopic Management of Posterior-Inferior Shoulder Instability: a systematic review comparing beach chair and lateral decubitus approaches. Arthrosc J Arthrosc Relat Surg. 2019;35(1):214–224.e3. [cited 2022 Jun 17]. Available from: https://linkinghub.elsevier.com/retrieve/pii/S0749806318305929.
4. DeLong JM, Jiang K, Bradley JP. Posterior instability of the shoulder. Am J Sports Med. 2015;43(7):1805–17.
5. Wagner ER, Gottschalk MB. Editorial commentary: open posterior shoulder stabilization—when is it needed? Glenoid bone loss patterns are not created equal. Arthrosc J Arthrosc Relat Surg. 2019;35(10):2785–7.
6. Bäcker HC, Galle SE, Maniglio M, Rosenwasser MP. Biomechanics of posterior shoulder instability – current knowledge and literature review. World J Orthop. 2018;9(11):245–54.
7. Murphy CP, Frangiamore SJ, Mannava S, Sanchez A, Beiter E, Whalen JM, et al. Effect of posterior glenoid labral tears at the NFL combine on future NFL performance. Orthop J Sports Med. 2018;6(10):232596711878746.
8. Shah N, Tung GA. Imaging signs of posterior Glenohumeral instability. Am J Roentgenol. 2009;192(3):730–5.
9. Smith PA, Nuelle CW, Bradley JP. Arthroscopic repair of a posterior bony humeral avulsion of the Glenohumeral ligament with associated Teres minor avulsion. Arthrosc Tech. 2014;3(1):e89–94.
10. Seebauer L, Keyl W. Posterior glenohumeral instability. Orthopade. 1998;27(8):542–55.
11. Moroder P, Tauber M, Scheibel M, Habermeyer P, Imhoff AB, Liem D, et al. Defect characteristics of reverse hill-Sachs lesions. Am J Sports Med. 2016;44(3):708–14.
12. Marcaccio SE, O'Donnel RM, Schilkowsky R, Owens MBD, Bokshan SL. Posterior glenoid osteotomy with Capsulolabral repair improves resistance forces in a critical glenoid bone loss model. Orthop J Sport Med. 2022;10(3):232596712210835.
13. Nacca C, Gil JA, Badida R, Crisco JJ, Owens BD. Critical glenoid bone loss in posterior shoulder instability. Am J Sports Med. 2018;46(5):1058–63.
14. Meyer DC, Ernstbrunner L, Boyce G, Imam MA, El Nashar R, Gerber C. Posterior acromial morphology is significantly associated with posterior shoulder instability. J Bone Joint Surg Am. 2019;101(14):1253–60. [cited 2022 Jun 20]. Available from: https://pubmed.ncbi.nlm.nih.gov/31318804/
15. Lavender CD, Hanzlik SR, Pearson SE, Caldwell PE. Arthroscopic reverse Remplissage for posterior instability. Arthrosc Tech. 2016;5(1):e43–7.
16. Lacheta L, Singh TSP, Hovsepian JM, Braun S, Imhoff AB, Pogorzelski J. Posterior open wedge glenoid osteotomy provides reliable results in young patients with increased glenoid retroversion and posterior shoulder

instability. Knee Surg Sports Traumatol Arthrosc. 2019;27(1):299–304.
17. Servien E, Walch G, Cortes ZE, Edwards TB, O'Connor DP. Posterior bone block procedure for posterior shoulder instability. Knee Surg Sport Traumatol Arthrosc. 2007;15(9):1130–6.
18. Checchia SL, Santos PD, Miyazaki AN. Surgical treatment of acute and chronic posterior fracture-dislocation of the shoulder. J Shoulder Elb Surg. 1998;7(1):53–65.
19. DeLong JM, Jiang K, Bradley JP. Posterior instability of the shoulder: a systematic review and Meta-analysis of clinical outcomes. Am J Sports Med. 2015;43(7):1805–17.
20. Bokshan SL, Marcaccio SE, Lemme NJ, Owens BD. Open Bankart repair for anterior shoulder instability. Oper Tech Orthop. 2020;30(3):100822.
21. Konda SR, Fisher N, Gage M, Egol KA. Posterior fracture dislocation of the shoulder: A modified McLaughlin procedure. J Orthop Trauma. 2017;31(3):S36–7.
22. Sánchez Novas D, Biscaiburo JP, Terrasa S, Vescovo A. Patient satisfaction and opioid requirements after ultrasound-guided interscalene block for arthroscopic shoulder surgery among operators with different levels of experience: A prospective observational study. J Clin Anesth. 2020;62. [cited 2022 Jun 20]. Available from: https://pubmed.ncbi.nlm.nih.gov/31978842/.
23. Bambaren IA, Dominguez F, Elias Martin ME, Domínguez S. Anesthesia and analgesia in the patient with an unstable shoulder. Open Orthop J. 2017;11(1):848–60. [cited 2022 Jun 20]. Available from: https://pubmed.ncbi.nlm.nih.gov/29114334/.
24. Higgins JD, Frank RM, Hamamoto JT, Provencher MT, Romeo AA, Verma NN. Shoulder arthroscopy in the beach chair position. Arthrosc Tech. 2017;6(4):e1153–8.
25. Mannava S, Jinnah AH, Plate JF, Stone AV, Tuohy CJ, Freehill MT. Basic shoulder arthroscopy: beach chair patient positioning. Arthrosc Tech. 2016;5(4):e731–5.
26. Provencher MT, McIntire ES, Gaston TM, Frank RM, Solomon CDJ. Avoiding complications in shoulder arthroscopy: pearls for lateral decubitus and beach chair positioning. Tech Shoulder Elbow Surg. 2010;11(1):1–3.
27. Skyhar MJ, Altchek DW, Warren RF, Wickiewicz TL, O'Brien SJ. Shoulder arthroscopy with the patient in the beach-chair position. Arthrosc J Arthrosc Relat Surg. 1988;4(4):256–9.
28. Gelber PE, Reina F, Caceres E, Monllau JC. A comparison of risk between the lateral decubitus and the beach-chair position when establishing an Anteroinferior shoulder portal: A cadaveric study. Arthrosc J Arthrosc Relat Surg. 2007;23(5):522–8.
29. Li X, Eichinger JK, Hartshorn T, Zhou H, Matzkin EG, Warner JP. A comparison of the lateral decubitus and beach-chair positions for shoulder surgery: advantages and complications. J Am Acad Orthop Surg. 2015;23(1):18–28.
30. Peruto CM, Ciccotti MG, Cohen SB. Shoulder arthroscopy positioning: lateral decubitus Versus Beach chair. Arthrosc – J Arthrosc Relat Surg. 2009;25(8):891–6.
31. Paxton ES, Backus J, Keener J, Brophy RH. Shoulder arthroscopy: basic principles of positioning, anesthesia, and portal anatomy. J Am Acad Orthop Surg. 2013;21(6):332–42.
32. Rains DD, Rooke GA, Wahl CJ. Pathomechanisms and complications related to patient positioning and anesthesia during shoulder arthroscopy. Arthrosc – J Arthrosc Relat Surg. 2011;27(4):532–41.
33. Murphy GS, Greenberg SB, Szokol JW. Safety of beach chair position shoulder surgery: A review of the current literature. Anesth Analg. 2019;129(1):101–18.
34. Fulle G. Les sources d'influence des pratiques d'emploi instaurées par les entreprises multinationales originaires des pays européens dans leurs filiales québécoises. 2014;120(1):176–85.
35. Koh JL, Levin SD, Chehab EL, Murphy GS. Neer Award 2012: cerebral oxygenation in the beach chair position: A prospective study on the effect of general anesthesia compared with regional anesthesia and sedation. J Shoulder Elbow Surg. 2013;22(10):1325–31. https://doi.org/10.1016/j.jse.2013.01.035.
36. Moerman AT, De Hert SG, Jacobs TF, De Wilde LF, Wouters PF. Cerebral oxygen desaturation during beach chair position. Eur J Anaesthesiol. 2012;29(2):82–7.
37. Paul RW, Zareef U, Streicher S, Osman A, Erickson BJ, Freedman KB, et al. Beach-chair versus lateral decubitus positioning for arthroscopic posterior shoulder labral repair: A retrospective comparison of clinical and patient-reported outcomes. Am J Sports Med. 2022; https://doi.org/10.1177/03635465221095243.
38. Moeller EA, Houck DA, McCarty EC, Seidl AJ, Bravman JT, Vidal AF, et al. Outcomes of arthroscopic posterior shoulder stabilization in the beach-chair versus lateral decubitus position: a systematic review. Orthop J Sports Med. 2019;7(1):2325967118822452.
39. Lizzio VA, Meta F, Fidai M, Makhni EC. Clinical evaluation and physical exam findings in patients with anterior shoulder instability. Curr Rev Musculoskelet Med. 2017;10(4):434–41. [cited 2022 Jun 20]. Available from: https://pubmed.ncbi.nlm.nih.gov/29043566/.
40. Cvetanovich GL, Hamamoto JT, Campbell KJ, McCarthy M, Higgins JD, Verma NN. The use of accessory portals in Bankart repair with posterior extension in the lateral decubitus position. Arthrosc Tech. 2016;5(5):e1121–8. [cited 2022 Jun 20]. Available from: http://www.arthroscopytechniques.org/article/S2212628716300652/fulltext.
41. Provencher MT, Leclere LE, King S, McDonald LS, Frank RM, Mologne TS, et al. Posterior instability of the shoulder: diagnosis and management. Am J Sports Med. 2011;39(4):874–86. [cited 2022 Jun 20]. Available from: https://pubmed.ncbi.nlm.nih.gov/21131678/.

42. DeFroda SF, Owens BD. Arthroscopic load-shift technique for intraoperative assessment of shoulder translation. Arthrosc Tech. 2018;7(3):e211–4.
43. Bokshan SL, DeFroda SF, Gil JA, Badida R, Crisco JJ, Owens BD. The 6-o'clock anchor increases labral repair strength in a biomechanical shoulder instability model. Arthroscopy. 2019;35(10):2795–800. [cited 2022 Jun 20]. Available from: https://pubmed.ncbi.nlm.nih.gov/31395394/.
44. Kim SH, Ha KI, Park JH, Kim YM, Lee YS, Lee JY, et al. Arthroscopic posterior labral repair and capsular shift for traumatic unidirectional recurrent posterior subluxation of the shoulder. J Bone Joint Surg Am. 2003;85(8):1479–87. [cited 2022 Jun 22]. Available from: https://pubmed.ncbi.nlm.nih.gov/12925627/.
45. Owens BD, Tucker CJ, Zacchilli M. Surgical management of posterior shoulder instability. Curr Orthop Pract. 2011;22(6):474–82.
46. Murrell GA, Warren RF. The surgical treatment of posterior shoulder instability. Clin Sports Med. 1995;14(4):903–15.
47. Tibone JE, Bradley JP. The treatment of posterior subluxation in athletes. Clin Orthop Relat Res. 1993;291:124–37.
48. Pollock RG, Bigliani LU. Recurrent posterior shoulder instability. Diagnosis and treatment. Clin Orthop Relat Res. 1993;291:85–96.
49. Savoie FH 3rd, Holt MS, Field LD, Ramsey JR. Arthroscopic management of posterior instability: evolution of technique and results. Arthrosc J Arthrosc Relat Surg. 2008;24(4):389–96.
50. DiMaria S, Bokshan SL, Nacca C, Owens B. History of surgical stabilization for posterior shoulder instability. JSES Open Access. 2019;3(4):350–6.
51. Antosh IJ, Tokish JM, Owens BD. Posterior shoulder instability. Sports Health. 2016;8(6):520–6.
52. Leivadiotou D, Ahrens P. Arthroscopic treatment of posterior shoulder instability: a systematic review. Arthrosc J Arthrosc Relat Surg. 2015;31(3):555–60.
53. Jain SR, Sayampanathan AA, Hwee Chye Tan A. Arthroscopic management of posterior instability of the shoulder: a systematic review of predictive factors associated with poorer surgical outcomes. J Orthop Surg (Hong Kong). 2017;25(3):2309499017743102.
54. Galvin JW, Morte DR, Grassbaugh JA, Parada SA, Burns SH, Eichinger JK. Arthroscopic treatment of posterior shoulder instability in patients with and without glenoid dysplasia: a comparative outcomes analysis. J Shoulder Elb Surg. 2017;26(12):2103–9.
55. Weishaupt D, Zanetti M, Nyffeler RW, Gerber C, Hodler J. Posterior glenoid rim deficiency in recurrent (atraumatic) posterior shoulder instability. Skeletal Radiol. 2000;29(4):204–10.
56. Brelin A, Dickens JF. Posterior shoulder instability. Sports Med Arthrosc. 2017;25(3):136–43.
57. Matar RN, Shah NS, Gardner TJ, Grawe BM. Return to sport after surgical treatment for posterior shoulder instability: a systematic review. JSES Int. 2020;4(4):797–802.
58. McClincy MP, Arner JW, Bradley JP. Posterior shoulder instability in throwing athletes: A case-matched comparison of throwers and non-throwers. Arthroscopy. 2015;31(6):1041–51.
59. Radkowski CA, Chhabra A, Baker CL 3rd, Tejwani SG, Bradley JP. Arthroscopic capsulolabral repair for posterior shoulder instability in throwing athletes compared with nonthrowing athletes. Am J Sports Med. 2008;36(4):693–9.
60. Gouveia K, Kay J, Memon M, Simunovic N, Bedi A, Ayeni OR. Return to sport after surgical Management of Posterior Shoulder Instability: a systematic review and Meta-analysis. Am J Sports Med. 2022;50(3):845–57.

RHAGL: Arthroscopic Approach

28

Misty Suri, Jordan Nester, and Arjun Verma

Introduction

Posterior shoulder instability is a well-known pathology. It is most often described as traumatic or associated with seizure or electric shock events. The shoulder is stabilized by its capsuloligamentous complex, humeral head and glenoid articulation, capsular attachments, and the dynamic stabilizers. The posterior inferior glenohumeral ligament (PIGHL), as well as the posterior labrum and capsule, is the primary restraint to posterior translation when the arm is in a position of flexion, abduction, and internal rotation [1, 2]. As seen in anterior shoulder instability with humeral avulsion of glenohumeral ligament (HAGL) injuries [3], posterior HAGL injuries have been described [4–6].

Illustrative Clinical Case

HPI A 17-year-old right-hand-dominant male football player (quarterback) presented to the clinic with right shoulder pain after a lineman landed on top of him and drove his right throwing shoulder into the ground during a game. He was not able to return to play at the time. He did not feel his shoulder dislocate and had never had an injury to this shoulder before. He denied any numbness or tingling in the right upper extremity. He denied any neck or back pain.

He was able to continue playing after a few days of rest and improvement in his pain. He had symptomatic treatment at that time, including over-the-counter pain medications, kinesiotaping of the shoulder, and bio-freeze gel. However, after 6 weeks of the above symptomatic treatment methods, he had a recurrence of symptoms and so was re-evaluated.

Exam Well-developed, well-nourished male. Neck exam demonstrated no tenderness to palpation and no pain with flexion/extension or lateral rotation to either side.

Right Upper Extremity (RUE) No obvious deformity present. The active range of motion (AROM) and passive range of motion (PROM) of both shoulders were symmetric in all planes. Forward elevation was 170 (AROM) and 175 (PROM), external rotation in adduction was 60 (AROM) and 65 (PROM), external rotation at 90 degrees of abduction was 90 (AROM) and 90 (PROM), internal rotation in adduction was to the T10 spine level, and internal rotation in 90

M. Suri (✉)
Ochsner Andrews Sports Medicine Institute, Department of Orthopedic Surgery, Ochsner Health System, New Orleans, LA, USA
e-mail: msuri@ochsner.org

J. Nester · A. Verma
Oschner Orthopedic Surgery, New Orleans, LA, USA

© The Author(s), under exclusive license to Springer Nature Switzerland AG 2026
R. M. Frank, J. M. Tokish (eds.), *Management of Shoulder Instability*,
https://doi.org/10.1007/978-3-032-18089-6_28

degrees of abduction was 40 (PROM). There was no weakness in the testing of the rotator cuff musculature. Shoulder stability testing demonstrated no increase in anterior translation when compared to the contralateral side, but the right shoulder did demonstrate grade 2 translation on posterior translation testing. Apprehension testing in abduction and external rotation was negative bilaterally with no change on relocation. The Jerk test and Kim test were positive for reproduction of symptoms on the right shoulder and negative on the left shoulder.

Imaging

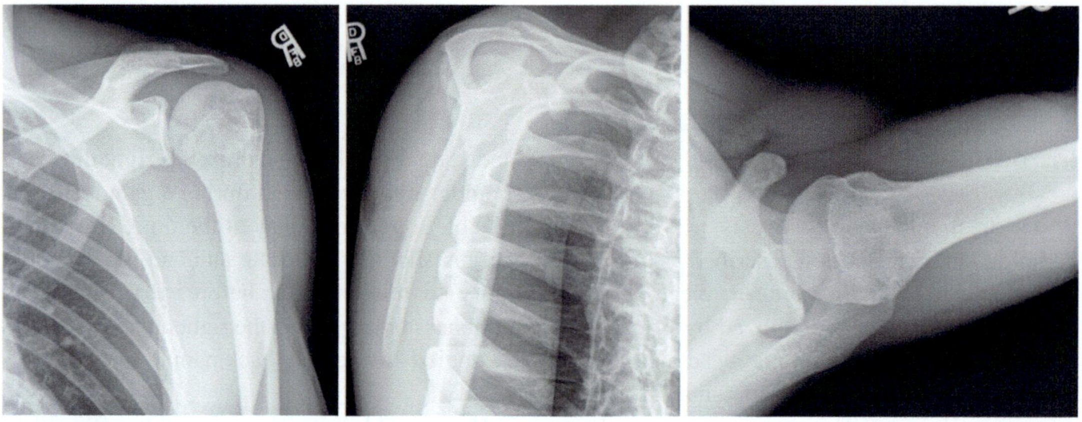

X-rays obtained were normal.

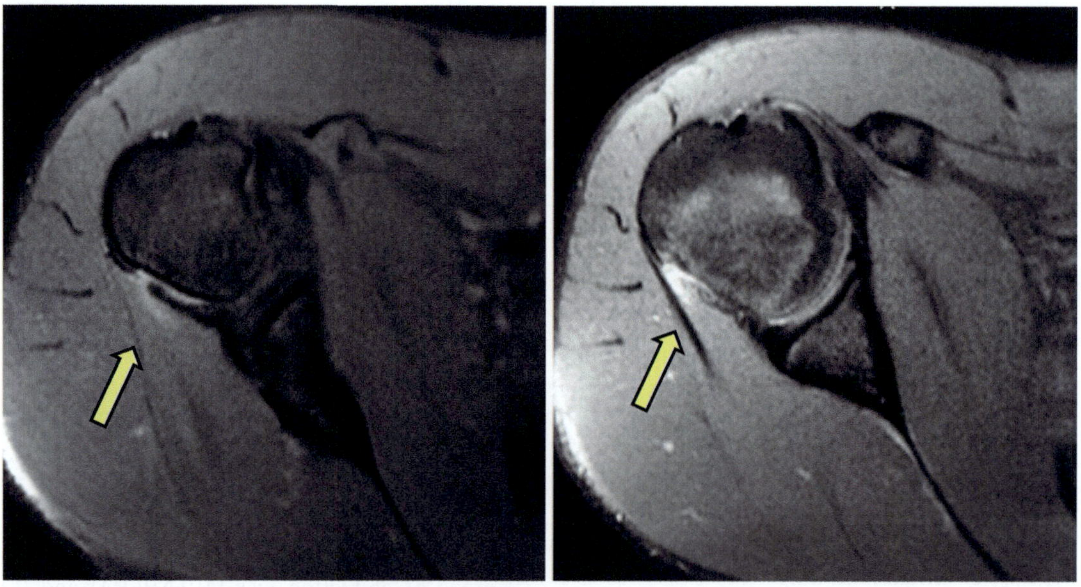

MRI of the right shoulder demonstrates avulsion of the posterior band of the inferior glenohumeral ligament from its humeral attachment with stripping of the periosteum.

Assessment/Plan

Diagnosis: Right shoulder posterior humeral avulsion of the inferior glenohumeral ligament (posterior HAGL).

Plan: Shoulder arthroscopy with repair of the posterior HAGL.

Posterior HAGL Repair Technique

The authors' preferred technique begins with the patient being placed in the lateral decubitus position with the operative shoulder up. The arm is placed in traction in a slightly more abducted position than is typical to allow for improved visualization. The standard posterior portal is made, followed by the anterior portal under direct visualization. Diagnostic arthroscopy is performed to identify any additional lesions that could be present. Once it is confirmed that the posterior HAGL is an isolated lesion, we proceed with the repair. An accessory posteroinferior portal is created about 2.5 cm distal to the standard posterosuperior portal, under direct visualization with the use of a spinal needle and blunt trocar, carefully protecting the axillary nerve, which lies medial. The avulsed inferior band of the posterior glenohumeral ligament complex may need to be mobilized if it is scarred back to a nonanatomic location. Mobilization is performed using a 15° elevator, electrocautery, and blunt dissection. The bony attachment site on the humerus is debrided and prepared using a shaver and burr to create a bleeding surface. Two 5.5-mm screw-in anchors are placed approximately 1 cm apart. Horizontal mattress sutures are placed through the posterior IGHL using a standard shuttling technique. The posterior IGHL (PIGHL) is reduced to its anatomic insertion with the arm in slight abduction and external rotation. The sutures are then tied from inferior to superior using modified Westin knots. The PIGHL is then visualized in its anatomic location prior to cycling of the shoulder through full internal and external rotation without any suture breakage or failure. The portal incisions are then closed using subcutaneous inverted 4-0 monocryl suture. The dressings are applied, and the operative shoulder is placed in a shoulder immobilizer (Figs. 28.1, 28.2, 28.3, 28.4, 28.5, 28.6, 28.7 and 28.8).

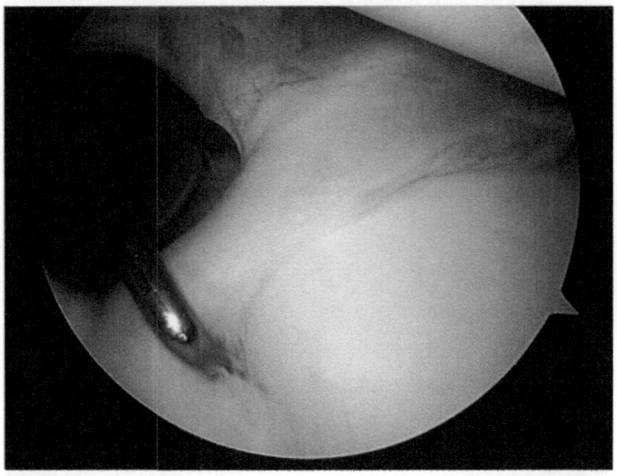

Fig. 28.1 A probe is used to evaluate the integrity of the posterior labrum

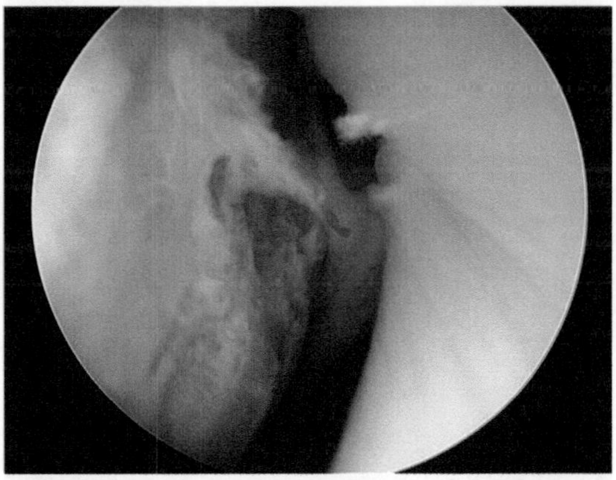

Fig. 28.2 Visualization of the humeral avulsion of the posterior inferior glenohumeral ligament

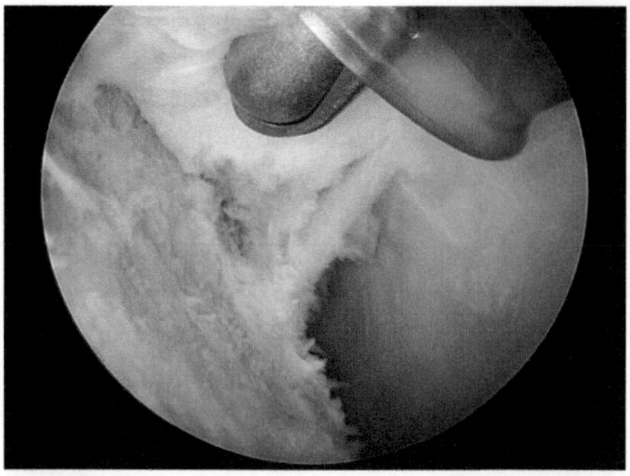

Fig. 28.3 Arthroscopic shaver and burr are utilized to debride the site of insertion of the avulsed glenohumeral ligament on the humerus

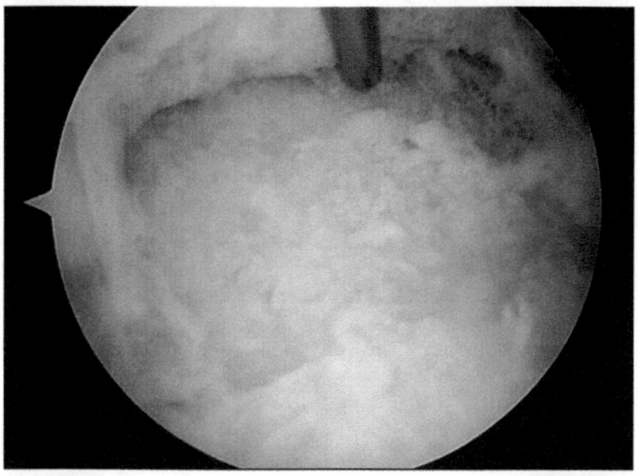

Fig. 28.4 The bony bed is prepared for anchor punch placement

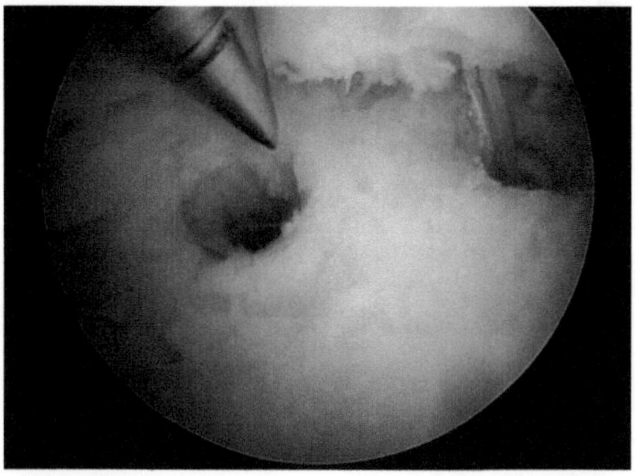

Fig. 28.5 Two 5.5-mm screw-in anchors are placed about 1 cm apart at the insertion site for the glenohumeral ligament on the humerus

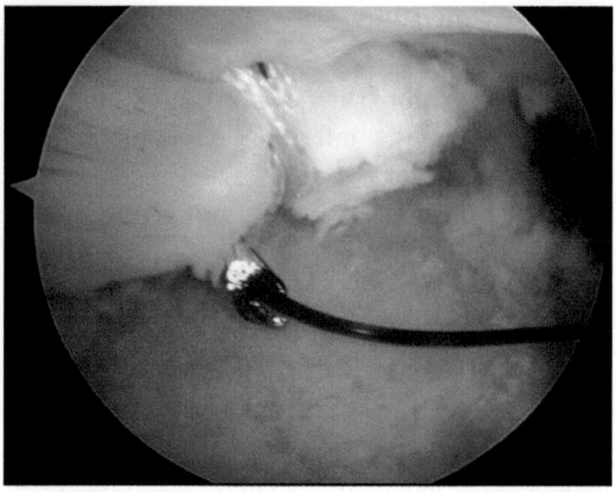

Fig. 28.6 A standard shuttling technique is used to capture the PIGHL

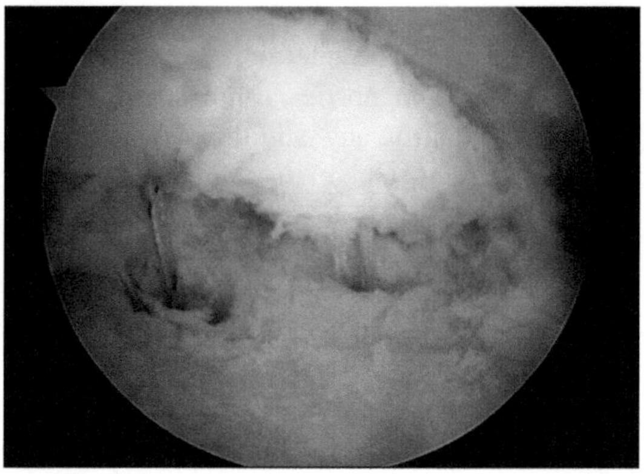

Fig. 28.7 The PIGHL is reduced to its anatomic insertion on the humerus

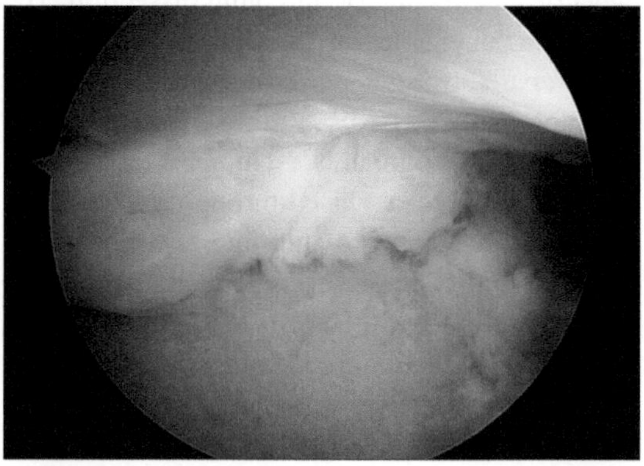

Fig. 28.8 The PIGHL is visualized in its anatomic location

Etiology

There are generally three main causes of posterior shoulder instability. The most common mechanism is repetitive microtrauma [2]. This can occur with the arm in positions of flexion, adduction, and internal rotation, as seen in football linemen, tennis, swimming, and other overhead sports, such as throwers in baseball. The repetitive loading of the posterior capsuloligamentous static shoulder stabilizers in this "active" position can cause significant laxity in these structures and lead to posterior instability of the shoulder.

Additionally, posterior shoulder instability can be seen in cases of acute trauma [7]. An axial load seen by the humerus in a posterior direction when the arm is in flexion, adduction, and internal rotation can cause acute traumatic injury to the posterior capsuloligamentous structures [8]. Additionally, a direct blow to the anterior shoulder, or an indirect force as seen with seizures or electrocution, can cause acute injury to these structures as well. If these structures are disrupted and do not heal, or heal in a nonanatomic position, this can cause significant laxity such that the shoulder experiences instability in the posterior direction.

There are atraumatic cases where, in the absence of trauma, it is presumed that posterior shoulder instability is caused by stretching of the posterior capsule and passive shoulder stabilizers. One must be sure to evaluate for multidirectional Instability and evaluate the shoulder in all potential provocative positions [9].

Diagnosis/Imaging

The physical examination begins with visual inspection of the shoulder, palpation, and active and passive ROM—all in comparison to the contralateral side. There may be subtle differences side to side, but largely this examination is often within normal limits [10]. Findings such as posterior subluxation, a positive sulcus sign, and a positive stress test may be found in patients with posterior shoulder instability [11]. The Jerk test is used to detect posterior labrum lesions in the shoulder. It is performed by placing the affected arm in 90° of elevation in the scapular plane with internal rotation and loading the glenohumeral joint with an axial load across the humerus while stabilizing the humerus. Then, the examiner adducts the arm across the body with a "clunk" or pain, denoting a positive test (there may or may not be pain associated with this examination) [12]. The Kim test is a maneuver used to specifically detect posteroinferior labrum pathology [13]. The Kim test is performed with the patient in a seated position by placing the affected humerus in 90° of abduction and placing an axial load on the humerus. Then, the examiner elevates the arm an additional 45° while still axially loading the humerus posteriorly and inferiorly, with reproduction of pain denoting a positive test.

The evaluation for shoulder instability should begin with radiographs of the shoulder to include a minimum of three views, with orthogonal views included [14]. A standard series may include AP, True AP (Grashey), Scapular Y view, Axillary, Internal, and External rotation views [15]. Other special views may include a glenoid profile view (West-Point), Bernageau, or Stryker notch view to evaluate for glenoid bone loss or humeral head lesions, respectively.

Advanced imaging may include computed tomography (CT) or magnetic resonance imaging (MRI). It is our experience that the axial cuts on MRI are of particular importance in the diagnosis of a PIGHL injury. These imaging modalities can help identify labral or capsuloligamentous injuries [9]. Additionally, other more subtle findings that otherwise may not be identified, such as posterior glenoid fractures, glenoid dysplasia, or anterior humeral head impression fractures (reverse Hill-Sachs), can be seen on CT imaging. In the case of a patient with significant glenoid retroversion or significant bone loss, this may cause an increased risk of failure when considering operative management of a capsuloligamentous injury [16].

Surgical Management

Surgical management is indicated in patients who have failed nonsurgical management or those who have a clear, identifiable soft tissue or bony pathology [10]. Surgical treatment can be divided into two main categories: soft tissue and bony repair/reconstruction. The associated pathoanatomy will guide treatment decisions. In the case of excessive posterior capsulolabral laxity, a capsular shift procedure is sometimes indicated. Posterior labral lesions can be treated with a labral repair either through an open or arthroscopic approach. A benefit of the arthroscopic approach allows the surgeon to address concomitant intra-articular pathology [9]. If there is significant posterior glenoid bone loss, a large reverse Hill-Sachs lesion, or excessive glenoid retroversion, then bone grafting or posterior opening wedge osteotomy may be indicated [9, 10]. When a reverse HAGL lesion is present, its anatomic restoration becomes critical in restoring stability to the affected shoulder.

Post-op/Additional Considerations

The patient is placed into a sling postoperatively. Gentle passive ROM is typically begun at 1 week postoperatively. From weeks 2 to 4, gentle passive external rotation to 30°, abduction to 45°, and forward flexion to 45 degrees are permitted. After 4 weeks, gentle passive external rotation to 45°, abduction, and forward flexion to 90° are permitted. Importantly, internal rotation is limited to no more than the forearm against the abdomen with the arm at the side for the first 6 weeks. After 6 weeks, the patient can begin gentle active and passive ROM against resistance, with the exception of internal rotation, which is still limited to a maximum of 45° until 3 months postoperatively. After 3 months, the patient continues to work to regain their pre-injury passive ROM. They begin an interval throwing program at 3 months, with progression toward unrestricted throwing at 4 months.

References

1. O'Brien SJ, Schwartz RS, Warren RF, Torzilli PA. Capsular restraints to anterior-posterior motion of the abducted shoulder: a biomechanical study. J Shoulder Elb Surg. 1995;4(4):298–308.
2. Provencher MT, LeClere LE, King S, McDonald LS, Frank RM, Mologne TS, Ghodadra NS, Romeo AA. Posterior instability of the shoulder: diagnosis and management. Am J Sports Med. 2011;39(4):874–86.
3. Wolf EM, Cheng JC, Dickson K. Humeral avulsion of glenohumeral ligaments as a cause of anterior shoulder instability. Arthroscopy. 1995;11:600–7.
4. Ames JB, Millett PJ. Combined posterior osseous bankart lesion and posterior humeral avulsion of the glenohumeral ligaments: a case report and pathoanatomic subtyping of "floating" posterior inferior glenohumeral ligament lesions. J Bone Joint Surg. 2011;93A:e1181–4.
5. Bokor DJ, Fritsch BA. Posterior shoulder instability secondary to reverse humeral avulsion of the glenohumeral ligament. J Shoulder Elb Surg. 2010;19:853–8.
6. Hill JD, Lovejoy JJF, Kelly RA. Combined posterior Bankart lesion and posterior humeral avulsion of the glenohumeral ligaments associated with recurrent posterior shoulder instability. Arthroscopy. 2007;23:327e1–3.
7. Doehrmann R, Frush TJ. Posterior shoulder instability. [Updated 2022 May 1]. In: StatPearls [Internet]. Treasure Island (FL): StatPearls Publishing; 2022.
8. Robinson CM, Aderinto J. Recurrent posterior shoulder instability. J Bone Joint Surg Am. 2005;87(4):883–92.
9. Antosh IJ, Tokish JM, Owens BD. Posterior shoulder instability. Sports Health. 2016;8(6):520–6. https://doi.org/10.1177/1941738116672446. Epub 2016 Oct 4. PMID: 27697889; PMCID: PMC5089362.
10. Frank RM, Romeo AA, Provencher MT. Posterior Glenohumeral instability: evidence-based treatment. J Am Acad Orthop Surg. 2017;25(9):610–23.
11. Pollock RG, Bigliani LU. Recurrent posterior shoulder instability. Diagnosis and treatment. Clin Orthop Relat Res. 1993;291:85–96.
12. Kim SH, Park JC, Park JS, Oh I. Painful jerk test: a predictor of success in nonoperative treatment of posteroinferior instability of the shoulder. Am J Sports Med. 2004;32(8):1849–55. https://doi.org/10.1177/0363546504265263. PMID: 15572311

13. Kim SH, Park JS, Jeong WK, Shin SK. The Kim test: a novel test for posteroinferior labral lesion of the shoulder–a comparison to the jerk test. Am J Sports Med. 2005;33(8):1188–92.
14. Ruiz Santiago F, Martínez Martínez A, Tomás Muñoz P, Pozo Sánchez J, Zarza Pérez A. Imaging of shoulder instability. Quant Imaging Med Surg. 2017;7(4):422–33. https://doi.org/10.21037/qims.2017.08.05. PMID: 28932699; PMCID: PMC5594016.
15. Brelin A, Dickens JF. Posterior shoulder instability. Sports Med Arthrosc Rev. 2017;25(3):136–43.
16. Millett PJ, Clavert P, Rick Hatch GF III, Warner JJP. Recurrent posterior shoulder instability. J Am Acad Orthop Surg. 2006;14(8):464–76.

29 Posterior Instability with the Reverse Hill-Sachs Lesion: The Arthroscopic McLaughlin (Reverse Remplissage) and Open Humeral Head Elliptical Osteochondral Allograft (BioHumi)

Colin J. Burgess and Paul Caldwell

Introduction

Posterior shoulder instability is an uncommon event that is often associated with electric shock or seizures. Posterior shoulder dislocations are reported to comprise 5% of all glenohumeral dislocations [1] and have a 50–79% incidence of delayed diagnosis due to their infrequent occurrence [2]. Similar to anterior instability, a humeral head defect can occur following a posterior dislocation. These are more commonly known as reverse Hill-Sachs lesions (RHSLs). An RHSL may contribute to recurrent posterior instability during internal rotation of the shoulder due to the engaging nature of the lesion on the posterior glenoid [1]. Treatment options for RHSLs range from interpositional procedures for smaller defects to osteochondral allograft implantation and, ultimately, arthroplasty for larger defects. The McLaughlin or modified McLaughlin procedures are the most traditional interpositional methods described and involve transferring the subscapularis with or without the lesser tuberosity into the RHSL using an arthroscopic or open technique [3]. More recently, the arthroscopic reverse remplissage technique has gained popularity due to its increased use for anterior instability. For larger defects of the humeral head, osteochondral restoration has become more accepted for younger patients and hemiarthroplasty for older patients [4]. This chapter will focus on our preferred arthroscopic and open methods of treatment of RHSLs.

C. J. Burgess
Department of Orthopaedic Surgery, Orthopaedic Research of Virginia, Richmond, VA, USA

P. Caldwell (✉)
Department of Orthopaedic Surgery, Orthopaedic Research of Virginia/Tuckahoe Orthopaedics Associates, Richmond, VA, USA

Case Presentation 1 (Arthroscopic Remplissage)

A 46-year-old, right-hand-dominant electrician presented to the clinic after an electric shock that he sustained at work. He was initially evaluated and treated in the emergency room and diagnosed with a shoulder strain. He was placed in a sling until follow-up in the clinic. Upon presentation to the clinic, he complained of significant right shoulder pain and limited range of motion. Right shoulder radiographs performed in the office demonstrated a posteriorly subluxated humeral head with a large anterior humeral head defect. The patient was referred for a computed tomography (CT) scan that subsequently demonstrated similar findings with an engaging reverse Hill-Sachs lesion (Figs. 29.1, 29.2 and 29.3).

© The Author(s), under exclusive license to Springer Nature Switzerland AG 2026
R. M. Frank, J. M. Tokish (eds.), *Management of Shoulder Instability*,
https://doi.org/10.1007/978-3-032-18089-6_29

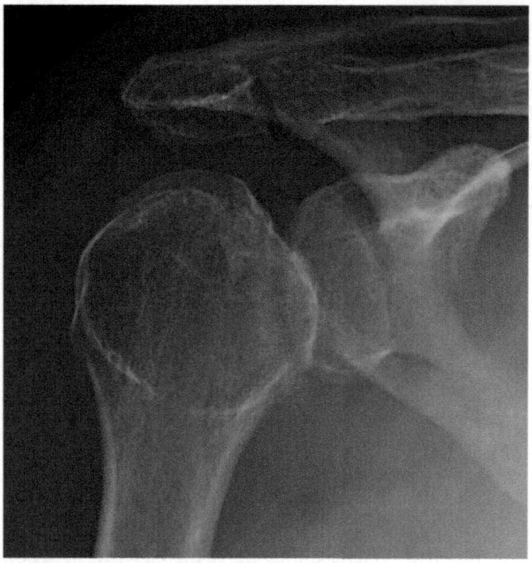

Fig. 29.1 Anteroposterior (AP) radiographic view of the right shoulder

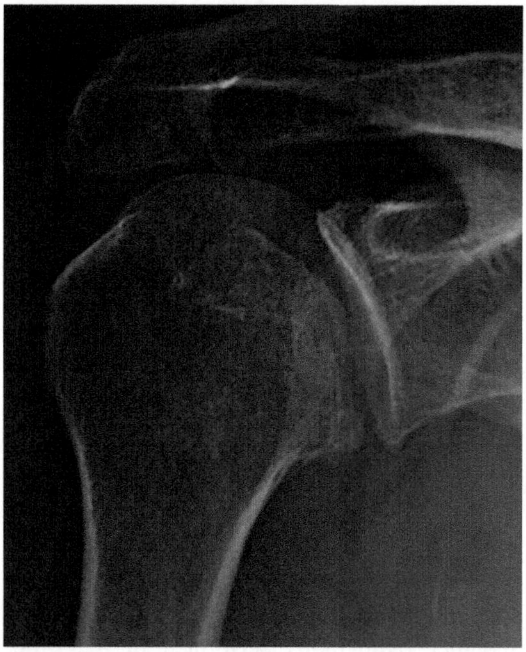

Fig. 29.2 Grashey radiographic view of the right shoulder

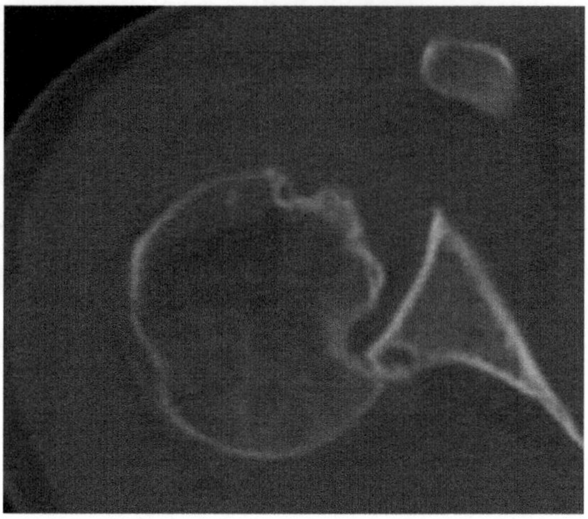

Fig. 29.3 Axial CT scan of the right shoulder demonstrating an engaged reverse Hill-Sachs lesion

After discussion with the patient, the decision was made to proceed with an arthroscopic reverse remplissage procedure to address the reverse Hill-Sachs lesion. Postoperative films demonstrated adequate reduction of the humeral head on the glenoid. At the 6-month follow-up visit, radiographs demonstrated a well-reduced glenohumeral joint and non-engaging reverse Hill-Sachs lesion (Figs. 29.4 and 29.5).

Surgical Technique Our technique uses the traditional lateral decubitus position for shoulder arthroscopy. A standard posterior portal is created, and a diagnostic arthroscopy is performed. An outside-in technique, with an 18-gauge spinal needle, is used to establish an anteroinferior portal just superior to the subscapularis tendon and an anterosuperior portal just inferior to the biceps tendon. Special attention is directed toward confirming an adequate working distance between the two portals. We recommend using a 70-degree arthroscope through the posterior portal to adequately visualize the reverse Hill-Sachs lesion and subscapularis tendon (Fig. 29.6). The poste-

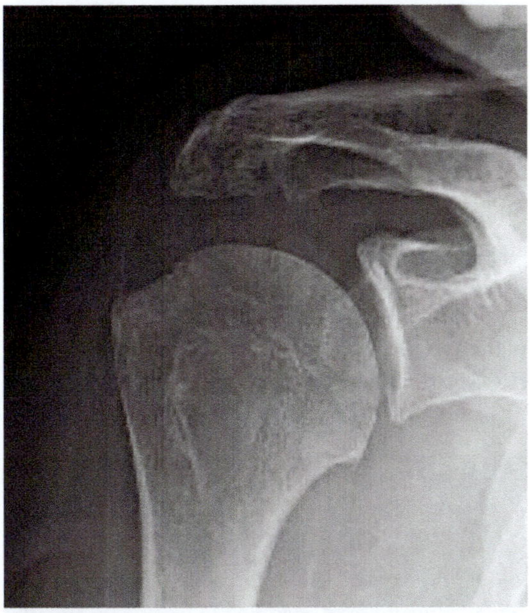

Fig. 29.4 Grashey radiographic view of the right shoulder status after reverse remplissage procedure

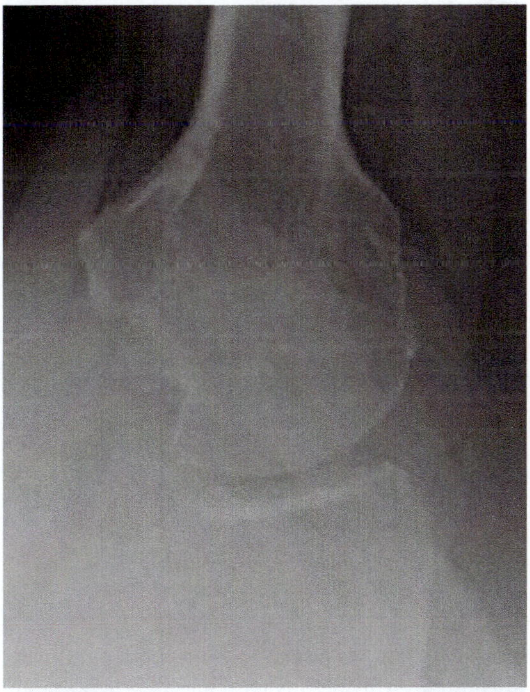

Fig. 29.5 Axillary radiographic view of the right shoulder status after reverse remplissage procedure

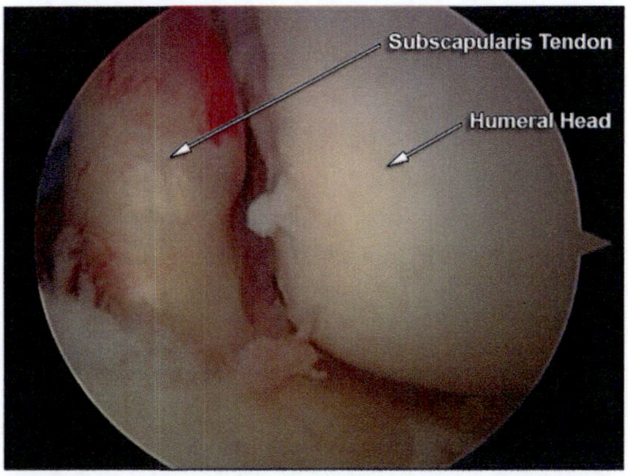

Fig. 29.6 Arthroscopic view of the right shoulder in the lateral decubitus position from the posterior portal with a 70-degree arthroscope visualizing the subscapularis tendon and humeral head

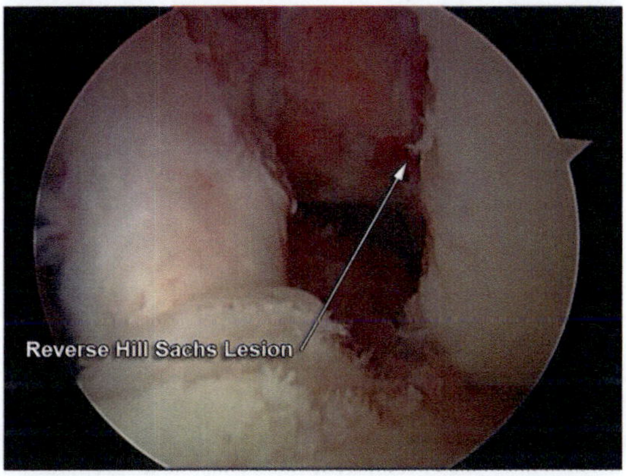

Fig. 29.7 Arthroscopic view of the right shoulder in the lateral decubitus position from the posterior portal with a 70-degree arthroscope visualizing the reverse Hill-Sachs lesion

rior portal is the primary viewing portal throughout the procedure to allow for maximal working space anteriorly. An assistant with knowledge of the "posterior lever push" is recommended for optimal visualization of the reverse Hill-Sachs lesion (Fig. 29.7). The lesion is first debrided of all soft tissue with an oscillating shaver to evaluate its size and location. A bur or open-ringed curette is used to lightly decorticate the lesion in preparation for repair. Two double-loaded suture anchors are placed within the defect (Figs. 29.8 and 29.9). A tap is uniformly used for insertion because the bone is dense due to the impaction injury. The anterosuperior portal is used for suture management and debridement of all soft tissue anterior to the subscapularis tendon, which is essential for adequate visualization. The sutures are then retrieved through the subscapularis tendon in a retrograde fashion (Fig. 29.10) from inferior to superior in a mattress configuration by use of a suture passer device. The sutures are retrieved in pairs from interior to superior through the anteroinferior portal (Fig. 29.11) and tied using a sliding-locking arthroscopic knot backed up with three reverse half-hitches. All sutures are retrieved before tying, and knot tying is carried out from inferior to superior for adequate visualization of the filling of the defect (Fig. 29.12). Once knot tying is completed, the portals are closed in the standard fashion, and the shoulder is immobilized in external rotation using a brace for 6 weeks before formal physical therapy is initiated. The patient is instructed on elbow range of motion (ROM), scapular positioning, and bathing.

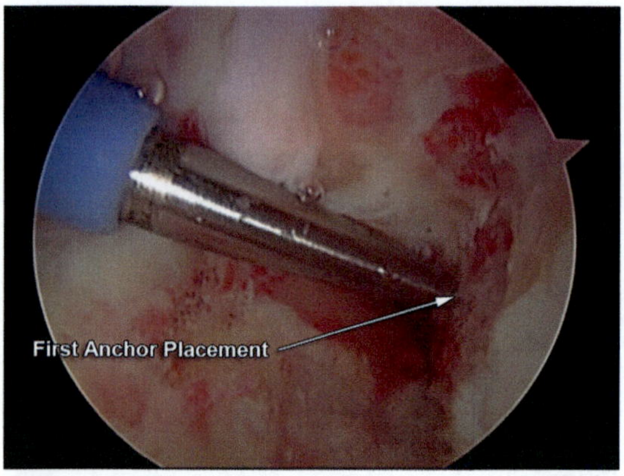

Fig. 29.8 Arthroscopic view of the right shoulder in the lateral decubitus position from the posterior portal with a 70-degree arthroscope visualizing the first anchor placement within the reverse Hill-Sachs lesion in preparation for a reverse remplissage procedure

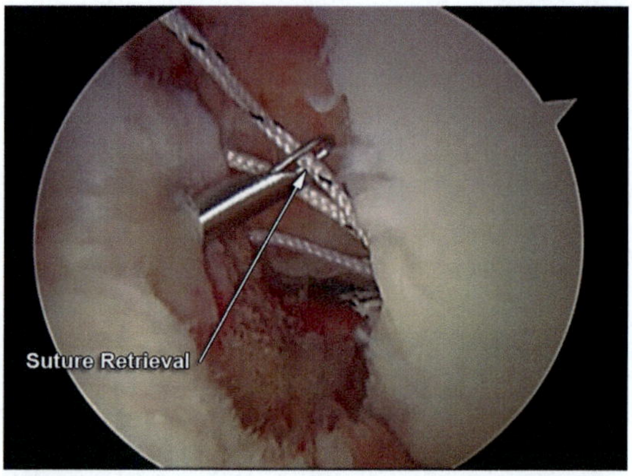

Fig. 29.10 Arthroscopic view of the right shoulder in the lateral decubitus position from the posterior portal with a 70-degree arthroscope visualizing suture retrieval in a retrograde fashion through the subscapularis tendon in preparation for a reverse remplissage procedure

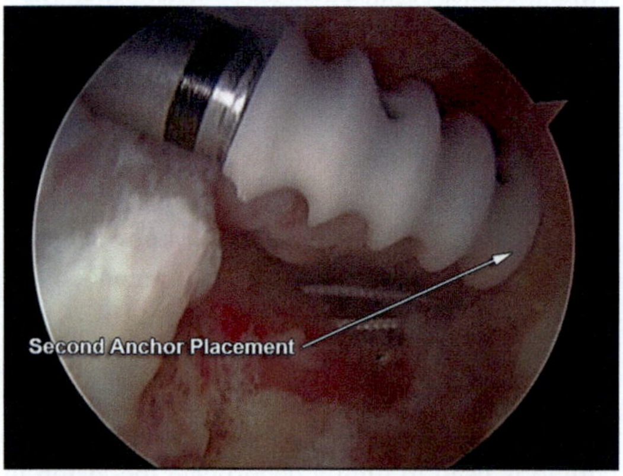

Fig. 29.9 Arthroscopic view of the right shoulder in the lateral decubitus position from the posterior portal with a 70-degree arthroscope visualizing the second anchor placement within the reverse Hill-Sachs lesion in preparation for a reverse remplissage procedure

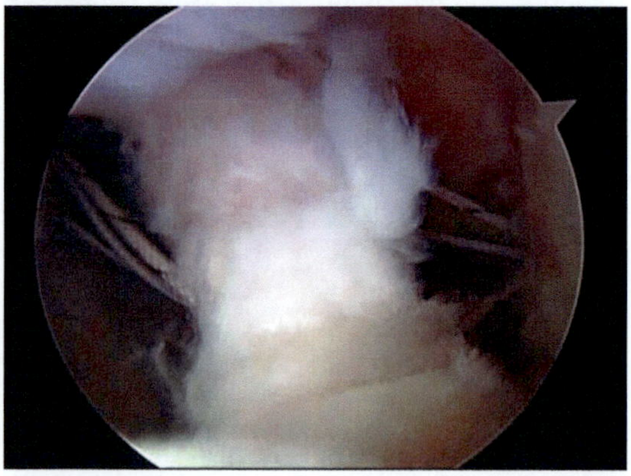

Fig. 29.11 Arthroscopic view of the right shoulder in the lateral decubitus position from the posterior portal with a 70-degree arthroscope visualizing sutures passed through the subscapularis tendon in preparation for a reverse remplissage procedure

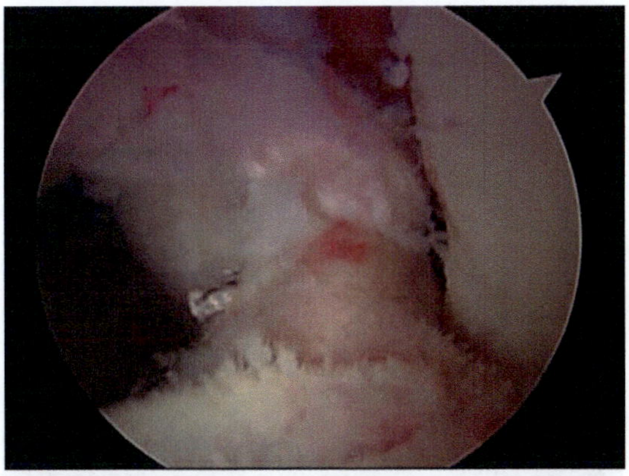

Fig. 29.12 Arthroscopic view of the right shoulder in the lateral decubitus position from the posterior portal with a 70-degree arthroscope visualizing sutures tied on the anterior aspect of the subscapularis tendon after completion of a reverse remplissage procedure

Case Presentation 2 (Open Elliptical Osteochondral Allograft)

A 33-year-old, right-hand-dominant male construction worker presented for evaluation of his right shoulder pain after sustaining his first seizure. He was initially evaluated in the emergency room and found to have a posteriorly dislocated shoulder. He underwent a closed reduction of the shoulder under sedation and was immobilized in a sling in internal rotation. He presented to the clinic in significant pain and with limited external rotation of the shoulder on exam.

Radiographs of his right shoulder demonstrated a posterior glenohumeral dislocation with a large bony defect in the anterior humeral head. A neurology consult was obtained, and a CT scan was ordered to evaluate the size of the reverse Hill-Sachs lesion that was engaging the posterior glenoid (Figs. 29.13, 29.14 and 29.15).

Due to the size of the lesion, the decision was made to perform a humeral head reconstruction using a humeral head osteochondral allograft. Initial postoperative films demonstrated adequate filling of the defect with no obvious impingement. At 4 months post-operation, radiographs revealed interval incorporation of the allograft into the native humeral head with a well-reduced glenohumeral joint (Figs. 29.16 and 29.17).

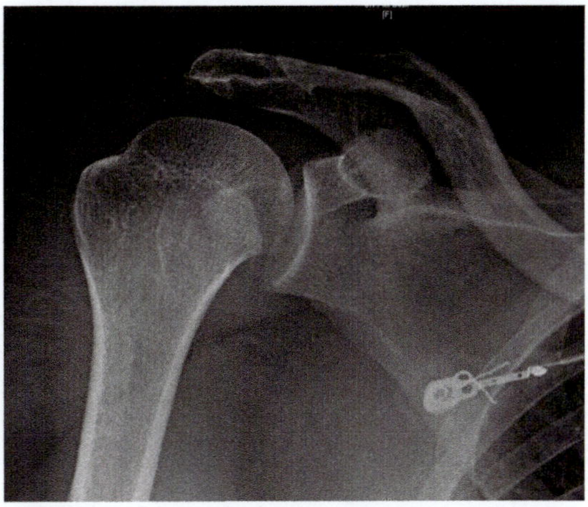

Fig. 29.13 Anteroposterior (AP) radiograph demonstrating a locked right shoulder posterior dislocation with a large engaging reverse Hill-Sachs lesion

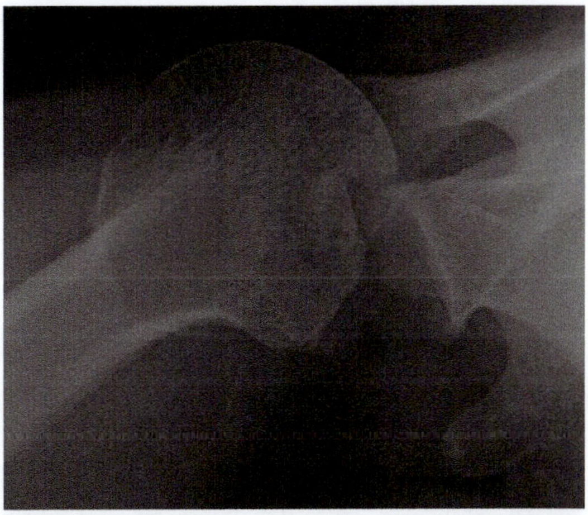

Fig. 29.14 Axillary radiographs demonstrating a locked right shoulder posterior dislocation with a large engaging reverse Hill-Sachs lesion

Surgical Technique This open procedure is performed in the modified beach chair position. Care is taken to position the patient on the edge of the bed to ensure that the elbow can be dropped off the side and the arm can be externally rotated to achieve adequate exposure of the humeral head. We also advocate for placing a bump behind the medial border of the scapula to stabilize and elevate the scapula. We recommend a standard deltopectoral approach to the shoulder. Our preference is to perform a subscapularis tenotomy to expose the humeral head, but a subscapu-

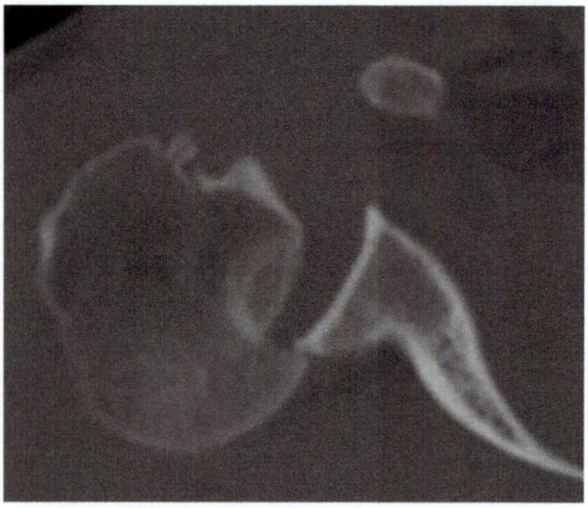

Fig. 29.15 Axial CT scan demonstrating locked right shoulder posterior dislocation with a large engaging reverse Hill-Sachs lesion

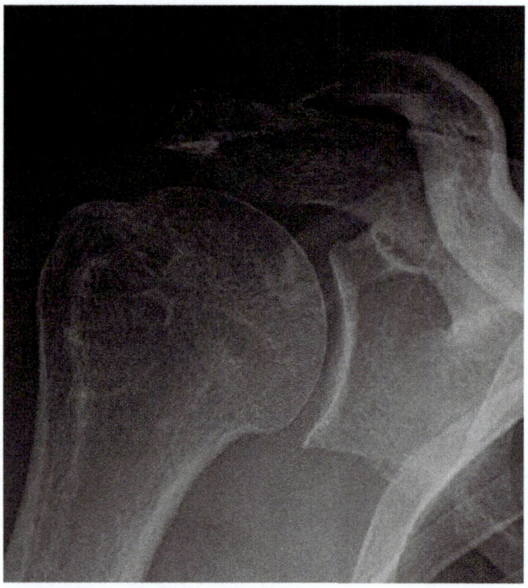

Fig. 29.16 Grashey radiographic view of the right shoulder 4 months after osteochondral allograft implantation using the BioHumi technique for treatment of a reverse Hill-Sachs lesion after a locked posterior dislocation

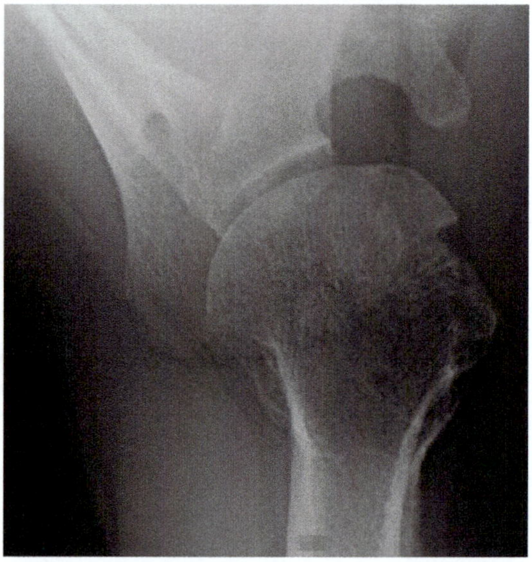

Fig. 29.17 Axillary radiographic view of the right shoulder 4 months after osteochondral allograft implantation using the BioHumi technique for treatment of a reverse Hill-Sachs lesion after a locked posterior dislocation

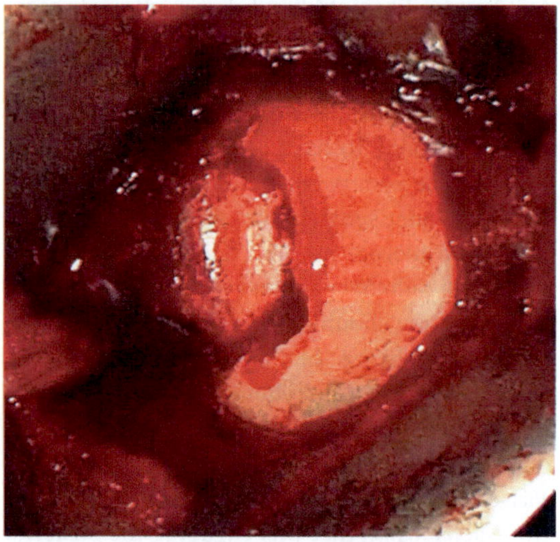

Fig. 29.18 An open approach of the right shoulder with a large reverse Hill-Sachs lesion of the humeral head from a locked posterior shoulder dislocation

laris peel or lesser tuberosity osteotomy may be used as well.

Once the humeral head has been exposed, the reverse Hill-Sachs lesion is evaluated for length, width, and depth, as well as the health of the surrounding cartilage (Fig. 29.18). Reverse Hill-Sachs lesions are typically elongated, wedge-shaped osteochondral fractures, and our preference is to use the elliptically shaped osteochondral allograft (OCA) instrumentation set for larger oval defects. Standard sizing methods are employed to select the appropriate sizer/drill guide to cover the defect and match the natural curvature of the humeral head (Fig. 29.19). Care is taken to ensure that all sides of the sizer are flush with the intact articular surface and that the sizer contains the entire defect. A surgical marking pen is used to trace the outline of the selected sizer/drill guide onto the humeral head, and attention is then turned to the preparation of the osteochondral graft (Fig. 29.20).

Prior to mounting the graft in the OCA workstation, the selected sizer is placed on the proposed harvest site to ensure conformity (Fig. 29.21). The osteochondral humeral head allograft is mounted and secured into the workstation, and a marking pen is again used to outline the sizer on the graft (Fig. 29.22). The marking pen is also used to mark the superior aspect of the graft for orientation. The oblong cutter is assembled onto the impactor handle, and a mallet is then used to drive the cutter into the allograft using constant adjustments to the cutter by slightly angling the impactor handle to ensure that the cutter is advanced evenly.

A sagittal saw blade is placed through the sagittal saw guide and advanced until it is through the humeral head to finish the harvest.

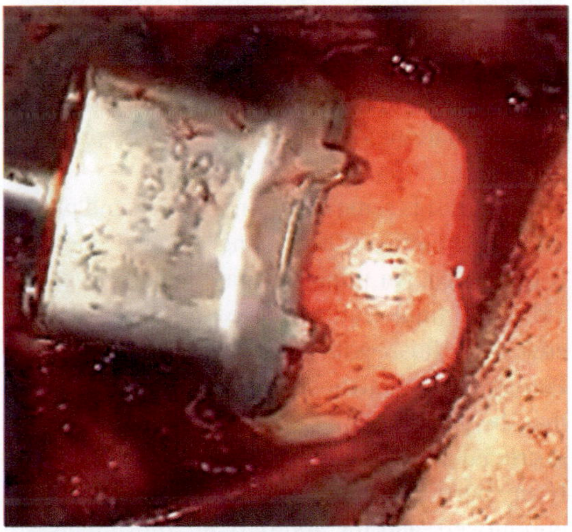

Fig. 29.19 An open approach of the right shoulder with sizing of a large reverse Hill-Sachs lesion of the humeral head from a locked posterior dislocation in preparation for osteochondral allograft transplantation using the BioHumi technique

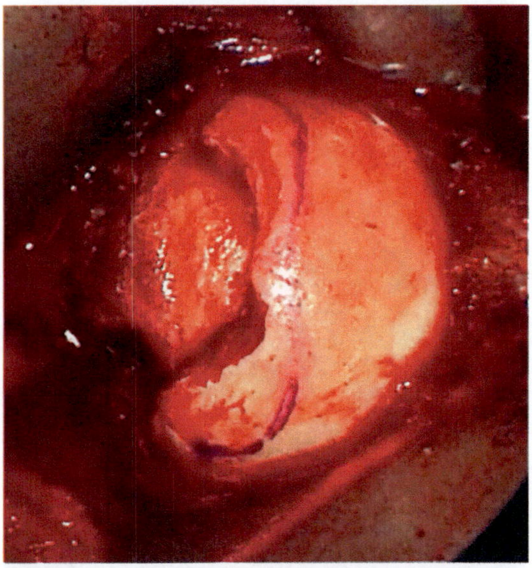

Fig. 29.20 An open approach of the right shoulder of a large reverse Hill-Sachs lesion of the humeral head from a locked posterior dislocation, with the planned recipient site outlined after sizing in preparation for osteochondral allograft transplantation using the BioHumi technique

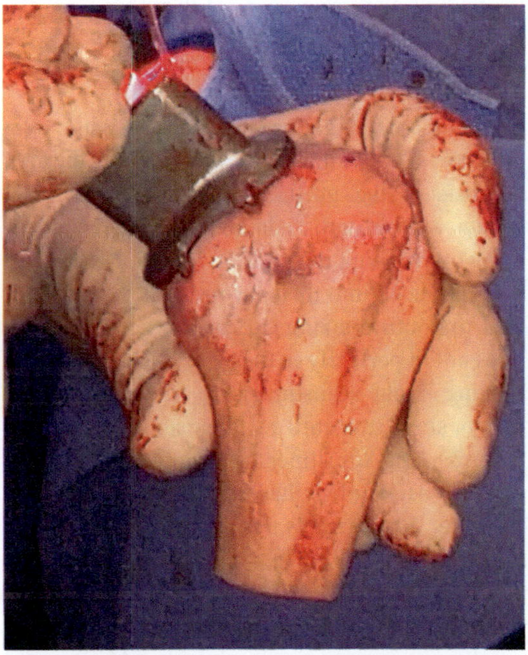

Fig. 29.21 The sizing of the proposed harvest site using a sizer from a right fresh humeral osteochondral allograft in preparation for osteochondral allograft transplantation using the BioHumi technique

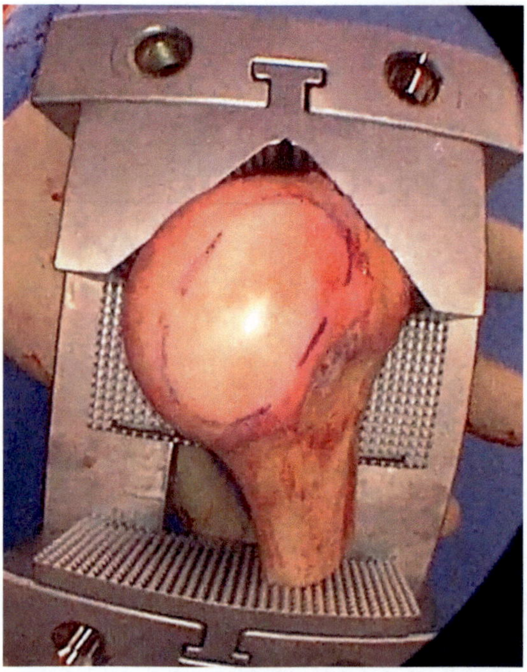

Fig. 29.22 A right fresh humeral osteochondral allograft within the graft station, with the proposed harvest site outlined in preparation for osteochondral allograft transplantation using the BioHumi technique

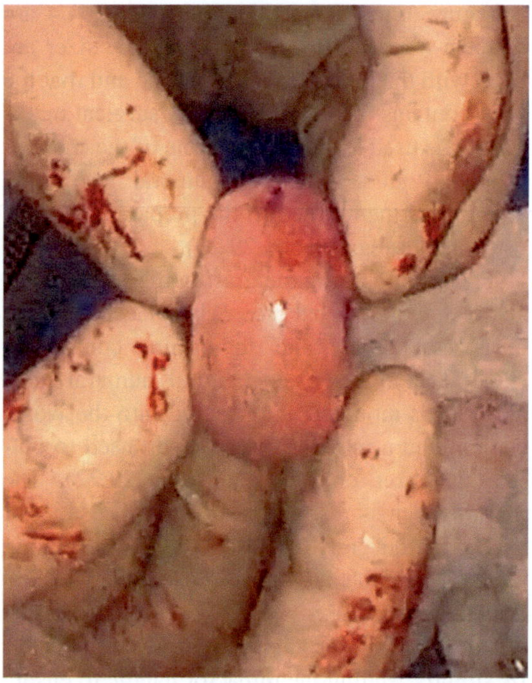

Fig. 29.23 The donor elliptical graft after harvest from the right humeral head osteochondral allograft in preparation for osteochondral allograft transplantation using the BioHumi technique

Dripping cold irrigation with a bulb syringe over the saw blade minimizes the risk of thermal necrosis to the graft. Extraction of the graft within a basin will reduce the risk of mishandling or dropping the graft on the floor. The graft is then placed into the appropriately sized donor trial to confirm sizing. In cases where the graft does not fit perfectly in the sizer, we advocate for making slight adjustments to the graft with a rasp or small saw until an adequate fit is achieved (Fig. 29.23). Adjustments to the graft are much easier to accomplish than alterations to the recipient site. A rongeur is then used to chamfer the edges of the graft to facilitate insertion into the recipient site. Pulse irrigation is used to remove marrow elements, and the graft is soaked in autologous conditioned plasma (ACP) until implantation.

Attention is then turned to the preparation of the humeral recipient site by placing the sizer/drill guide onto the previously outlined defect. The surgeon confirms that the sizer covers the entirety of the defect and that all four sides are flush with the healthy chondral surface. The recipient site is prepared using standard surgical fashion, using a scoring guide, reamer, box cutter, and dilatator to match the previously prepared graft (Fig. 29.24).

The graft is removed from the ACP and placed into the recipient site using manual pressure (Fig. 29.25). An impactor may be used to gently aid in the final seating of the graft to ensure the edges are flush with the surrounding cartilage. Palpating the graft-recipient interface to confirm that the graft edges are flush or slightly recessed is crucial to the allograft implantation technique. If any portion of the graft is proud, then the graft is removed, and the appropriate adjustments are made to ensure proper fit. Care is taken to avoid forceful impaction of the graft to prevent potential iatrogenic chondral injury. Once the graft is well seated, the shoulder is taken through a full range of motion to ensure the security and chondral continuity of the graft.

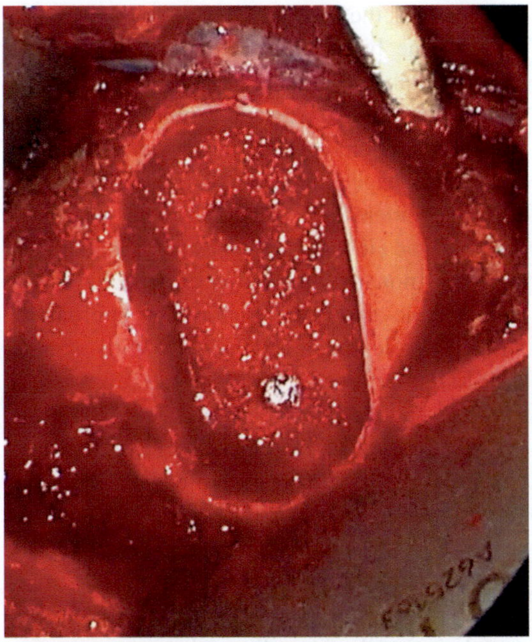

Fig. 29.24 An open approach of the right shoulder of a large reverse Hill-Sachs lesion of the humeral head from a locked posterior dislocation, with the recipient site prepared for graft implantation, in preparation for osteochondral allograft transplantation using the BioHumi technique

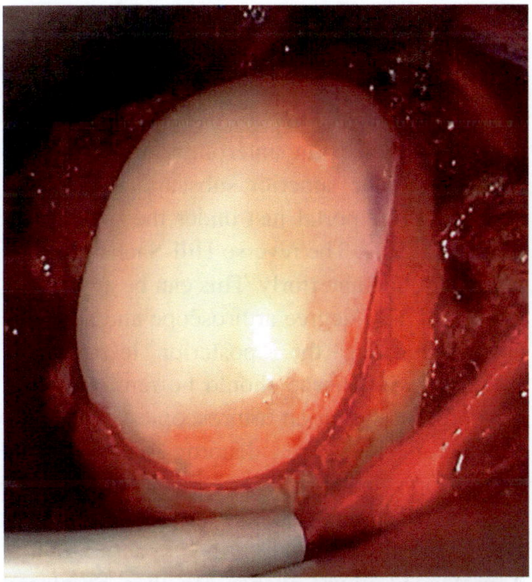

Fig. 29.25 An open approach of the right shoulder of a large reverse Hill-Sachs lesion of the humeral head from a locked posterior dislocation, with final implantation of the elliptical-shaped fresh humeral head osteochondral allograft using the BioHumi technique

The shoulder is irrigated copiously, and the subscapularis is repaired using suture anchors. The incision is closed in layers, and a dry, sterile dressing is applied. The patient is placed in a sling postoperatively. The patient is seen 1 week after surgery and begins a physical therapy program to achieve full passive ROM while protecting the subscapularis repair. Strengthening is initiated at 3 months postoperatively, and return to sports is considered at 6 months if ROM and strength goals are achieved. The graft incorporation is followed radiographically during the rehabilitative process.

Etiology

The spectrum of posterior instability of the shoulder ranges from chronic, repetitive microtrauma of the posterior capsulolabral complex to acute traumatic posterior dislocation. Acute posterior dislocations are typically associated with extreme forces to the arm in a position of flexion, adduction, and internal rotation. The humeral head dislocates postero-inferiorly, and the anterior aspect of the head can impact the posterior glenoid [5]. This mechanism often results in an impaction fracture of the anterior aspect of the humeral head, known as a reverse Hill-Sachs lesion. More than 50% of posterior shoulder dislocations are missed on initial presentation, and subsequent locked dislocations with larger RHSLs are more difficult to manage and more likely to require surgical management[2]. These larger defects are known to be a significant risk factor for recurrent instability along with a younger age at the time of an initial dislocation, glenoid retroversion, dislocation from seizures, and athletes who participate in contact sports [6]. The primary goal for management of these lesions is to prevent engagement of the defect on the glenoid to decrease the chance of recurrent instability.

Diagnosis/Imaging

Initial evaluation of suspected posterior instability begins with a thorough history and physical exam. The resting position of the arm is often a key to the diagnosis, as the arm is classically held in an internally rotated and adducted position. Upon inspection of the skin, the coracoid process may be prominent in addition to a palpable posterior fullness of the axilla [7]. Von Raebrox et al. performed a study that showed skin dimpling over the posteromedial aspect of the shoulder to have 67% sensitivity and 92% specificity for the diagnosis of posteromedial instability [8]. Active and passive ROM of the affected and unaffected shoulder should also be assessed. Patients with an engaging RHSL often present with restricted ROM and pain with attempted ROM [9]. In the case of a locked posterior dislocation, the fundamental exam finding is the lack of external rotation of the arm by the side with active and passive ROM. In these instances, instability and strength testing are compromised due to the lack of ROM and pain.

A complete radiographic series of the shoulder should be obtained, including anteroposterior (AP), scapular-Y, and axillary views. The axillary X-ray is particularly important as the RHSL is best evaluated with this view [10]. As in our case examples, an axillary view is not commonly obtained upon initial evaluation due to providers often overlooking locked posterior dislocations. A CT scan is a more accurate diagnostic test to confirm the diagnosis of a posterior shoulder dislocation and should be performed in cases when an axillary view is not definitive [11]. Thin-sliced axial CT cuts best define the size of RHSL and the extent of the articular surface of the humeral head involved. MRI is not typically utilized in the setting of a locked traumatic posterior glenohumeral dislocation, but it can be beneficial for identifying any soft tissue structures that may prevent reduction in addition to concomitant injuries to the posterior capsulolabral complex and rotator cuff [10].

Surgical Management

With an acute posterior glenohumeral dislocation, closed reduction should be attempted. Nonoperative treatment with immobilization in external rotation followed by physical therapy is attempted if the RHSL is less than or equal to 20% of the humeral head and if the shoulder remains stable following reduction [10]. If the shoulder remains unstable despite reduction and/or the RHSL engages on the posterior glenoid, surgical management is warranted.

Management of posterior shoulder instability with reverse Hill-Sachs lesions has evolved from historic nonanatomic open procedures to arthroscopic and joint restoration approaches. For older, less active patients with smaller RHSLs, an arthroscopic soft tissue reverse remplissage should be considered. This procedure utilizes the subscapularis tendon to fill the anterior defect in a similar fashion to the common technique employed to address anterior instability. There are many advantages to using the arthroscopic reverse remplissage technique. It utilizes standard arthroscopic shoulder setup and portals, as well as familiar arthroscopic passing and shuttling techniques. It allows the surgeon the ability to address common posterior pathology arthroscopically and alleviates the need for special equipment or grafts. It is minimally invasive and reduces the potential for recurrent instability.

In brief, the author's preferred technique for this procedure involves performing a standard diagnostic shoulder arthroscopy with the patient in the lateral decubitus position. Care should be used to establish an anteroinferior portal just proximal to the superior subscapularis and an anterosuperior portal just under the biceps tendon (Fig. 29.7). The reverse Hill-Sachs lesion is then identified anteriorly. This can be aided with the use of a 70-degree arthroscope and an assistant performing the "posterior lever push" maneuver. Soft tissue should be removed from the defect utilizing an arthroscopic shaver. The bone can then be decorticated with an arthroscopic bur to prepare the lesion for the repair. The surgeon should note that this bone may be dense as a result of the impaction injury. A preloaded suture anchor can then be placed into the defect after utilizing the appropriate tap. The sutures should then be passed retrograde through the subscapularis tendon. The paired sutures can then be retrieved and tied in an inferior-to-superior manner using a sliding arthroscopic knot reinforced with three reverse half-hitches. This method of tying from inferior to superior allows for adequate visualization of filling the defect [12].

For younger, more active patients with larger RHSLs, an open elliptical osteochondral allograft implantation (OAT) is preferred to restore the osteochondral integrity of the humeral head. Although reports of treatment of oblong or elliptical chondral or osteochondral lesions in the humeral head using a single, elongated osteochondral graft are limited, there are numerous advantages of this technique compared to traditional open procedures. Osteochondral lesions of the humeral head from posterior instability are seldom circular in shape, and this technique offers considerable advantages to restoring the osteochondral contour for larger, oblong defects while minimizing disruption of normal surrounding cartilage. Multiple circular grafts in a "snowman" or "Mastercard" configuration have been the traditional option for treatment of longer, narrow lesions in the knee. Unfortunately, this technique in the knee has been shown to be inferior to single-graft transplantation, with a reoperation rate of 44% and failure rate of 33% compared to 20% and 6% for single grafts [13]. The authors concluded that multiple graft constructs demonstrate inferior clinical outcomes, graft incorporation, and graft survival due to articular incongruity and subsequent "cobble stoning" with fibrocartilage filling in the spaces between the grafts. Given the recent emphasis on the importance of subchondral bone in the treatment of chondral lesions, multiple graft constructs are less advantageous in restoring this critical foundation for long-term cartilage survival. In addition, treatment with multiple grafts adds considerable operative time and often requires graft fixation, often through the cartilage, to minimize the risk of loosening. The ability to harvest a larger, single graft is also beneficial due to the paucity of surface area available to harvest multiple grafts. Other techniques to address large humeral head defects have been described [14–20], but the "free-hand" nature of these techniques can be difficult to replicate, and it is challenging to adequately restore the chondral surface and subchondral bone of the humeral head. The "Elliptical BioHumi" technique for OAT of the humeral head simplifies a technically demanding procedure with a reproducible method for addressing large, oblong osteochondral defects and potentially offers improved patient outcomes.

References

1. Blasier RB, Burkus JK. Management of posterior fracture-dislocations of the shoulder. Clin Orthop Relat Res. 1988;232:197–204.
2. Kelly MJ, Holton AE, Cassar-Gheiti AJ, Hanna SA, Quinlan JF, Molony DC. The aetiology of posterior glenohumeral dislocations and occurrence of associated injuries: a systematic review. Bone Joint J. 2019;101-B:15–21. https://doi.org/10.1302/0301-620X.101B1.BJJ-2018-0984.R1.
3. Martetschläger F, Padalecki JR, Millett PJ. Modified arthroscopic McLaughlin procedure for treatment of posterior instability of the shoulder with an associated reverse Hill-Sachs lesion. Knee Surg Sports Traumatol Arthrosc. 2013;21:1642–6. https://doi.org/10.1007/S00167-012-2237-6.
4. Provencher MT, Sanchez G, Schantz K, Ferrari M, Sanchez A, Frangiamore S, et al. Anatomic humeral head reconstruction with fresh osteochondral talus allograft for recurrent glenohumeral instability with reverse Hill-Sachs lesion. Arthrosc Tech. 2017;6:e255–61. https://doi.org/10.1016/j.eats.2016.10.017.
5. Frank RM, Romeo AA, Provencher MT. Posterior glenohumeral instability: evidence-based treatment. J Am Acad Orthop Surg. 2017;25:610–23. https://doi.org/10.5435/JAAOS-D-15-00631.
6. Owens BD, Campbell SE, Cameron KL. Risk factors for posterior shoulder instability in young athletes. Am J Sports Med. 2013;41:2645–9. https://doi.org/10.1177/0363546513501508.
7. Schliemann B, Muder D, Gessmann J, Schildhauer TA, Seybold D. Locked posterior shoulder dislocation: treatment options and clinical outcomes. Arch Orthop Trauma Surg. 2011;131(8):1127–34. https://doi.org/10.1007/S00402-011-1310-9.
8. von Raebrox A, Campbell B, Ramesh R, Bunker T. The association of subacromial dimples with recurrent posterior dislocation of the shoulder. J Shoulder Elb Surg. 2006;15:591–3. https://doi.org/10.1016/J.JSE.2005.11.003.
9. Bell RH, Noble JS. An appreciation of posterior instability of the shoulder. Clin Sports Med. 1991;10:887–99.
10. Rouleau DM, Hebert-Davies J, Robinson CM. Acute traumatic posterior shoulder dislocation. J Am

Acad Orthop Surg. 2014;22:145–52. https://doi.org/10.5435/JAAOS-22-03-145.

11. Wadlington VR, Hendrix RW, Rogers LF. Computed tomography of posterior fracture-dislocations of the shoulder: case reports. J Trauma. 1992;32:113–5. https://doi.org/10.1097/00005373-199201000-00024.
12. Lavender CD, Hanzlik SR, Pearson SE, Caldwell PE 3rd. Arthroscopic reverse remplissage for posterior instability. Arthrosc Tech. 2016;5:e43–7. https://doi.org/10.1016/j.eats.2015.09.005.
13. Patrizio L, Sabetta E. Acute posterior shoulder dislocation with reverse Hill-Sachs lesion of the epiphyseal humeral head. ISRN Surg. 2011;2011:1–4. https://doi.org/10.5402/2011/851051.
14. Diklic ID, Ganic ZD, Blagojevic ZD, Nho SJ, Romeo AA. Treatment of locked chronic posterior dislocation of the shoulder by reconstruction of the defect in the humeral head with an allograft. J Bone Joint Surg Br. 2010;92:71–6. https://doi.org/10.1302/0301-620X.92B1.22142.
15. Marcheggiani Muccioli GM, Rinaldi VG, Lullini G, Ritali A, Mosca M, Romagnoli M, et al. Mid-term outcomes following fresh-frozen humeral head osteochondral allograft reconstruction for reverse Hill Sachs lesion: a case series. BMC Musculoskelet Disord. 2021;22:1–8. https://doi.org/10.1186/S12891-021-04657-Z/TABLES/3.
16. Mastrokalos DS, Panagopoulos GN, Galanopoulos IP, Papagelopoulos PJ. Posterior shoulder dislocation with a reverse Hill-Sachs lesion treated with frozen femoral head bone allograft combined with osteochondral autograft transfer. Knee Surg Sports Traumatol Arthrosc. 2017;25:3285–8. https://doi.org/10.1007/S00167-016-4220-0.
17. Provencher MT, LeClere LE, Ghodadra N, Solomon DJ. Postsurgical glenohumeral anchor arthropathy treated with a fresh distal tibia allograft to the glenoid and a fresh allograft to the humeral head. J Shoulder Elb Surg. 2010;19:e6–e11. https://doi.org/10.1016/j.jse.2010.03.006.
18. Gerber C, Lambert SM. Allograft reconstruction of segmental defects of the humeral head for the treatment of chronic locked posterior dislocation of the shoulder. J Bone Joint Surg Am. 1996;78:376–82. https://doi.org/10.2106/00004623-199603000-00008.
19. Zhuo H, Xu Y, Zhu F, Pan L, Li J. Osteochondral allograft transplantation for large Hill-Sachs lesions: a retrospective case series with a minimum 2-year follow-up. J Orthop Surg Res. 2019;14:1–7. https://doi.org/10.1186/S13018-019-1366-8/FIGURES/4.
20. DiPaola MJ, Jazrawi LM, Rokito AS, Kwon YW, Patel L, Pahk B, et al. Management of humeral and glenoid bone loss associated with glenohumeral instability: results with anatomical bone grafting. Bull NYU Hosp Jt Dis. 2010;68:245–50.

Posterior Shoulder Instability with Bone Deficiency: Distal Tibia/Distal Clavicle/ICBG/Scapular Spine

30

Tucker Morey, Matthew L. Vopat, Ryan J. Whalen, and Matthew T. Provencher

Introduction

The anatomy of the glenohumeral joint allows for a large range of motion and rotation, inherently predisposing it to an increased risk of instability. Glenohumeral instability is a relatively common musculoskeletal pathology, occurring most often in young athletes, military personnel, and physically active populations. Studies report that military personnel are at a 20x increased risk of shoulder instability compared to the general population [31]. While anterior shoulder instability accounts for the majority of cases, posterior shoulder instability represents 10% of instability events in active patients [42]. Postsurgical outcomes for posterior instability, including failed management, remain a significant challenge [14]. While patients with anterior instability have a primary complaint of joint instability, patients with posterior instability, with or without bone loss, have more vague findings, with the primary complaint being pain with provocative activities [4, 36]. It is important to recognize patients at risk for not only primary instability events but recurrent events of instability as well, as numerous studies have reported a correlation between not only increased activity level and instability recurrence but also the presence and severity of posterior glenoid bone loss and the recurrence of instability following surgical treatment [43].

Whereas anterior glenoid bone loss management has well-defined surgical algorithms, posterior bone loss is still evolving. Studies show that patients with posterior shoulder instability have bone loss that is sloped 30° relative to the glenoid fossa, increased retroversion, and a lack of posterior bony concavity; furthermore, for every 1-degree increase in glenoid retroversion, there was a 17% increased risk of developing repeat instability [3, 30]. Likewise, an 11% posterior glenoid bone loss implicated a 10× higher surgical failure rate, while a 15% loss related to a 25× higher failure rate for patients undergoing arthroscopic posterior capsulolabral repair [1]. Additionally, patients with as little as 13.5% glenoid bone loss have worse functional outcomes following surgical stabilization. Furthermore, 5°

T. Morey
University of Kansas School of Medicine,
Kansas City, KS, USA
e-mail: tmorey@kumc.edu

M. L. Vopat
Department of Orthopedic Surgery and Sports Medicine, University of Kansas Medical Center,
Kansas City, KS, USA
e-mail: mvopat@kumc.edu

R. J. Whalen
Center for Outcomes Based Orthopaedic Research,
Steadman Philippon Research Institute,
Vail, CO, USA
e-mail: rwhalen@sprivail.org

M. T. Provencher (✉)
Department of Orthopaedic Surgery and Sports Medicine, The Steadman Clinic and the Steadman Philippon Research Institute, Vail, CO, USA
e-mail: mprovencher@thesteadmanclinic.com

© The Author(s), under exclusive license to Springer Nature Switzerland AG 2026
R. M. Frank, J. M. Tokish (eds.), *Management of Shoulder Instability*,
https://doi.org/10.1007/978-3-032-18089-6_30

of posterior glenoid bone loss and 2.5° of retroversion significantly increase the amount of posterior humeral head translation [8]. Numerous osseous grafts and augmentations have been proposed to reduce the risk of recurrent instability, such as the iliac crest bone graft (ICBG), distal tibial allograft (DTA), distal clavicular autograft (DCA), and the scapular spine autograft (SSA), for patients with symptomatic posterior bone loss.

Illustrative Clinical Case

A 35-year-old male presented with right shoulder pain secondary to persistent posterior shoulder instability. He experienced his first dislocation event when he was 12 years old while wrestling with his brother and has suffered from chronic instability and shoulder pain that has increased within the last 6 months. He continued to have instability events into his adulthood and experienced a dislocation 6 months ago while lifting a box overhead. He can no longer lift any weight overhead due to his pain and fear of experiencing another instability event. He has tried extensive physical therapy but now has more persistent pain and wakes up at night due to his pain, as well as catching and weakness. He is unable to hunt, fish, kayak, or play golf, but he wants to be able to do his hobbies as he likes. Physical examination demonstrated limited and painful forward flexion range of motion (ROM) to 160°; painful end of abduction ROM to 160°; apprehension at end ROM for external rotation with the arm at his side and with the arm in abduction; scapular winging; 4/5 strength in his deltoid, rotator cuff, biceps, and triceps; positive posterior load and shift; positive posterior apprehension with subluxation; and the ability to subluxate his shoulder on command. His imaging (Figs. 30.1, 30.2 and 30.3) revealed 25–30% posterior glenoid bone loss, cystic formation changes, inferior humeral head osteophyte, and anterior Hill-Sachs lesions.

The patient underwent a posterior glenoid reconstruction with a distal tibia allograft (DTA). The DTA was fashioned to the posterior glenoid with two 3.75-mm fully threaded cannulated screws (Fig. 30.4).

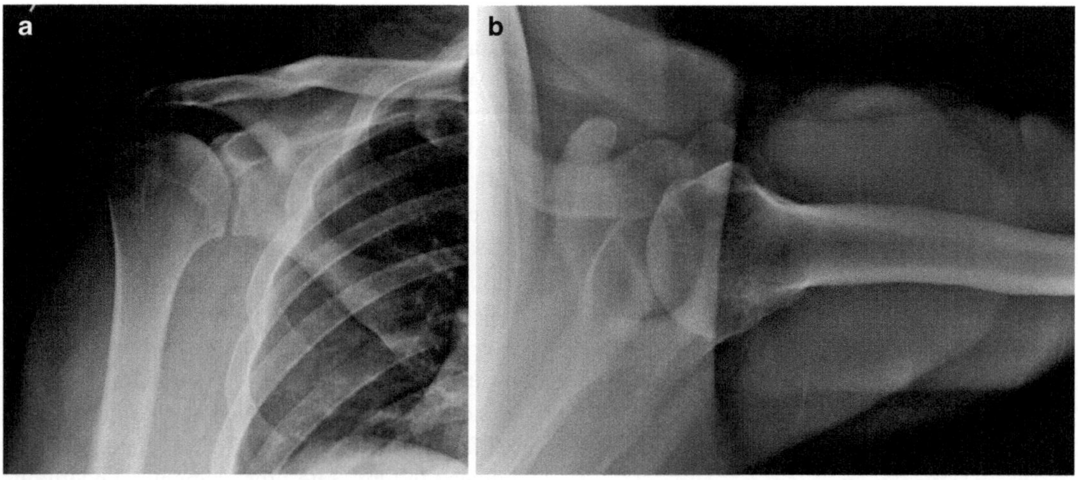

Fig. 30.1 (**a**, **b**) Preoperative radiographs (X-rays) for a patient with posterior glenoid bone loss. (**a**) AP Grashey view. (**b**) Axillary view

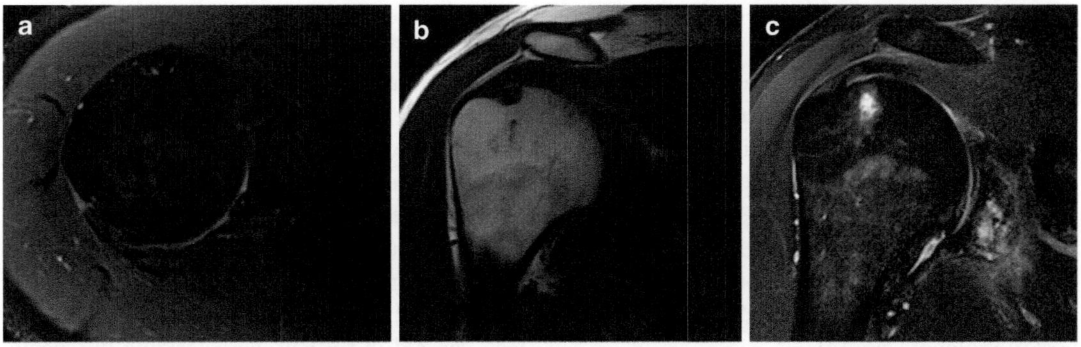

Fig. 30.2 (**a**–**c**) Preoperative magnetic resonance imaging (MRI). (**a**) Axial proton density fat suppressed. (**b**) Coronal T1-weighted image. C) Coronal T2 fat suppressed

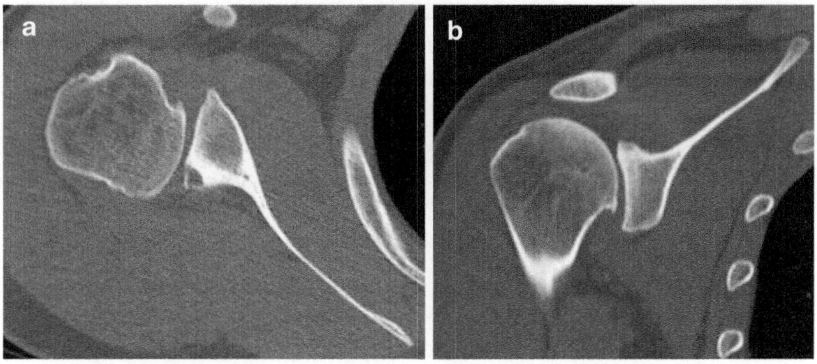

Fig. 30.3 (**a**, **b**) Preoperative computed tomography (CT) scan. (**a**) Axial view. (**b**) Coronal view

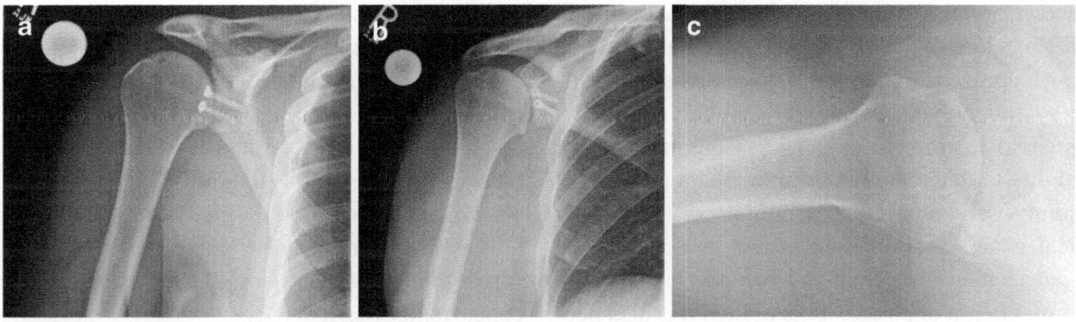

Fig. 30.4 (**a**–**c**) Postoperative radiographs following DTA stabilization procedure. (**a**) AP view. (**b**) AP Grashey view. (**c**) Axillary view

Etiology

Posterior glenohumeral joint instability often presents in young athletes involved in collision sports and military populations, commonly without an identified mechanism of injury. There are three main causes of posterior instability: repetitive microtrauma, atraumatic events, and acute traumatic events. Posterior shoulder stabilization is dependent upon both osseous and soft tissue stabilizers. The dynamic posterior loading onto shoulders that are flexed and internally rotated, such as the shoulders of football linemen, military personnel, and weightlifters, can result in repetitive microtrauma due to decreased functioning and tearing of the posterior band of the inferior glenohumeral ligament and posterior capsulolabral complex [3, 4, 36]. Atraumatic events leading to instability commonly involve generalized laxity of the glenohumeral ligaments. An acute posterior dislocation is a distinct event, presenting with frank dislocation and more traumatic injury to the posterior tissues, seen in patients with epileptic seizures, electrocution, or direct anterior to posterior shoulder force, leading to shearing of the humeral head across the posterior glenoid rim [4].

Studies on risk factors for posterior shoulder instability are limited. A study found that risk factors for failure of surgical management and recurrent instability included female sex, dominant shoulder, concomitant rotator cuff injury, use of three or fewer anchors, and decreased glenoid bone width [7].

Diagnosis

Physical Exam

Due to the nature of posterior shoulder instability primarily arising from recurrent microtrauma secondary to subluxation, damage to the bony architecture of the humeral head and glenoid can develop over time. In contrast, shoulder instability commonly arising from a Bankart tear of the glenoid labrum often lacks osseous injury. The ability to detect bony injury to the glenohumeral joint based on thorough patient history and physical exam is critical to ensure proper surgical management, especially given the nonspecific presentation of posterior instability. It is also necessary to understand the pathogenesis of shoulder instability and additionally assess clinical factors such as age, activity level, gender, and episodes of recurrent instability, as these findings will aid in guiding the surgical or nonsurgical treatment plan and help predict the likelihood of recurrent instability or further osseous deterioration.

The physical examination should always include a detailed neurovascular evaluation of the entire upper extremity, evaluation of rotator cuff strength, testing for active and passive range of motion, and provocative labral signs. It is essential that both shoulders be examined in order to identify physical deformities, prior surgical scarring, scapular winging, muscular atrophy, and/or rotator cuff abnormalities. By comparing the bilateral shoulders, both the direction and magnitude of glenohumeral laxity and instability symptoms in the affected arm can be appreciated. Physical manipulations of the shoulder, such as the posterior drawer test, the load and shift test, the Kim test, the jerk test, and the posterior stress test, can aid in further characterizing this posterior instability.

The Kim test is performed with the patient in the seated position, and the affected arm is abducted to 90°. While simultaneously holding the patient's elbow in one hand, an axial force is applied to the lateral aspect of the patient's proximal arm with the other hand. During further elevation of the arm to 45° above the horizontal, a downward and posterior force is applied to the patient's proximal arm. The sudden sensation of pain indicates a positive exam. The jerk test is performed with the physician positioned behind the standing patient's affected arm. The clavicle and scapular spine are grasped in one hand, while the lateral aspect of the patient's elbow is grasped in the other hand. The arm is held at 90° abduction with internal rotation. The humerus is posteriorly loaded, and the scapula is pushed anteriorly while the arm is moved horizontally across the body. A positive test occurs if a sudden jerk is associated with pain as the translocated humeral head repositions within the glenoid. A 97% sensitivity for posterior instability has been reported in cases where both the jerk and the Kim test are concurrently positive [22].

Imaging

Patients exhibiting signs of significant posterior glenoid bone loss, such as posterior or inferior translation of the humeral head, warrant advanced imaging investigations. Both CT and MRI arthrograms have proven to be equivocal in providing the high-resolution views needed to determine the extent of glenoid bone loss [3]. Utilizing a 3D reconstruction, the surface area method models the inferior two-thirds of the glenoid as a true circle when reformatting from the en face view. The bone loss can then be quantified by dividing the surface area of loss by the total area of the true glenoid circle. If the image was not reformatted to the correct en face view, bone loss could be overestimated by up to 5–8%, potentially affecting clinical and surgical approaches [1]. While using the en face view, both the superior-inferior height and the anterior-posterior width can be assessed. While the S-I height measures the maximal and minimal points of the bony defect, the A-P width was measured at five equal intervals, ranging over the inferior two-thirds of the glenoid surface. The anterior-posterior width of a healthy glenoid was used to determine the width lost.

Further imaging can be used to calculate the glenoid vault version and slope. The vault method [26] utilizes axial cross-sections taken perpendicular to the glenoid face. Glenoid version was represented by the angle between the line perpendicular to the glenoid vault axis and the glenoid line, with a positive number indicating retroversion. The bony defect slope is determined as the angle between the glenoid line and the line parallel to the surface of the bone defect. Multiple studies have noted that posterior bone loss occurs at an angle of 30–40° slope away from the long axis of the glenoid, as opposed to anterior bone loss, which is nearly perpendicular to the long axis [13]. The amalgamation of these imaging findings promotes a more thorough understanding of the osseous defect leading to posterior shoulder instability.

Surgical Management

Nonoperative treatments should be the initial treatment of choice for posterior shoulder instability, focusing on proprioception and strength training programs. Studies show that pain and/or instability were reported in roughly 66% of patients with posterior or multidirectional instability. Although physical therapy can be helpful in patients with instability as a result of recurrent microtrauma or joint paucity, patients with trauma-induced instability were less likely to benefit [9, 16]. Special attention to the main dynamic stabilizer for posterior shoulder stability, the subscapularis, as well as the scapular muscles and position, is key. Prior to surgical intervention, a preoperative strengthening program should be initiated to improve the scapular stabilizers and allow a smoother postoperative rehabilitation process.

Iliac Crest Bone Graft

For patients with glenoid bone loss with recurrent posterior shoulder instability, iliac crest bone grafts (ICBGs) have been the most commonly reported bony augmentation technique. The graft has historically been used as a nonanatomic bone block with the goal of preventing posterior translation. Long-term clinical outcomes are inconsistent, with high rates of inability to return to their previous activity level, patient dissatisfaction, and instability recurrence [2, 24, 27, 40, 41]. Although an ICBG can be customized to match the curvature of the glenoid, there is still a concern for glenohumeral arthritis due to the disruption of the articular surface of the joint [43]. Rohman et al. [38] reported that the radius of curvature (ROC) of the ICBG had congruence with the native glenoid ROC. Even with the lack of anatomical properties of the ICBG, it remains a prominent source of autograft due to the ample amount of graft available and the ease with which it is harvested. Biomechanical studies displayed that the iliac crest bone graft provided a comparable contact pressure and peak force to the intact native glenoid [18]. The significant harvest area of an ICBG is preferred when compared to distal clavicular autografts or scapular spine autografts in the setting of large glenoid bone loss due to the potentially limited size of the clavicular and scapular grafts. Even more, ICBG provides some versatility by allowing surgeons to choose between bicortical and tricortical grafts. However, the patient should be told about notable donor site morbidity at the ICBG site.

Preoperative workup should include a history and physical examination, paying close attention to areas of tenderness, range of motion, strength, and neurovascular status, and the patient should demonstrate signs of posterior instability. Standard shoulder radiographs (AP/Grashey/scapular Y/axillary lateral) in addition to 3D CT to determine the amount of glenoid bone loss should be obtained. The senior author uses the circle method on an en face view of the reformatted CT scan to quantify bone loss.

Operative Technique

Arthroscopic and open techniques have been described for posterior bone grafting in the setting of posterior shoulder instability with glenoid bone loss. The arthroscopic approach is becoming the dominant treatment for patients without significant glenoid bone loss or damage to the anterior humeral head. This can be attributed to the smaller incision sites and the ease with which the capsulolabral complex can be accessed from the posterior side [34]. Both grafts may be performed either arthroscopically or open and affixed both ways.

Patient Positioning

Following induction of anesthesia, an interscalene regional block, and local anesthetic at the site of bone graft harvest, the patient is set up in a lateral decubitus position, resting on the nonoperative side. Ensuring adequate access to the ipsilateral iliac crest harvest site, the arm can be supported by an arm holder in either anterior elevation or in neutral rotation, leaving the forearm to rest on the arm support.

Approach

Using a posterior approach of the glenohumeral joint, a 6-cm vertical incision is made, starting 2 cm medial to the posterolateral acromial tip and extending inferiorly toward the axillary fold. The deltoid is either elevated or split in line with the posterior/middle third fibers. With the deltoid retracted, the infraspinatus fascia is readily identified by internal rotation of the shoulder, causing tension of the muscle. The infraspinatus is horizontally split in line with the fibers at the junction of the lower and middle thirds, exposing the posterior aspect of the capsule and posterior glenoid. With two angled retractors placed on the upper and lower borders of the joint line, a third angled retractor is inserted laterally in the subacromial bursa. A "T"-shaped arthrotomy is made with the horizontal incision at the level of the glenoid equator extending laterally, with the vertical incision located at the edge of the posterior labrum. A specialized deep Gelpi retractor is placed within the joint and onto the anterior glenoid rim to laterally retract the humeral head for joint exploration, and any posterior labral lesions are excised. A burr is then utilized to prepare the posterior cortex of the glenoid until a smooth and bleeding surface is achieved. A high-speed powered rasp is used as well.

ICBG Harvesting

A linear 3-cm curvilinear incision is made starting 2 cm posterior to the anterior superior iliac spine along the iliac crest. Electrocautery is used to perform a subperiosteal dissection in the medial and lateral directions to expose the inner and outer tables of the iliac wings. Blunt retractors positioned on the inner and outer tables further allow for graft harvest. Using the electrocautery to mark the graft dimensions (typically 2.5 cm superior to inferior x 2 cm deep), an oscillating saw and an osteotome are implemented to remove the graft en bloc. With the graft removed from the inner iliac table and secured, the surgical site is thoroughly irrigated, and bone wax is administered to prevent hematoma formation.

Graft Fixation

After the posterior capsule and labrum are interposed between the head of the humerus and graft, 4.5-mm malleolar screws are implemented to affix the bone block to the posteroinferior quadrant of the glenoid, ensuring that the screws are parallel to the surface of the glenoid. The first screw is then placed in the inferiorly located predrilled hole. The second screw is placed about 1 cm higher, once again aligned parallel to the glenoid surface, and the two are fastened alternatively to avoid damaging the graft. It is imperative that the screws have sufficient purchase into the anterior glenoid cortex for strong fixation. The bone graft is then shaped to avoid humeral head impingement, leaving a lateral extension of roughly 10 mm and a posterior extension of 5–10 mm from the posterior glenoid. The wound is then closed in layers. Depending on the degree of retroversion, some patients may require an osteotomy of the glenoid as well.

Distal Tibial Allograft

Distal tibial allografts (DTAs) provide an anatomically congruent articular surface that is not seen with an iliac crest or scapular spine autograft. Frank et al. [15] reported that compared to ICBG, DTAs demonstrated at least equivalent biomechanical properties immediately postoperatively. Furthermore, Nacca et al. [29] proved in cadaveric studies that DTA showed no statistical difference from native glenoid joints when comparing peak force or lateral displacement. Other studies have further shown that DTA improves joint congruency and lowers the peak forces in the ABER position and in 60° of abduction, compared to the Latarjet procedure [5]. Further studies have shown that the distal tibial allografts' radius of curvature (ROC) is similar to the ROC of native glenoid bone [12].

Although the DTA provides many beneficial properties that are lacking from other traditional graft options, there remain many associated downsides when using cadaveric allografts. With wait times exceeding 6 months, or even no availability in some regions of the country, fresh allografts can cost up to tens of thousands of dollars. Furthermore, there is a concern for increased infection risk and antigenic reactions [43].

Allograft Preparation

Sourced from a donor cadaver, a fresh bone graft was obtained from the lateral one-third of the distal tibia. Preparation occurs on the back table of the operating room, where the graft is cut to size to match the defective posterior glenoid bone. Constant irrigation covers the allograft with saline to keep the graft cool and prevent thermal damage. Utilizing a small sagittal saw, the superior and inferior aspects of the graft are rounded to mimic the shape of the glenoid. Using a graft holder for a guide, two 4.0-mm drill holes are bored into the graft, followed by lavage to remove all bone marrow elements for 60 s. The graft can additionally be soaked in patient-derived platelet-rich plasma for another 60 s. While using a graft holder for guidance, two parallel 3.5-mm holes are drilled into the graft to expedite the lag-by-technique fixation.

Graft Fixation

The distal tibial graft is temporarily fashioned in place against the posterior glenoid rim using two K-wires. With two fully threaded 3.5-mm cortical screws of appropriate length, the graft is fixed to the posterior glenoid. A meticulous assessment of a smooth transition between the native and allograft cartilage is crucial. Following satisfactory graft fixation, the posterior capsule is reattached, and nonabsorbable sutures are implemented to approximate the infraspinatus and teres minor. The deltoid fascia is closed using absorbable suture, and the wound is closed in a layered fashion [11, 35].

Distal Clavicular Autograft

The use of distal clavicular autograft (DCA) in the setting of recurrent shoulder instability with associated glenoid bone loss was first described by Tokish et al [43] The DCA provides a cartilaginous surface to the glenoid, able to articulate with the humeral head, giving it this distinct advantage over iliac crest bone grafts and scapular spine autografts, which still encounter concerns over their predisposition to early onset osteoarthritis of the glenohumeral joint. Although both distal clavicular autografts and distal tibial allographs provide an articular surface to replace the damaged glenoid, the DCA is more readily available and cost-effective because the graft is taken from the patient, given that no existing acromioclavicular arthritis exists. Autografts also provide less antigenicity and have been reported with lower infection rates compared to allografts [10].

Many authors have suggested 20–25% as the critical value where bone loss should be operatively restored, yet the value of bone loss that requires osseous augmentation is still debated [17, 21, 43]. Larouche et al. [23] studied the DCA and found that the graft is able to restore 22% of the glenoid face. One of the main limiting factors of a distal clavicular autograft is the amount of bone loss needing to be restored, as resection of as little as 2.6 mm and 2.3 mm in men and women, respectively, can contribute to acromioclavicular instability [33]. Another study provided that resections of more than 1.5 cm of the distal clavicle increased the risk of AC joint instability [6]. Even so, large DCA grafts also increase the risk of complications and failure during iatrogenic AC joint instability repair due to the distorted anatomy. Given the insufficient data on the amount of glenoid bone loss that can be restored using DCA, further studies are needed.

In line with patients receiving an iliac crest bone graft, preoperative workup should include a history and physical examination, paying close attention to areas of tenderness, range of motion, strength, and neurovascular status, and the patient should demonstrate signs of posterior instability. Standard shoulder radiographs (AP/Grashey/scapular Y/axillary lateral) in addition to 3D CT to determine the amount of glenoid bone loss should be obtained. The senior author uses the circle method on an en face view of the reformatted CT scan to quantify bone loss. In the case of distal clavicular grafts, the AP radiograph should be inspected to rule out arthritis of the acromioclavicular joint. Arthritis at the AC joint would be a contraindication due to the potential destruction of the articular surface of the graft.

Operative Technique

Approach

As first outlined by Tokish et al. [43] the first objective when performing a DCA augmentation for glenoid bone loss is an arthroscopic inspection of the glenohumeral joint. Starting 2 cm distal and 1 cm medial to the posterolateral acromial border, a posterior portal is created. Using an outside-in technique, the arthroscope and a switching stick navigate the establishment of anterosuperior, mid-glenoid, and posterolateral portals. With the arthroscope in the anterosuperior portal, a 3-mm graduated probe confirms imaging estimates of bone loss. With the joint thoroughly evaluated, a high-speed burr creates a smooth and readily bleeding bony surface, situated perpendicular to the glenoid.

DCA Harvesting

Along the midline of the clavicular long axis, a 3-cm dissection is made horizontally over the subcutaneous border of the acromioclavicular joint. With a single periosteal flap raised to expose the joint and distal 8 mm of the clavicle, a 1-cm saw is used to excise the distal clavicle.

Graft Preparation and Fixation

After measuring to match the width of the glenoid bone loss, the graft is cut perpendicular to its articular surface, paying attention to closely match the curvature of the glenoid fossa. Using two cannulated, 3.75-mm screws, the graft is then arthroscopically fixed to the posterior aspect of the glenoid. The labrum is attached to the new articular surface, the arthroscopic tools are removed, and the wounds are sterilely dressed.

Scapular Spine Autograft

For patients with posterior glenoid bone loss in the setting of recurrent instability, scapular spine autografts (SSAs) have been proposed as an alternative to the more common iliac crest bone graft. Both grafts have been used as extracapsular bone blocks with the goal of preventing posterior translation. Compared to the ICBG, the superficial nature and anatomical proximity of the scapular spine graft to the posterior glenohumeral joint make the SSA a convenient alternative. The SSA graft has minimal soft tissue attachments and lacks the nearby neurovascular structures that can increase operative complications, as seen in other graft options [38]. Additionally, iliac crest bone grafts require a second surgery site inferior to the glenohumeral joint site, which has been reported to increase complications, such as donor site morbidity, postoperative pain, immobilization, nerve injury, blood loss, and infection [19, 25, 28, 39]. As preoperative imaging is often recommended prior to surgical intervention, the preoperative CT imaging used to evaluate glenoid surface area can simultaneously evaluate potential scapular harvest area dimensions due to the proximity of the graft to the shoulder joint, thus limiting costs associated with additional imaging series [38].

Conflicting reports on the size of glenoid bone loss that can be corrected in the setting of SSA leave the literature ambiguous. To optimize the dimensions of the SSA, harvesting should occur around the scapular spine midpoint, which is 49.6 mm lateral to the medial scapular border. Rohman et al. [38] reported that 96 out of 100 scapular spine allografts fit the minimal requirement of 20 mm × 8 mm × 8 mm to be a suitable graft and could restore an average glenoid width of 44%. In this same study, 100% of iliac crest bone grafts qualified for the minimal requirements. In contrast, Rodriguez et al. [37] reported the SSA to restore an average of 28.2%, with only 66% and 28% of scapular spine grafts able to restore 20% and 30% of glenoid bone loss, respectively. Additionally, the radius of curvature (ROC) of the scapular spine graft, although concave, was dissimilar to the ROC of the glenoid fossa [38]. Even so, the smaller graft size of the scapular spine does allow for easier transfer and manipulation within the joint during graft fixation.

Operative Technique

Graft Harvesting

Starting 5 cm laterally from the medial border of the scapula, a 5-cm incision is made horizontally along the scapular spine. The trapezius fascia and posterior deltoid are dissected to expose the scapular spine. Using an oscillating saw, a tricortical graft with a minimum thickness of 8 mm is extracted. The width of the graft is limited by the maximal width of the spine. Once removed, the graft can be resized to fit the glenoid defect as needed.

Graft Fixation

Graft fixation for scapular spine autografts is performed in the same fashion as the fixation of ICBG, as described above.

Arthroscopic Bone Block Fixation for Posterior Instability and Posterior Glenoid Bone Loss

Emerging techniques have been developed to address posterior glenoid bone loss arthroscopically. There are a variety of graphs that have been described, including iliac crest autograft, posterior scapular spine, distal tibial allograft, and distal clavicle [11, 19, 28, 32, 41, 43, 44]. The arthroscopic techniques have some benefits in terms of excellent visualization of the procedure [19, 20, 41, 43, 44]; the ability to fully prepare the posterior glenoid under direct visualization with a high-speed burr, as well as a motorized arthroscopic rasp; and the ability to insert the graft using a variety of commercially available guides and implants.

Traditionally, the bone blocks have been fixed with cannulated versus non-cannulated screw fixation and/or washers to help with the bone compression of the glenoid construct. However, recently, techniques of arthroscopic bone grafting using a button and a suture construct have been described, and sutures, suture tapes, and cortical buttons and tapes have all been utilized with an all-arthroscopic approach to fix the bone graft posteriorly [20, 32, 44]. The advantages of these are that they avoid metal and screws from the graft and into the glenoid; however, there could be some potential pitfalls in terms of graft loosening, shear force stability (mediolateral stability of the graft), and ultimate healing. These techniques are starting to be employed more frequently with a variety of fixation constructs. However, it remains too early to determine the overall efficacy and ultimate healing of these graphs and constructs. Regardless, the arthroscopic approach, especially fixed with metal screws and/or washers, has proven to be a very solid construct and a viable option for consideration in fixing posterior glenoid bone deficiency.

Here are some images of the arthroscopic bone grafting type of procedure (Fig. 30.5). In this example, a DTA procedure is performed to repair the bone loss on the posterior glenoid.

This is an emerging technology but an exciting field for bone grafting. One has to be cautious with posterior bone grafting in regards to the

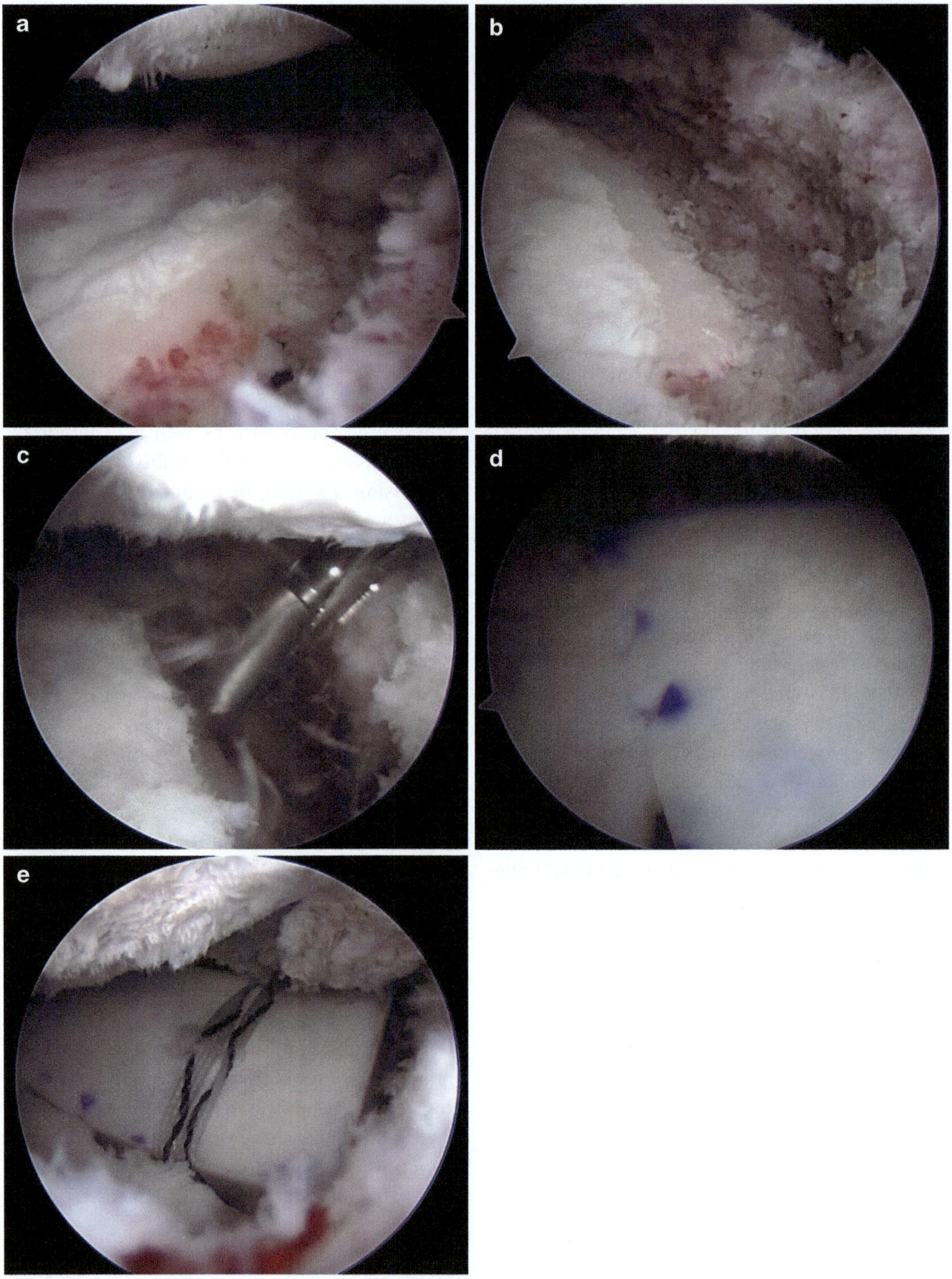

Fig. 30.5 (**a–e**) Intraoperative arthroscopic images from a posterior stabilization procedure using a DTA. (**a**) Posterior glenoid lesion prior to the bone preparation. (**b**) Posterior glenoid following initial bone preparation. (**c**) Final preparation of the posterior glenoid. (**d**) DTA lined up with the posterior glenoid. (**e**) Final fixation of the DTA to the posterior glenoid construct

suprascapular nerve, as it is in a superior but medial location, in terms of any bone grafting to the glenoid, and we need to monitor this. Visualizing the nerve arthroscopically or knowing the anatomic location is imperative to avoid the suprascapular nerve as it comes around posteriorly in the glenoid track. Overall, these arthroscopic techniques for bone grafting with a variety of fixation constructs are very promising and an exciting field for grafting posterior bone blocks for posterior glenoid bone loss.

Postoperative Rehabilitation

Following surgery, the patient is placed in a neutral rotation sling with a 30° abduction pillow for 4–6 weeks. Some have proposed external rotation bracing, thus limiting internal rotation and preventing the application of stress to the freshly repaired posterior capsule. Throughout the initial 6-week recovery period, active elbow and wrist motion, gentle passive scapular plane motion, and passive pendulum movements are encouraged. Passive movements of the glenohumeral joint are initiated within the first postoperative week, with flexion up to 120° and abduction up to 90°. Internal rotation and adduction should be restricted for the first 6 weeks. Active motion and strengthening regimen of the shoulder joint can be initiated as early as 4 weeks, and the timeframe is dependent on both the magnitude of the injury and the extent of the repair. Between 4 and 6 months, most patients are cleared to return to full activities following the completion of individually tailored training programs. Final imaging studies should be obtained to confirm proper graft fixation to the glenoid.

References

1. Arner JW, Ruzbarsky JJ, Midtgaard K, et al. Defining critical glenoid bone loss in posterior shoulder Capsulolabral repair. Am J Sports Med. 2021;49(8):2013–9.
2. Barbier O, Ollat D, Marchaland JP, Versier G. Iliac bone-block autograft for posterior shoulder instability. Orthop Traumatol Surg Res. 2009;95(2):100–7.
3. Beaulieu-Jones BR, Peebles LA, Golijanin P, et al. Characterization of posterior glenoid bone loss morphology in patients with posterior shoulder instability. Arthroscopy. 2019;35(10):2777–84.
4. Bernhardson AS, Murphy CP, Aman ZS, LaPrade RF, Provencher MT. A prospective analysis of patients with anterior versus posterior shoulder instability: a matched cohort examination and surgical outcome analysis of 200 patients. Am J Sports Med. 2019;47(3):682–7.
5. Bhatia S, Van Thiel GS, Gupta D, et al. Comparison of glenohumeral contact pressures and contact areas after glenoid reconstruction with Latarjet or distal tibial osteochondral allografts. Am J Sports Med. 2013;41(8):1900–8.
6. Blazar PE, Iannotti JP, Williams GR. Anteroposterior instability of the distal clavicle after distal clavicle resection. Clin Orthop Relat Res. 1998;348:114–20.
7. Bradley JP, Arner JW, Jayakumar S, Vyas D. Revision arthroscopic posterior shoulder Capsulolabral repair in contact athletes: risk factors and outcomes. Arthroscopy. 2020;36(3):660–5.
8. Bryce CD, Davison AC, Okita N, et al. A biomechanical study of posterior glenoid bone loss and humeral head translation. J Shoulder Elb Surg. 2010;19(7):994–1002.
9. Burkhead WZ Jr, Rockwood CA Jr. Treatment of instability of the shoulder with an exercise program. J Bone Joint Surg Am. 1992;74(6):890–6.
10. Choate WS, Kwapisz A, Tokish JM. Distal clavicle autograft—I would like to use my own osteochondral graft please. Ann Joint. 2017;2(12):27.
11. Cooper JD, Ruzbarsky JJ, Nolte PC, Elrick BP, Millett PJ. Posterior glenoid reconstruction using a distal Tibial allograft. Arthrosc Tech. 2021;10(5):e1227–32.
12. Dehaan A, Munch J, Durkan M, Yoo J, Crawford D. Reconstruction of a bony Bankart lesion: best fit based on radius of curvature. Am J Sports Med. 2013;41(5):1140–5.
13. Dekker TJ, Peebles LA, Goldenberg BT, et al. Location of the glenoid defect in shoulders with recurrent posterior Glenohumeral instability. Am J Sports Med. 2019;47(13):3051–6.
14. Forsythe B, Ghodadra N, Romeo AA, Provencher MT. Management of the failed posterior/multidirectional instability patient. Sports Med Arthrosc Rev. 2010;18(3):149–61.
15. Frank RM, Shin J, Saccomanno MF, et al. Comparison of glenohumeral contact pressures and contact areas after posterior glenoid reconstruction with an iliac crest bone graft or distal tibial osteochondral allograft. Am J Sports Med. 2014;42(11):2574–82.
16. Fronek J, Warren RF, Bowen M. Posterior subluxation of the glenohumeral joint. J Bone Joint Surg Am. 1989;71(2):205–16.
17. Gerber C, Nyffeler RW. Classification of glenohumeral joint instability. Clin Orthop Relat Res. 2002;400:65–76.
18. Ghodadra N, Gupta A, Romeo AA, et al. Normalization of glenohumeral articular contact pres-

sures after Latarjet or iliac crest bone-grafting. J Bone Joint Surg Am. 2010;92(6):1478–89.
19. Gupta AK, Chalmers PN, Klosterman E, et al. Arthroscopic distal tibial allograft augmentation for posterior shoulder instability with glenoid bone loss. Arthrosc Tech. 2013;2(4):e405–11.
20. Hachem AI, Rondanelli SR, Costa D'O G, Verdalet I, Rius X. Arthroscopic "Bone Block Cerclage" technique for posterior shoulder instability. Arthrosc Tech. 2020;9(8):e1171–80.
21. Itoi E, Lee SB, Berglund LJ, Berge LL, An KN. The effect of a glenoid defect on anteroinferior stability of the shoulder after Bankart repair: a cadaveric study. J Bone Joint Surg Am. 2000;82(1):35–46.
22. Kim SH, Park JS, Jeong WK, Shin SK. The Kim test: a novel test for posteroinferior labral lesion of the shoulder--a comparison to the jerk test. Am J Sports Med. 2005;33(8):1188–92.
23. Larouche M, Knowles N, Ferreira L, Tokish JM, Athwal GS. Osteoarticular distal clavicle autograft for the management of instability-related glenoid bone loss: an anatomic and cadaveric study. J Shoulder Elb Surg. 2020;29(8):1615–20.
24. Levigne C, Garret J, Walch G. Posterior bone block for posterior instability. Tech Shoulder Elbow Surg. 2005;6(1):26.
25. Loeffler BJ, Kellam JF, Sims SH, Bosse MJ. Prospective observational study of donor-site morbidity following anterior iliac crest bone-grafting in orthopaedic trauma reconstruction patients. J Bone Joint Surg Am. 2012;94(18):1649–54.
26. Matsumura N, Ogawa K, Ikegami H, et al. Computed tomography measurement of glenoid vault version as an alternative measuring method for glenoid version. J Orthop Surg Res. 2014;9(1):17.
27. Meuffels DE, Schuit H, van Biezen FC, Reijman M, Verhaar JA. The posterior bone block procedure in posterior shoulder instability: a long-term follow-up study. J Bone Joint Surg Br. 2010;92(5):651–5.
28. Moroder P, Kathi T, Lacheta L, et al. Arthroscopic bone block Cerclage technique using a Tricortical scapular spine autograft for glenoid reconstruction in patients with anterior shoulder instability. Arthrosc Tech. 2022;11(3):e379–83.
29. Nacca C, Gil JA, DeFroda SF, Badida R, Owens BD. Comparison of a distal Tibial allograft and scapular spinal autograft for posterior shoulder instability with glenoid bone loss. Orthop J Sports Med. 2018;6(7):2325967118786697.
30. Owens BD, Campbell SE, Cameron KL. Risk factors for posterior shoulder instability in young athletes. Am J Sports Med. 2013;41(11):2645–9.
31. Owens BD, Duffey ML, Nelson BJ, et al. The incidence and characteristics of shoulder instability at the United States Military Academy. Am J Sports Med. 2007;35(7):1168–73.
32. Parada SA, Shaw KA. Graft transfer technique in arthroscopic posterior glenoid reconstruction with distal tibia allograft. Arthrosc Tech. 2017;6(5):e1891–5.
33. Peebles LA, Dekker TJ, Akamefula RA, et al. Distal clavicular augmentation with acromioclavicular and Coracoclavicular ligament reconstruction in the setting of iatrogenic induced acromioclavicular instability. Arthrosc Tech. 2019;8(12):e1583–9.
34. Provencher MT, Bell SJ, Menzel KA, Mologne TS. Arthroscopic treatment of posterior shoulder instability: results in 33 patients. Am J Sports Med. 2005;33(10):1463–71.
35. Provencher MT, Ghodadra N, LeClere L, Solomon DJ, Romeo AA. Anatomic osteochondral glenoid reconstruction for recurrent glenohumeral instability with glenoid deficiency using a distal tibia allograft. Arthroscopy. 2009;25(4):446–52.
36. Provencher MT, LeClere LE, King S, et al. Posterior instability of the shoulder: diagnosis and management. Am J Sports Med. 2011;39(4):874–86.
37. Rodriguez S, Mancini MR, Kakazu R, et al. Comparison of the coracoid, distal clavicle, and scapular spine for autograft augmentation of glenoid bone loss: a radiologic and cadaveric assessment. Am J Sports Med. 2022;50(3):717–24.
38. Rohman E, Gronbeck K, Tompkins M, et al. Scapular spine dimensions and suitability as a glenoid bone graft donor site. Am J Sports Med. 2019;47(10):2469–77.
39. Schaaf H, Lendeckel S, Howaldt HP, Streckbein P. Donor site morbidity after bone harvesting from the anterior iliac crest. Oral Surg Oral Med Oral Pathol Oral Radiol Endod. 2010;109(1):52–8.
40. Servien E, Walch G, Cortes ZE, Edwards TB, O'Connor DP. Posterior bone block procedure for posterior shoulder instability. Knee Surg Sports Traumatol Arthrosc. 2007;15(9):1130–6.
41. Smith T, Goede F, Struck M, Wellmann M. Arthroscopic posterior shoulder stabilization with an iliac bone graft and capsular repair: a novel technique. Arthrosc Tech. 2012;1(2):e181–5.
42. Song DJ, Cook JB, Krul KP, et al. High frequency of posterior and combined shoulder instability in young active patients. J Shoulder Elb Surg. 2015;24(2):186–90.
43. Tokish JM, Fitzpatrick K, Cook JB, Mallon WJ. Arthroscopic distal clavicular autograft for treating shoulder instability with glenoid bone loss. Arthrosc Tech. 2014;3(4):e475–81.
44. van Spanning SH, Picard K, Buijze GA, et al. Arthroscopic bone block procedure for posterior shoulder instability: updated surgical technique. Arthrosc Tech. 2022;11(10):e1793–9.

31 Glenoid Osteotomy for Severe Glenoid Retroversion and Posterior Instability

Maximilian Hinz, Jonas Pogorzelski, and Andreas B. Imhoff

Introduction

Glenoid retroversion has been identified as a risk factor for the onset of posterior shoulder instability (PSI) [1–4]. Both biomechanical and clinical studies have reported unsatisfactory results in patients with PSI and increased glenoid retroversion (greater than 15°) if solely treated by arthroscopic posterior capsulolabral repair [1, 5, 6]. Consequently, surgical procedures that aim to reduce increased glenoid retroversion have been developed. The first reports of surgical techniques for posterior open-wedge glenoid osteotomy (POWGO) were published in the last century, and more recent publications have refined these techniques and reported satisfying results with a low rate of postoperative instability recurrence [7].

Besides describing the authors' preferred technique for performing a POWGO, the article aims to provide the reader with a detailed guide on the diagnostic work-up necessary when treating patients with PSI, as well as postoperative rehabilitation recommendations following POWGO.

M. Hinz · A. B. Imhoff (✉)
Department of Sports Orthopaedics, Technical University of Munich, Munich, Germany
e-mail: maximilian.hinz@tum.de; imhoff@tum.de

J. Pogorzelski
Department of Sports Orthopaedics, Technical University of Munich, Munich, Germany

OC Erlangen, Erlangen, Germany
e-mail: jonas.pogorzelski@tum.de

Illustrative Clinical Case

A 19-year-old male patient presented at our department with bilateral chronic PSI, recurrent posterior shoulder subluxations, and failed conservative treatment. These bilateral posterior subluxations occurred involuntarily during activities of daily living. During physical examination, a reduced range of motion with positive signs of posterior instability as well as hyperlaxity was evident. The X-ray imaging suggested increased glenoid retroversion, and through MRI, a hypoplastic posterior labral complex was determined. Because of the suspected increased glenoid retroversion, a CT scan was performed, which revealed pathological glenoid retroversion (26° of retroversion bilaterally).

Due to the patient's increased glenoid retroversion and history of failed conservative treatment, POWGO was selected for treatment of the right side first. The same procedure was performed on the left side 5 months after. Glenoid retroversion was corrected successfully (14.5° retroversion on the right side, 13.5° retroversion on the left side).

At each three-month postoperative check-up, a full range of motion was regained, and the patient reported no signs of recurrent instability.

© The Author(s), under exclusive license to Springer Nature Switzerland AG 2026
R. M. Frank, J. M. Tokish (eds.), *Management of Shoulder Instability*,
https://doi.org/10.1007/978-3-032-18089-6_31

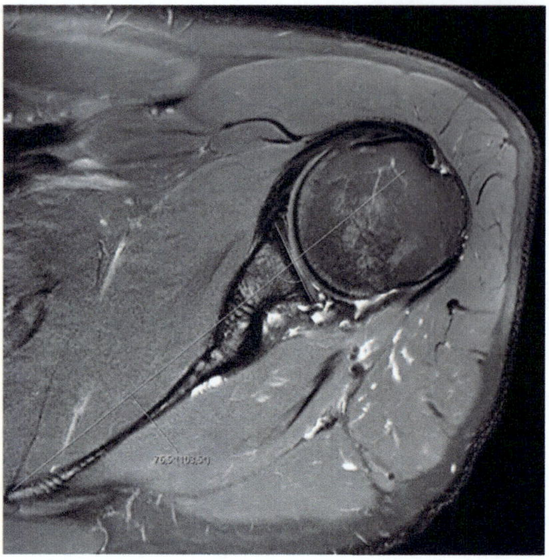

Fig. 31.1 MRI of the left shoulder 7.5 years after POWGO. Glenoid retroversion was reduced from 26° to 13.5°. Additionally, no full-thickness cartilage damage and sufficient bone healing were evident at follow-up

At a second, 8-year (right side) and 7.5-year (left side) postoperative check-up, the patient reported high satisfaction with the postoperative result and had no further signs of instability and very little pain (Visual Analog Scale for pain—right side: five preoperatively versus two at follow-up; left: six preoperatively versus two at follow-up). An MRI was obtained on the left side, which showed a centered humeral head and no relevant progression of osteoarthritis (Fig. 31.1).

Patient History

Posterior shoulder instability most often affects male patients between the ages of 20 and 30 years who report a singular traumatic posterior shoulder subluxation or dislocation preceding PSI [8, 9]. In patients with increased glenoid retroversion, however, an atraumatic, gradual onset of PSI is seen more frequently [10]. Full dislocations are rare, and the governing symptoms usually encompass posterior subluxations and/or insidious pain in the later phases of sporting activities when muscle fatigue occurs and dynamic stability is compromised, including aching pain along the posterior aspect of the shoulder or even anterior shoulder pain [5, 11–13].

Classification

In 2017, the ABC classification was proposed by Moroder et al., which may help guide the treatment for patients with PSI [14]. In brief, three different types of PSI are categorized based on the type of instability: A (first time), B (dynamic), and C (static). Each group is then further differentiated based on its specific pathomechanism.

Group A includes all patients with an acute, first-time subluxation (A1) or dislocation (A2). Group B encompasses patients with recurrent dynamic PSI. These patients suffer from PSI events during motion due to functional (B1) or structural instability (B2). Group C comprises patients with static PSI, either caused by constitutional structural deficiencies (C1) or acquired structural defects (C2).

Patients suffering from recurrent or chronic PSI, classified as Type B2 or C according to Moroder et al., who show an associated increased glenoid retroversion, may be considered for POWGO. Type B1 instability is associated with a pathological activation pattern of the rotator cuff and periscapular muscles, which causes mostly posterior dislocations during motion [15]. While this type of PSI may be associated with structural deficiencies such as increased glenoid retroversion, structural damage is often absent. Surgery is contraindicated in these patients, and conservative treatment is recommended instead [14, 16].

Lastly, a constitutional static posterior humeral subluxation—apparent in Type C1 instability—is considered a borderline indication as static posterior humeral subluxation may be caused by imbalances of the transverse force couple [17]. Although increased glenoid retroversion may be apparent in these patients, mixed results—including no postoperative change in static posterior humeral subluxation—have previously been reported following POWGO [17–19].

Physical Assessment

Posterior shoulder instability may be detected using the Jerk [20], Kim [21], and load-and-shift tests [22]. Additionally, general hyperlaxity should be assessed using the Beighton score [23], and shoulder-specific hyperlaxity may be evaluated using the sulcus [24] and Gagey [25] signs. The presence of hyperlaxity may indicate the degree to which a posterior capsular shift may be performed, which is explained further in the section *Surgical Management.*

Lastly, posterior positional functional shoulder instability, which may result from pathological muscle activation patterns of the external rotators and periscapular muscles, should be ruled out, as conservative treatment may be indicated in such cases [16].

Imaging

Anteroposterior, Y-view, and axillary-view X-rays should be performed routinely when treating a patient with suspected PSI. By doing so, concomitant bony pathologies can be ruled out, and the general state of the joint may be assessed. Even though glenoid retroversion may be assessed on the axillary view, it is not recommended as glenoid retroversion is often overestimated on plain radiographs when compared to computed tomography (CT) scans with a mean difference of more than 6° [26].

Next, magnetic resonance imaging (MRI) should be performed. Posterior labral and cartilage defects, lack of glenoid concavity, humeral and glenoid bone defects, glenoid dysplasia, and humeral head subluxation may be present in cases with PSI. As MRI is usually performed in a supine position, the degree to which posterior humeral head subluxation may be observed should not be overestimated. It has been shown that MRI may reliably assess glenoid retroversion only within 5° of accuracy when compared to CT [27].

Glenoid retroversion should be measured as accurately as possible, necessitating the visualization of the whole scapular body. Consequently, a CT scan should be routinely undertaken to evaluate the degree of glenoid retroversion. This is typically done using Friedman's line (Fig. 31.2) [28].

Physiological glenoid retroversion ranges between −9° and 13° (mean 1° ± SD 3°) [29], but the threshold for pathological values is still unclear, as patients with PSI and glenoid retroversion of greater than 10° may already be at a higher risk for failure following capsulolabral repair. As mentioned earlier, it was shown biomechanically that capsulolabral repair may be insufficient in the presence of glenoid retroversion greater than 15°. Because no clear cut-off value exists to date, careful patient selection is paramount, and POWGO should only be considered as a salvage procedure in young patients suffering from Type B2 or C

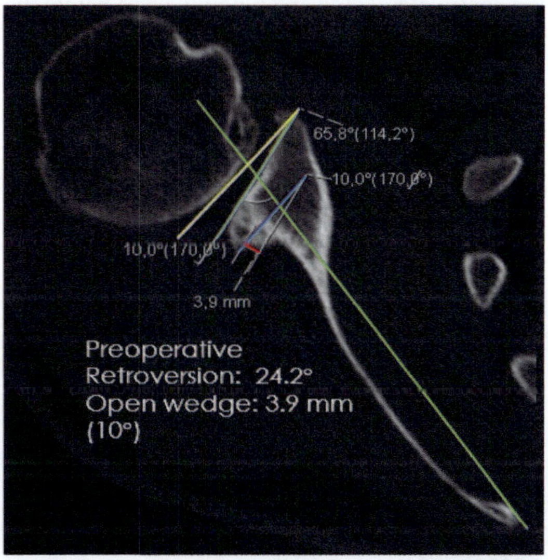

Fig. 31.2 Glenoid retroversion is measured on a preoperative CT scan. The Friedman line (green line) is drawn from the tip of the medial border of the scapula to the center of the glenoid fossa. Glenoid retroversion is measured as the angle between a line along the glenoid fossa (the Friedman line or green line) and a line perpendicular to the Friedman line. Next, a line is drawn that indicates physiological retroversion (yellow line). Following that, the glenoid line and the one which represents physiological retroversion are translated approximately 5 mm medially to the location of the planned osteotomy. The distance between the two lines of the correction angle, measured at the posterior glenoid cortex (red line), represents the width of the bone block that should be inserted surgically. CT computed tomography. (Figure from Lacheta et al. [7])

instability without glenoid or humeral bone loss who have failed nonoperative treatment and/or soft-tissue procedures [7, 14].

For young patients with PSI and increased retroversion (greater than 15°), preoperative planning for POWGO is done according to a previously described method (Fig. 31.2) [7]. It is the opinion of the authors that the correction of glenoid retroversion should not exceed 10° of retroversion to limit the interference with the individual's anatomy.

Surgical Management

The patient is placed in a prone position on a carbon fiber table with the affected arm placed in a supportive arm (Fig. 31.3a). By tilting the table to the contralateral side and placing a pad below the affected shoulder, an exposure adjacent to the glenohumeral joint line may later be achieved which is paramount in performing a precise osteotomy [7, 30].

A 7-cm longitudinal skin incision is made 3 cm medial and 2 cm distal to the posterolateral acromion toward the posterior axillary fold (Fig. 31.3b). Next, an incision through subcutaneous tissue is made to visualize the scapular spine 5 cm medial to the posterolateral acromion, and an approximately 3 cm area of the dorsolateral deltoid insertion is released. Using an oscillating saw or chisel, a rectangular, monocortical bone block (according to the size measured on the preoperative CT scan) is harvested. The fibers of the deltoid muscle that were detached earlier may be refixated transosseously, and the bone block may be prepared on the back table to create a wedge-shaped graft of the size determined via the preoperative CT scan [7, 30].

Next, the posterior fibers of the deltoid and infraspinatus muscles are split along their fibers, and the posterior capsule is incised in a T-shaped fashion to allow for a posterior capsular shift at the end of surgery. A Fukuda retractor is then placed between the now-exposed humeral head and glenoid. Two 1.6-mm Kirschner wires are placed approximately 10 mm medial to the glenoid and parallel to the Fukuda retractor to determine the osteotomy direction parallel to the glenohumeral joint line. A 20-mm chisel is then placed medial to the Kirschner wires. Thereafter, the osteotomy is performed according to the preplanned distance in a posteroanterior direction under careful protection of the anterior glenoid

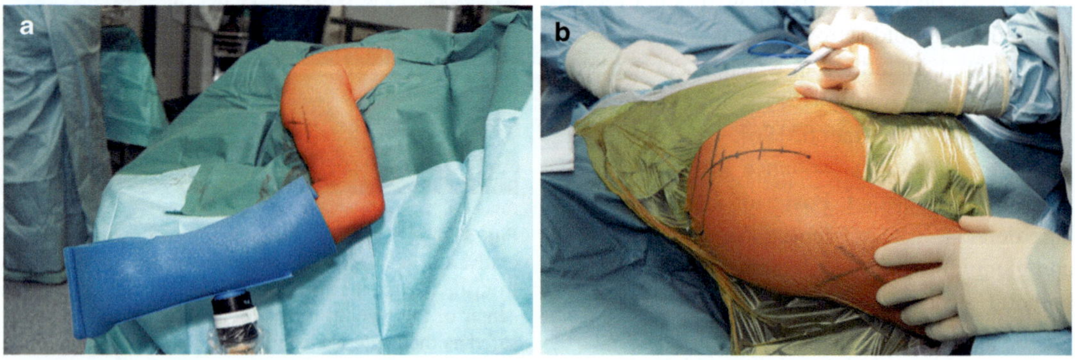

Fig. 31.3 Patient positioning (**a**) and surgical approach (**b**)

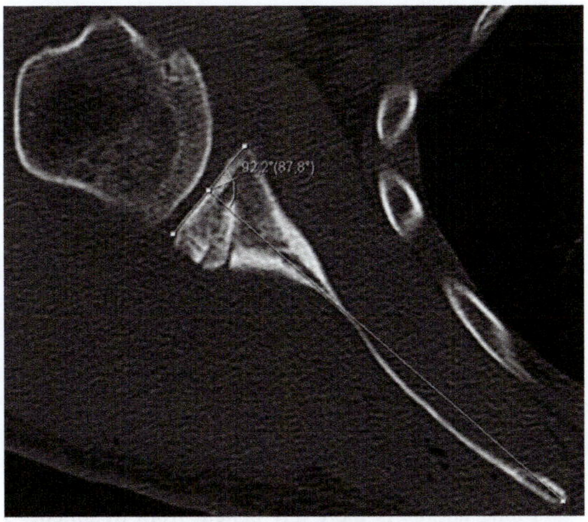

Fig. 31.4 Postoperative CT scan showing the correct graft placement and physiological retroversion. (Figure from Pogorzelski et al. [30])

cortex to avoid a hinge fracture. Further, chisels are carefully added adjacent to the first chisel until the calculated osteotomy gap is established. The graft is then inserted into the triangular gap with the use of a spreader in a press-fit fashion. Through this process, an implant-free osteotomy with a thin anterior pole and a thick posterior base is performed, and the retroversion is reduced. Finally, the wound may be irrigated, a T-shaped shift of the posterior capsule may be performed (with the arm in neutral rotation), and the wound is closed [7, 30].

On the first postoperative day, CT imaging may be obtained to evaluate the change in glenoid retroversion and to rule out perioperative complications such as hinge fractures (Figs. 31.4 and 31.5).

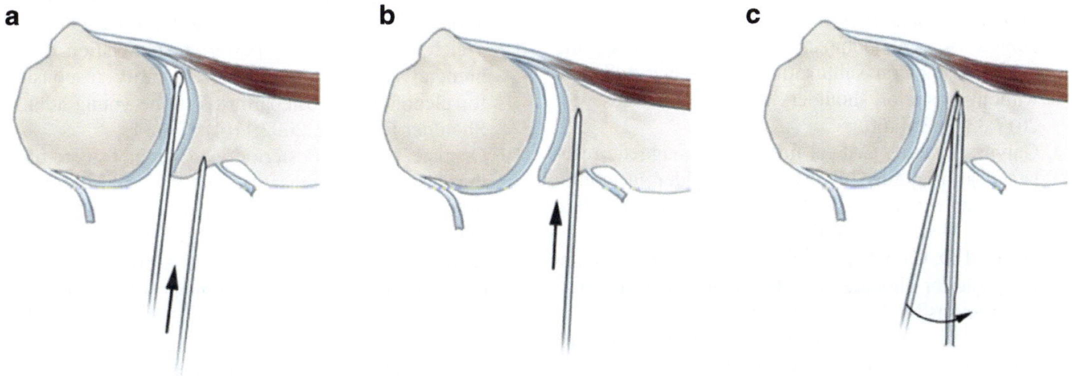

Fig. 31.5 Insertion of two 1.6-mm Kirschner wires approximately 10 mm medially to the glenoid and parallel to the Fukuda retractor (**a**). A 20-mm chisel is used to perform the osteotomy under careful protection of the anterior cortex of the glenoid (**b**). Further chisels are introduced into the joint until the desired width is achieved (**c**). (Figure from Pogorzelski et al. [30])

Postoperative Management

Postoperatively, the operated shoulder is secured immediately in neutral rotation using a shoulder brace (e.g., SLK 90, medi GmbH & Co. KG, Germany). Passive external rotation should be limited to 60°, passive internal rotation limited to 30°, and abduction limited to 45° for the first 3 weeks. Following this period, weaning from the orthosis and active-assisted motion are approved. Active range of motion is permitted after 6 weeks. Finally, full return to activity is permitted at approximately 6 months postoperatively.

References

1. Imhoff FB, et al. Glenoid retroversion is an important factor for humeral head centration and the biomechanics of posterior shoulder stability. Knee Surg Sports Traumatol Arthrosc. 2019;27(12):3952–61.
2. Parada SA, et al. Comparison of glenoid version and posterior humeral subluxation in patients with and without posterior shoulder instability. Arthroscopy. 2017;33(2):254–60.
3. Galvin JW, et al. Critical findings on magnetic resonance arthrograms in posterior shoulder instability compared with an age-matched controlled cohort. Am J Sports Med. 2016;44(12):3222–9.
4. Owens BD, Campbell SE, Cameron KL. Risk factors for posterior shoulder instability in young athletes. Am J Sports Med. 2013;41(11):2645–9.
5. Wolfe JA, et al. Effect of posterior glenoid bone loss and retroversion on arthroscopic posterior glenohumeral stabilization. Am J Sports Med. 2020;48(11):2621–7.
6. Eichinger JK, et al. Glenoid dysplasia: pathophysiology, diagnosis, and management. J Bone Joint Surg Am. 2016;98(11):958–68.
7. Lacheta L, et al. Posterior open wedge glenoid osteotomy provides reliable results in young patients with increased glenoid retroversion and posterior shoulder instability. Knee Surg Sports Traumatol Arthrosc. 2019;27(1):299–304.
8. Williams RJ 3rd, et al. Arthroscopic repair for traumatic posterior shoulder instability. Am J Sports Med. 2003;31(2):203–9.
9. Wolf EM, Eakin CL. Arthroscopic capsular plication for posterior shoulder instability. Arthroscopy. 1998;14(2):153–63.
10. Katthagen JC, et al. Association of traumatic and atraumatic posterior shoulder instability with glenoid retroversion and outcomes after arthroscopic capsulolabral repair. Arthroscopy. 2017;33(2):284–90.
11. Galvin JW, et al. High incidence of anterior shoulder pain in young athletes undergoing arthroscopic posterior labral repair for posterior shoulder instability. Arthrosc Sports Med Rehabil. 2021;3(5):e1441–7.
12. Millett PJ, et al. Recurrent posterior shoulder instability. J Am Acad Orthop Surg. 2006;14(8):464–76.
13. Robinson CM, Aderinto J. Recurrent posterior shoulder instability. JBJS. 2005;87(4):883–92.
14. Moroder P, Scheibel M. ABC classification of posterior shoulder instability. Obere Extrem. 2017;12(2):66–74.
15. Takwale VJ, Calvert P, Rattue H. Involuntary positional instability of the shoulder in adolescents and young adults. Is there any benefit from treatment? J Bone Joint Surg Br. 2000;82(5):719–23.
16. Moroder P, et al. Shoulder-pacemaker treatment concept for posterior positional functional shoulder instability: a prospective clinical trial. Am J Sports Med. 2020;48(9):2097–104.
17. Mitterer M, et al. Muscle volume imbalance may be associated with static posterior humeral head subluxation. BMC Musculoskelet Disord. 2021;22(1):279.
18. Walch G, et al. Static posterior subluxation of the humeral head: an unrecognized entity responsible for glenohumeral osteoarthritis in the young adult. J Shoulder Elb Surg. 2002;11(4):309–14.
19. Ortmaier R, et al. Posterior open wedge osteotomy of the scapula neck for the treatment of advanced shoulder osteoarthritis with posterior head migration in young patients. J Shoulder Elb Surg. 2017;26(7):1278–86.
20. Kim SH, et al. Painful jerk test: a predictor of success in nonoperative treatment of posteroinferior instability of the shoulder. Am J Sports Med. 2004;32(8):1849–55.
21. Kim SH, et al. The Kim test: a novel test for posteroinferior labral lesion of the shoulder–a comparison to the jerk test. Am J Sports Med. 2005;33(8):1188–92.
22. Baker CL, Merkley MS. Clinical evaluation of the athlete's shoulder. J Athl Train. 2000;35(3):256–60.
23. Beighton P, Solomon L, Soskolne CL. Articular mobility in an African population. Ann Rheum Dis. 1973;32(5):413–8.
24. Neer CS 2nd, Foster CR. Inferior capsular shift for involuntary inferior and multidirectional instability of the shoulder. A preliminary report. J Bone Joint Surg Am. 1980;62(6):897–908.
25. Gagey OJ, Gagey N. The hyperabduction test. J Bone Joint Surg Br. 2001;83(1):69–74.
26. Nyffeler RW, et al. Measurement of glenoid version: conventional radiographs versus computed tomography scans. J Shoulder Elb Surg. 2003;12(5):493–6.

27. Parada SA, et al. Magnetic resonance imaging correlates with computed tomography for glenoid version calculation despite lack of visibility of medial scapula. Arthroscopy. 2020;36(1):99–105.
28. Friedman RJ, Hawthorne KB, Genez BM. The use of computerized tomography in the measurement of glenoid version. J Bone Joint Surg Am. 1992;74(7):1032–7.
29. Matsumura N, et al. Morphologic features of humeral head and glenoid version in the normal glenohumeral joint. J Shoulder Elb Surg. 2014;23(11):1724–30.
30. Pogorzelski J, et al. Open-wedge-Glenoidosteotomie als Therapie bei posteriorer Schulterinstabilität aufgrund vermehrter Glenoidretroversion. Oper Orthop Traumatol. 2016;28(6):438–48.

32 Posterior Instability Outcomes Over the Last 20 Years: Where Are We Now?

Daniel J. Kaplan, Garrett R. Jackson, Christopher M. Brusalis, and Nikhil N. Verma

Case

HPI A 27-year-old righ- hand-dominant male presented with 4 years of posterior-based right shoulder pain. He denied an acute inciting trauma; however, he noted exacerbated symptoms with weightlifting and overhead activities. He denied any episodes of overt shoulder dislocations. His pain occurs most commonly with his arm flexed and slightly adducted. His symptoms have persisted despite prolonged activity modification and a physical therapy rehabilitation program. A prior ultrasound-guided intra-articular corticosteroid injection provided significant, albeit transient, relief. He has not experienced any neurovascular deficits in his right upper extremity.

PMHx No past medical or surgical history

Focused Right Shoulder Physical Exam
Range of Motion

Forward elevation: 180°
Abduction: 180°
External rotation with the arm in adduction: 70°
Functional internal rotation to T10
No tenderness to palpation at the acromioclavicular joint, sternoclavicular joint, greater tuberosity, or biceps tendon.
Strength: 5/5 supraspinatus/infraspinatus/teres minor/subscapularis

Positive Jerk Test, Positive Kim Test
Negative apprehension sign, negative anterior load and shift, negative posterior load and shift, and negative sulcus sign

Neurovascularly intact (Figs. 32.1, 32.2, 32.3, and 32.4)

D. J. Kaplan
NYU Langone Health, New York University Langone Medical Center, New York, NY, USA

G. R. Jackson · N. N. Verma (✉)
Department of Orthopaedic Surgery, Rush University Medical Center, Chicago, IL, USA
e-mail: nikhil.verma@rushortho.com

C. M. Brusalis
Sports Medicine Institute, Hospital for Special Surgery, New York, NY, USA

© The Author(s), under exclusive license to Springer Nature Switzerland AG 2026
R. M. Frank, J. M. Tokish (eds.), *Management of Shoulder Instability*,
https://doi.org/10.1007/978-3-032-18089-6_32

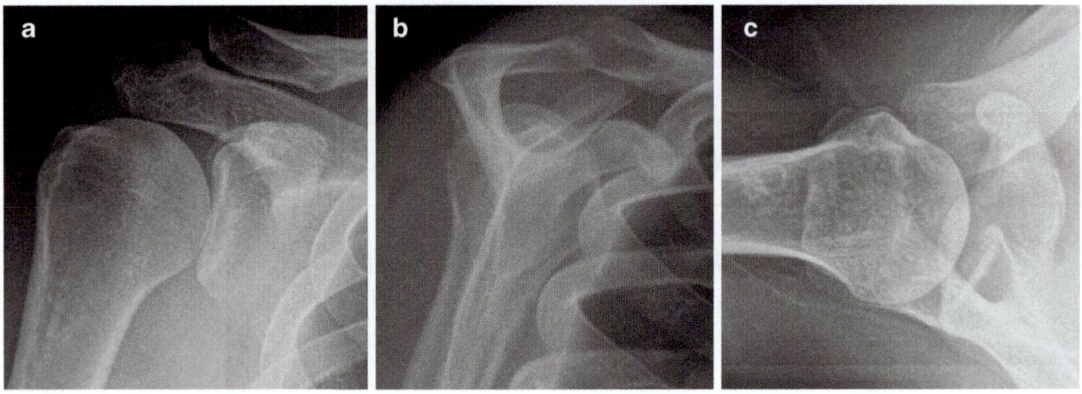

Fig. 32.1 Grashey (**a**), scapular Y (**b**), and axillary (**c**) radiographic views of a right shoulder do not demonstrate any obvious pathology, such as fractures, dislocations, reverse Hill-Sachs lesions, or significant glenoid version abnormalities

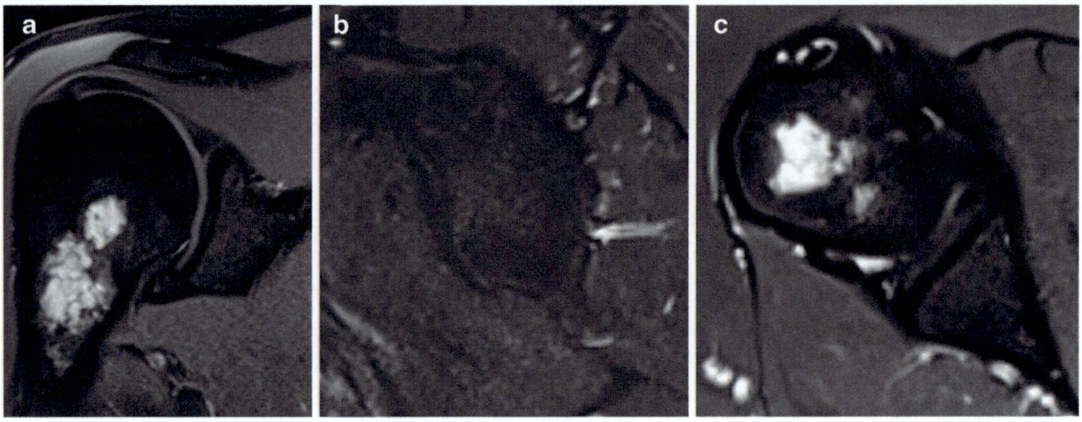

Fig. 32.2 Coronal (**a**), sagittal (**b**), and axial (**c**) T2-weighted MRI of a right shoulder demonstrating a posteroinferior labral tear, along with cystic changes within the humeral head

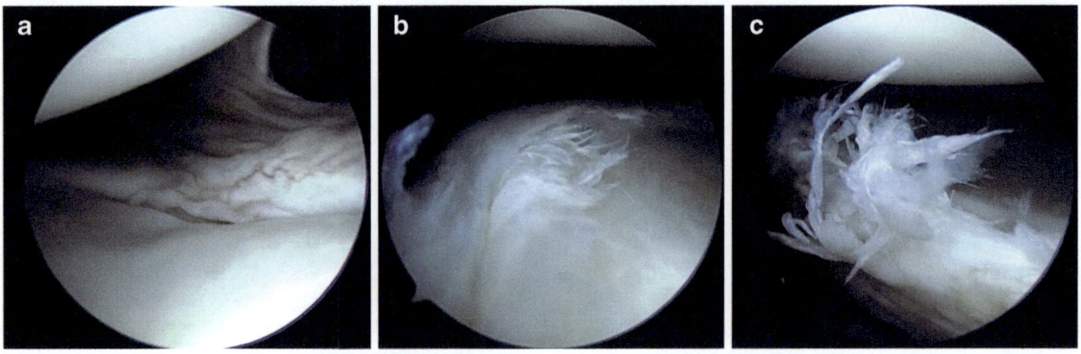

Fig. 32.3 Intraoperative arthroscopic images of a right shoulder viewing from the anterior portal (**a**) and posterior portal (**b** and **c**) demonstrating a torn posteroinferior labrum

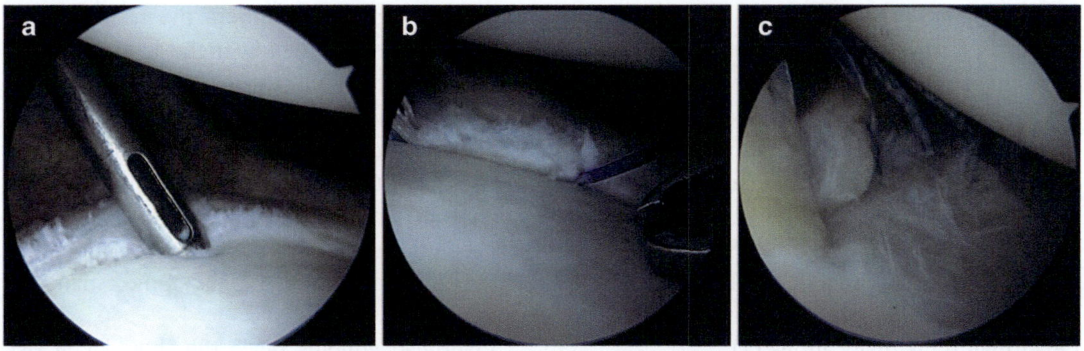

Fig. 32.4 Intraoperative arthroscopic images of a right shoulder viewed from the anterior portal. A guide is placed on the glenoid rim for proper anchor placement (**a**). Followed by the insertion of a soft tissue anchor, a suture passing device is placed under the labrum to allow shuttling of the working stitch from the anchor (**b**). Posterior labrum with bumper restored after three anchors were placed. Suture limbs are still in place, allowing final tightening (**c**)

Anatomy

Similar to the anterior shoulder, the posterior aspect of the shoulder is stabilized by a combination of static and dynamic stabilizers, working in concert throughout the range of motion (ROM). The primary static stabilizers include the bony buttress imparted by the geometry of the glenoid as well as the capsulolabral complex [1–4]. The most important ligament for posterior shoulder stability is the posterior inferior glenohumeral ligament (PIGHL), which is placed under tension when the shoulder is loaded posteriorly with forward flexion and internal rotation [5]. The middle glenohumeral ligament (MGHL) and superior glenohumeral ligament (SGHL) contribute to resisting posterior translation with the arm in midrange abduction and shoulder adduction, respectively [6].

The labrum augments the static stability provided by the bony constraints of the glenoid-humeral head relationship by increasing the depth of the humeral articulation, as well as increasing the concavity-compression mechanism of the humeral head in the glenoid socket [4]. It has been demonstrated that patients with recurrent shoulder instability have a loss of chondrolabral containment, which includes both an increase in bony retroversion of the glenoid as well as a loss of the posteroinferior labral height [7].

The role of anterior structures in providing static posterior instability is controversial. A biomechanical study by Cole et al. found that when the arm was in an adducted position, both the SGHL and the rotator interval limited posterior humeral head translation [8]. Similarly, Wellman et al. found that a deficient rotator interval increased glenohumeral translation [9]. Conversely, more recent work has not found any contribution of the rotator interval and questions the utility of closing it to further reduce posterior instability at the risk of diminished external rotation [10].

The subscapularis is the primary dynamic stabilizer, supporting the action of the PIGHL. However, all four rotator cuff muscles, in addition to those of the scapula, contribute to the cavity compression of the shoulder, limiting posterior translation. The infraspinatus and teres minor, in particular, act as posterior compressors [7].

Important anatomic differences exist between the posterior and anterior shoulder, which must be considered when approaching posterior pathology. The posterior capsule and posterior inferior glenohumeral ligament have substantially less tensile strength than their analogous anterior counterparts. While this weaker restraint is usually sufficient to resist the comparatively lower posteriorly directed forces transmitted to the humeral head, the posterior capsule is susceptible to attenuation from repetitive stresses. This anatomic discrepancy between anterior and posterior capsulolabral structures is, in part, responsible for why patients with PSI present more frequently with a primary complaint of pain due to microinstability or recurrent subluxations rather than frank dislocations [7].

Pathophysiology

Posterior shoulder instability can be categorized broadly into three groups based on pathophysiology: pure atraumatic, repetitive microtraumatic, and acute traumatic. As the underlying anatomic disruptions are different for each pathology, it is crucial to determine the nature of the instability to treat it appropriately.

Patients presenting with acute traumatic posterior instability have a distinct injury immediately preceding symptom onset, typically with a frank shoulder subluxation or dislocation. While seizure and electrocution are possible etiologies for posterior shoulder dislocations, the most common cause of acute traumatic posterior instability is due to a direct blow to an adducted, internally rotated arm in the forward flexed position [11]. This may occur after a fall onto an outstretched hand, after falling forward on a bicycle, falls during rugby or American football, or a lineman injured while blocking with the arm in the forward flexed and internally rotated position.

The most common cause of posterior shoulder pain is repetitive microtrauma to the posteroinferior shoulder complex [7]. This occurs with activities that place the shoulder in a flexed and internally rotated position. When the shoulder is loaded in this position, the PIGHL, as well as associated posterior restraints, may become stretched or injured. With repeated loads, the labrum and PIGHL may become incompetent or frankly torn, leading to posterior laxity [12, 13]. This repetitive pathology is prevalent in football linemen, weightlifters, golfers, overhead athletes, and swimmers [11]. Unlike in the acute traumatic setting, where the patient may sustain a discrete capsulolabral detachment (such as a reverse Bankart lesion), recurrent posterior subluxations often stretch the capsulolabral complex, leading to labrum detachment and capsular incompetence. In these patients, the primary complaint is often posterior shoulder pain, rather than true instability.

Overhead athletes place the shoulder at risk for posterior dislocation in two positions during the throwing motion. First, during the late cocking phase with the shoulder fully externally rotated and abducted to 90°, the posterosuperior humerus may impinge on the posterior articular portion of the rotator cuff, the posterosuperior glenoid, and the labrum. This unique pathophysiologic cascade is known as "internal impingement." In addition to direct injury from the impingement, this same motion can cause injury through a traction-type mechanism. Pitchers may gain increased external rotation at the expense of decreased internal rotation due to physiologic anatomic adaptations, such as increased humeral retroversion. These changes may become pathologic if the posterior capsule contracts, limiting the total arc of motion [14]. Posterior contracture may shift the fulcrum of the glenohumeral joint posterosuperior to clear the anteroinferior labroligamentous restraints [15]. Excessive external rotation with the arm in an abducted position may expose the posterosuperior labrum, biceps tendon, and undersurface of the rotator cuff to excessive rotatory forces, resulting in the peel-back phenomenon [11]. This pathology is distinct from recurrent shoulder instability in that it results primarily in posterosuperior labral tears, whereas recurrent shoulder instability typically causes anteroinferior labral tears [11]. Additionally, initial treatment for thrower's etiology related to a tight posterior capsule is focused on posteroinferior capsular stretching, as opposed to surgery to tighten that area of the joint. The second throwing phase, placing the posterior shoulder at risk, is the follow-through phase, during which the humerus continues to rapidly adduct, flex, and internally rotate, which places significant stress across the posterior capsulolabral complex [16].

The least common etiology of PSI is atraumatic. It is most often found in patients with generalized ligamentous laxity and is primarily due to capsular redundancy rather than a discrete tear [7]. In addition, it is often associated with instability in other directions, most commonly inferior.

One point to emphasize is that, in contrast to anterior shoulder instability and its pathognomonic anteroinferior labral injury, PSI lacks an "essential lesion." In a retrospective review of 92 shoulders in 90 patients treated surgically for posterior instability, Savoie et al. found varied pathologies, including ligament tears, without a consistent posteroinferior labral tear. As a result, the authors emphasize a thorough diagnostic evaluation of the intra-articular space for any patient being treated for posterior instability, as multiple structures may be injured [17].

Patient Evaluation

Presenting symptoms will vary based on etiology. Patients with an acute traumatic event will describe a specific injury mechanism and potentially associated instability. Patients with microinstability, however, may have a more subtle presentation, with vague symptoms of posterior shoulder pain, commonly associated with the offending action (such as blocking for linemen or bench pressing for weight lifters) [18]. There may also be impaired athletic performance or a decrease in weightlifting capacity. Patients with atraumatic posterior instability may similarly have vague pain complaints, possibly with associated complaints in other joints related to generalized laxity. Clicking, popping, or slipping may be described. Patients also note difficulty loading the shoulder in the affected plane. Providers should try to clarify the first time the patient felt pain or instability, the number of subluxations/dislocations (if present), the nature of traumatic events (if they occurred), and the direction of instability.

Examination begins with inspection, primarily to assess for atrophy of the rotator cuff or scapular dyskinesia, which can contribute to posterior shoulder pain. Palpation along the posterior joint line can elicit tenderness. Range of motion, particularly the total arc of rotation, should be evaluated, looking for a decrease in the total arc of motion in comparison to the contralateral shoulder. Rotator cuff strength should be assessed, as concomitant rotator cuff pathology may occur, particularly in overhead athletes, if there is a component of internal impingement.

Special provocative maneuvers for the posterior shoulder begin with an assessment of instability. With the arm abducted to 120° and in neutral rotation, a posterior load and shift maneuver can be performed by applying axial load and a posterior force on the proximal humerus. Translation of the humeral head is graded on a 0–3 scale [11]. A jerk test can be performed with the patient seated. While stabilizing the scapula, a posteriorly directed force is applied to the arm in a 120° abducted, adducted, and internally rotated position. Pain or subluxation is considered a positive test. Often, posterior labral clicking or catching can be appreciated. A Kim test is similar; however, the arm is also forward flexed 45°. A posterior load applied in this position adds more stress to the posteroinferior labrum [19].

Imaging

An initial imaging evaluation should begin with a routine set of shoulder radiographs, including Grashey anterior-posterior X-ray, scapular Y, and axillary views. X-rays are typically normal but should be scrutinized, as subtle signs of posterior instability may be appreciated, such as a reverse Hill-Sachs sign or a posteriorly translated humeral head (Fig. 32.5). Most importantly, one should confirm that a posterior dislocation was not missed during the patient's prior work-up.

A computed tomography (CT) is not always necessary and should be ordered if concerned for osseous pathology. CT imaging is particularly

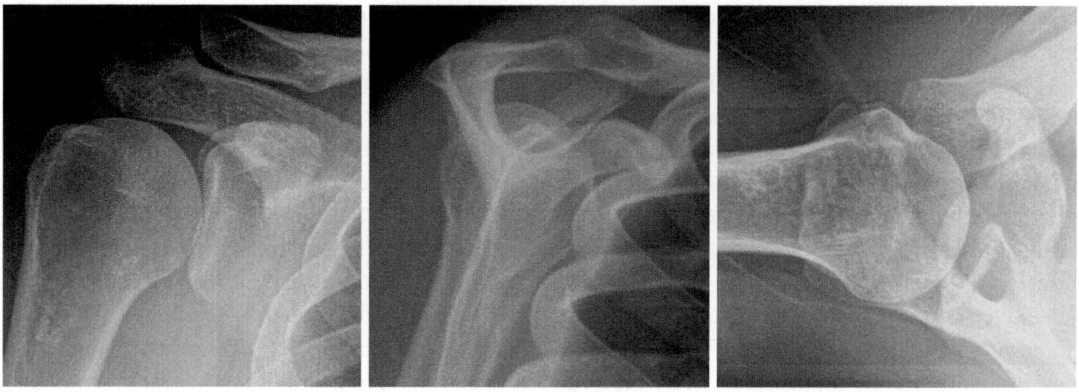

Fig. 32.5 Grashey, scapular Y, and axillary X-rays of a right shoulder in a patient with posterior instability. These do not demonstrate any obvious pathology, including fractures, dislocations, or reverse-Hill-Sachs lesions

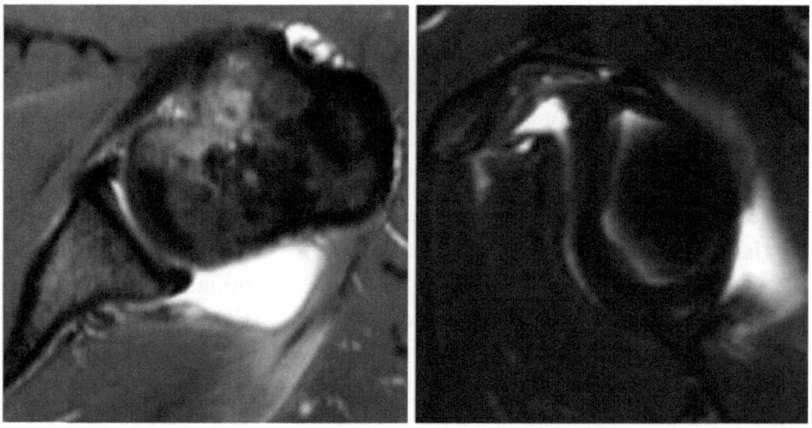

Fig. 32.6 Axial and sagittal MRI of a left shoulder, demonstrating a bone bruising pattern associated with a posterior instability event. Additionally, a posterior labral tear can be appreciated in the axial plane, with a suggestion of one in the posteroinferior position on the sagittal imaging

useful to assess for posterior bone loss, glenoid version, and the size of a reverse Hill-Sachs lesion.

Magnetic resonance imaging (MRI) and magnetic resonance arthrograms (MRAs) are essential for evaluating the status of the posterior labrum and capsule. While MRA has historically been the gold standard, improvements in MRI, particularly the increasing availability of 3T MRI, have largely obviated the requirement for MRA (Fig. 32.6). However, in revision settings or if there is ambiguity in the MRI, an MRA can be extremely useful in detecting subtle labral pathology. The posterior labrum often has much less conspicuous tears than do tears of the anterior labrum, and an MRA can help elucidate this. In throwers, the ABER position is helpful in evaluating the posterior superior labrum and posterior rotator cuff for evidence of internal impingement.

A measurement being increasingly utilized to assess the reverse Hill-Sachs is the modified gamma angle [20]. Using an axial plane CT or MRI, a best-fit circle is placed centered over the humeral head. The angle is formed from a line drawn from the posterior margin of the reverse Hill-Sachs defect to the center of the circle, and a second line is drawn from the bicipital groove to the center of the circle. While strict cut-offs are still being developed, an increased modified gamma angle has been associated with an increased risk of instability [20].

Outcomes of Posterior Shoulder Instability Treatment

Much has changed over the last two decades regarding the management approach, techniques, and ultimately outcomes of PSI. As understanding of the anatomy and biomechanical forces on the posterior shoulder restraints has evolved, so too has the ability to restore function to these patients.

Nonoperative Management

The decision to proceed to surgery is complex and dependent on a multitude of factors, including patient age, sports participation/time in season, and underlying pathology/symptomology. A 2019 retrospective study by Woodmass et al. evaluating 143 patients with posterior instability (not subcategorized as recurrent microinstability vs. acute) found that 45% of patients underwent surgery at presentation [21]. Of the remaining 55% of patients who were treated nonoperatively (for at least 1 year), 46% of patients were later converted to surgery for persistent PSI symptoms over the next 10 years. The authors postulated that the high conversion rate could be primarily due to two reasons: 1) changes in the literature supporting the efficacy of capsulo labral repair over the study period and 2) the progressive nature of microinstability (the most common form of PSI), which is fundamentally different from traumatic anterior instability and may continue to get incrementally worse with time [21].

A subsequent 2022 multicenter retrospective study by Festbaum et al. of 28 patients with first-time acute posterior shoulder dislocations (traumatic type) treated nonoperatively found that only 31% of patients subsequently underwent surgery [22]. Though it did not reach significance (likely due to the small sample size), patients in the failed nonoperative group had a higher modified gamma angle, which was larger than 90° in all patients who failed conservative management. Similarly, there was a trend toward increased posterior humeral head subluxation among patients who failed nonoperative treatment [22]. The authors attributed their much lower surgical conversion rate relative to the Woodmass study to their study population—namely, acute first-time traumatic injuries as opposed to the microinstability included in the 2019 study. They suggest that differences between anteriorly directed and posteriorly directed shoulder loading account for the lower recurrence rate for acute posterior instability and higher success rate with nonoperative management [22].

A single comparative study exists comparing operative and nonoperative management. In 2017, Cruz-Ferreira et al. retrospectively compared a heterogenous group of 51 patients with multiple types of PSI, with 19 receiving nonoperative management and 32 undergoing one of several surgical correction methods (labral repair, bone defect filling, posterior bone block) [23]. Patients treated operatively had significantly higher Constant, Rowe, and Walch Duplay scores. However, the study's retrospective analysis, low sample size, and heterogeneity of both patient populations and surgical interventions limit the conclusions that can be drawn from its findings. Future prospective, randomized controlled trials are needed to better elucidate which patients may be successfully treated nonoperatively.

Operative Management Outcomes

Pre-Modern Techniques (Pre-2000)

While techniques have improved over the last 20 years (Tables 32.1 and 32.2), the ultimate aim of PSI surgery remains the same: restoration of both the posterior labral buttress as well as tension on the posterior capsulolabral complex [24]. Prior to 2000, several small case series exploring arthroscopic posterior labral repair were published [25–28], demonstrating promising results; however, these early studies included small sample sizes, heterogeneous posterior pathologies, patients treated with multiple surgical procedures, and a wide array of techniques (including anterior capsularrhaphy).

Table 32.1 Eras of posterior labral repair outcome research

Years	Grouping	Contribution
Pre-2000s	Pre-modern techniques	Demonstrated potential efficacy of capsulolabral repair
2003–2006	Modern techniques	Established modern arthroscopic techniques—labral repair with capsular shift using multiple suture anchors
2006–2015	Larger, homogenous studies	Introduction of prospective studies, with large sample sizes, allowing for a better understanding of outcomes
2016 to present	Evaluation of specific outcome factors	Identification of specific factors related to outcomes
2018 to present	Revision risk	Follow-up of previous studies allows evaluation of risk factors for undergoing revision
2021 to present	Non-labral repair techniques	Evaluation of techniques, including posterior bone blocks and glenoid osteotomies

Table 32.2 Studies evaluating operative techniques and outcomes

Study (Year)	No. of patients	Return to play, %	Failures/ revisions, %	Mean postoperative outcome scores	Key takeaways
Pre-modern techniques (pre-2000)					
Papendick and Savoie 3rd. [25]	41	–	–	Neer-Foster rating scale: 95% ($n = 39/41$ patients) satisfactory	Small sample sizes, with heterogenous pathologies, but promising early results
McIntyre et al. [26]	19 ($n = 20$ shoulders)	–	15 ($n = 3/20$)	Athletic shoulder outcome rating scale: 83	Small sample sizes, with heterogenous pathologies, but promising early results
Wolf and Eakin [27]	14	90 ($n = 9/10$)	7.1 ($n = 1/14$)	–	Small sample sizes, with heterogenous pathologies, but promising early results
Wirth et al. [28]	10	66.7 ($n = 6/9$)	10 ($n = 1/10$)	–	Small sample sizes, with heterogenous pathologies, but promising early results
Misamore et al. [54]	14	85.7 ($n = 12/14$)	7.1 ($n = 1/14$)	Rowe grading system: 13 of 14 patients achieved excellent results	Small sample sizes, with heterogenous pathologies, but promising early results
Modern techniques (2003–2006)					
Williams 3rd et al. [24]	27	–	7.4 ($n = 2/27$)	L'Insalata shoulder score: 90 ± 13.9; SF-36 PCS: 50.4 ± 7; SF-36 MCS: 53.9 ± 9	Capsulolabral repair with bioabsorbable suture tacks used No ROM deficits

(continued)

Table 32.2 (continued)

Study (Year)	No. of patients	Return to play, %	Failures/ revisions, %	Mean postoperative outcome scores	Key takeaways
Kim et al. [30]	15	93.3 (*n* = 14/15)	6.7 (*n* = 1/15)	All patients showed improved UCLA, ASES, and Rowe scores	Success attributed to the use of suture anchors, nonabsorbable suture, and large capsular shift Identified, "Kim Lesion"
Larger, homogenous studies (2006–2015)					
Bradley et al. [12]	91 (*n* = 100 shoulders)	89 (*n* = 89/100)	11 (*n* = 11/100)	ASES score: 85.66	First large-scale homogoenous cohort study -failures associated with a low number of suture anchors and isolated capsular plication
Savoie 3rd et al. [17]	90 (*n* = 92 shoulders)	–	2.2 (*n* = 2/92)	Neer-Foster rating scale: 97% (*n* = 89/92 shoulders) success	Absence of any "essential lesion"
Bradley et al. [16]	200	90 (*n* = 180/200)	9.5 (*n* = 19/200)	ASES score: 85.1	Reinforced the importance of anchor-based fixation and associated decreased failure rates
McClincy et al. [32]	96	Throwers: 8.45 (*n* = 41/48) Non-throwers: 87.5 (*n* = 42/48)	Throwers: 6.3 (*n* = 3/48) Non-throwers 8.3 (*n* = 4/48)	ASES score: 84.6 ± 15 (throwers), 85.7 ± 17 (non-throwers)	No difference in failure rate or PRO scores between throwers and non-throwers, but lower RTP in throwers
Katthagen et al. [34]	38 (*n* = 41 shoulders)	Atramautic: 72.2 (*n* = 13/18) traumatic: 90 (*n* = 9/10)	Atramautic: 5.6 (*n* = 1/18) traumatic: 10 (*n* = 1/10)	ASES score: 95.8 (atraumatic), 99.9 (traumatic); QuickDASH score: 5.7 (atraumatic), 1.1 (traumatic); SANE score: 86.5 (atraumatic), 98 (traumatic); SF-12 PCS: 54.5 (atraumatic), 56.8 (traumatic)	Patients with traumatic etiology had significantly improved PRO scores compared to nontraumatic etiology

(continued)

Table 32.2 (continued)

Study (Year)	No. of patients	Return to play, %	Failures/ revisions, %	Mean postoperative outcome scores	Key takeaways
Evaluation of specific factors related to outcomes (2016 to present)					
Glenoid characteristics					
Mauro et al. [35]	183 shoulders	–	11.7 (n = 13/111)	Patients with wider glenoids reported better pain and ASES scores	Posterior instability patients had increased glenoid retroversion compared with controls Wider glenoids associated with better PRO scores
Bradley et al. [36]	281 (n = 297 shoulders)	–	6.4 (n = 19/297)	ASES score: 88 ± 14.5	Increased glenoid retroversion did not increase the risk of revision surgery Patients requiring revision had narrower glenoids
Hines et al. [39]	32	<13.5% bone loss: 92 (n = 23/25) >13.5% bone loss: 85.7 (n = 6/7)	6.3 (n = 2/32)	SANE score: 50 (<13.5% bone loss), 69 (>13.5% bone loss); WOSI score: 1066 (<13.5% bone loss), 1020 (>13.5% bone loss)	Patients with >13.5% posterior bone loss had lower return to duty, but no differences in reoperation rate, complications, or PROs
Concomitant pathology					
Nourissat et al. [40]	144	–	–	Constant score: 86.2 ± 14.5; Walch-Duplay score: 79.8 ± 24.2	Of several factors analzyed, only the presence of a glenoid cartilage lesion was associated w/worse PROs
Ferrando et al. [41]	26	70 (n = 7/10)	11.5 (n = 3/26)	SANE score: 90*; WOSI score: 385*	Patients with more severe cartilage injury had decreased PROs at follow-up
Arner et al. [42]	56	Concomitant RCTs: 91.7 (n = 22/24) No RCTs: 84.4 (n = 27/32)	Concomitant RCTs: 0 No RCTs: 9.4 (n = 3/32)	ASES score: 41.8 (concomitant RCTs); 49.7 (no RCTs)	No significant differences between patients with associated partial thickness rotator cuff tears and controls
Revision risk (2018 to present)					
Bradley et al. [52]	149	Revision: 50 (n = 4/8) Nonrevision 93.6 (132/141)	5.4 (n = 8/149)	ASES score: 75.1 (revisions), 87.8 (nonrevisions)	Postoperative instability and decreased glenoid bone width associated w/ failure in contact athletes

(continued)

Table 32.2 (continued)

Study (Year)	No. of patients	Return to play, %	Failures/ revisions, %	Mean postoperative outcome scores	Key takeaways
Vaswani et al. [53]	105	Revision: 14.3 Nonrevision 83.7	8.6 (*n* = 9/105)	ASES score: 74.7 ± 19.3 (revisions), 80.4 ± 15.2 (nonrevisions); KJOC score: 52.6 ± 28.7 (revisions), 51.9 ± 21.8 (nonrevisions)	Female sex associated with failure
Techniques other than labral repair (2021 to present)					
Struck et al. [43]	13 (*n* = 15 shoulders)	83.3 (*n* = 10/12)	33.3 (*n* = 5/15)	Constant score: 82; Rowe score: 88; Walch-Duplay score: 81	Reoperation in 5/15 patients (four due to hardware irritation, one for recurrent instability)
Meuffels et al. [44]	11	–	–	Rowe score: 60*; WOSI score: 60*	45% of patients would not have chosen to have the operation again
Lacheta et al. [47]	11 (*n* = 12 shoulders)	–	0	ROWE score: 90*; Oxford instability score: 44	4 cases of intraoperative glenoid neck fracture
Waltenspul et al. [49]	6 (*n* = 7 shoulders)	Return to work: 100 (*n* = 7/7)	42.9 (*n* = 3/7)	Constant score: 68;	86% recurrent instability with 6/7 shoulders developing arthritis at follow-up
Mi et al. [50]	10	Return to work: 100 (*n* = 10/10)	10 (*n* = 1/10)	Constant-Murley score: 40.6 ± 10.3; VAS: 0.61 ± 0.21	Reverse Hill-Sachs treated with bone grafting and internal fixaion
Cohen et al. [51]	10	–	0	Constant-Murley score: 65 ± 21.5; UCLA score: 27 ± 9.7; VAS: 2.4 ± 2.3	Patients treated with the modified McLaughlin –80% satisfaction rate

Legend: No. number, *SF-12 PCS* Short-Form 12 Physical Component Summary, *SF-12 MCS* Short-Form Mental Component Summary, *ASES* American Shoulder and Elbow Surgeons, *QuickDASH* Quick Disabilities of the Arm, Shoulder, and Hand, SANE, Single Assessment Numeric Evaluation, *WOSI* Western Ontario Shoulder Instability Index, *KJOC* Kerlan-Jobe Orthopaedic Clinic, *RCTs* rotator cuff tears, *PRO* patient-reported outcome, * median

In 2000, Misamore et al. reported on a small series of traumatic, unidirectional PSI treated with open posterior capsulorrhaphy. At 45-month follow-up, 13/14 patients were pain-free, with an 85/7% RTP. While these early papers helped establish the efficacy of capsulolabral repair for treating PSI, it would be several more years before outcomes of patients treated with techniques resembling those commonly employed today would be published.

Modern Techniques (2003–2006)

Two studies published in 2003 exclusively utilized what would become staples of contemporary practice. Such techniques included labral repair with a capsular shift using suture anchors, as well as the use of accessory posterior portals.

Kim et al. published a retrospective review of 27 patients treated for unidirectional acute traumatic PSI [29]. At a mean follow-up of 39 months, all had significant improvement in pain and were able to return to sport, aside from one patient who had residual symptoms of instability. There was, however, a loss of mean one vertebral level of internal rotation. The authors attributed their success to the use of suture anchors, nonabsorbable suture, and a large capsular shift. Of note, the authors also highlighted an important difference between anterior and posterior labral injuries—namely, a common apparent superficial "crack" at the chondrolabral junction, which may appear benign, but upon probing would reveal a deep partial detachment of the labrum from the glenoid. The authors strongly advocated completing this avulsion and repairing it. This lesion would ultimately be named a "Kim Lesion" after a 2004 paper published by the same group further discussed it [30].

Williams et al. treated patients with acute traumatic PSI with arthroscopic capsulolabral repair (though using bioabsorbable suture tacks) and found no patient with a ROM deficit, no instability, and 92% of patients without persistent pain at a mean follow-up of 5 years [24]. Two patients had 4 out of 5 strength in external rotation. Similar to the Kim et al. study, the group emphasized the pre-eminent role of the PIGHL in resisting posterior translation and the importance of restoring tension on the ligament (in addition to the posteroinferior labrum) to achieve optimal results [24].

In a precursor to several studies that would come out about a decade later, a 2005 study by Kim et al. compared patients with atraumatic posterior shoulder instability (or recurrent posterior subluxation [RPS]) with matched controls in an attempt to uncover native anatomic risk factors [31]. The group found that both osseous (4.6° vs. 1.4°) and chondrolabral version (7.0° vs. 2.3°) were greater in the RPS group compared with controls, with the greatest difference being in the chondrolabral version. Posteroinferior labral height was also shallower posteriorly in the RPS group (3.5 mm vs. 5.0 mm) [31]. The authors suggest that this constellation of findings ultimately leads to decreased containment of the humeral head with a posteriorly directed force.

Larger, Homogenous Studies (2006–2015)

Building off the foundation laid by the Kim and Williams studies, the next decade of research focused on larger studies with more homogenous patient samples, including prospective data collection.

In a 2006 landmark study, Bradley et al. published their prospective data of 100 patients with both traumatic and atraumatic PSI [12]. Importantly, three surgical techniques were utilized based on the underlying pathology: (1) capsulolabral plication without suture anchors (tied knots to an intact labrum), (2) capsulolabral plication with suture anchors, or (3) capsulolabral plication with suture anchors and additional plication sutures. At 27-month follow-up, investigators found that patients significantly improved their ASES scores (50 to 86) without a difference between contact and noncontact athletes. Furthermore, instability scores significantly decreased from 7.36 to 1.9. Neither pain nor instability scores were significantly different between contact and noncontact athletes. Additionally, 89% of athletes were able to return to sport (85% for contact athletes), with 67% able to return to the same level (74% for contact) [12]. Interestingly, not only were the clinical metrics similar between contact and noncontact athletes, but there was also no significant difference in terms of surgical pathology identified (similar capsulolabral tears, similar degree of capsular laxity).

Patients were also compared to controls for radiologic risk factors. Similar to the 2005 Kim study [31], Bradley et al. found significantly increased chondrolabral (10.7° vs. 5.5°) and osseous (7.1° vs. 3.5°) retroversion in the instability group.

Finally, due to the size of the study, the Bradley group was to provide analysis of failures, which included 8% of patients, based on whether the patient was satisfied with surgery (9% based on ASES scoring, 11% based on residual instability). This rate was not worse in contact athletes. Importantly, the majority of patients who failed did not have suture anchors used and rather had isolated capsular plication for perceived intact labrums with patulous capsules. The authors hypothesize that more aggressive capsular plication with suture anchor repairs may decrease the failure rate [12].

Two years later, Savoie et al. published a large retrospective series of 92 shoulders in 90 patients treated surgically for PSI from 1989–2001 [17]. Due to the long study period, the authors note that techniques evolved, so it is difficult to interpret efficacy; however, the authors found 97% of shoulders to be stable and considered a "success" at follow-up. As mentioned earlier, what was consistent throughout their experience was the lack of an analogous posterior, "essential lesion." The authors noted most cases had multiple "breaks in the ring of the shoulder" and stressed the evaluation and treatment of all supporting structures (including rotator interval closure). They also emphasized the importance of a vertical/superior capsular shift, which adequately tightens the posterior constraints of the shoulder, regardless of the specific technique used [17].

Bradley et al. followed up their 2006 study in 2013, now with 200 patients prospectively evaluated following arthroscopic treatment for PSI [16]. Updated ASES, instability, ROM, and pain scores were similar to those in the prior study. Return-to-play (RTP) statistics were also similar, with 90% of patients returning to their sport and 64% returning to the same level (again with no difference between contact and noncontact athletes). Failure rates were lower compared to their 2006 study, which the authors attributed to their increased use of suture anchors based on the results of the first study. Crystalizing the importance of anchor fixation, the authors note that 14% of anchorless repairs went on to failure vs. just 4% of anchor repairs. There was also a significantly higher RTP with anchor fixation. The authors concluded that anchor fixation with capsular labral repair can be considered the gold standard [16]. Lastly, the authors noted no difference in outcomes for patients treated for acute traumatic or RPS. They attribute this to the standardization in repair techniques utilized based on the results of their prior study.

A 2015 study by McClincy et al. used the same database from the 2013 Bradley study to compare PSI, specifically in throwers and non-throwers. Interestingly, they did not find any difference in failure rate between throwers (6%) and non-throwers (8%). There were also no differences in PRO scores between pitchers and non-pitchers; however, there was a lower RTP for pitchers (50%) compared to 60% in non-pitching throwers [32]. The authors attribute the discrepancy in similar PRO scores between pitchers and other throwers with the differing RTP rates to the repetitive high-stress demands of overhand pitching on the postoperative shoulder [32]. Similar to the 2013 Bradley study, throwers treated with suture anchors (92%) had higher RTP compared to anchorless repairs (55%). The authors postulated that this was due to either less aggressive capsular shifts in patients with intact labrums due to a fear of compromising rotation or the low number of suture anchors used, as the only patients treated without suture anchors had intact labrums [32].

A 2015 systematic review by the same group reported that, while throwers overall had similar outcomes scores and objective measures of shoulder function as other athletes, throwers had lower RTP rates (91.8% vs. 83.9% [33]). Open procedures were found to have higher levels of recurrence (19% vs. 8%), subjective stability (91% vs. 80%), patient satisfaction (94% vs. 86%), and RTP (92% vs. 66%). The authors also highlighted the importance of delineating between unidirectional and multidirectional instability. Repair failure was found to be related to an initial diagnosis of unidirectional instability, with follow-up examination at the time of revision surgery noting multidirectional [33].

Lastly, a 2016 retrospective review by Katthagen et al. of 41 shoulders treated with arthroscopic labral repair for either traumatic or atraumatic posterior instability found that while both groups had significantly improved ASES scores, only those with a traumatic etiology had significantly improved with Single Assessment Numeric Evaluation (SANE); Quick Disabilities of the Arm, Shoulder and Hand; and Short-Form 12 Physical Component Summary scores [34].

Evaluation of Specific Factors Related to Outcomes (2016 to Present)

Armed with the results of the previous decade demonstrating that arthroscopic capsulolabral repair with multiple suture anchors was a reliable procedure for both functional outcomes and RTP, recent research has focused on identifying specific risk factors for unsatisfactory outcomes.

Glenoid Characteristics

Glenoid anatomic factors, which can be identified preoperatively on imaging, have garnered interest, as they are easily identifiable and have a major impact on outcomes.

Glenoid version has been extensively studied, as far back as 2005 with the Kim group [31], which found that both chondrolabral and glenoid bone retroversion increased in patients with posteroinferior labral tears compared to native controls; however, they did not correlate this with outcomes. Relatedly, the Katthagen et al. study aforementioned found that atraumatic PSI patients had significantly higher glenoid retroversion compared to traumatic PSI patients [34]. A 2016 study retrospective review by Mauro et al. of 183 consecutive PSI patients treated with capsulolabral repair similarly found that PSI patients had increased glenoid retroversion compared to controls, suggesting that this may be a risk factor for PSI; however, glenoid version did not correlate with outcomes at 2-year follow-up [35]. These findings were corroborated in 2018 by Bradley et al., who reviewed 297 patients who underwent arthroscopic posterior capsulolabral repair and found that increased glenoid retroversion did not increase the risk of revision surgery [36]. Similarly, a 2021 retrospective review by Arner et al. compared 19 patients who failed arthroscopic labral repair with 56 matched controls, again finding that retroversion did not increase risk for failure [37]. One interesting point to consider is the causality of retroversion. As the above studies were retrospective, they are not able to inform us if the retroversion is itself a cause of instability or a result similar to bone loss with anterior dislocations. A 2013 prospective study by Owens et al. of military recruits, however, did find significantly increased glenoid retroversion in patients that subsequently went on to develop PSI, helping to establish that retroversion is a cause, not a sequela of PSI [38]. This body of evidence ultimately indicates that while increased glenoid retroversion increases the risk of developing PSI, it does not affect outcomes after patients undergo repairs.

Conversely, glenoid width has been shown to affect outcomes. Mauro et al. found an average glenoid bone width of 28.9 mm in their cohort and that at final follow-up, patients with wider glenoids had significantly better American Shoulder and Elbow Surgeon (ASES) scores compared to those with narrow glenoids [35]. Bradley et al. similarly found that patients requiring revision had significantly narrower glenoids compared to those who did not require revision

(26.0 vs. 29.0) [36]. Most recently, Arner et al. again found that PSI patients who required revision had significantly narrow glenoid compared to those who did not (25.5 vs. 28.8 mm) [37]. The group also found that female sex had a small, albeit negative, effect on outcomes.

Related to glenoid width is bone loss, with the distinction being that glenoid width is an absolute value, whereas bone loss is a relative value, calculated as a ratio of missing posterior bone and presumed native glenoid width (with multiple techniques used to determine the patient's native glenoid width). In a retrospective review of posterior capsulolabral repair patients, Hines et al. reported that patients with more than 13.5% bone loss (measured using the perfect circle technique) were less likely to return to duty (14.3% vs. 8%) than those with less than 13.5%; however, there was no significant difference in reoperation rate, complications, or functional outcome scores [39]. The authors were unsure how to explain the discrepancy between similar functional outcomes, but worse return to duty. Importantly, they found relatively less bone loss (mean 7%) in posterior rather than anterior instability. They attribute this to the different etiology in posterior vs. anterior instability—namely, PSI is typically caused by low-level microinstability rather than frank dislocations. In trying to define the critical bone loss value, analogous to that studied in anterior instability, [37] study found two inflection points after performing linear regression. Patients with 11% bone loss had an approximately 10× higher failure rate, and patients with 15% bone loss had a nearly 25× higher failure rate than patients without bone loss. The overall mean loss in the cohort was 5.2% [37]. When taken together, these studies suggest that both absolute value and relative bone loss affect the risk of failure.

Concomitant Pathology

The effect of concomitant pathology on outcomes of posterior labral repair has undergone extensive study over the last 5 years. A 2020 retrospective review by Nourissat et al. analyzed outcomes of 150 patients treated for isolated PSI at ten centers. Patients were treated with bone-block procedures (45%), posterior labral repair (47%), and capsular plication (8%). Among several factors evaluated, including type of procedure, prior trauma, presence of a reverse Hill-Sachs lesion, and age, only the presence of a glenoid cartilage lesion was associated with worse Constant scores on multivariable regression analysis [40]. The authors suggest that providers should consider early intervention to prevent the development of cartilage injury prior to repair. A 2022 study by Ferrando et al. compared PSI patients with an elevated cartilage wear index (a novel measurement established by the group) with those who did not have any signs of cartilage injury. They also found that patients with more severe cartilage damage had significantly worse Western Ontario Shoulder Instability Index (WOSI) and SANE scores [41].

Partial-thickness rotator cuff tears may occur with posterior labral tears, particularly if there is an element of internal impingement. Arner et al. investigated if presence of these lesions affected posterior labral repairs in throwers. Of 56 throwing athletes studied, 24 were found to have partial rotator cuff pathology (<50% tearing). When compared to the isolated PSI group, there were no significant differences found for ASES score, stability score, ROM, strength, RTP, or failure rate following surgical repair [42]. However, a 2018 study by Bradley et al. found presence of a partial rotator cuff tear contributed to the risk of revision surgery [36].

Revision Risk (2018 to Present)

With the increase in posterior stabilization procedures over the last two decades, several recent studies have been able to evaluate risk factors for revision. [36] study mentioned earlier found a 6.4% revision rate at a 9-year follow-up of 297 shoulders. When patients who required revision were compared to those who did not, female sex, dominant shoulder involved, use of three or fewer anchors, smaller glenoid bone width, and concomitant rotator cuff injury all increased risk. Conversely, participation in contact sports, level of sport, and glenoid/labral version did not contribute to revision risk [36]. Unsurprisingly, patients requiring revision did not have decreased instability following index surgery and had significantly worse ASES and pain scores compared to non-revision patients [36].

In 2020, the Bradley group published two studies, one on risk factors for revision surgery in contact athletes [52] and an analogous study focused on throwing athletes [53]. In contact athletes, factors predictive of revision surgery included postoperative stability and decreased glenoid bone width (26.4 mm vs. 29.1 mm). Factors that were not predictive included cartilage, labral, and bony version, sex, and level of sport [52]. Importantly, patients who required revision labral repair had significantly worse RTP rates following their revision than those who only had a primary repair (50.0% vs. 93.1%) [52]. In their study of 105 throwing athletes, 8.6% of patients required revision. Unlike contact athletes, the only factor that increased the risk of needing a revision was female gender. However, patients requiring revision again had a significantly lower RTP rate compared with those who only had a primary repair (14.3% vs. 83.6%). The authors hypothesized that glenoid width was not a risk factor for throwers, as the mechanism for capsulolabral instability in this group is related to repetitive microtrauma, minimizing the protective effect of a larger glenoid [53].

Techniques Other than Labral Repair (2021 to Present)

While arthroscopic labral repair has been shown to consistently result in excellent clinical outcomes in most cases of PSI, there are instances, such as with substantial bone loss, where failure rates have been found to be significantly higher. In response, investigators have attempted to utilize techniques to improve outcomes in these challenging presentations. Small case series have been published over the last 10–20 years, but enough data for quality analysis has been available for approximately 2 years.

Analogous to the Latarjet procedure in anterior shoulder surgery, posterior bone block procedures have been employed in cases of posterior glenoid bone loss. Some earlier examples of studies with positive results exist, such as a 2016 study by Struck et al. evaluating 15 patients with hyperlaxity treated with either scapular spine autograft or distal tibial allograft, with significantly improved Constant, Rowe, and WOSI scores at 42-month follow-up. However, even this study, which is often referenced as an example of the potential value of posterior bone block surgery, had four instances of hardware irritation necessitating reoperation [43]. More studies have been similar to a 2010 study by Meuffels et al., who presented 18-year follow-up data on 11 patients. They found that 45% of patients would not have chosen the operation again, 36% had subsequent posterior dislocations, and all 11 patients had glenohumeral arthritis at follow-up [44]. A recent 2021 systematic review of posterior bone block procedure outcomes by Mojica et al. crystallized the challenges with the various types of glenoid augmentation procedures. Of 225 shoulders, recurrent instability was found in 9.8%, with an overall complication rate of 13.8%. The majority of these complications were related to hardware irritation. The authors note that there were relatively high functional outcome scores (WOSI) 68, Visual Analogue Pain Scale (VAS) 1.8, Constant 7, and Walch-Duplay 8 and opined that there may be a steep learning curve with the technique [45]. A second systematic review published in 2022 by Cognetti also found an unacceptably high complication (instability from 0% to 73%; revision procedures 0–67%) with heterogenous outcome scores across studies. Importantly, they did not find any superiority among graft types (iliac crest, scapular spine, acromion, distal tibial allograft) [46].

In response to increased glenoid retroversion, glenoid osteotomies have also been investigated as a means to decrease the shear force on the capsulolabral complex. Lacheta et al. published a relatively encouraging case series on 12 shoulders in 11 patients, with mean preoperative glenoid retroversion decreasing from 23.3 degrees to 13 degrees postoperatively. At a relatively short follow-up time of 19.8 months, there were no re-dislocations or revision surgeries. However, one patient had "signs of recurrent instability," and four had intraoperative glenoid neck fractures (though these did not require additional fixation or surgery beyond the osteotomy) [47]. Two years later, Malik et al. published a systematic review on posterior glenoid osteotomies, finding a recurrence rate of 22% (though this dropped to 11% once two studies from the 1980s were excluded) and a complication rate of 18.3%. The most common complications were glenohumeral joint degeneration (7.3%) and iatrogenic fracture (5.5%). The authors concluded that glenoid osteotomies were a potential option, but they carried a significant risk [48]. Most recently, Waltenspul et al. published a case series on seven shoulders (six patients) treated with glenoid osteotomy with concerning results. They found a recurrent symptomatic PSI rate of 86%, with one necessitating revision with a posterior bone block procedure. Constant score did not significantly increase, and pain did not decrease. At a mean follow-up of 15 years, six patients had developed osteoarthritis (all had none previously) [49]. Given the lack of effect of version on outcomes following labral repair, as well as the significant complication risk, glenoid osteotomy appears to be an unfavorable option.

With traumatic PSI, the anterior aspect of the humeral head can impact on the posterior glenoid rim, creating a reverse Hill-Sachs lesion. In addition to the rarity of these lesions, their clinical significance is still evolving. Accordingly, clinical outcomes data remains limited. A retrospective review of ten patients treated with bone grafting and internal fixation of reverse Hill-Sachs lesions occupying >25% of the humeral head was published in 2021 by Mi et al. At follow-up of 22.5 months, CT evidence of fracture healing was observed by 8 weeks in all cases. Additionally, Constant scores improved from 40.6 preoperatively to 91.7 postoperatively, and no recurrent dislocations were reported [50]. The more traditional technique for treating reverse Hill-Sachs lesions is the modified McLaughlin, which transfers an osteotomized lesser tuberosity into the defect. At present, only scattered case series exist on the success of this technique. A 2022 study by Cohen et al. reported on ten patients treated with a modified McLaughlin for treatment of a chronic locked posterior dislocation of the shoulder (6 weeks to 14 months duration). At a minimum 2-year follow-up, Constant and VAS scores significantly improved, and 80% of patients were satisfied with the procedure. The unsatisfied patients each had a >6 months delay in treatment and developed severe osteoarthritis. There were no complications or recurrent dislocations in the remaining patients [51].

Authors' Preferred Technique

Setup

Both beach chair position and lateral decubitus position may be used for the procedure; however, the authors believe that the lateral position affords a greater amount of distraction, which permits greater access to the inferior glenoid for anchor placement. Accordingly, the patient is placed laterally and stabilized with a bean bag positioner. Importantly, the patient is brought to the top of the table, as it is recommended for the surgeon to operate from the top of the bed (rather than from the posterior position). The patient is rotated posteriorly about 20 degrees, as the arm holder will pull the patient slightly anteriorly. After standard prepping and draping, a distraction device is applied to the arm. The optimal position of the arm is about 20 degrees of abduction (more than this may close the glenohumeral space) and 20 degrees anteriorly (Fig. 32.7).

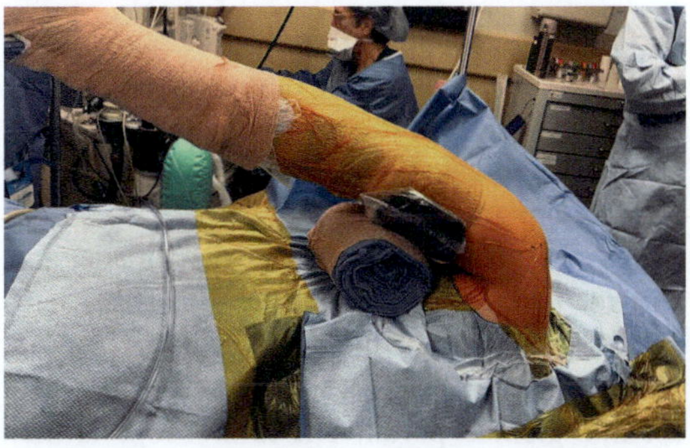

Fig. 32.7 Lateral decubitus position for the posterior labral repairs

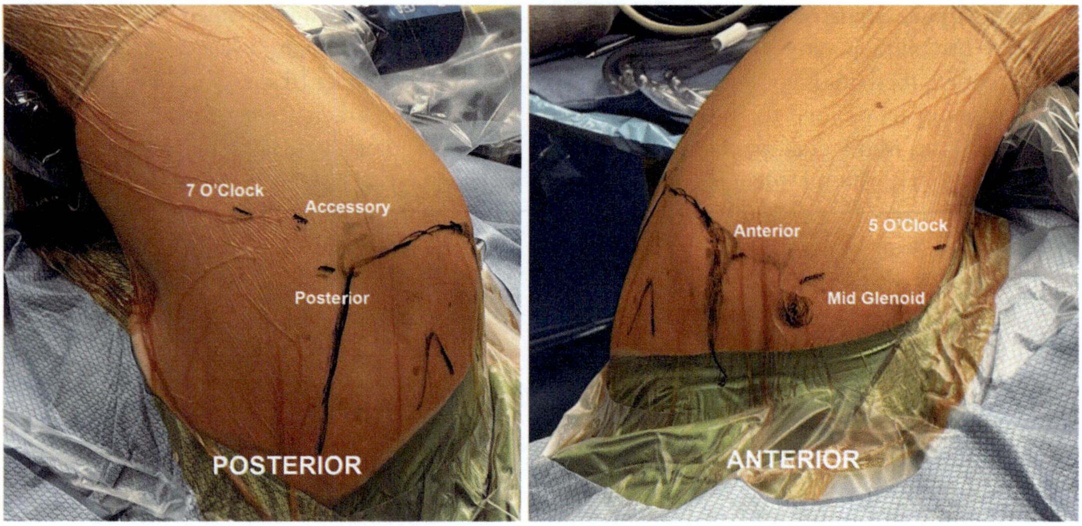

Fig. 32.8 Landmarks for portal locations for posterior labral repair

Diagnostic Scope

A posterior portal is placed, just 1/2 centimeter distal and medial to the posterolateral corner (Fig. 32.8). This more superior and lateral posterior portal position improves the view of the glenoid face and helps avoid posterior portal crowding. A routine diagnostic scope is performed, with particular attention to the biceps tendon, entirety of the labrum, and undersurface of the posterior-superior rotator cuff (Fig. 32.9)

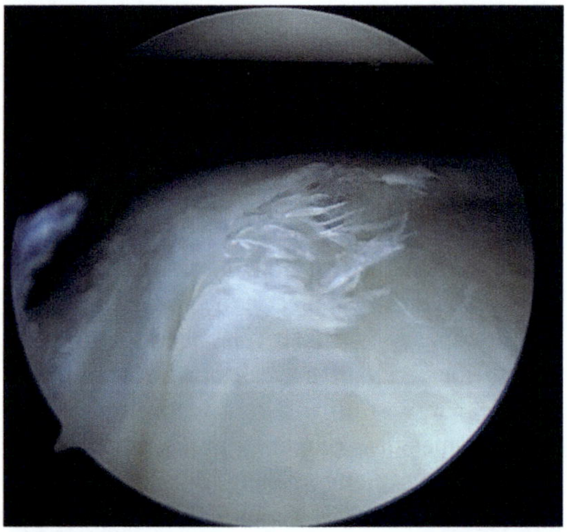

Fig. 32.9 Viewing from the posterior portal of a left shoulder, a diagnostic scope is performed, demonstrating a posteroinferior labral tear

Additional Portal Creation

Next, a mid-glenoid portal is made about 1 cm lateral to the coracoid. Intra-articularly, this should be low in the rotator interval, immediately above the subscapularis tendon. A twist-in 8-mm cannula is placed.

An anterosuperior portal is then made, just anterior to the anterolateral corner of the acromion. This should be high in the rotator interval, above the biceps tendon, to avoid crowding with the mid-glenoid portal. The arthroscope is then switched to this portal. From here, portal creation is dictated by the tear pattern.

For a routine posterior-inferior labral tear, a 7 o'clock portal is made, which provides an excellent trajectory for inferior anchor placement. This portal is made roughly 2–4 cm lateral from the posterosuperior portal, under spinal needle localization. Finally, an accessory posterior portal may be required, placed between the posterosuperior portal and the 7 o'clock portal, slightly posterior to the 7 o'clock portal.

Glenoid Preparation

The labrum is initially debrided with a shaver, placed from the mid-glenoid portal, with care not to resect any healthy tissue that can be used for the repair. Next, an elevator is used to help develop the interval between the labrum and glenoid, which will facilitate recreation of the bumper. This will be placed from whichever portal permits ease of access around the glenoid posteroinferior corner, but the authors find that this is typically from the anterior midglenoid portal working across the glenoid. Finally, the glenoid rim is decorticated with a bone cutting shaver or burr to create bleeding bone to augment the biologic healing response.

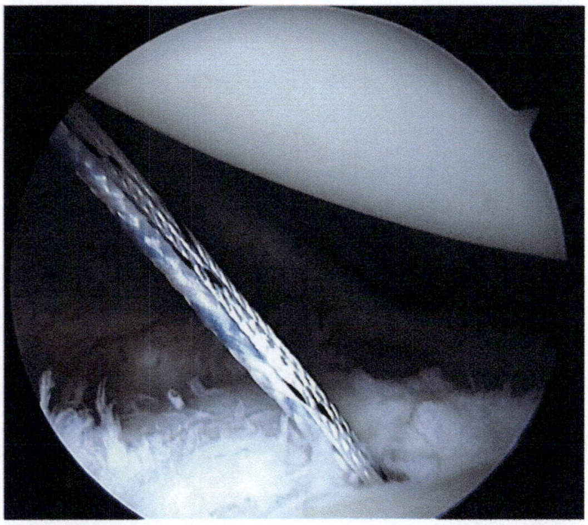

Fig. 32.10 Knotless suture anchor placed on glenoid, deep to labrum

Labral Repair

A number of anchor types are available, which generally have similar efficacy when used appropriately. The authors' preferred implant is the knotless Fibertak (Arthrex, Naples, FL), which is an all-suture knotless device. All-suture anchors provide a smaller pilot hole, allowing multiple anchors to be used in the same area as larger anchors, affording multiple points of fixation. A drill is placed through the corresponding guide from the 7 o'clock portal along the glenoid rim, between the glenoid and the labrum. The anchor is then inserted, taking care to achieve an acute angle to the glenoid to avoid injury to the articular cartilage (Fig. 32.10).

A suture passing device (the authors prefer one with a 45-degree angle) is then used, typically inserted from the posterosuperior portal. Most commonly, the device is placed percutaneously to avoid overcrowding in the shoulder with cannulas. This is used to first penetrate the capsule and then exit under the labrum (Fig. 32.11). The number of capsules included is dictated by the patient's pathology and degree of laxity. Taking more capsules may result in less instability or a lower risk of recurrence but comes with the consequences of limiting internal rotation.

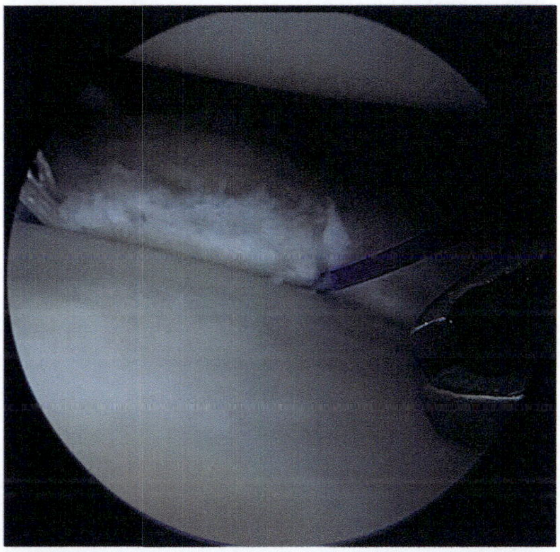

Fig. 32.11 Suture passing device placed under the labrum, to allow the shuttling of the working stitch from the anchor

The suture passing device is then used to shuttle the working stitch from the anchor under the labrum and through the capsular tissue. The working stitch and the passing stitch are then retrieved from the posterior accessory portal. The working stitch is then passed around the labrum and locked into the anchor using the passing stitch. One advantage of this construct is that it can still be tensioned at this point, allowing final tightening after all anchors are placed.

Additional anchors are placed using the same technique, with anchors from 6 o'clock to 9

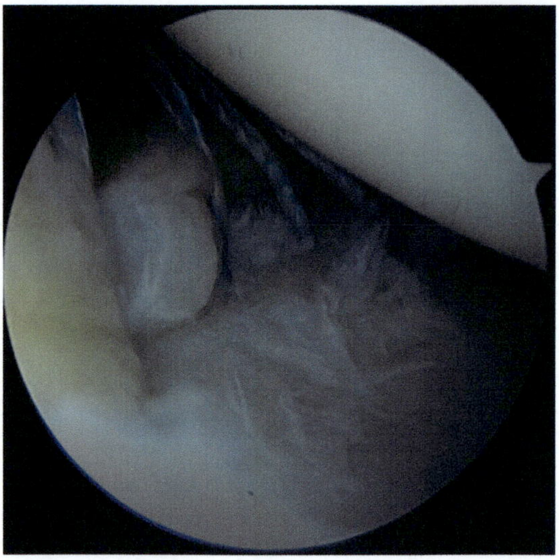

Fig. 32.12 Posterior labrum with bumper restored after three anchors were placed. Suture limbs are still in place, allowing final tightening

o'clock generally placed from the 7 o'clock portal. More proximal anchors may be placed from the accessory posterior portal. Once all anchors are placed, the anchors are sequentially tightened (Fig. 32.12), and the suture limbs are cut, completing the repair. Typically, a minimum of four anchors is used for a standard repair.

Postoperative Rehab

Patients are initially placed in a sling for 6 weeks, with formal physical therapy focusing on passive range of motion. Active range of motion may begin at 4 weeks, under supervision by a physical therapist. Starting at 6 weeks, strengthening exercises are initiated, focusing on the rotator cuff, deltoid, and scapula. From 12 weeks to 1 year, the patient should work toward a goal of full, painless ROM.

Conclusion

Due to its lower incidence, research on posterior shoulder instability lagged behind that of anterior shoulder instability, particularly in the 1990s and early 2000s. However, over the last two decades, results of outcome studies have helped sports surgeons continue to improve and refine techniques for treating posterior shoulder instability. While multiple etiologies exist, today, results are increasingly predictable, with patients obtaining excellent functional outcome scores and high return-to-play rates.

References

1. McLaughlin H. Posterior dislocation of the shoulder. J Bone Joint Surg Am. 1952;24A(3):584–90.
2. Antoniou J, Duckworth DT, Harryman DT 2nd. Capsulolabral augmentation for the management of posteroinferior instability of the shoulder. J Bone Joint Surg Am. 2000;82(9):1220–30.
3. Boyd HB, Sisk TD. Recurrent posterior dislocation of the shoulder. J Bone Joint Surg Am. 1972;54(4):779–86.
4. Matsen FA 3rd, Chebli C, Lippitt S, American Academy of Orthopaedic S. Principles for the evaluation and management of shoulder instability. J Bone Joint Surg Am. 2006;88(3):648–59.
5. Blasier RB, Soslowsky LJ, Malicky DM, Palmer ML. Posterior glenohumeral subluxation: active and passive stabilization in a biomechanical model. J Bone Joint Surg Am. 1997;79(3):433–40.
6. Bradley JP, Forsythe B, Mascarenhas R. Arthroscopic management of posterior shoulder instability: diagnosis, indications, and technique. Clin Sports Med. 2008;27(4):649–70.
7. Provencher MT, LeClere LE, King S, et al. Posterior instability of the shoulder: diagnosis and management. Am J Sports Med. 2011;39(4):874–86.
8. Cole BJ, Rodeo SA, O'Brien SJ, et al. The anatomy and histology of the rotator interval capsule of the shoulder. Clin Orthop Relat Res. 2001;390:129–37.
9. Wellmann M, Blasig H, Bobrowitsch E, et al. The biomechanical effect of specific labral and capsular lesions on posterior shoulder instability. Arch Orthop Trauma Surg. 2011;131(3):421–7.
10. Provencher MT, Mologne TS, Hongo M, Zhao K, Tasto JP, An KN. Arthroscopic versus open rotator interval closure: biomechanical evaluation of stability and motion. Arthroscopy. 2007;23(6):583–92.
11. Bradley J, Tjoumakaris FP. Posterior shoulder instability. In: Miller MD, Thompson SR, editors. DeLee Drez and Miller's orthopaedic sports medicine. Elsevier; 2020. p. 463–75.
12. Bradley JP, Baker CL 3rd, Kline AJ, Armfield DR, Chhabra A. Arthroscopic capsulolabral reconstruction for posterior instability of the shoulder: a prospective study of 100 shoulders. Am J Sports Med. 2006;34(7):1061–71.

13. Robinson CM, Aderinto J. Recurrent posterior shoulder instability. J Bone Joint Surg Am. 2005;87(4):883–92.
14. Burkhart SS, Lo IK. The cam effect of the proximal humerus: its role in the production of relative capsular redundancy of the shoulder. Arthroscopy. 2007;23(3):241–6.
15. Burkhart SS, Morgan CD, Kibler WB. The disabled throwing shoulder: spectrum of pathology. Part II: evaluation and treatment of SLAP lesions in throwers. Arthroscopy. 2003;19(5):531–9.
16. Bradley JP, McClincy MP, Arner JW, Tejwani SG. Arthroscopic capsulolabral reconstruction for posterior instability of the shoulder: a prospective study of 200 shoulders. Am J Sports Med. 2013;41(9):2005–14.
17. Savoie FH 3rd, Holt MS, Field LD, Ramsey JR. Arthroscopic management of posterior instability: evolution of technique and results. Arthroscopy. 2008;24(4):389–96.
18. Millett PJ, Clavert P, Hatch GF 3rd, Warner JJ. Recurrent posterior shoulder instability. J Am Acad Orthop Surg. 2006;14(8):464–76.
19. Tannenbaum E, Sekiya JK. Evaluation and management of posterior shoulder instability. Sports Health. 2011;3(3):253–63.
20. Moroder P, Tauber M, Scheibel M, et al. Defect characteristics of reverse Hill-Sachs lesions. Am J Sports Med. 2016;44(3):708–14.
21. Woodmass JM, Lee J, Johnson NR, et al. Nonoperative Management of Posterior Shoulder Instability: an assessment of survival and predictors for conversion to surgery at 1 to 10 years after diagnosis. Arthroscopy. 2019;35(7):1964–70.
22. Festbaum C, Minkus M, Akgun D, et al. Conservative treatment of acute traumatic posterior shoulder dislocations (Type A) is a viable option especially in patients with centred joint, low gamma angle, and middle or old age. Knee Surg Sports Traumatol Arthrosc. 2022;30(7):2500–9.
23. Cruz-Ferreira E, Abadie P, Godeneche A, et al. Posterior shoulder instability: prospective non-randomised comparison of operative and non-operative treatment in 51 patients. Orthop Traumatol Surg Res. 2017;103(8S):S185–8.
24. Williams RJ 3rd, Strickland S, Cohen M, Altchek DW, Warren RF. Arthroscopic repair for traumatic posterior shoulder instability. Am J Sports Med. 2003;31(2):203–9.
25. Papendick LW, Savoie FH 3rd. Anatomy-specific repair techniques for posterior shoulder instability. J South Orthop Assoc. 1995;4(3):169–76.
26. McIntyre LF, Caspari RB, Savoie FH 3rd. The arthroscopic treatment of posterior shoulder instability: two-year results of a multiple suture technique. Arthroscopy. 1997;13(4):426–32.
27. Wolf EM, Eakin CL. Arthroscopic capsular plication for posterior shoulder instability. Arthroscopy. 1998;14(2):153–63.
28. Wirth MA, Groh GI, Rockwood CA Jr. Capsulorrhaphy through an anterior approach for the treatment of atraumatic posterior glenohumeral instability with multidirectional laxity of the shoulder. J Bone Joint Surg Am. 1998;80(11):1570–8.
29. Kim SH, Ha KI, Park JH, et al. Arthroscopic posterior labral repair and capsular shift for traumatic unidirectional recurrent posterior subluxation of the shoulder. J Bone Joint Surg Am. 2003;85(8):1479–87.
30. Kim SH, Ha KI, Yoo JC, Noh KC. Kim's lesion: an incomplete and concealed avulsion of the posteroinferior labrum in posterior or multidirectional posteroinferior instability of the shoulder. Arthroscopy. 2004;20(7):712–20.
31. Kim SH, Noh KC, Park JS, Ryu BD, Oh I. Loss of chondrolabral containment of the glenohumeral joint in atraumatic posteroinferior multidirectional instability. J Bone Joint Surg Am. 2005;87(1):92–8.
32. McClincy MP, Arner JW, Bradley JP. Posterior shoulder instability in throwing athletes: a case-matched comparison of throwers and non-throwers. Arthroscopy. 2015;31(6):1041–51.
33. DeLong JM, Jiang K, Bradley JP. Posterior instability of the shoulder: a systematic review and meta-analysis of clinical outcomes. Am J Sports Med. 2015;43(7):1805–17.
34. Katthagen JC, Tahal DS, Montgomery SR, Horan MP, Millett PJ. Association of Traumatic and Atraumatic Posterior Shoulder Instability with Glenoid Retroversion and Outcomes After Arthroscopic Capsulolabral Repair. Arthroscopy. 2017;33(2):284–90.
35. Mauro CS, McClincy MP, Bradley JP. Effect of glenoid version and width on outcomes of arthroscopic posterior shoulder stabilization. Am J Sports Med. 2016;44(4):941–7.
36. Bradley JP, Arner JW, Jayakumar S, Vyas D. Risk factors and outcomes of revision arthroscopic posterior shoulder Capsulolabral repair. Am J Sports Med. 2018;46(10):2457–65.
37. Arner JW, Ruzbarsky JJ, Midtgaard K, Peebles L, Bradley JP, Provencher MT. Defining critical glenoid bone loss in posterior shoulder Capsulolabral repair. Am J Sports Med. 2021;49(8):2013–9.
38. Owens BD, Campbell SE, Cameron KL. Risk factors for posterior shoulder instability in young athletes. Am J Sports Med. 2013;41(11):2645–9.
39. Hines A, Cook JB, Shaha JS, et al. Glenoid bone loss in posterior shoulder instability: prevalence and outcomes in arthroscopic treatment. Am J Sports Med. 2018;46(5):1053–7.
40. Nourissat G, Hardy MB, Garret J, Mansat P, Godeneche A, Societe Francophone dA. Glenoid cartilage lesions compromise outcomes of surgical treatment for posterior shoulder instability. Orthop J Sports Med. 2020;8(1):2325967119898124.
41. Ferrando A, Aguilar J, Valencia M, Novo U, Calvo E. The cartilage Wear index: a new evaluation method

to improve patient selection in surgical treatment of recurrent posterior glenohumeral instability. JSES Int. 2022;6(3):368–73.

42. Arner JW, McClincy MP, Bradley JP. In throwers with posterior instability, rotator cuff tears are common but do not affect surgical outcomes. Am J Orthop (Belle Mead NJ). 2018;47(1). https://doi.org/10.12788/ajo.2018.0005.
43. Struck M, Wellmann M, Becher C, Pastor MF, Smith T. Results of an open posterior bone block procedure for recurrent posterior shoulder instability after a short- and long-time follow-up. Knee Surg Sports Traumatol Arthrosc. 2016;24(2):618–24.
44. Meuffels DE, Schuit H, van Biezen FC, Reijman M, Verhaar JA. The posterior bone block procedure in posterior shoulder instability: a long-term follow-up study. J Bone Joint Surg Br. 2010;92(5):651–5.
45. Mojica ES, Schwartz LB, Hurley ET, Gonzalez-Lomas G, Campbell KA, Jazrawi LM. Posterior glenoid bone block transfer for posterior shoulder instability: a systematic review. J Shoulder Elb Surg. 2021;30(12):2904–9.
46. Cognetti DJ, Hughes JD, Kay J, et al. Bone block augmentation of the posterior glenoid for recurrent posterior shoulder instability is associated with high rates of clinical failure: a systematic review. Arthroscopy. 2022;38(2):551–563 e555.
47. Lacheta L, Singh TSP, Hovsepian JM, Braun S, Imhoff AB, Pogorzelski J. Posterior open wedge glenoid osteotomy provides reliable results in young patients with increased glenoid retroversion and posterior shoulder instability. Knee Surg Sports Traumatol Arthrosc. 2019;27(1):299–304.
48. Malik SS, Jordan RW, Tahir M, MacDonald PB. Does the posterior glenoid osteotomy reduce the rate of recurrence in patients with posterior shoulder instability – a systematic review. Orthop Traumatol Surg Res. 2021;107(1):102760.
49. Waltenspul M, Haller T, Ernstbrunner L, Wyss S, Wieser K, Gerber C. Long-term results after posterior open glenoid wedge osteotomy for posterior shoulder instability associated with excessive glenoid retroversion. J Shoulder Elb Surg. 2022;31(1):81–9.
50. Mi M, Zhang JM, Jiang XY, Huang Q. Management of locked posterior shoulder dislocation with reverse hill-Sachs lesions via anatomical reconstructions. Orthop Surg. 2021;13(7):2119–26.
51. Cohen M, Fonseca R, Galvao Amaral MV, Monteiro MT, Motta Filho GR. Treatment of chronic locked posterior dislocation of the shoulder with the modified McLaughlin procedure. J Shoulder Elb Surg. 2022;31(1):100–6.
52. Bradley JP, Arner JW, Jayakumar S, Vyas D. Revision arthroscopic posterior shoulder Capsulolabral repair in contact athletes: risk factors and outcomes. Arthroscopy. 2020;36(3):660–5.
53. Vaswani R, Arner J, Freiman H, Bradley JP. Risk factors for revision posterior shoulder stabilization in throwing athletes. Orthop J Sports Med. 2020;8(12):2325967120967652.
54. Misamore GW, Facibene WA. Posterior capsulorrhaphy for the treatment of traumatic recurrent posterior subluxations of the shoulder in athletes. J Shoulder Elbow Surg. 2000 Sep-Oct;9(5):403–8. https://doi.org/10.1067/mse.2000.108963. PMID: 11075324.

Part IV

Multidirectional Instability

The Open Inferior Capsular Shift for MDI (Multidirectional Instability)

33

Andrew Assenmacher and Jeffrey S. Abrams

Introduction

Shoulder instability is a common condition generally seen following trauma [1]. The description of multidirectional instability (MDI) originally appeared in Neer and Foster's case series from 1980 [2]. Patients with a unique subset of shoulder instability presented with inferior symptomatic excessive translation [3]. The typical anterior or posterior stabilization repairs were at high risk of failing, as they did not address the enlarged inferior pouch. In addition to the inferior symptoms, patients had associated increases in glenohumeral translation in anterior and/or posterior directions that interfered with sporting and daily activities. Matsen et al. differentiated this classification further with the definition of AMBRI or atraumatic multidirectional instability, which commonly affects patients bilaterally and is best approached with rehabilitation and potentially an inferior capsular shift [4]. While traumatic instability generally disrupts the glenoid labral attachments, the MDI patient has a stretched capsular pouch. An additional subset of these patients has collagen syndromes such as Marfan's or Ehlers-Danlos. These more severe cases often need additional measures to stabilize their shoulders using allograft or bone grafting [5–8]. We can conclude that MDI patients have increased inferior translation due to a combination of inherited characteristics and acquired changes due to repetitive activities.

There is a difference between patients with laxity and instability. While some laxity may be advantageous for gymnasts or swimmers, it also puts the joints at a higher risk of creating instability with repetitive use or trauma. Commonly seen, poor scapulothoracic and glenohumeral rhythm in this population can reverse, and a large number of patients will do well with conservative management like therapy working on neuromuscular control [9]. Biofeedback with electrical muscle stimulation has been shown to maintain positive results at a 2-year follow-up [10]. However, conservative treatment has shown poor results in athletes, especially if they display no response to 3 months of conservative rehabilitation. In Misamore et al., a third of patients at 8-year follow-up required surgery, a third had persistent instability, and only half rated their shoulder function as improved with a rehabilitation program alone [11].

The sulcus sign has been a hallmark physical finding in this group of patients for demonstrating excessive inferior translation [2] (Fig. 33.1). The load-and-shift maneuver introduced by Hawkins and Abrams [12, 13] can also reproduce the patient's symptoms in tested directions

A. Assenmacher
Department of Orthopedic Surgery, ProMedica Health System, Toledo, OH, USA

J. S. Abrams (✉)
Department of Orthopedic Surgery, Princeton Orthopedic Associates, Princeton, NJ, USA

© The Author(s), under exclusive license to Springer Nature Switzerland AG 2026
R. M. Frank, J. M. Tokish (eds.), *Management of Shoulder Instability*,
https://doi.org/10.1007/978-3-032-18089-6_33

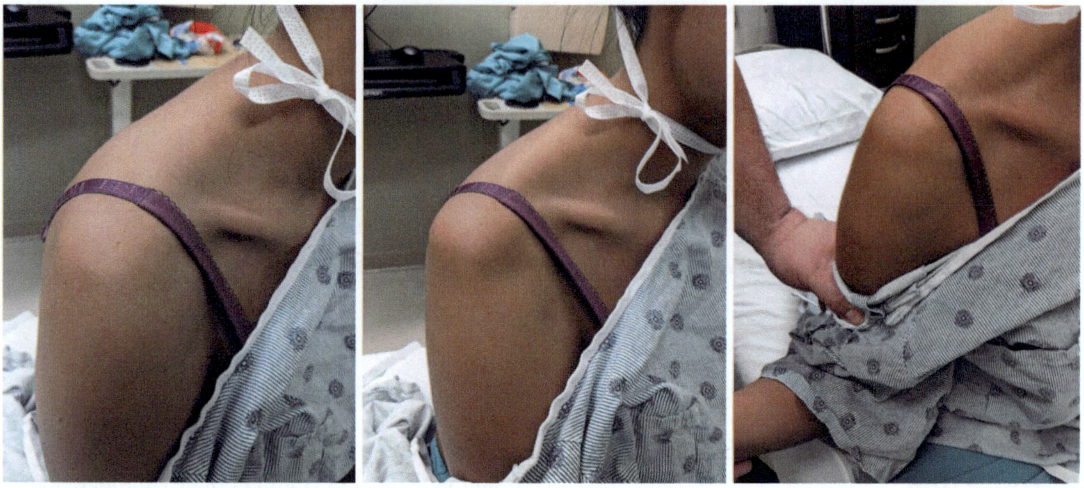

Fig. 33.1 Inferior sulcus test (left: at rest; middle: test applied in neutral rotation; right: test applied in external rotation)

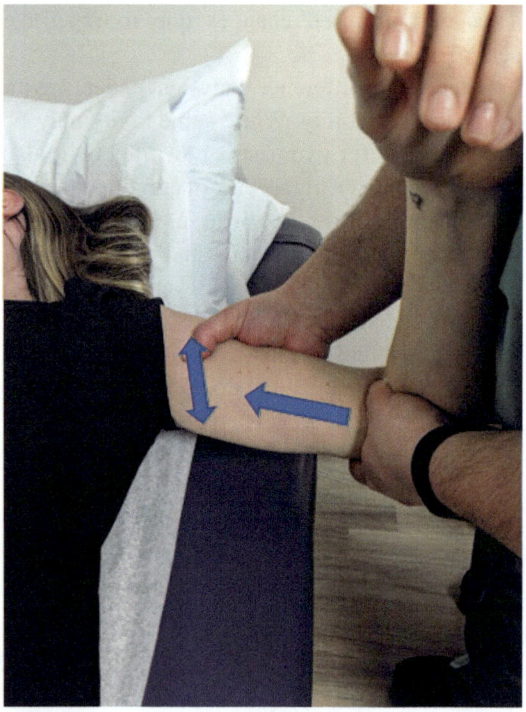

Fig. 33.2 Load-and-shift test

and with varying degrees of abduction and rotation (Fig. 33.2). A grading system can be helpful to communicate the severity of the translation, such as translation to the edge of the glenoid, over the edge, or locking out when forces are removed.

Articular findings can range from an enlarged and stretched capsule to a combination of labral flattening or tears, mild chondral changes of the humeral head, widened rotator interval, and superior labral tears. Although arthroscopy can readily address the labral pathology, the lateral capsular tissue is difficult to address. The open shift procedure permits a greater degree of repositioning of the lateral capsule, creating overlapping flaps and providing additional reinforcement to reduce translation.

The advantages of the open capsular shift procedure include its ability to allow for direct repair of the labral and lateral capsular tears, creation of laterally based flaps, and repositioning to optimize tension and recreate additional tissue thickness with overlapping flaps. During the procedure, the arm can be repositioned in varying degrees of abduction, rotation, and flexion to visualize and add desired correction to the repair. This flexibility can improve the repair of the static stabilizers, limiting inferior and additional directions of increased translation.

There is continued interest in complex subgroups, including genetic "collagenopaths." Tissue healing may not be adequate for humeral restraint, and additional soft tissue grafting may be needed to provide improved selective stiffness. The dynamic nature of stability also continues to be an important factor. Additional feedback treatments with physical therapy can improve functional outcomes [10].

Humeral head translation can be affected by medial labrum bumper restraint and attached capsular integrity and tensioning with positions of abduction and rotation. The MDI patient can be symptomatic with their arm at their side and an inferior force applied. Here, the capsule is lax, and the cuff muscles in the front and back of the shoulder are not in an optimal position to restrain. Superior and inferior structures are better positioned to limit translation as proposed by the circle concept of Warren [14]. The open capsular shift provides the opportunity to reduce the inferior pouch, reinforce the rotator interval from the bursal perspective, and anatomically repair labral tears if needed.

Illustrative Clinical Case

A 19-year-old, right-hand-dominant female presents with recurrent complaints of pain and popping of her right shoulder. She reports a sensation of her shoulder shifting but denies a history of dislocation requiring reduction. More than a year ago, she underwent an arthroscopy and biceps tenodesis at an outside hospital. The patient reports no improvement following surgery and rehabilitation. Examination shows a positive sulcus sign, load-and-shift test, and apprehension in both abduction and external rotation.

Etiology

The common presentation of MDI is in patients undergoing repetitive motions for their sport or occupation, complicated by a superimposed traumatic event. The trauma can be low impact and relatively innocuous but is often identified as the onset of symptoms. The stretching that occurs over time is an adaptation to activities such as gymnastics, swimming, and overhead throwing motions. Interestingly, there is often a similar degree of laxity and translation in their asymptomatic opposite shoulder. The painful condition with complaints of instability can be exacerbated by altered compensation mechanisms. This condition is a combination of injured static and dynamic stabilization of the shoulder. Shoulders with deficient capsular restraint have additional loss of proprioceptive skills, making self-correction a difficult process [14].

Rodeo et al. suggested an underlying connective tissue abnormality in a study analyzing collagen and elastic fibers in the shoulder [15]. In the general population, generalized ligamentous laxity has been seen at rates of 5–15% [16, 17]. In the pediatric population, 10% of males and 15% of females had Beighton's criteria greater than five, indicating generalized ligamentous laxity [18]. Patients who suffer a shoulder dislocation have up to a 6.8 times greater incidence of ligamentous laxity in that shoulder compared to age-matched controls [19]. Ehlers-Danlos syndrome (EDS) is a disorder of collagen that affects multiple organs, including the skin, soft tissues, and vessels. A hypermobile subtype of EDS (hEDS) affects the joints and can be diagnosed by the criteria in Table 33.1. A joint hypermobility syndrome can be diagnosed, as in Table 33.2, with the presentation of two major criteria, one major and two minor, four minor, or two minor criteria with a known first-degree relative who has joint

Table 33.1 Diagnostic criteria for hEDS (hypermobile Ehlers-Danlos syndrome) [20]

Requirements	Finding
1	Generalized joint hypermobility
2	Two or more of the following must be present: 1. Systemic manifestations of a more generalized connective tissue disorder (5 out of 12 must be present): Unusually soft or velvety skin; mild skin hyperextensibility; unexplained striae; bilateral piezogenic papules of the heel; recurrent or multiple hernias; atrophic scarring of at least 2 sites; pelvic, rectal, or uterine prolapse; dental crowding and high or narrow palate; arachnodactyly; arm span-to-height $\geq$1.05; mitral valve prolapse; and aortic root dilatation 2. Positive family history with one or more confirmed hEDS first-degree relatives 3. Musculoskeletal complications
3	Must not have unusual skin fragility, any other heritable or acquired connective tissue disorder, or autoimmune disorder must be ruled out, as well as other causes of hypermobility

Table 33.2 Diagnostic criteria for joint hypermobility syndrome [20]

Major criteria	Minor criteria
1. Beighton score ≥ 4/9	1. Beighton score 1–3/9
2. Arthralgia for >3 months in 4 or more joints	2. Arthralgia for >3 months in 1–3 joints or back, including spondylopathy
	3. Dislocation of more than one joint or recurrent dislocation in one joint
	4. Three or more soft tissue lesions (bursitis, tendinitis, etc.)
	5. Marfanoid habitus
	6. Skin changes (abnormal scarring, thin or extendable, striae)
	7. Eye signs (drooping lid, myopia, antimongoloid slant)
	8. Varicose veins, hernia, or uterine/rectal prolapse

hypermobility syndrome [20]. These patients have an increased risk of failure with arthroscopic management; an open approach to stabilization is preferred. The patient in the illustrative case example met several of these criteria for JHS but did not meet hEDS criteria.

Diagnosis/Imaging

As is the case in many shoulder instability diagnoses, the patient's history leads to a strong suspicion of the patient's condition. The event that begins the onset of symptoms can often tip the scale from a well-tolerated loose joint to a disabling condition. Subluxation and spontaneous reduction are more common than requiring assistance with reduction.

The physical examination begins with the patient reproducing the most symptomatic postures. Their range of motion and strength testing is often normal. While apprehension is uncommon, a patient may report that their discomfort can be reproduced with various postures and movements. Additionally, posterior visualization of the scapula may demonstrate abnormal scapulothoracic mechanics.

An inferior sulcus sign is the hallmark of diagnosis (Fig. 33.1). In a relaxed seated patient, the proximal humerus is drawn inferiorly, creating a dimpling effect above the humeral head. Many patients do not complain of discomfort but may appreciate this same translation if the head is pressed toward the glenoid during the inferior translation. A second maneuver includes placing the arm in external rotation during the same movement. If the same degree of inferior translation is present, then the rotator interval is felt to be widened and less effective at reducing the inferior drawer.

The patient is then placed in the supine position with slight abduction and neutral rotation for the load-and-shift exam (Figs. 33.2 and 33.3). Pressing the humeral head into the glenoid vault and translating anteriorly, posteriorly, and inferiorly may reproduce the complaints in the affected shoulder. Quantification of the shift to the glenoid edge (I), over the edge with spontaneous reduction (II), and dislocation over the edge without spontaneous reduction (III) can be recorded for each of the directions. This test can be repeated in 40 degrees of abduction and 45 degrees of external rotation (anteriorly) or 30 degrees of internal rotation (posteriorly) for specific ligament testing. The apprehension signs and reduction maneuvers can be variable with this diagnosis.

Plain radiographic imaging is often normal. Advanced imaging consists of an MRI and a 3D CT scan. In the illustrative patient, the MRI (Figs. 33.4 and 33.5) shows an anchor within the bicipital groove consistent with the previous tenodesis. There is blunting of the anterior and posterior labrum without an obvious tear. Increased axillary volume seen on coronal view may be seen with capsular redundancy. The 3D CT reconstructions (Fig. 33.6) show a mild amount of anteroinferior bone loss but less than 15%. In the setting of instability with a history of previous shoulder surgery, a 3D CT scan is recommended to evaluate any bone loss. Beighton's criteria were a six out of nine. Moreover, EMG testing did not indicate abnormalities, specifi-

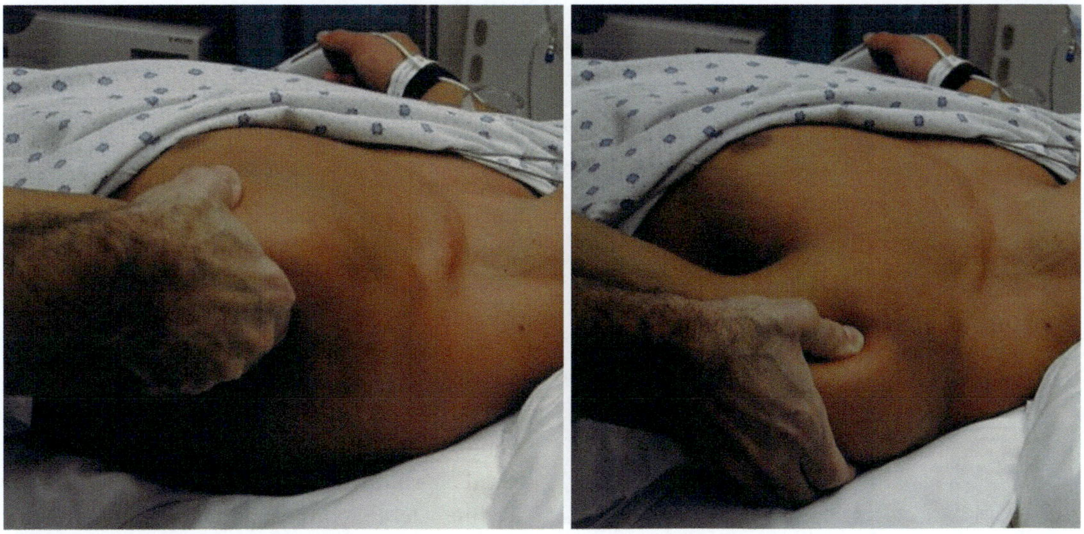

Fig. 33.3 Positive load-and-shift examination

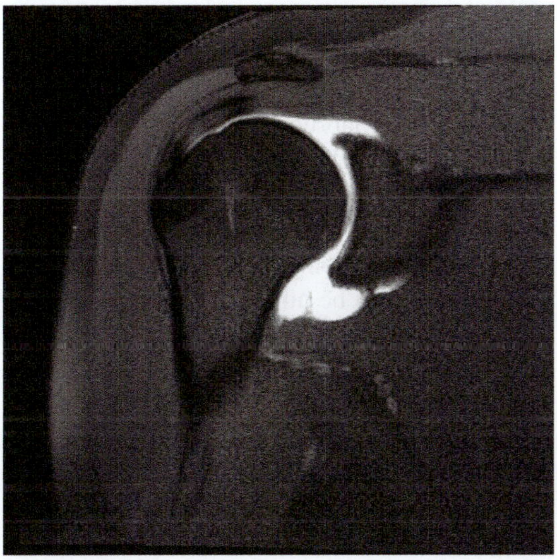

Fig. 33.4 Coronal MRI showing inferior capsular redundancy. (With permission of Joaquin Sanchez-Sotelo, M.D. [Mayo Clinic])

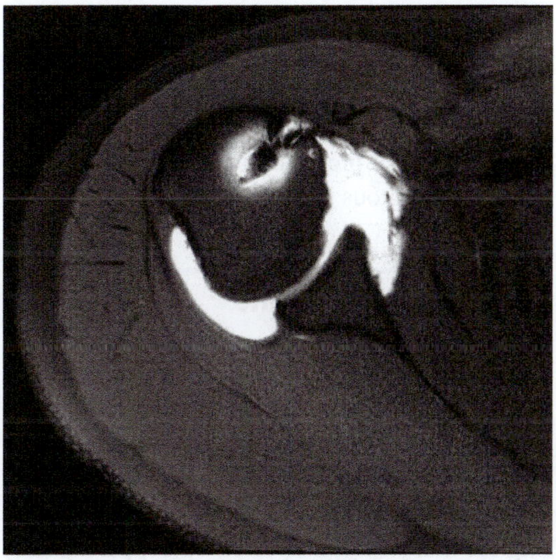

Fig. 33.5 Axillary MRI shows screw from previous biceps tenodesis, blunting of labrum without obvious tear. (With permission of Joaquin Sanchez-Sotelo, M.D. [Mayo Clinic])

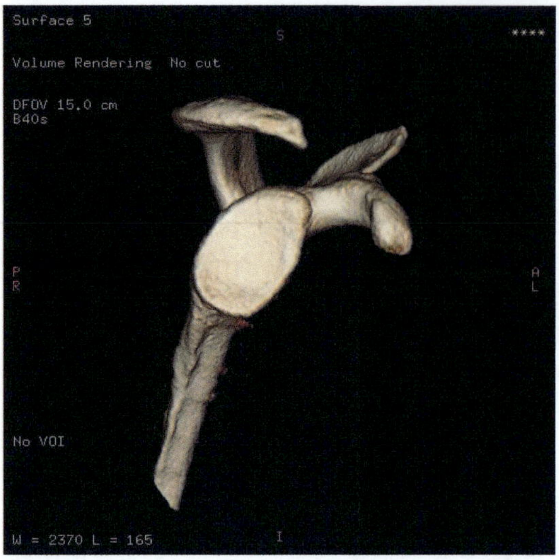

Fig. 33.6 3D CT recon showing mild anteroinferior bone loss. (With permission of Joaquin Sanchez-Sotelo, M.D. [Mayo Clinic])

cally in the long thoracic and suprascapular nerves.

The patient from the illustrative case was diagnosed with recurrent shoulder instability with a history of previous arthroscopy and generalized ligamentous laxity.

Surgical Management

We perform surgical stabilization on patients with continued instability who have failed adequate symptom resolution after at least 3 months of conservative management. However, surgical stabilization may also be used in the primary setting for many MDI suspected cases, particularly as an index procedure in patients with instability on exam and ligamentous laxity as tested using Beighton's criteria but without a labral tear. We also consider the use of the open technique in the revision setting with minimal bone loss or post-thermal capsulorrhaphy. A collision athlete may also benefit from an open procedure due to the added tensioning and reinforcement of the repair.

The technique has undergone some modifications since it was first described by Neer and Foster. A deltopectoral approach is used, and the subscapularis may undergo a partial L-shaped tenotomy or split. The authors generally perform a tenotomy to allow for improved visibility and access to the capsular tissue, as seen in Figs. 33.7 and 33.8. We prefer a lateral-based T-shaped tenotomy; however, intermediate [21] or medial-based capsulotomies have been utilized [22]. We feel the lateral approach and tenotomy allow for a larger amount of capsular tissue for plication, greater access to the inferior pouch, and pose less risk to the axillary nerve. A Fukuda is placed, and the joint is inspected, addressing any labral pathology as needed. Suture anchors are then placed along the glenoid rim/labrum junction after bony preparation. Suture is passed through the capsule and labrum and tied exterior to the articulation for a glenoid-based repair. The inferior leaf of the capsulotomy is then mobilized, including the inferior pouch, and attached superiorly with nonabsorbable suture, although suture anchors may also be utilized. The arm is held in 30° external rotation. Tensioning can be assessed by attempting to place a finger in the axillary pouch. With the pouch obliterated, the finger should not fit. Sutures are passed and tied down. The superior leaf is then pulled inferiorly over the top and sutured into place. Tenotomy repair is performed with nonabsorbable sutures at anatomic subscapularis length. A load-and-shift exam can be retested to confirm that multiple directions of laxity have been addressed.

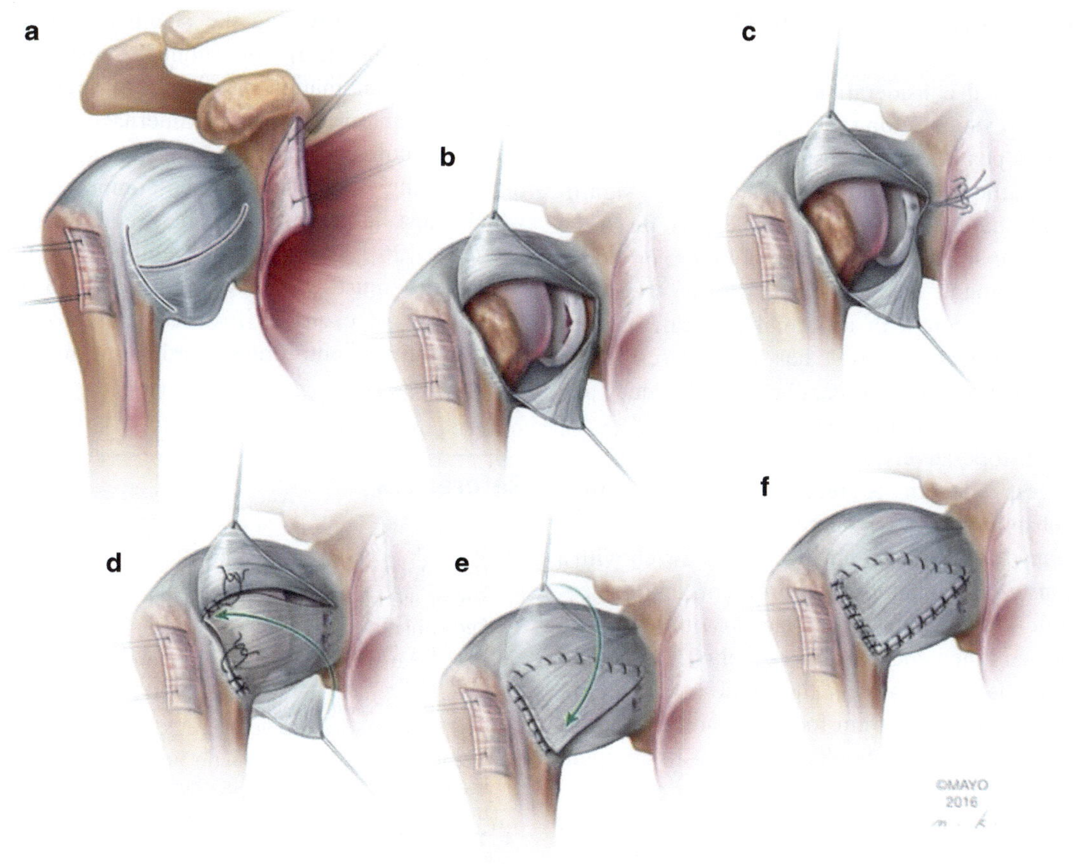

Fig. 33.7 The steps for open capsular shift. (**a**) The subscapularis tendon has been divided and peeled off of the anterior capsule. (**b**) A T shaped arthrotomy at the midline of the anterior capsule. (**c**) Medial suture anchors place in the glenoid incorporate the capsule and labrum to the glenoid rim. (**d**) The inferior capsule is mobilized and reatteched to the lateral capsular stump with superior shift to reduce the inferior and posterior pouches. (**e**) The superior capsule is oversewn tofurthe tighten the rotator interval and thicken the anterior capsule. (**f**) The capsular shift has created a reduced volume and reinforced capsular thickness. (With permissions from Joaquin Sanchez-Sotelo, M.D. [Mayo Clinic])

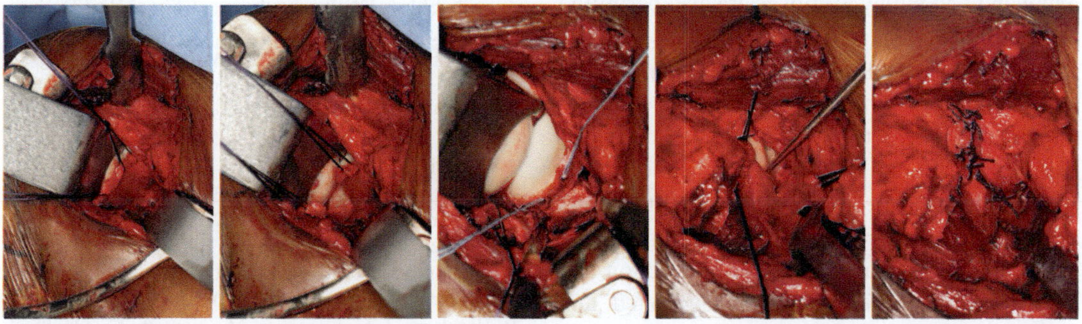

Fig. 33.8 Sequence from left to right of lateral capsulotomy, capsular split, glenoid-based capsular fixation, inferior capsular leaf shifted superior, and superior plication of the capsule over the top of the inferior leaf. (With permission of Joaquin Sanchez-Sotelo, M.D. [Mayo Clinic])

Post-Op/Additional Considerations

Additional considerations may arise, especially in the revision setting. Significant collagen disorder or post-thermal capsulorrhaphy can weaken the quality of the anterior capsule, and a significantly damaged anterior capsule may place the capsular shift at a higher risk of failure or reduce the amount of sufficient tissue available. Augmentation with a dermal allograft anterior capsular reconstruction has been described in conjunction with subscapularis insufficiency and may be useful in this setting [23].

Postoperatively, in patients with MDI, the largest concern is recurrence of instability. Rehabilitation after surgery progresses slowly. Many MDI patients may be managed well with a nonsurgical rehabilitation program, and in general, a large emphasis is placed on the return to normal kinematics postoperatively [24]. As ligamentous laxity affects the static stabilizers, a rehabilitation program focusing on the dynamic stabilizers of the shoulder may act to compensate and improve neuromuscular control [25].

The author's preferred protocol is 6 weeks of sling immobilization and protection of the subscapularis and capsular repair. At this time, elbow and wrist active range of motion and scapular isometrics are allowed. For the first 6 weeks, passive shoulder range of motion of forward elevation (FE) is allowed to 90° and external rotation (ER) to neutral. After 6 weeks, the sling is discontinued, and active-assisted motion is started, with FE increased to 120° and ER to 45°. Internal rotation and wand and pulley exercises are also permitted at this time. Patients continue to progress motion in FE and ER to tolerance at 8 weeks, with special focus on restoring scapulothoracic and glenohumeral kinematics. Closed-chain exercises like wall and table slides may help recruit the serratus anterior. Pectoralis minor and the short head of the biceps may develop postsurgical contracture that may cause scapular protraction and recurrence, and this should be evaluated and treated in the postoperative phase. Many MDI patients can have associated scapular dyskinesis either as a learned component adapted from chronic shoulder instability or as part of the ligamentous laxity affecting the stabilizers of the shoulder blade [26]. In shoulder instability patients, a combination of scapular protraction, increased anterior tilt, and internal rotation decreases cuff activation and muscle coordination, causing fatigue and learned compensation, which must be addressed through rehabilitation exercises [26]. The dynamic stabilizers of the rotator cuff must also be strengthened, and the final phase of exercises focuses on improving neuromuscular control and coordinating muscle activation.

References

1. Kraeutler MJ, McCarty EC, Belk JW, Wolf BR, Hettrich CM, Ortiz SF, et al. Descriptive epidemiology of the MOON shoulder instability cohort. Am J Sports Med. 2018;46(5):1064–9.
2. Neer CS 2nd, Foster CR. Inferior capsular shift for involuntary inferior and multidirectional instability of the shoulder. A preliminary report. J Bone Joint Surg Am. 1980;62(6):897–908.
3. Neer CS 2nd. Involuntary inferior and multidirectional instability of the shoulder: etiology, recognition, and treatment. Instr Course Lect. 1985;34:232–8.
4. Thomas SC, Matsen FA 3rd. An approach to the repair of avulsion of the glenohumeral ligaments in the management of traumatic anterior glenohumeral instability. J Bone Joint Surg Am. 1989;71(4):506–13.
5. Schoorl TJ, Nguyen NTV, van Noort A, Alta TDW, Sanchez-Sotelo J. Capsulorraphy with Achilles allograft augmentation for shoulder instability in patients with Ehlers-Danlos syndrome. J Shoulder Elb Surg. 2021;30(4):865–70.
6. Chaudhury S, Gasinu S, Rodeo SA. Bilateral anterior and posterior glenohumeral stabilization using Achilles tendon allograft augmentation in a patient with Ehlers-Danlos syndrome. J Shoulder Elb Surg. 2012;21(6):e1–5.
7. Iannotti JP, Antoniou J, Williams GR, Ramsey ML. Iliotibial band reconstruction for treatment of glenohumeral instability associated with irreparable capsular deficiency. J Shoulder Elb Surg. 2002;11(6):618–23.
8. Armstrong MD, Smith B, Coady C, Wong IH. Arthroscopic anterior and posterior glenoid bone augmentation with capsular plication for Ehlers-Danlos syndrome with multidirectional instability. Arthrosc Tech. 2018;7(5):e541–e5.
9. Brostrom LA, Kronberg M, Nemeth G, Oxelback U. The effect of shoulder muscle training in patients with recurrent shoulder dislocations. Scand J Rehabil Med. 1992;24(1):11–5.

10. Moroder P, Plachel F, Van-Vliet H, Adamczewski C, Danzinger V. Shoulder-pacemaker treatment concept for posterior positional functional shoulder instability: a prospective clinical trial. Am J Sports Med. 2020;48(9):2097–104.
11. Misamore GW, Sallay PI, Didelot W. A longitudinal study of patients with multidirectional instability of the shoulder with seven- to ten-year follow-up. J Shoulder Elb Surg. 2005;14(5):466–70.
12. Hawkins RJ, Abrams JS, Schutte JP. Multidirectional instability of the shoulder: an approach to diagnosis. Orthop Trans. 1987;11:246.
13. Abrams JS. Special shoulder problems in the throwing athlete: pathology, diagnosis, and nonoperative management. Clin Sports Med. 1991;10(4):839–61.
14. Warren RF. Subluxation of the shoulder in athletes. Clin Sports Med. 1983;2(2):339–54.
15. Rodeo SA, Suzuki K, Yamauchi M, Bhargava M, Warren RF. Analysis of collagen and elastic fibers in shoulder capsule in patients with shoulder instability. Am J Sports Med. 1998;26(5):634–43.
16. Juul-Kristensen B, Rogind H, Jensen DV, Remvig L. Inter-examiner reproducibility of tests and criteria for generalized joint hypermobility and benign joint hypermobility syndrome. Rheumatology (Oxford). 2007;46(12):1835–41.
17. Remvig L, Jensen DV, Ward RC. Epidemiology of general joint hypermobility and basis for the proposed criteria for benign joint hypermobility syndrome: review of the literature. J Rheumatol. 2007;34(4):804–9.
18. Cahill SV, Sharkey MS, Carter CW. Revisiting the beighton criteria: does ligamentous laxity testing correlate with shoulder range of motion norms in a north American, pediatric population? J Pediatr Orthop. 2020;40(9):536–42.
19. Chahal J, Leiter J, McKee MD, Whelan DB. Generalized ligamentous laxity as a predisposing factor for primary traumatic anterior shoulder dislocation. J Shoulder Elb Surg. 2010;19(8):1238–42.
20. Castori M, Tinkle B, Levy H, Grahame R, Malfait F, Hakim A. A framework for the classification of joint hypermobility and related conditions. Am J Med Genet C Semin Med Genet. 2017;175(1):148–57.
21. Wirth MA, Blatter G, Rockwood CA Jr. The capsular imbrication procedure for recurrent anterior instability of the shoulder. J Bone Joint Surg Am. 1996;78(2):246–59.
22. Altchek DW, Warren RF, Skyhar MJ, Ortiz G. T-plasty modification of the Bankart procedure for multidirectional instability of the anterior and inferior types. J Bone Joint Surg Am. 1991;73(1):105–12.
23. Rogers JP, Kwapisz A, Tokish JM. Anterior capsule reconstruction for irreparable subscapularis tears. Arthrosc Tech. 2017;6(6):e2241–e7.
24. Burkhead WZ Jr, Rockwood CA Jr. Treatment of instability of the shoulder with an exercise program. J Bone Joint Surg Am. 1992;74(6):890–6.
25. Barden JM, Balyk R, Raso VJ, Moreau M, Bagnall K. Dynamic upper limb proprioception in multidirectional shoulder instability. Clin Orthop Relat Res. 2004;420:181–9.
26. Kibler WB, Sciascia A. The role of the scapula in preventing and treating shoulder instability. Knee Surg Sports Traumatol Arthrosc. 2016;24(2):390–7.

The Arthroscopic Pan Capsular Plication for Multidirectional Shoulder Instability

34

Zachary Salas, Liam A. Peebles, Felix H. Savoie III, and Michael J. O'Brien

Introduction

Multidirectional instability (MDI) is a term first coined in 1980 by Charles Neer and Craig Foster to describe a large redundant inferior capsule with rotator interval laxity as seen by bulging of the rotator interval on arthrogram [1]. Neer and Foster described MDI as anterior and posterior instability associated with involuntary inferior subluxation or dislocation. The diagnosis can be challenging due to the lack of standardized criteria to define MDI and to variations in patient symptoms and presentation. Some patients will describe feelings of instability, while others will only present with shoulder pain. This can be compounded by the need to distinguish laxity from instability, which underscores the current challenges and misconceptions of MDI. We define multidirectional instability as symptomatic instability in two or more directions, one of which is inferior, with or without associated hyperlaxity.

Rehabilitation focusing on scapular stabilizing exercises and rotator cuff strengthening remains the mainstay of treatment. Surgical intervention is reserved for those who fail an extensive nonoperative rehabilitation program. While open inferior capsular shift has long been considered the gold standard and remains a viable surgical option to treat MDI, arthroscopic techniques, including pan capsular plication, are effective and less invasive options that allow the surgeon to address all areas of the capsule in one approach. Advantages of arthroscopy include decreased morbidity; access to the entire shoulder capsule; visual confirmation of decreased capsular volume; avoidance of subscapularis detachment; addressing of capsular redundancies and deficiencies anteriorly, posteriorly, and inferiorly; and closure of the rotator interval all at the same setting [2–6].

Illustrative Clinical Case

The patient is a 23-year-old, right-hand-dominant female who presented with a longstanding history of progressively worsening left shoulder pain and instability. The patient had initially injured her shoulder in high school 5 years prior and experienced traumatic reinjury 6 months before presenting to the senior authors. She failed extensive conservative treatment with rest, physical therapy for 6 months, bracing and taping of the shoulder, and home exercises with continued left posterior shoulder pain and multiple sublux-

Z. Salas · F. H. Savoie III · M. J. O'Brien (✉)
Department of Orthopaedic Surgery, Tulane University School of Medicine, New Orleans, LA, USA
e-mail: fsavoie@tulane.edu; mobrien@tulane.edu

L. A. Peebles
Tulane University School of Medicine, New Orleans, LA, USA

© The Author(s), under exclusive license to Springer Nature Switzerland AG 2026

R. M. Frank, J. M. Tokish (eds.), *Management of Shoulder Instability*,
https://doi.org/10.1007/978-3-032-18089-6_34

ations. Physical examination revealed generalized ligamentous laxity of the shoulders, with anterior, posterior, and inferior laxity, with posterior laxity being the primary direction of her pain and instability. An MRI arthrogram was obtained, which revealed a potential posterior labral tear and patulous posterior capsule. Due to her continued pain and recurrent instability, surgery was offered for left shoulder arthroscopy with posterior labral repair and capsulorrhaphy. The risks and benefits of the procedure were described in detail. She understood the risks and agreed to proceed with surgery.

Etiology

Neer and Foster first described multidirectional instability (MDI) in 1980 [1]. It is defined by symptomatic involuntary shoulder laxity in more than one direction [7–10]. It is critical to differentiate instability from laxity. The term "laxity" describes the physiological looseness or tightness of the shoulder with variation between individuals. It is measured on exam under anesthesia and should be equal bilaterally. In contrast, the term "instability" is used to describe a pathologic condition in which there is abnormal movement of the humeral head on the glenoid, producing *symptoms* of pain and functional impairment. It represents a change from normal with multiple causes, including but not limited to traumatic injury, overuse, tissue attenuation, and posture [11]. MDI most often occurs in the shoulders with inherent laxity in multiple directions that becomes symptomatic in one or more directions because of muscle imbalance or loss of proprioception. Most authors believe that inferior instability combined with posterior instability, anterior instability, or both is required to be considered MDI [7, 8, 12, 13].

Neer and Foster described three groups of patients with MDI. The first group included those with anterior and inferior dislocation and posterior subluxation. The second group included individuals with posterior and inferior dislocation with anterior subluxation. The third included those with recurrent dislocation in all directions [14].

The precise incidence of MDI is unknown due to the challenge of diagnosing this condition, but Blomquist et al. reported that 7% of the operations for shoulder instability in Norway during 2008 were attributed to MDI [15]. It typically presents during the second or third decade of life [16]. It is less common after the age of 40 due to the natural stiffening of tissues around the shoulder [17]. Current literature supports that MDI occurs equally among males and females [18, 19].

There appear to be two separate populations with MDI: those with congenital, generalized hyperlaxity and those who develop MDI secondary to repetitive microtrauma to the primary and secondary stabilizers of the glenohumeral joint. This second group usually includes athletes who repetitively load the shoulder joint in a flexed and internally rotated position during overhead sports such as gymnastics, baseball, softball, volleyball, rowing, and swimming. MDI from overt trauma may be seen in rugby players, collision and contact sports, and people who have been involved in motor vehicle accidents and explosions.

MDI secondary to trauma may be due to a single or multiple traumatic dislocations. It is important to note that patients with significant trauma are more likely to have structural lesions to the glenoid labrum or joint capsule. Traumatic MDI will have one predominant direction of instability and may have better outcomes with early surgical stabilization. In contrast, patients with an atraumatic or repetitive microtraumatic MDI, especially from overhead activities, are more likely to have an intact but attenuated capsule associated with globally increased capsular volume, signs of poor motor control, scapular dyskinesis, and instability in multiple directions. They generally respond well to nonoperative management and rehabilitation. In both groups, the laxity of the capsule must be addressed to restore native stability. It should be noted that all groups share similar characteristics: scapular dyskinesia, rotator cuff inflammation, and a lack of spatial awareness of the position of the shoulder.

MDI can also develop secondary to collagen tissue disorders. Patients with congenital conditions such as Ehlers-Danlos syndrome (EDS), Marfan syndrome, osteogenesis imperfecta, and benign joint hypermobility syndrome may be predisposed to developing MDI [20–24]. These connective tissue disorders affect the rate of collagen formation, the number of collagen fibrils and crosslinks, and the type of collagen in tissues, which may contribute to glenohumeral joint instability.

Pathogenesis

MDI is caused by alterations between the static (glenoid concavity and version, labral height, and glenohumeral ligaments and capsule) and dynamic stabilizers (rotator cuff, scapulothoracic muscles, proprioceptive and neuromuscular control), causing symptoms in two or more directions. Patients become symptomatic due to pain from rotator cuff tendonitis. Laxity in the glenohumeral ligaments and joint capsule leads to shoulder instability, and the rotator cuff becomes overworked trying to provide dynamic stability to the shoulder, which causes rotator cuff swelling, tendonitis, and pain. This pain leads to the development of scapular protraction with dyskinesia, as the patient tries to splint the arm in a position of comfort, which produces trapezial pain, weakness, and spasms.

Poor posture and scapular protraction place an increased strain on the rotator cuff, producing more pain. The resulting rotator cuff weakness thereby increases shoulder subluxation, which creates a worsening cycle of instability, dyskinesia, tendonitis, and pain. This ultimately manifests as pain at rest and with any activities, as the inflamed rotator cuff struggles to provide stability to the dyskinetic and unbalanced shoulder.

Athletes may exhibit symptoms if they have shoulder inferior subluxation at rest, especially in circumstances of poor core and hip strength. These patients are typically asymptomatic once a balance among shoulder muscle stabilizers is achieved. The progression of MDI can be thought of as a cyclical exacerbation of the disease process with initial rotator cuff tendonitis leading to shoulder pain and protraction, which causes further rotator cuff weakness, increases shoulder subluxation, and thereby worsens the initial rotator cuff tendonitis. The final pathway results in shoulder pain and dysfunction. The glenohumeral joint remains subluxated inferiorly at rest, with the inflamed rotator cuff unable to provide dynamic stability to the joint and severe pain that impairs all function.

Diagnosis and Examination

Patient History

A detailed history and physical exam are extremely important for the evaluation of the patient with MDI. Patients may present with confounding symptoms, ranging from vague shoulder pain to outright instability. The usual multidirectional instability patient will be in their teens or twenties and complain of nonspecific pain, decreased athletic performance, and loss of strength [1, 25]. Patients will complain of feelings of instability with shoulder shifting or clunking. This may occur while lying in bed or in their sleep. They may also report subluxation events that occur during sleep.

Pain and instability can occur with simple activities such as walking, as is worsened with lifting, overhead function, and any athletic activities. Pain may occur at rest when rotator cuff inflammation is severe. The presence of impingement syndrome and rotator cuff tendonitis on Neer and Hawkins impingement maneuvers in patients under the age of 20 should raise suspicion of possible MDI. Pain is more pronounced during the midrange of glenohumeral motion due to rotator cuff activation. Patients may report their shoulder "falls out the bottom." Symptoms that present when carrying heavy objects at one's side are indicative of inferior instability. Patients may experience transient neurologic symptoms from shoulder subluxation and neuropraxia. The shoulder pain described with MDI is consistent with pain exhibited secondary to rotator cuff tendonitis, as there is an imbalance between shoulder muscles, scapular dyskinesia, and loss of proprioception.

Physical Examination

Patients will commonly present with a severely protracted shoulder, poor posture, and scapular protraction with shoulders rolled forward. Scapular dyskinesia is distinctly apparent in all cases by viewing scapular mechanics from the posterior during active arm elevation. The shoulder may have a "squared off" appearance due to the prominence of the acromion secondary to an inferiorly translated humeral head and disuse atrophy of the deltoid.

Both shoulders should be examined as part of the physical examination of the patient. One can then compare symmetry, scapular motion, swelling, and scapular winging. Apprehension with range of motion and tenderness along the medial angle of the scapula and anterior rotator cuff are associated with MDI [12]. Internal rotation strength can be reduced up to 30%, emphasizing the dynamic muscular dysfunction in this condition [26]. The most common physical finding in symptomatic MDI is a loss of spatial awareness of the shoulder [8].

When palpating the shoulder, tenderness is present on the distal supraspinatus tendon as well as the coracoid, with typical tightness over the pectoralis minor tendon. Range of motion may be limited secondary to pain. Pay particular attention to hyper-external rotation and hyper-abduction. Shoulder stability and strength can be assessed with the patient sitting or supine but may be easier to perform supine for patient comfort. Patients may have diminished rotator cuff (supraspinatus) and periscapular muscle strength due to inflammation and rotator cuff tendonitis.

A sulcus sign must reproduce symptoms in order to indicate MDI. One should check for a symptomatic sulcus sign in neutral rotation and external rotation and abduction to evaluate the degree of dysfunction of the superior glenohumeral and coracohumeral ligaments of the rotator interval. Beighton criteria, or signs of generalized ligamentous laxity, should be examined in every patient. Common physical exam findings of a patient with generalized ligamentous laxity include the ability to touch the thumb to the ipsilateral forearm, hyperextend the elbow greater than 5 degrees, and/or place the palm of the hand flat on the floor with legs fully extended [3].

When assessing anterior and posterior instability, the *load-and-shift test* can provide critical information about instability in multiple directions. Perform the load-and-shift test with the patient supine for patient comfort. The shoulder usually can be subluxated over the rim of the glenoid (Grade 3 laxity) anteriorly, posteriorly, and inferiorly or dislocated outright [10]. Generalized laxity may be present in all three directions; however, it is important to determine the primary direction of instability that elicits pain and symptoms.

When assessing inferior instability, it is important to assess for a positive *sulcus sign*. While applying a downward traction force to the elbow of the patient with the arm resting at the side in a neutral position, greater than a fingerbreadth of depression under the lateral acromion is created. It is important to note that the positive sulcus does not diminish with external rotation and is increased in comparison to the contralateral shoulder when the shoulder is in adduction.

When suspecting MDI, assess for a positive *Whipple test* with and without scapula stabilization. The arm is placed in 90° of forward flexion with neutral forearm rotation, and the patient resists a downward force. A positive test recreates pain and weakness, indicating scapular dyskinesis.

Pain with inferior subluxation of the arm in adduction is indicated with a positive *Gagey test*. To perform the Gagey test, the patient sits in an upright position in front of the examiner. Stabilize the patient's shoulder girdle by placing one hand on the clavicle and scapula to prevent the shoulder from elevating. Use the other hand to passively move the patient's arm into end-range abduction. A normal shoulder will abduct to 90°, while a positive Gagey test will abduct greater than 105°, indicating inferior glenohumeral instability.

The *Lafosse hyperextension-internal rotation (HERI) test* is a method that can evaluate the integrity of the inferior glenohumeral ligament (IGHL) by measuring the glenohumeral extension angle [27]. The patient stands in front of the examiner facing away. To perform the HERI test and to measure the glenohumeral extension angle of the right shoulder, the examiner places the left elbow against the patient's left scapula and maximally elevates the patient's left arm to lock the thoracic spine and prevent the patient from bending forward while also locking both scapulothoracic joints. The examiner then grasps the patient's right forearm, pulling it backwards and in pronation with the elbow extended, thereby inducing hyperextension and internal rotation of the patient's right glenohumeral joint. Internal rotation of the glenohumeral joint prevents anterior subluxation and apprehension. The examiner increases the degree of hyperextension until a hard resistance is felt, indicating maximal glenohumeral extension. When the right glenohumeral joint is maximally extended, the extension angle is measured, and any pain or apprehension reported by the patient is recorded. The HERI test should be performed on both sides and the results of the two tests compared. A side-to-side difference greater than 15° increase in the glenohumeral angle during maximal extension indicates IGHL injury in the affected extremity.

Examine for scapular dyskinesis to gain additional information about alterations to muscle activation via the *scapular assistance test* and *scapular retraction test*. The *scapular assistance test* is performed by stabilizing the patient's shoulder girdle by placing a hand on the clavicle and scapular spine. The other hand is used to grasp the inferior angle of the scapula on the same side. Ask the patient to abduct their arm and assist the movement of the scapula. A positive scapular assistance test is seen when a patient experiences less pain during the assisted movement in comparison to non-assisted movement due to weakness of scapular stabilizers. The *scapular retraction test* can also be utilized to evaluate scapular dyskinesis by stabilizing the retracted scapula to test the rotator cuff. This is done by placing your hand over the patient's clavicle and scapular spine with your forearm supporting the medial border of the scapula. Ask the patient to perform an empty can test while providing resistance and a downward force with your other hand. A positive test is seen when a patient's rotator cuff strength is restored during the scapular retraction test.

Imaging

Standard radiographs of the shoulder are obtained, including anteroposterior (AP), scapular Y, and axillary lateral views. These views should be obtained to evaluate for any bony deficiency of the glenoid or humeral head. They may also reveal subluxation, indicating a failure of the resting tension of the muscles of the rotator cuff to be sufficient to keep the shoulder in place. Additional subluxation in the various views may also reveal a lack of spatial awareness of the shoulder at rest, a common finding in the symptomatic MDI shoulder. It should be noted that plain radiographs are usually normal in MDI patients.

Advanced imaging modalities include computerized arthrotomography (CT arthrogram) and magnetic resonance imaging (MRI) with intra-articular contrast (MRA). CT is the best modality to evaluate glenoid bone loss, version, and dysplasia. MRA is the imaging modality of choice in MDI to define soft tissue (labrum, ligament, cartilage, and tendon) pathology. The typical MRA findings include a large capsular volume that can appear as an "upside-down bubble" extending inferiorly to the glenoid on the coronal view. The pathognomonic hallmark of MDI, as described by Neer, is bulging of the rotator interval with contrast [14]. One may also see the entire silhouette of the intra-articular portion of the biceps tendon with significant rotator interval laxity. The axial sections will demonstrate laxity of both the anterior and the posterior capsule, commonly in the inferior sections of the glenoid. In addition to examination of the capsule, one should always evaluate the MRI for labral pathology and the integrity of the rotator cuff.

Nonoperative Management

Due to altered proprioception and neuromuscular control of the glenohumeral joint and scapulothoracic articulation, treatment always begins with nonoperative management of symptomatic MDI with shoulder rehabilitation in all patients. The initial goal of nonoperative treatment is focused on reducing inflammation and correcting scapular position through proprioceptive training. Inflammation is controlled with nonsteroidal anti-inflammatory medications and selective corticosteroid injections. Static bracing, dynamic bracing, and McConnell taping may be employed to correct dyskinesis and place the shoulder back into the correct position.

Pain-free rotator cuff exercises are initiated only after the correct scapular position has been reestablished. Physical therapy is aimed at not only improving the strength of the rotator cuff and dynamic stabilizers, but also improving neuromuscular control by retraining the pattern of shoulder muscle activation through exercise in order to compensate for static deficiencies. The scapula in MDI patients is typically protracted; therefore, the rehabilitation protocol is directed toward restoring correct motor control of the scapulothoracic stabilizers. Coordination and strength of both the rotator cuff muscles and the periscapular musculature should be achieved to provide stability. Moreover, during the early rehabilitation course, closed-chain kinetic exercises will provide patients with safe co-contraction of the scapular and rotator cuff muscles during muscle activation training. Core and hip abduction strengthening exercises should be added to provide additional core stability. Patients typically follow this regimen for 3–6 months. Devices such as scapular posture shirts, bracing, taping, and electrical stimulation may provide additional support during rehabilitation.

Operative Management

Indications and Contraindications

The symptomatic pattern of the instability (anterior, posterior, inferior, or a combination thereof) should be clearly documented prior to surgical intervention. The shoulder may demonstrate laxity in many directions and have symptomatic primary instability in only one direction. One must be mindful of the fact that laxity does not necessarily correlate with instability [11]. Asymptomatic, normal laxity does not usually need to be surgically addressed. Indications for surgical management of MDI may include continued pain, functional impairment in acts of daily living, and a failure of adequate rehabilitation that included postural correction and scapular stabilization. Surgical options include an open capsular shift or arthroscopic shift with capsulorrhaphy and capsular plication.

Relative contraindications to arthroscopic capsular shift procedures in the MDI patient include failure to complete a structured rehabilitation program, voluntary dislocators who may seek secondary gain following soft tissue stabilization, and those with known connective tissue disorders. EDS is a well-documented example of such conditions. Although there are multiple genetic variants that account for the different subtypes of EDS, they all interfere with the proper formation of Type I and Type III procollagens in some respect. With abnormal Type I and Type III collagen production, healing and scar tissue formation occur normally, but this tissue is replaced by the patients' own normal, poor-quality ligaments. Laxity and capsular redundancy can thereby redevelop soon after surgical shift of the tissue and yield variable success rates. In the setting of EDS and other collagen tissue disorders, an allograft capsular reconstruction may be performed. Surgeons should use their best judgment in providing solutions for MDI patients and may opt for continued nonoperative management rather than early surgical intervention if there is any doubt.

Patient Positioning and Approach

Arthroscopic pan capsular plication may be performed with the patient in either the beach chair or lateral decubitus position. The senior authors (F.H.S and M.J.O.) prefer the lateral decubitus position due to the ease of access provided to the inferior capsule and the avoidance of additional inferior portals. The arm is suspended with 5–10 lbs. of balanced suspension and positioned in 45° of abduction with 15–20° of forward flexion. The lateral decubitus setup also allows for the arm to be positioned in 90° of external rotation when shifting the anterior capsule and closing the rotator interval to avoid overtightening of the shoulder.

Surgery is performed under general anesthesia with an interscalene nerve block. After the induction of adequate anesthesia, it is imperative to perform an examination under anesthesia in every case to determine the direction and degree of shoulder laxity. After positioning, prepping, and draping have been achieved, diagnostic arthroscopy should follow.

Diagnostic arthroscopy should be performed through a standard posterior portal. On diagnostic arthroscopy, it is imperative to critically assess for a widened rotator interval (Fig. 34.1), a loose patulous capsule (Fig. 34.2), and possible associated labral tears, capsular tears, or humeral avulsion of the glenohumeral ligaments (HAGL lesions). The anterior, inferior, and posterior capsules should be evaluated for laxity and/or tearing, along with inspection of the rotator cuff. Initially, the shoulder may appear reduced in a native position. After the application of 5–10 lbs. of balanced suspension, the shoulder will subluxate or dislocate in an inferior direction into the axillary pouch due to the attenuated rotator interval, coracohumeral ligament (CHL), and superior glenohumeral ligament (SGHL) (Fig. 34.3). An arthroscopic "drive-through sign" of the glenohumeral joint is easily performed due to capsular laxity and attenuation. The arthroscope can be placed in the anterior-superior portal to view the entire glenohumeral joint and evaluate for anterior or posterior capsular redundancy. If the aforementioned structures appear to be in their native state, surgeons may proceed with arthroscopic MDI stabilization.

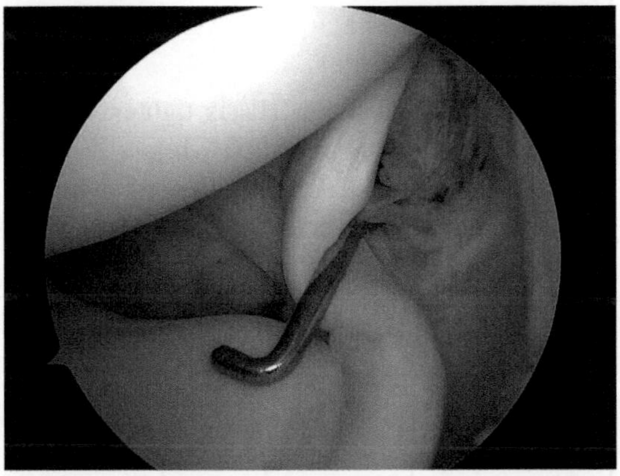

Fig. 34.1 Posterior view of the left shoulder demonstrating a widened rotator interval, an intact biceps tendon, and a biceps anchor without evidence of SLAP tear

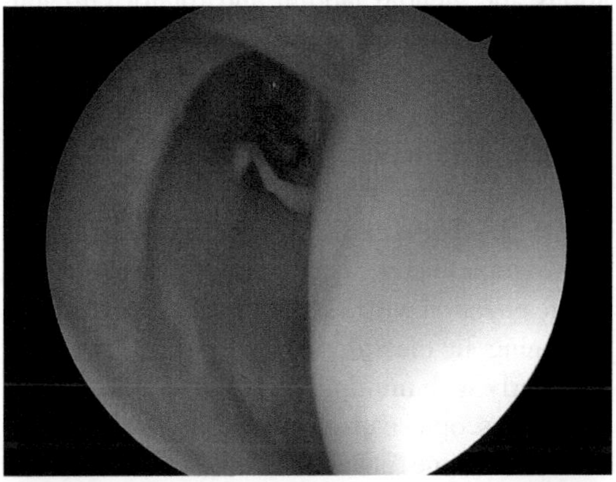

Fig. 34.2 View of the left shoulder from the anterosuperior portal demonstrating a patulous posterior capsule with an intact posterior labrum

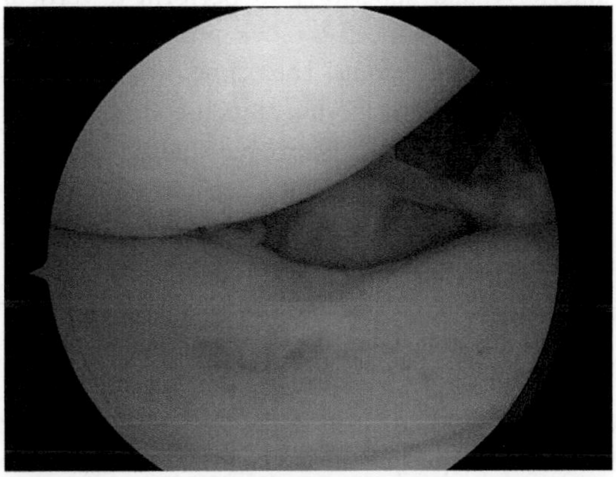

Fig. 34.3 View of the left shoulder from the posterior portal showing the humeral head sitting subluxated in an anterior and inferior position

Surgical Technique

In true MDI patients, key pathologic structures requiring surgical management commonly include the inferior joint capsule, the anterior and posterior capsule, and the rotator interval. The inferior capsule will demonstrate increased laxity and poorly defined bands of the inferior glenohumeral ligament (IGHL) in either the anterior or posterior pouches or both. Similarly, the widened rotator interval will exhibit excessive laxity and may have a "bulged out" appearance through which the coracohumeral ligament, superior glenohumeral ligament, and joint capsule can be visualized [28]. Secondary to chronic subluxations, the glenoid labrum and rotator cuff tendons may also appear atrophic with possible complete or partial tears that will need to be addressed during the operation.

When performing a capsulorrhaphy for MDI, capsular abrasion is performed prior to the capsular shift. This can be completed with an arthroscopic shaver or rasp. Subsequently, a suture plication with a superior shift is performed, beginning in the inferior capsule and working superiorly with multiple plication sutures.

Arthroscopic capsular plication begins with the arthroscope posteriorly. A suture hook or retriever is then passed through the inferior capsule at the 6 o'clock position, approximately 1 cm from the labrum at the bottom of the capsule's "valley of laxity." The capsule is pulled anteriorly and superiorly to perform a vertical shift to at least the 5 o'clock position until the capsule appears taut. The same hook is then passed through the labrum at its junction with the articular margin. An absorbable suture (usually 0 PDS) is shuttled through the capsule and glenoid labrum (Fig. 34.4). If the labrum is found to be detached from the glenoid or deficient, use of a suture anchor may be indicated. With a stable labral bone interface, the suture is shuttled, and the two ends of the suture are tied with a sliding, self-locking knot, shifting the capsule superiorly with an oblique plication. The suture knot must be placed on the capsular side, avoiding placement of the knot on the articular cartilage. As the plication suture is tied, redundant capsular tissue is diminished, and the IGHL is tightened. This suturing technique is repeated while advancing superiorly up the face of the glenoid, with the second stitch starting at the 5 o'clock position and being pulled taut to near 4 o'clock. Additional plication sutures are placed as needed until the anterior laxity has been eliminated entirely (Fig. 34.5).

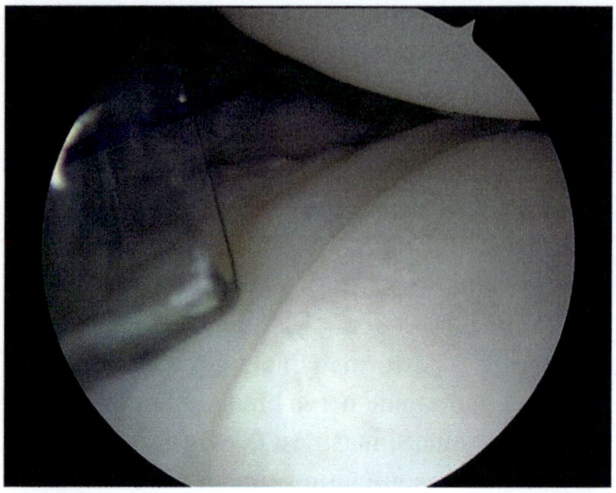

Fig. 34.4 Anterosuperior view of the left shoulder with posterior capsulorrhaphy being performed using four PDS sutures placed from the 6 o'clock to 10 o'clock position

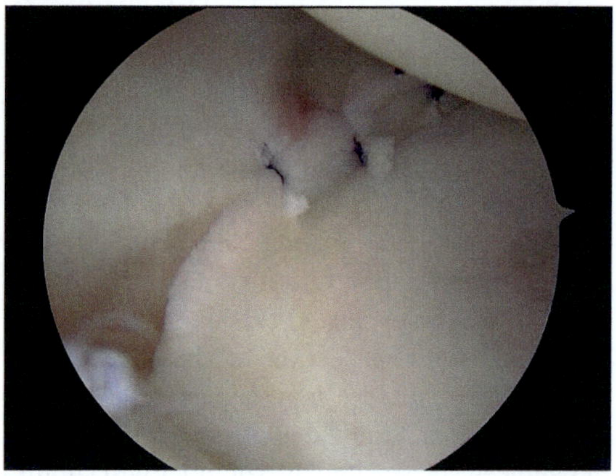

Fig. 34.5 Anterosuperior view of completed posterior capsulorrhaphy in the left shoulder that successfully decreased redundancy of the posterior and inferior capsular pouch

The arthroscope is then placed anteriorly, and plication of the posterior capsule is performed in a similar fashion. In the setting of MDI, it is not uncommon to have a degenerative posterior capsule that is insufficient to hold plication sutures.

In such cases, sutures may be passed through the infraspinatus tendon to provide a more stable plication construct. This technique begins by piercing the lateral capsule near its insertion on the humerus with an 18-G spinal needle and threading a suture through the needle into the joint. The initial stitch should be placed at the 7 o'clock position. The suture is grasped while the spinal needle is removed, and a suture-retrieving device is then used to pierce the capsule adjacent to the labrum and hold the percutaneously placed suture. The suture is pulled through the posterior portal, and the canula is retracted until outside the infraspinatus tendon. The cannula is advanced into the subacromial space using a switching stick, and a crochet hook is used to grasp the suture while watching from inside the joint. Once the suture is tied and the degree of capsular tightening is assessed, these steps are repeated until the excessive posterior laxity has been corrected.

If there is evidence of an absent, hypotrophic, or dysfunctional labrum, then a suture anchor must be placed for the capsulorrhaphy. The suture anchor is placed into the glenoid between the glenoid and the labrum, taking care not to place the suture anchor through the labrum.

After completion of the capsulorrhaphy, the arthroscope is placed back in the posterior portal, and attention is turned to the rotator interval for plication. In the setting of MDI, complete closure of the rotator interval (RI) with a wide plication of the superior glenohumeral ligament and coracohumeral ligament is required to effectively stabilize the shoulder posteriorly and inferiorly. The rotator interval closure is performed by placing two to three permanent plication sutures in an oblique medial-to-lateral fashion between the supraspinatus and subscapularis, taking care not to incarcerate the long head of the biceps tendon. This is accomplished by tightening both the inner and outer layers of the rotator interval. RI closure begins by placing a spinal needle percutaneously approximately 1 cm from the humeral articular cartilage margin, anterior to the edge of the supraspinatus tendon. A permanent suture is then passed through the needle, and the anterior canula is retracted just anterior to the subscapularis tendon and the rotator interval's outer layer. Through the anterior layer of the rotator interval tissue, a suture retriever is placed through the capsule to enter the joint. At this point, the upper border of the subscapularis tendon and the middle glenohumeral ligament may be incorporated into the closure. The percutaneously passed suture is pulled through the anterior canula, and a switching stick is used to pass the canula around the subscapularis tendon into the subacromial space. A crochet hook grasps the suture from the subacromial space and retrieves it out the anterior canula. Finally, a sliding locking knot is used to close the interval. Working progressively medially with each stitch, additional sutures may be placed in a similar manner. Typically, two to three rotator interval sutures will be placed. The sutures are tied while holding the arm in 90° of external rotation to prevent over-tensioning. When the arm begins to internally rotate, the rotator interval closure and MDI reconstruction are complete.

Postoperative Rehabilitation and Additional Considerations

Postoperatively, rehabilitation protocols should be tailored to patients based on the individual's primary direction of instability and robustness of repair and progressed based on activity level and sport. In these patients, the shoulder is immobilized in either a gunslinger-type brace or an abduction sling in neutral rotation for 6 weeks postoperatively. Scapular repositioning exercises are done within the brace, and it is removed during showers and dressing. Active-assisted range of motion exercises are performed at home 4–6 weeks postoperatively. At 6 weeks postoperative, the brace is removed, and gentle physical therapy emphasizing scapular retraction and awareness of the shoulder's position in space is initiated. The use of static and dynamic bracing, as well as scapular taping, is often quite useful during this phase of rehabilitation. The therapist is not allowed to stretch the shoulder at any point during the rehabilitation of MDI surgery.

At 3 months postoperative, the rehabilitation has progressed to include overhead exercises and progressive rotator cuff strengthening, along with continued progression of the core strengthening and periscapular exercises. It is critical, as the exercises are progressed, that scapular position is continually monitored to maintain its retracted, balanced position. Usually, at 4–6 months postoperative, functional rehabilitation and sport-specific conditioning are continued and advanced, with continued progression of Kibler-type integrated scapular rehabilitation. At 6 months postoperative, the patient is allowed to resume normal activities as tolerated. Stretching by the therapist is avoided in these patients until at least 6 months have passed and is seldom necessary in the ideal patient with MDI.

Results

In 1980, Neer and Foster first reported satisfactory results in 16 of 17 shoulders (94%) following an open inferior capsular shift technique with at least 2-year follow-up [1]. Since Neer's original paper, treatment of MDI has progressed with the advent of arthroscopic techniques. Functional outcomes for MDI are typically measured using a variety of shoulder scoring systems, including but not limited to the Rowe scale, Constant score, Neer score, UCLA score, American Shoulder and Elbow Society (ASES) score, and the Western Ontario Shoulder Instability (WOSI) index.

Using laser-assisted capsulorrhaphy for MDI, Lyons reported that 96% of patients remained stable and asymptomatic at a minimum of 2 years postoperatively [29]. Thermal capsulorrhaphy has been largely abandoned due to capsular thermal necrosis and high failure rates.

Gartsman demonstrated that 91% of patients had successful outcomes according to the Rowe score with arthroscopic plication surgery during a 2–5-year follow-up [30]. In a 5-year follow-up study of MDI treated with arthroscopic shift, Treacy reported that 88% of patients had a satisfactory Neer score with maintained shoulder stability [31]. In a 4–10-year follow-up, Marquardt reported that 89% of patients treated with an open inferior capsular shift procedure had successful results according to the Rowe scale [32]. Pollock reported a favorable outcome in 94% of patients and 96% stability of MDI shoulders after an open inferior capsular shift at a mean 61-month follow-up [33]. Wichman and Snyder demonstrated satisfactory results in 79% of patients with the Neer criteria at a minimum follow-up of 2 years with the use of arthroscopic capsular plications for MDI [5].

Complications

Recurrence of MDI has been reported to range between 8% and 30% following surgical repairs and plication [19, 34–36]. The high rate of recurrence is thought to be due to the inability to change the structural integrity of collagen, which contributes to future laxity. It is unknown if chondrolysis may be associated with MDI. A foreseen complication is postsurgical arthritis and capsulorrhaphy arthropathy. Due to the close proximity of the axillary nerve to the inferior glenohumeral pouch, axillary nerve injury may occur after open, thermal, and arthroscopic procedures. Great care must be taken while placing inferior plication sutures to not overpenetrate the inferior capsule and injure the axillary nerve. Although rare, stiffness and loss of motion may also be seen. Additionally, subscapularis insufficiency may result when an open procedure is performed. In cases of failure, a modified Gallie allograft reconstruction procedure may be performed, especially in Ehlers-Danlos patients. In the authors' experience, this has maintained stability in the setting of collagen tissue disorders for 7–8 years.

Conclusion

Multidirectional instability is a complex disorder that is suspected when a patient presents with shoulder pain and instability in two or more directions (anterior, posterior, or inferior). Physical examination confirms the diagnosis and the primary direction of instability. Although plain radiographs may provide some insight into traumatic injury, MRI arthrogram is the imaging modality of choice and provides a definitive assessment of the shoulder by identifying capsular laxity with a patulous inferior capsule. The mainstay of treatment is rehabilitation and physical therapy aimed at reducing inflammation and restoring scapular position and mechanics. Strengthening of shoulder stabilizers, rotator cuff, and periscapular musculature should only be initiated after pain is reduced and correct scapular positioning is achieved. Surgery is only considered when there is a failure of 6 months of rehabilitation, which must have included scapular stabilization exercises and scapular support with bracing and taping. Surgical options include open and arthroscopic stabilization procedures, including capsular shift, rotator interval closure, and plication of capsular tissue. Posterior plication with the addition of infraspinatus may be used to repair a thin posterior capsule. Results of surgical stabilization are promising, with 85% and greater success rates at mid-term and long-term follow-up.

References

1. Neer CS 2nd, Foster CR. Inferior capsular shift for involuntary inferior and multidirectional instability of the shoulder. A preliminary report. J Bone Joint Surg Am. 1980;62(6):897–908.
2. Abrams JS, Savoie FH 3rd, Tauro JC, Bradley JP. Recent advances in the evaluation and treatment of shoulder instability: anterior, posterior, and multidirectional. Arthroscopy. 2002;18(9 Suppl 2):1–13. https://doi.org/10.1053/jars.2002.36504.
3. Frangiamore SJ, Ramkumar PN, Fritz EM, Mannava S, Millett PJ. Pancapsular shift for multidirectional instability. In: Millett PJ, Pogorzelski J, editors. Advanced techniques in shoulder arthroscopy. Cham, Switzerland: Springer; 2019.
4. Schamblin ML, Snyder SJ. Arthroscopic capsular plication techniques. Tech Shoulder Elbow Surg. 2004;5(4):193–9.
5. Wichman MT, Snyder SJ. Arthroscopic capsular plication for multidirectional instability of the shoulder. Op Tech Sports Med. 1997;5(4):238–43.
6. Wolf EM, Eakin CL. Arthroscopic capsular plication for posterior shoulder instability. Arthroscopy. 1998;14(2):153–63. https://doi.org/10.1016/s0749-8063(98)70034-9.
7. Duncan R, Savoie FH 3rd. Arthroscopic inferior capsular shift for multidirectional instability of the shoulder: a preliminary report. Arthroscopy. 1993;9(1):24–7. https://doi.org/10.1016/s0749-8063(05)80340-8.
8. Lephart SM, Warner JJ, Borsa PA, Fu FH. Proprioception of the shoulder joint in healthy, unstable, and surgically repaired shoulders. J Shoulder Elb Surg. 1994;3(6):371–80. https://doi.org/10.1016/S1058-2746(09)80022-0.
9. Provencher MT, Romeo AA. Posterior and multidirectional instability of the shoulder: challenges associated with diagnosis and management. Instr Course Lect. 2008;57:133–52.
10. Schenk TJ, Brems JJ. Multidirectional instability of the shoulder: pathophysiology, diagnosis, and management. J Am Acad Orthop Surg. 1998;6(1):65–72. https://doi.org/10.5435/00124635-199801000-00007.
11. Fu FH, Burkhead WZ, Flatow EL. Controversies in reconstruction of the unstable shoulder: mobility vs instability. Contemp Orthop. 1993;26:301–22.
12. An YH, Friedman RJ. Multidirectional instability of the glenohumeral joint. Orthop Clin North Am. 2000;31(2):275–85. https://doi.org/10.1016/s0030-5898(05)70147-4.
13. Warner JJ, Micheli LJ, Arslanian LE, Kennedy J, Kennedy R. Patterns of flexibility, laxity, and strength in normal shoulders and shoulders with instability and impingement. Am J Sports Med. 1990;18(4):366–75. https://doi.org/10.1177/036354659001800406.
14. Neer CS 2nd. Dislocations. In: Neer CS, editor. Shoulder reconstruction. Philadelphia, PA: WB Saunders; 1990. p. 273–341.
15. Blomquist J, Solheim E, Liavaag S, Schroder CP, Espehaug B, Havelin LI. Shoulder instability surgery in Norway: the first report from a multicenter register, with 1-year follow-up. Acta Orthop. 2012;83(2):165–70. https://doi.org/10.3109/17453674.2011.641102.
16. VandenBerghe G, Hoenecke HR, Fronek J. Glenohumeral joint instability: the orthopedic approach. Semin Musculoskelet Radiol. 2005;9(1):34–43. https://doi.org/10.1055/s-2005-867097.
17. Longo UG, Rizzello G, Loppini M, Locher J, Buchmann S, Maffulli N, et al. Multidirectional instability of the shoulder: a systematic review. Arthroscopy. 2015;31(12):2431–43. https://doi.org/10.1016/j.arthro.2015.06.006.
18. Cameron KL, Duffey ML, DeBerardino TM, Stoneman PD, Jones CJ, Owens BD. Association of generalized joint hypermobility with a history of glenohumeral joint instability. J Athl Train. 2010;45(3):253–8. https://doi.org/10.4085/1062-6050-45.3.253.
19. Kiss J, Damrel D, Mackie A, Neumann L, Wallace WA. Non-operative treatment of multidirectional

shoulder instability. Int Orthop. 2001;24(6):354–7. https://doi.org/10.1007/s002640000202.
20. Kitagawa T, Matsui N, Nakaizumi D. Structured rehabilitation program for multidirectional shoulder instability in a patient with Ehlers-Danlos syndrome. Case Rep Orthop. 2020;2020:8507929. https://doi.org/10.1155/2020/8507929.
21. Malfait F, Hakim AJ, De Paepe A, Grahame R. The genetic basis of the joint hypermobility syndromes. Rheumatology (Oxford). 2006;45(5):502–7. https://doi.org/10.1093/rheumatology/kei268.
22. Maltz SB, Fantus RJ, Mellett MM, Kirby JP. Surgical complications of Ehlers-Danlos syndrome type IV: case report and review of the literature. J Trauma. 2001;51(2):387–90. https://doi.org/10.1097/00005373-200108000-00029.
23. Shirley ED, Demaio M, Bodurtha J. Ehlers-danlos syndrome in orthopaedics: etiology, diagnosis, and treatment implications. Sports Health. 2012;4(5):394–403. https://doi.org/10.1177/1941738112452385.
24. Zweers MC, Hakim AJ, Grahame R, Schalkwijk J. Joint hypermobility syndromes: the pathophysiologic role of tenascin-X gene defects. Arthritis Rheum. 2004;50(9):2742–9. https://doi.org/10.1002/art.20488.
25. Neer CS 2nd. Involuntary inferior and multidirectional instability of the shoulder: etiology, recognition, and treatment. Instr Course Lect. 1985;34:232–8.
26. Savoie FH. Multidirectional instability of the glenohumeral joint. In: Ryu RK, editor. The shoulder. Philadelphia, PA: Saunders Elsevier; 2010. p. 124–35.
27. Lafosse T, Fogerty S, Idoine J, Gobezie R, Lafosse L. Hyper extension-internal rotation (HERI): a new test for anterior Gleno-humeral instability. Orthop Traumatol Surg Res. 2016;102(1):3–12. https://doi.org/10.1016/j.otsr.2015.10.006.
28. O'Brien MJ, Savoie FH. Arthroscopic treatment for multidirectional instability. Oper Tech Sports Med. 2014;22(1):25–33.
29. Lyons TR, Griffith PL, Savoie FH 3rd, Field LD. Laser-assisted capsulorrhaphy for multidirectional instability of the shoulder. Arthroscopy. 2001;17(1):25–30. https://doi.org/10.1053/jars.2001.20663.
30. Gartsman GM, Roddey TS, Hammerman SM. Arthroscopic treatment of multidirectional glenohumeral instability: 2- to 5-year follow-up. Arthroscopy. 2001;17(3):236–43. https://doi.org/10.1053/jars.2001.21529.
31. Treacy SH, Savoie FH 3rd, Field LD. Arthroscopic treatment of multidirectional instability. J Shoulder Elb Surg. 1999;8(4):345–50. https://doi.org/10.1016/s1058-2746(99)90158-1.
32. Marquardt B, Potzl W, Witt KA, Steinbeck J. A modified capsular shift for atraumatic anterior-inferior shoulder instability. Am J Sports Med. 2005;33(7):1011–5. https://doi.org/10.1177/0363546504272685.
33. Pollock RG, Owens JM, Flatow EL, Bigliani LU. Operative results of the inferior capsular shift procedure for multidirectional instability of the shoulder. J Bone Joint Surg Am. 2000;82-A(7):919–28. https://doi.org/10.2106/00004623-200007000-00003.
34. Alpert JM, Verma N, Wysocki R, Yanke AB, Romeo AA. Arthroscopic treatment of multidirectional shoulder instability with minimum 270 degrees labral repair: minimum 2-year follow-up. Arthroscopy. 2008;24(6):704–11. https://doi.org/10.1016/j.arthro.2008.01.008.
35. Ide J, Maeda S, Yamaga M, Morisawa K, Takagi K. Shoulder-strengthening exercise with an orthosis for multidirectional shoulder instability: quantitative evaluation of rotational shoulder strength before and after the exercise program. J Shoulder Elb Surg. 2003;12(4):342–5. https://doi.org/10.1016/s1058-2746(02)86886-0.
36. Misamore GW, Sallay PI, Didelot W. A longitudinal study of patients with multidirectional instability of the shoulder with seven- to ten-year follow-up. J Shoulder Elb Surg. 2005;14(5):466–70. https://doi.org/10.1016/j.jse.2004.11.006.

Allograft Additions to the Multidirectional Shoulder

35

Stephen D. Daniels and Jonathan Bravman

Introduction

Shoulder instability is a prevalent pathology in the practice of sports and shoulder surgeons. The majority of patients present with unidirectional, anterior, or posterior instability, which has been extensively reported in the literature [1–3]. A small subset of patients with glenohumeral instability falls into a unique category of multidirectional instability (MDI). This complex pathology poses a challenging problem to the treating orthopedic surgeon. It has been reported that 5–15% of patients with shoulder instability will receive this diagnosis [4, 5]. Accordingly, there is far less literature to provide evidence-based treatment guidelines for MDI.

The first step in the management of MDI is an accurate diagnosis. MDI has been defined as symptomatic instability of the GH joint in at least two distinct planes of shoulder motion [6]. It is imperative that the surgeon responsible for managing the patient with MDI establish the correct diagnosis and distinguish this disorder from similar pathologies along the spectrum of GH instability for which management will differ. Unidirectional instability is a far more prevalent condition and is typically accompanied by an associated unidirectional pathologic lesion resulting from a traumatic event. This patient population has been known to do well with surgical intervention. Unidirectional instability may be present in the setting of joint hypermobility or laxity, which should be differentiated from MDI, as treatment algorithms may differ [7, 8].

Multidirectional instability can be the direct result of trauma but is often atraumatic or the consequence of repetitive microtrauma in patients with pre-existing joint laxity—roughly 40–70% of patients with MDI [9–11]. Overhead athletes, particularly females, and patients with soft tissue disorders such as Marfan and Ehlers-Danlos syndrome (EDS), osteogenesis imperfecta (OI), and benign hypermobility syndrome are at increased risk. While the occasional presentation with an identifiable lesion may warrant acute surgical intervention, the mainstay of treatment for MDI is improvement in "dynamic stability" with physiotherapy focusing on rotator cuff and periscapular muscle strengthening and mechanics [4, 6]. This highlights the importance of appropriate diagnosis, as at least 6 months of conservative treatment is often recommended before consideration of operative intervention.

In cases of failed conservative therapy, there are a number of surgical options that have been reported in the literature. Addressing the pathologic hallmarks of MDI, such as a patulous capsule, increased joint capsular volume, widened rotator interval, and redundant inferior capsule, is the goal of surgical intervention. Open inferior

S. D. Daniels · J. Bravman (✉)
Department of Orthopedic Surgery, University of Colorado, Aurora, CO, USA
e-mail: jonathan.bravman@cuanschutz.edu

© The Author(s), under exclusive license to Springer Nature Switzerland AG 2026
R. M. Frank, J. M. Tokish (eds.), *Management of Shoulder Instability*,
https://doi.org/10.1007/978-3-032-18089-6_35

capsular shift, arthroscopic capsular plication, and rotator interval closure are common surgical strategies. While some studies have reported successful outcomes using these techniques, compromised integrity of collagen-based soft tissue interventions can result in variable outcomes. Consequently, additional considerations have been given to soft tissue augmentation. The focus of this chapter will be on allograft techniques for soft tissue reconstruction and augmentation options for surgical candidates with MDI.

Case Presentation

A 28-year-old female presented to the clinic with a history of recurrent right shoulder pain and glenohumeral instability. Seven years prior to presentation, she reported a traumatic instability event during a motor vehicle crash and was diagnosed with MDI. She subsequently underwent capsular plication and rotator interval closure. Three years postoperatively, she sustained a recurrent traumatic dislocation and underwent revision capsulorraphy. She reported an uncomplicated postoperative course until she sustained a third incidence of traumatic instability, 2 years after her revision surgery. Her past medical history was notable for anxiety and daily cigarette use. Radiographic and computed tomography images demonstrating glenoid dysplasia, osseous changes from prior stabilization procedures, and posterior humeral head subluxation are shown in Fig. 35.1. Magnetic resonance imaging was obtained, further demonstrating these findings. On physical assessment, the patient demonstrated

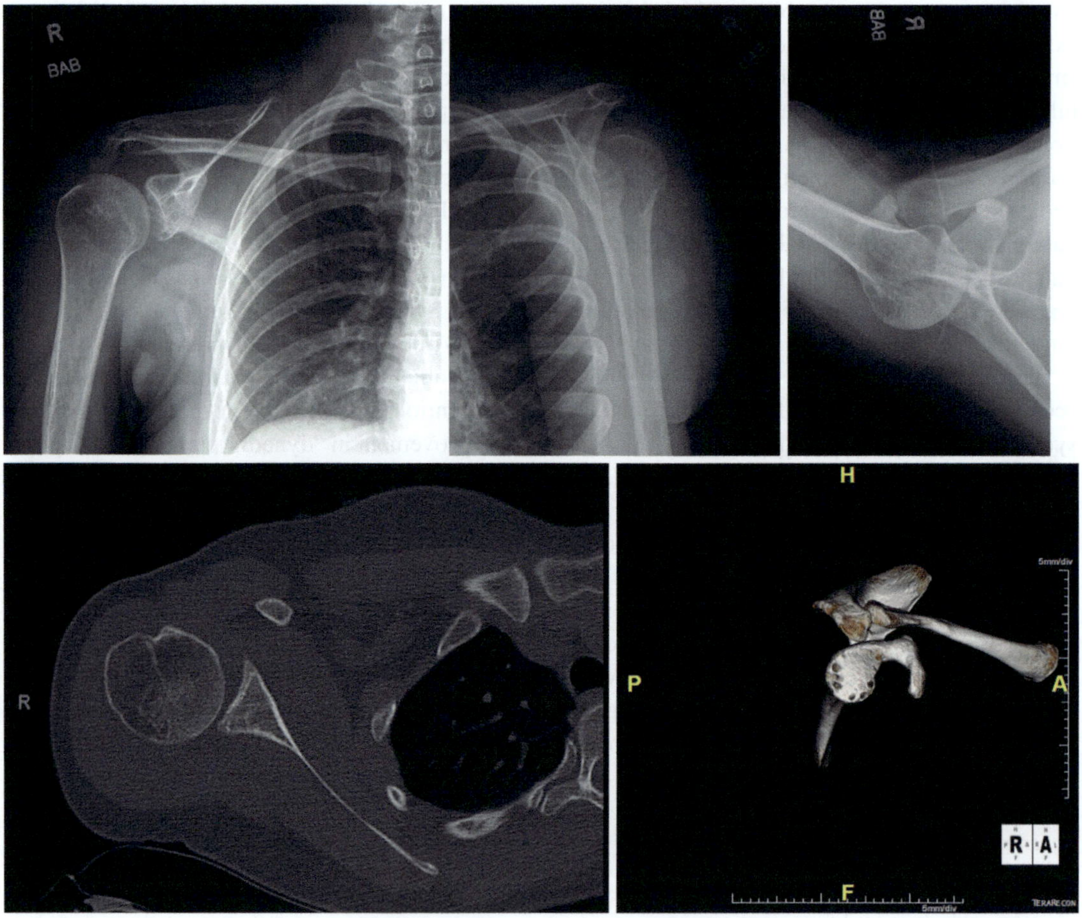

Fig. 35.1 Preoperative radiographic and CT imaging demonstrating glenoid dysplasia with posterior wear and humeral head subluxation. Osseous changes in the setting of prior surgical intervention are present

a full active range of motion with 5/5 strength testing of her rotator cuff and deltoid. A positive sulcus sign was noted, as well as static posterior humeral head subluxation, which was readily reducible.

A 6-month course of physical therapy focused on periscapular muscle training and trigger point injections greatly improved the acutely painful symptoms on presentation. Despite these conservative measures, she continued to report recurrent episodes of daily glenohumeral subluxation. Consequently, surgical intervention in the form of posterior bone block augmentation was offered to address her identifiable pathoanatomy.

In beach chair positioning, an examination under anesthesia on the day of surgery demonstrated 1+ anterior and 2+ posteroinferior translation, confirming the predominant direction of her instability. Diagnostic arthroscopy revealed intra-articular findings consistent with chronic posteroinferior labral tearing and capsular laxity, as well as posterior glenoid bone loss (Fig. 35.2). Through an open posterior approach, a posterior bone block established from a distal tibia allograft was secured from 6:00 to 3:00 on the posterior glenoid with two 3.5-mm cortical screws. The posterior capsule was then subsequently reconstructed with a dermal allograft with humeral head–based suture anchors, as depicted in Fig. 35.3. Intraoperative assessment of the shoulder demonstrated a stable glenohumeral joint throughout the arc of motion. Postoperatively, the patient was placed into an abduction sling and immobilized for 7 days. Gentle range of motion began 10 days postoperatively, with bracing out to 6 weeks.

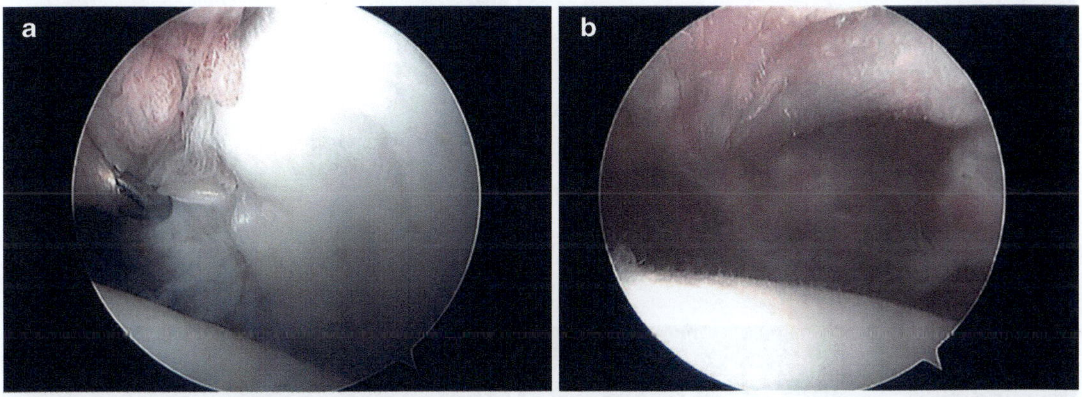

Fig. 35.2 (**a**) Diagnostic arthroscopic images highlighting posteroinferior labral tearing and bone loss. (**b**) Redundant capsule with increased capsular volume was evident

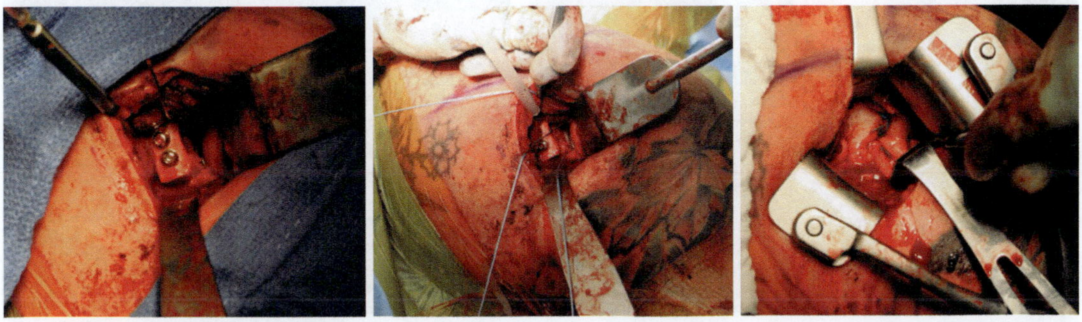

Fig. 35.3 Intraoperative photographs depicting the posterior bone block created from distal tibia allograft. The graft was fixed to the posterior glenoid with two 3.5-mm cortical screws. Reconstruction of the posterior capsule was then performed with dermal allograft

The patient reported a stable shoulder for nearly 3 years postoperatively, when an overhead activity caused a recurrent episode of posterior subluxation. CT would go on to demonstrate resorption of her bone graft and recurrent posterior humeral head subluxation (Fig. 35.4). She subsequently underwent revision stabilization with posterior glenoid bone block using iliac crest autograft. Six months postoperatively, the patient had no subjective reports of instability. Active range of motion demonstrated forward flexion to 120°, external rotation at neutral to 40°, 5/5 strength in external and internal rotation, and 4/5 strength on an empty can test, limited by mild discomfort.

This case was chosen to illustrate the challenging nature of managing the MDI patient. Importantly, informed, goal-oriented discussions

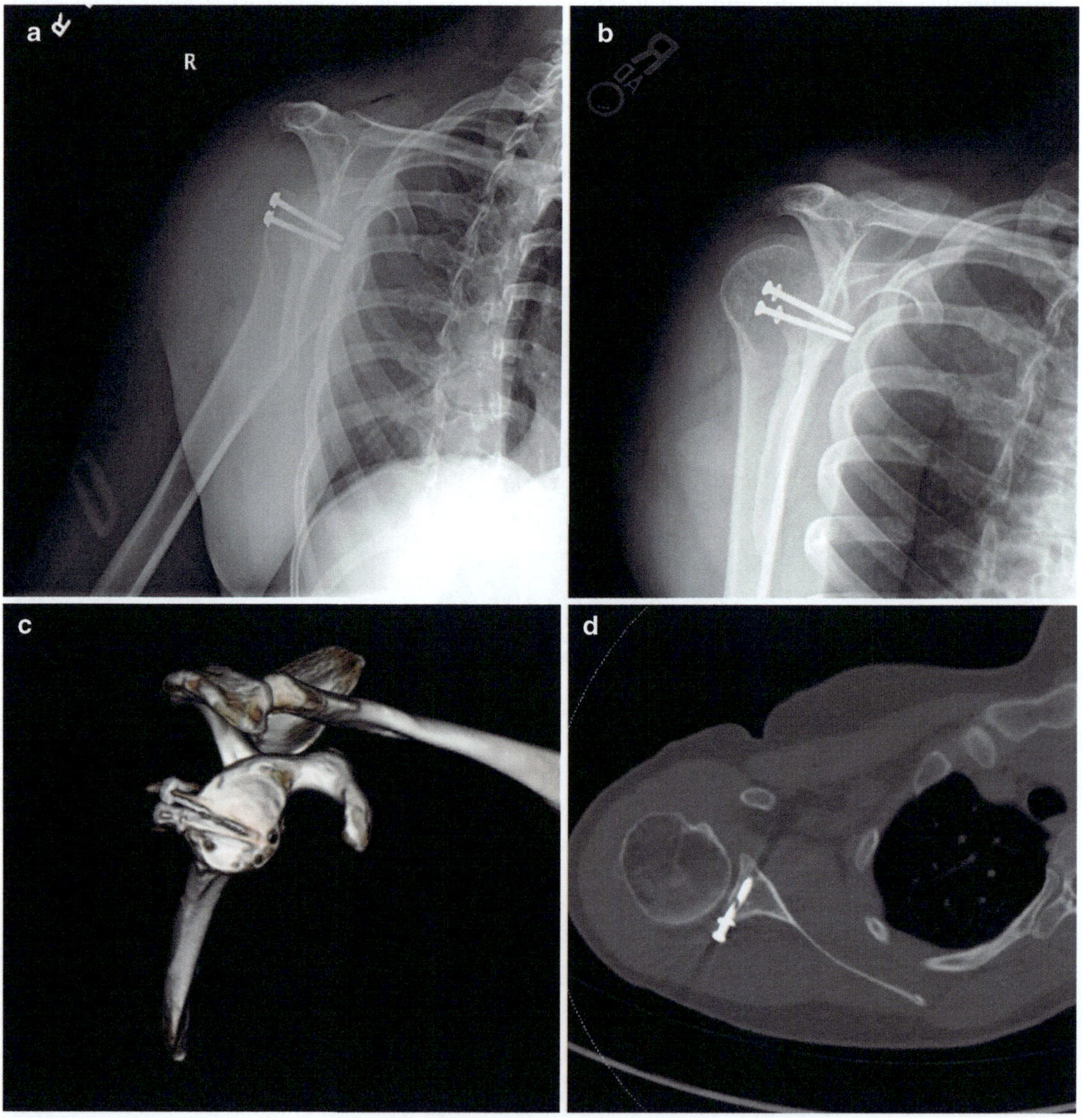

Fig. 35.4 (**a**) Immediate postoperative X-ray showing an intact posterior bone block. (**b**) Radiograph 3 years postoperatively depicting resorption of the graft with prominent screws and posterior decentering of the humeral head. (**c** and **d**) CT representation of the resorbed graft with posterior humeral head subluxation

are a critical component in the management of this patient population. Obtaining a "normal," entirely asymptomatic shoulder may be an unrealistic pursuit; rather, the goals of intervention are to provide the patient with a stable, functional shoulder to improve their quality of life.

Etiology and Diagnosis

Due to the significance of appropriate diagnosis, it is imperative to touch on the assessment and work-up of MDI. The presentation of MDI is typically of an insidious onset of shoulder complaints that can range from vague discomfort to symptomatic instability. The most common patient populations are patients of younger age (typically <40 years), overhead athletes, females, and patients exhibiting signs or history of soft tissue–related disorders [12]. These can be congenital, such as EDS, Marfan syndrome, and OI, and be unrelated to a particular syndrome but demonstrate objective joint laxity, as can be assessed with the Beighton score [13]. The majority of cases tend to be of atraumatic origin. Unlike unilateral instability, which is typically associated with an identifiable soft tissue or osseous pathology, MDI commonly presents in the absence of a discrete anatomic lesion. Further, it is imperative to distinguish MDI from unidirectional instability in the setting of hyperlaxity to afford appropriate treatment.

Imaging can aid in diagnosis. Plain radiographs may demonstrate increased acromial-humeral distance, indicating inferior subluxation of the humeral head. Magnetic resonance imaging (MRI) and more specifically MR arthrography (MRA) may reveal increased glenohumeral capsular volume, a widened rotator interval, and other nonspecific labral/capsuloligamentous abnormalities. While these findings may aid in diagnosis and guide targeted therapy, clinical assessment remains the cornerstone of diagnosis [6].

Physical exam should begin with observation to identify any gross asymmetry of the shoulders. This may reveal signs of muscular atrophy, static subluxation, and abnormal shoulder girdle kinematics if observed through a range of motion. Generalized laxity may be assessed with the Beighton score, which focuses on evidence of joint laxity at the elbow, knee, first metacarpal phalangeal joint, and fifth metacarpal phalangeal joint. Attention should be directed to shoulder-specific maneuvers to portend diagnosis.

A positive sulcus, or dimple sign, with adducted inferior traction of the humerus is considered abnormal if there is >2 cm of inferior humeral displacement from the acromion, indicating a high grade of inferior capsule redundancy. This may be tested in 90° of abduction—if positive, this suggests a high-grade laxity. The supine load-and-shift test assesses anterior and posterior translation of the humeral head relative to the glenoid. Gagey demonstrated that abduction of the affected shoulder >105°is associated with laxity of the inferior glenohumeral ligament [14]. The apprehension and relocation test can produce a sensation of instability with the arm abducted at 90° with external rotation and relief with a posterior force directed on the humeral head. Finally, a jerk test with the shoulder flexed, adducted, and internally rotated may produce a clunk and "uneasy feeling," indicative of posterior instability. One if not several of these maneuvers tend to produce the sensation of instability in multiple directions when performed on patients with MDI. This is critical in isolating the appropriate diagnosis from unidirectional instability. This further delineates true MDI patients from another category of individuals with psychological conditions that have the ability to voluntarily dislocate. These patients typically will not display apprehension when examined and are poor surgical candidates who benefit more greatly from appropriate psychiatric counseling [4, 15]. Once a patient with MDI has been accurately diagnosed, has failed conservative management, and, in some cases, has undergone a primary soft tissue procedure, options for surgical stabilization with allograft augmentation should be considered. The remainder of this chapter will focus on techniques and small patient reports focusing on the surgical technique of allograft augmentation for glenohumeral stabilization in patients with MDI. A summary of these techniques can be found in Table 35.1.

Table 35.1 Summary of surgical techniques to address multidirectional instability

Capsuloligamentous reconstruction	Graft	Technique	Remarks	Outcomes
Bouaicha, Moor (2013)	Hamstring autograft	Reconstruction of the anterior and inferior bands of IGHL	Can tension as needed Maintain anatomic shoulder range of motion	Cadaveric study—no outcomes reported
Dewing et al.	Tibialis anterior allograft	Open anterior labral, MGHL, and IGHL reconstruction with a single, multiple-limb graft. Imbrication of the rotator interval		70% of shoulders stable at a 3.8-year follow-up Overall, ASES increased from 43 at pre-op to 84 postoperatively Subgroups demonstrated Type III EDS to have lower postoperative ASES scores of 71 vs. 92 for patients with hyperlaxity syndrome
Gallie (1948)	IT band autograft	Reconstruction of the superior, middle, and inferior bands of IGHL		Reported a record of 175 cases over a 20-year period
Caspari, Lynch	Fascia Lata	IGHL ligamentoplasty		20% rate of instability recurrence
Cabo et al.	Tibialis anterior allograft	Arthroscopic IGHL ligamentoplasty—weaved through subscapularis, modification to capsular plication		No outcomes reported—technique report
Ianotti et al. (2002)	IT band auto ($n = 4$) or allograft ($n = 3$)	Triple limb graft—reconstruction of the rotator interval, MGHL, IGHL	Supplement to anterior capsular insufficiency Spans the entire anterior shoulder Individually tension reconstructed ligaments in varying degrees of abduction/external rotation	Results reported for 7 consecutive patients (failed a primary stabilization procedure) Pre-op ASES of 30–55 postoperatively Passive ER decreased from 72° pre-op to 35° post-operatively
MacDonald	Achilles tendon allograft	Reconstruct limbs of SGHL, MGHL, and IGHL with bone graft augment secured to the anterior glenoid	Robust origin site for anchoring of limbs	Four patients with diagnosed EDS, four post-traumatic MDI 31% recurrent instability rate WOSI improved from 14.2 pre-op to 42.0 postoperatively Improved ROM and functional capability

(continued)

Table 35.1 (continued)

Capsuloligamentous reconstruction	Graft	Technique	Remarks	Outcomes
Aman et al. (2019)		Coracohumeral ligament reconstruction	A good revision option when other primary techniques have failed	Technique paper—no outcomes
Maloney et al.	Gracilis allograft	Establish a posterior sling-like structure anchored to the glenoid and humeral head		Technique paper—no outcomes
Gallagher et al.	Human dermal allograft	All-arthroscopic anterior capsule augmentation, posterior capsular reconstruction	Incorporation of native tissues into reconstruction Maintain native ROM No donor site morbidity	Technique paper—no outcomes
Braun et al. (2011)	Tibialis anterior allograft	Open reconstruction of the MGHL and IGHL		Restricted postoperative shoulder ROM
Gervasi et al.	Porcine skin surgical mesh	Subequatorial graft on the perimeter of the glenoid that	Improves the depth of the glenoid, acting as a bumper to humeral translation Reduces tension on compromised capsuloligamentous structures with humeral translation	Technique paper—no outcomes
Schoorl et al.	Achilles allograft	Open suture anchor repair of labral and capsular lesions with incorporation of Achilles allograft for anterior capsular reconstruction		3.6-year follow-up ($n = 4$ patients, 5 shoulders) Improved pre- to post-op VAS pain scores from 7 to 2 Subjective shoulder value 84 American shoulder and elbow score 77.3

Surgical Management

Capsuloligamentous Reconstruction

Bouaicha et al. promoted the concept of reconstructing the anterior and posterior bands of the IGHL as a method to address recurrent, chronic anteroinferior instability. Using hamstring autograft from a cadaver, they reconstructed the anterior and posterior IGHL bands and demonstrated that this could be tensioned to appropriately resist anterior-inferior translation in shoulder abduction and external rotation, all the while maintaining anatomic shoulder range of motion [16].

In 1948, Gallie et al. were among the first to focus on pathology within the IGHL and the significance to anterior stability of the shoulder. They wrote the first description of a technique used to reconstruct the bands of the IGHL with multiple bone tunnels through the scapular neck, coracoid, and humeral head, fashioning a patch of IT fascia lata autograft over the anterior aspect of the GH joint [17]. Caspari and Lynch later modified this technique to perform an IGHL replacement ligamentoplasty with fascia lata but reported a 20% recurrence rate [18, 19]. Recently, Cabo et al. described an arthroscopic technique for IGHL ligamentoplasty to modify inferior capsular plication [20]. The authors utilized the tibialis anterior allograft by weaving the graft through the subscapularis tendon to provide stability while in the abducted and externally rotated position. The group had a recurrent instability rate of 31%. However, it should be noted that they had a patient population of eight subjects (four diagnosed with EDS, four with post-traumatic MDI), with a total of 16 procedures (ten primary allografts and six revisions). The patients reported improved pain and functional scores, and despite the high failure rate, the majority indicated they would repeat the procedure as a direct result of the temporary symptomatic relief.

Ianotti et al. described the use of IT band auto- or allograft for anterior capsular deficiency reconstruction [21]. The author's technique involved a triple-layered section of graft first anchored into the glenoid neck, followed by reconstruction of the rotator interval, middle glenohumeral ligament, and inferior glenohumeral ligament by folding the graft onto itself at the appropriate anatomic location with the arm in varying degrees of abduction for appropriate tensioning. The authors reported that the ability of the IT band graft to span the anterior shoulder and individually tension the reconstructed ligaments is an advantage over other graft options.

Similarly, MacDonald et al. reconstructed the limbs of the SGHL and middle-inferior glenohumeral ligament complex with an Achilles tendon allograft [22]. Additionally, the authors incorporated a bone block into the Achilles graft, secured to the anterior glenoid to provide an anchor site for the two reconstructive limbs.

Biomechanical studies have demonstrated the contributing role of the rotator interval to glenohumeral stability. Specifically, the coracohumeral ligament has been reported to have a role in the prevention of posterior and inferior instability [23–26]. Accordingly, Aman and colleagues reported a technique for CHL reconstruction in patients with soft tissue deficiency when primary stabilization techniques have failed [27].

While not as common as anterior-based techniques, posterior-based soft tissue procedures are a viable option supported by biomechanical studies for the treatment of GH instability. Maloney et al. describe the use of a gracilis tendon allograft to supplement the posterior soft tissues. The authors describe a technique that creates a "sling"-like structure anchored to the posterior glenoid and humeral head. Anecdotally, they state that this posterior augmentation has demonstrated improved stability without a restricted range of motion that may be seen with anteriorly based procedures [28]. The authors do mention some limitations of this technique, including the inability to address significant bone loss and the possibility of an intra-articular loose body if there is anchor failure at the graft-suture interface.

Similarly, Braun et al. described an open reconstruction technique utilizing tibialis anterior allograft to reconstruct the bands of the MGHL and IGHL in shoulders with recurrent anterior instability and soft tissue deficiency. While specific values are not reported, the authors did mention one potential disadvantage of this anteriorly based procedure to be the potential restricted shoulder ROM postoperatively [29]. Dewing et al. reported on the mid-term outcomes of 15 patients (20 shoulders) who underwent anterior capsuloligamentous reconstruction with tibialis anterior allograft. Thirteen shoulders were in patients diagnosed with chronic MDI (five with genetically confirmed Type III EDS). Specifically, the authors' technique involved open reconstruction of the anterior labrum with two additional limbs of the graft used to reconstruct the MGHL and anterior band of the IGHL. This was followed by imbrication of the rotator interval. Overall, 70% of the shoulders remained stable at a mean follow-up of 3.8 years. Six shoulders with MDI (30%) required a revision procedure for recurrent instability. Overall, the postoperative functional outcome scores were lower for patients diagnosed with EDS compared to those with generalized hyperlaxity [30].

Lastly, Gallagher and colleagues published on an all-arthroscopic technique for combined anterior capsule augmentation and posterior glenohumeral capsular reconstruction utilizing human dermal allograft. The authors noted several advantages with this graft to include incorporation into native tissues, maintenance of range of motion, and no donor site morbidity [31].

Capsulolabral Reconstruction

Capsuloligamentous structures play a critical role in ensuring shoulder stability. These structures become compromised in patients with underlying soft tissue disorders, and therefore, the labrum plays an increasing role in humeral head stability. Accordingly, Gervasi et al. described an arthroscopic technique of labral augmentation with resorbable surgical mesh from porcine skin to supplement capsuloplasty in patients with MDI [32]. Their described technique involves anchoring a subequatorial graft around the perimeter of the glenoid to improve glenoid depth and act as a large bumper to humeral translation. They mention the possibility of anterior or posterior extension of the graft as needed to manage specific directional instability. The authors theorize the importance of labral reconstruction to reduce tension during humeral translation on the already compromised capsuloligamentous structures to reduce surgical failure.

Commonly, there is significant attenuation of the labrum, which can readily compromise standalone repair. Accordingly, Schoorl et al. described a series of five shoulders (four patients) with EDS with multidirectional laxity and recurrent anterior shoulder instability refractory to conservative treatments. Through a deltopectoral approach, open suture anchor repair of an identifiable Bankart or capsular lesion was performed. The Achilles allograft was then subsequently incorporated into the repair utilizing the sutures from the glenoid anchors. Outcomes at ~3.5 years were reported, demonstrating an overall improvement in preoperative to postoperative pain. Objective outcome measures were collected postoperatively without preoperative data for comparison and are displayed in Table 35.1. One patient required reoperation for the development of posterior instability. The authors concluded that Achilles tendon allograft was a viable option for augmentation of repair when addressing anterior instability in patients with MDI [33].

Similarly, Chaudhury et al. presented a single patient case report, successfully managing a patient with bilateral MDI with an Achilles tendon allograft. The initial anterior-based procedure was an open repair of an identifiable Bankart/capsule lesion, combined with a capsular shift and incorporation of Achilles allograft into a capsular augmentation using the glenoid suture anchors from prior repair. Five years after this initial procedure, the patient went on to develop posterior instability and underwent a repeat procedure utilizing the same technique for posterior augmentation. The patient then went on to develop symptomatic instability of the contralateral shoulder for which she underwent simultaneous anterior and posterior stabilization with the same technique [34].

Conclusions

Multidirectional shoulder instability is a complex problem, most commonly seen in patient populations with underlying soft tissue disorders that further complicate management of this pathology. Conservative therapy is the first-line strategy and should be exhausted prior to discussion of surgical intervention. After an appropriate and accurate diagnosis has been made and nonoperative modalities have failed, there are a number of surgical strategies that may be pursued. In general, repair of any specific capsulolabral lesions should be performed; however, it is likely insufficient as the sole means of fixation/stabilization. We have discussed several options for soft tissue augmentation within this chapter. These procedures are technically demanding, and no strategy has been proven superior over others. With accurate diagnosis and surgical planning, there are several augmentation options available in the armamentarium of shoulder surgeons managing this complex pathology.

References

1. Brelin A, Dickens JF. Posterior shoulder instability. Sports Med Arthrosc Rev. 2017;25:136–45.
2. Witney-Lagen C, Hunter A. Diagnosis and management of shoulder instability. Br J Hosp Med. 2019;80:C34–8.
3. Tokish JM. Shoulder Instability. Sports Med Arthrosc Rev. 2020;28:121.
4. Warby SA, Watson L, Ford JJ, Hahne AJ, Pizzari T. Multidirectional instability of the glenohumeral joint: etiology, classification, assessment, and management. J Hand Ther. 2017;30:175–81.
5. Kraeutler MJ, McCarty EC, Belk JW, et al. Descriptive epidemiology of the MOON shoulder instability cohort. Am J Sports Med. 2018;46:1064–9.
6. Gaskill TR, Taylor DC, Millett PJ. Management of multidirectional instability of the shoulder. J Am Acad Orthop Surg. 2011;19:758–67.
7. Best MJ, Tanaka MJ. Multidirectional instability of the shoulder: treatment options and considerations. Sports Med Arthrosc Rev. 2018;26:113–9.
8. Millett PJ, Clavert P, Warner JJP. Arthroscopic management of anterior, posterior, and multidirectional shoulder instability: pearls and pitfalls. Arthroscopy. 2003;19:86–93.
9. Van Blarcum GS, Svoboda SJ. Glenohumeral instability related to special conditions: SLAP tears, pan-labral tears, and multidirectional instability. Sports Med Arthrosc Rev. 2017;25:e12–7.
10. Alpert JM, Verma N, Wysocki R, Yanke AB, Romeo AA. Arthroscopic treatment of multidirectional shoulder instability with minimum 270 degrees labral repair: minimum 2-year follow-up. Arthroscopy. 2008;24:704–11.
11. Jensen K. Posterior-inferior instability in the competitive swimmer. J Shoulder Elbow Surg. 2007;16
12. Rupp MC, Rutledge JC, Quinn PM, Millett PJ. Management of shoulder instability in patients with underlying hyperlaxity. Curr Rev Musculoskelet Med. 2023; https://doi.org/10.1007/S12178-023-09822-6.
13. Engelbert RH, Rombaut L. Clinimetrics: assessment of generalised joint hypermobility: the Beighton score. J Physiother. 2022; https://doi.org/10.1016/J.JPHYS.2022.02.004.
14. Gagey OJ, Gagey N. The hyperabduction test. J Bone Joint Surg Br. 2001;83:69–74.
15. Moroder P, Danzinger V, Maziak N, Plachel F, Pauly S, Scheibel M, Minkus M. Characteristics of functional shoulder instability. J Shoulder Elb Surg. 2020;29:68–78.
16. Bouaicha S, Moor BK. Arthroscopic autograft reconstruction of the inferior glenohumeral ligament: exploration of technical feasibility in cadaveric shoulder specimens. Int J Shoulder Surg. 2013;7:32–6.
17. Gallie WE, LE Mesurier AB. Recurring dislocation of the shoulder - PubMed. JBJS. 1948:9–18.
18. Caspari RB, Savoie FH, Meyers JF, et al. Arthroscopic shoulder reconstruction. J Orthop Transl. 1989;13:559.
19. Lynch GJ. Arthroscopic substitution of the anterior inferior glenohumeral ligament. Arthroscopy. 1991;7:325.
20. de Cabo G, Rubio JA, González-Martín D, Martínez de Aragón A, Leyes M. Anterior shoulder ligamentoplasty as a treatment for multidirectional shoulder instability. Arthrosc Tech. 2022;11:e2219–24.
21. Iannotti JP, Antoniou J, Williams GR, Ramsey ML. Iliotibial band reconstruction for treatment of glenohumeral instability associated with irreparable capsular deficiency. J Shoulder Elb Surg. 2002;11:618–23.
22. MacDonald PB, McRae S, Leiter J. Achilles allograft stabilization of the shoulder in refractory multidirectional Glenohumeral instability. Tech Shoulder Elb Surg. 2008;9:60–5.
23. Clark J, Sidles J, Matsen F. The relationship of the glenohumeral joint capsule to the rotator cuff. Clin Orthop Relat Res. 1990;254:29–34.
24. Clark J, Harryman D. Tendons, ligaments, and capsule of the rotator cuff. Gross and microscopic anatomy. J Bone Joint Surg Am. 1992;74:713–25.
25. Jost B, Koch PP, Gerber C. Anatomy and functional aspects of the rotator interval. J Shoulder Elb Surg. 2000;9:336–41.
26. Field LD, Warren RF, O'brien SJ, Altchek DW, Wickiewicz TL. Isolated closure of rotator interval defects for shoulder instability. Am J Sports Med. 1995;23:557–63.
27. Aman ZS, Peebles LA, Shubert D, Golijanin P, Dekker TJ, Provencher MT. Coracohumeral ligament reconstruction for patients with multidirectional shoulder instability. Arthrosc Tech. 2019;8:e561–5.
28. Maloney MD, Schaffer JC, Kenney RJ. Arthroscopic posterior Glenohumeral capsular augmentation with gracilis tendon allograft. Arthrosc Tech. 2019;8:e1277–82.
29. Braun S, Horan MP, Millett PJ. Open reconstruction of the anterior glenohumeral capsulolabral structures with tendon allograft in chronic shoulder instability. Oper Orthop Traumatol. 2011;23:29–36.
30. Dewing CB, Horan MP, Millett PJ. Two-year outcomes of open shoulder anterior capsular reconstruction for instability from severe capsular deficiency. Arthroscopy. 2012;28:43–51.
31. Gallagher F, Wong IHB. Anterior capsule augmentation and posterior Glenohumeral capsular reconstruction with human dermal allograft for multidirectional shoulder instability. Arthrosc Tech. 2020;9:e657–62.

32. Gervasi E, Sebastiani E, Spicuzza A. Multidirectional shoulder instability: arthroscopic labral augmentation. Arthrosc Tech. 2017;6:e219–25.
33. Schoorl TJ, Nguyen NTV, van Noort A, Alta TDW, Sanchez-Sotelo J. Capsulorraphy with Achilles allograft augmentation for shoulder instability in patients with Ehlers-Danlos syndrome. J Shoulder Elb Surg. 2021;30:865–70.
34. Chaudhury S, Gasinu S, Rodeo SA. Bilateral anterior and posterior glenohumeral stabilization using Achilles tendon allograft augmentation in a patient with Ehlers-Danlos syndrome. J Shoulder Elbow Surg. 2012;21:e1.

Part V

Special Cases

Instability Due to Subscapularis Deficiency: Reconstructive Options

36

Joseph T. Labrum IV, Yousif Atwan, and Joaquin Sanchez-Sotelo

Introduction

Instability resulting from chronic subscapularis deficiency represents a rare but challenging clinical problem that requires thorough patient evaluation and advanced surgical techniques for proper diagnosis and management. Surgical intervention is typically required to alleviate symptoms and restore stability. There are several reconstructive options available to orthopaedic surgeons treating this pathology, which include attempted subscapularis repair with augmentation, anterior capsular reconstruction, dynamic muscle tendon transfers, reverse shoulder arthroplasty, and shoulder arthrodesis. This chapter will highlight the etiology, diagnosis, reconstructive techniques, and postsurgical rehabilitation in the treatment of instability related to subscapularis deficiency.

Illustrative Clinical Case

A 59-year-old male presented with a three-year history of left shoulder pain and weakness following a snowmobile accident in which he injured his left shoulder. He had undergone a prior rotator cuff repair 13 years before on the same side and felt that his shoulder was normal prior to the snowmobile accident. His subjective shoulder value at presentation was 60%. Examination revealed 160° of forward elevation, 90° of external rotation, and internal rotation to L4. He had a positive bear-hug test and a positive belly press test with clear weakness in internal rotation when compared to the contralateral side. MR imaging, which can be found in Fig. 36.1, revealed a chronic subscapularis tear with retraction on axial T2 imaging and severe fatty infiltration of the subscapularis muscle on sagittal oblique T1 imaging, consistent with subscapularis deficiency. The patient was educated on his diagnosis and treatment options and elected to undergo an anterior transfer of the latissimus dorsi tendon for treatment of subscapularis deficiency. Figure 36.2 shows intraoperative images which highlight the surgical technique for anterior latissimus dorsi transfer as executed in this patient. At one-year follow-up, the patient was noted to have complete resolution of shoulder pain. Clinical examination at this time, as highlighted in Fig. 36.3, revealed 160° of forward elevation, 90° of external rotation, internal rotation to L4, and restoration of adequate internal rotation strength in the left shoulder.

J. T. Labrum IV · Y. Atwan · J. Sanchez-Sotelo (✉)
Department of Orthopaedic Surgery, Mayo Clinic, Rochester, MN, USA
e-mail: SanchezSotelo.Joaquin@mayo.edu

© The Author(s), under exclusive license to Springer Nature Switzerland AG 2026
R. M. Frank, J. M. Tokish (eds.), *Management of Shoulder Instability*,
https://doi.org/10.1007/978-3-032-18089-6_36

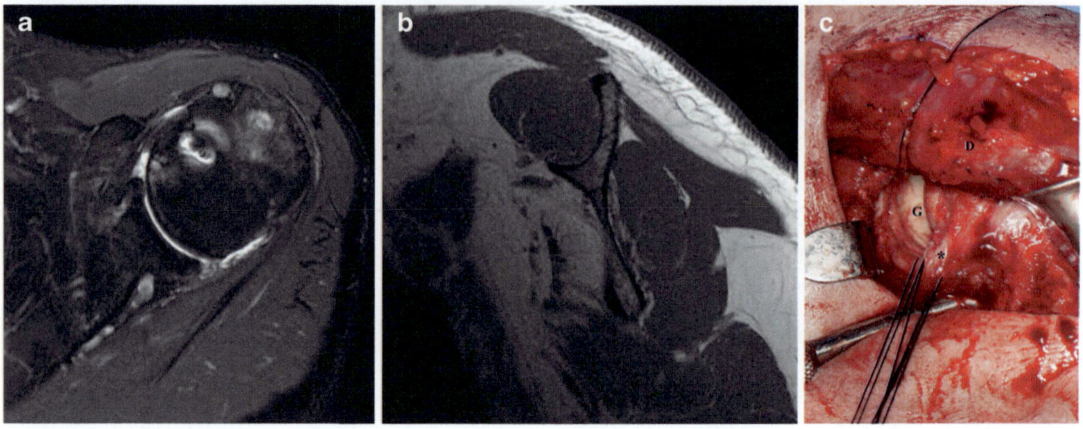

Fig. 36.1 MR imaging of the presented patient, with images highlighting a chronic subscapularis tear with retraction on axial T2 image (**a**) and severe fat infiltration of the subscapularis muscle on sagittal oblique T1 imaging (**b**), indicative of subscapularis deficiency. (**c**) Deltopectoral approach highlighting subscapularis deficiency (* insufficient subscapularis remnant, D deltoid, G glenoid articular cartilage)

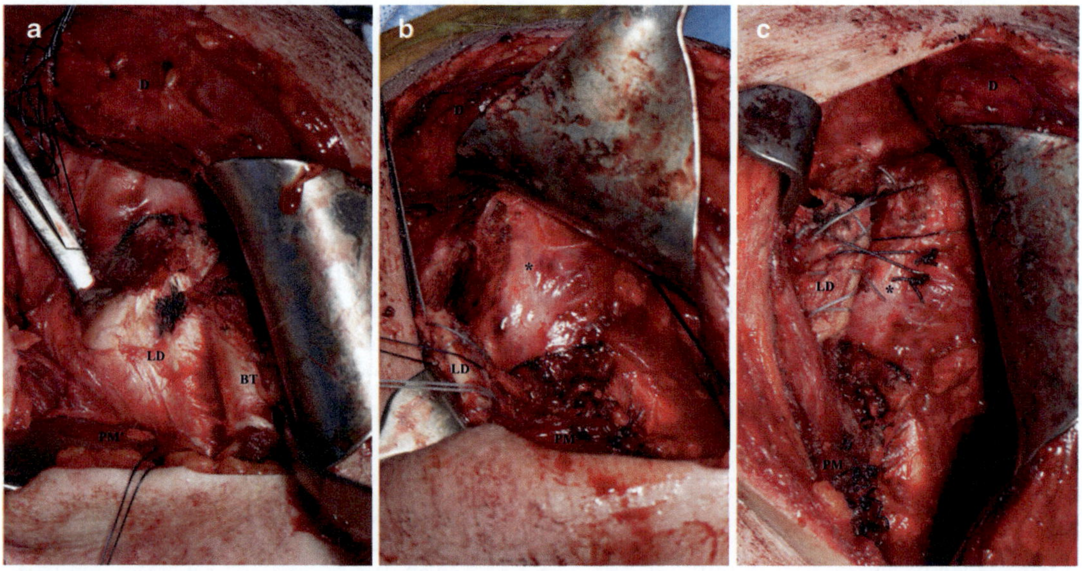

Fig. 36.2 Intraoperative images obtained at the time of anterior latissimus dorsi tendon transfer achieved through a standard deltopectoral approach. (**a**) Isolation of the latissimus dorsi tendon insertion on the proximal humerus, deep to the partially released pectoralis major and medial to the long head of the biceps tendon. (**b**) Mobilization of the latissimus dorsi tendon after identification and release. (**c**) Completed reconstruction with anterior transfer of the latissimus dorsi tendon to the lesser tuberosity (LD latissimus dorsi, * insufficient subscapularis remnant, BT long head biceps tendon, PM' pectoralis major following partial release, PM pectoralis major following repair, D deltoid)

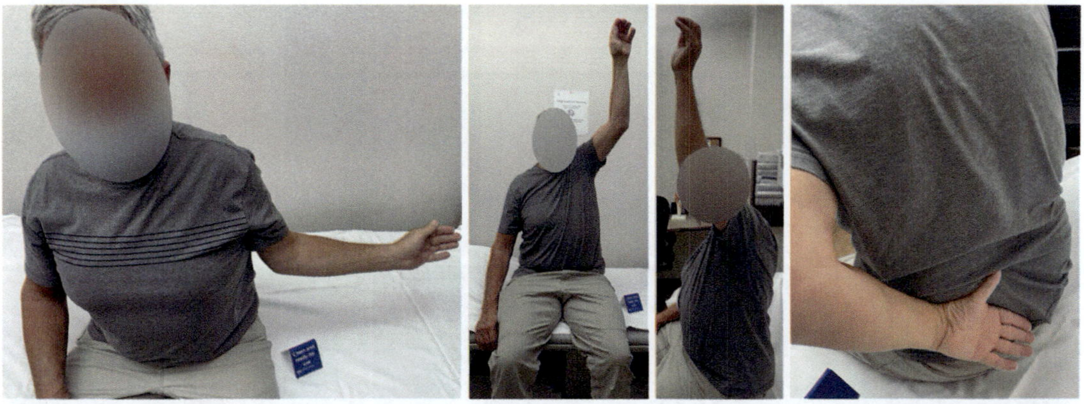

Fig. 36.3 Clinical images obtained at 1-year follow-up status after latissimus dorsi tendon transfer for subscapularis deficiency. The patient was noted to have no pain at follow-up, with examination revealing 160° forward elevation, 90° external rotation, and internal rotation to L4

Etiology

The subscapularis muscle functions as an internal rotator of the glenohumeral joint and works in concert with the supraspinatus, infraspinatus, and teres minor to provide concavity compression at the glenohumeral joint. In addition, the subscapularis is intimately related to the anterior shoulder capsule, especially in its inferior third, and acts as a dynamic and static restraint against excessive anterior translation of the glenohumeral joint. Traumatic or degenerative subscapularis tears may respond to conservative treatment or surgical repair, but some individuals may develop chronic subscapularis deficiency.

Chronic subscapularis deficiency typically arises in the setting of a subscapularis tear that goes untreated and develops irreversible retraction, atrophy, and fatty infiltration. Other etiologies include failed subscapularis repair and subscapularis deficiency following surgical subscapularis takedown for exposure, as can be seen in failed anterior open instability surgery or as a complication of anatomic total shoulder arthroplasty. Rarely, subscapularis deficiency can result from iatrogenic injury to the subscapularis nerves as a consequence of an aggressive surgical release at the conjoined tendon/subscapularis space (Table 36.1).

Table 36.1 Etiology of subscapularis deficiency leading to anterior instability

Untreated chronic subscapularis tears
Failed subscapularis repair
Failed subscapularis surgical takedown for exposure
Open anterior instability surgery
After anatomic shoulder arthroplasty
Iatrogenic subscapularis denervation

Diagnosis/Imaging

History and Physical Examination

Most patients with subscapularis deficiency complain of pain and weakness. Often, they also present with loss of active motion, especially internal rotation and elevation. Although irreparable subscapularis tears involving the whole subscapularis lead to anterior humeral head translation and dynamic instability, only a subset of patients recognize and complain of frank instability. Typically, these include (1) patients' status after unsuccessful open anterior stabilizing surgery with failed healing of the subscapularis takedown, (2) certain patients with subscapularis insufficiency after anatomic shoulder arthroplasty, and (3) elderly patients who suffer an irreparable cuff tear in the setting of a traumatic anterior dislocation with continued instability thereafter.

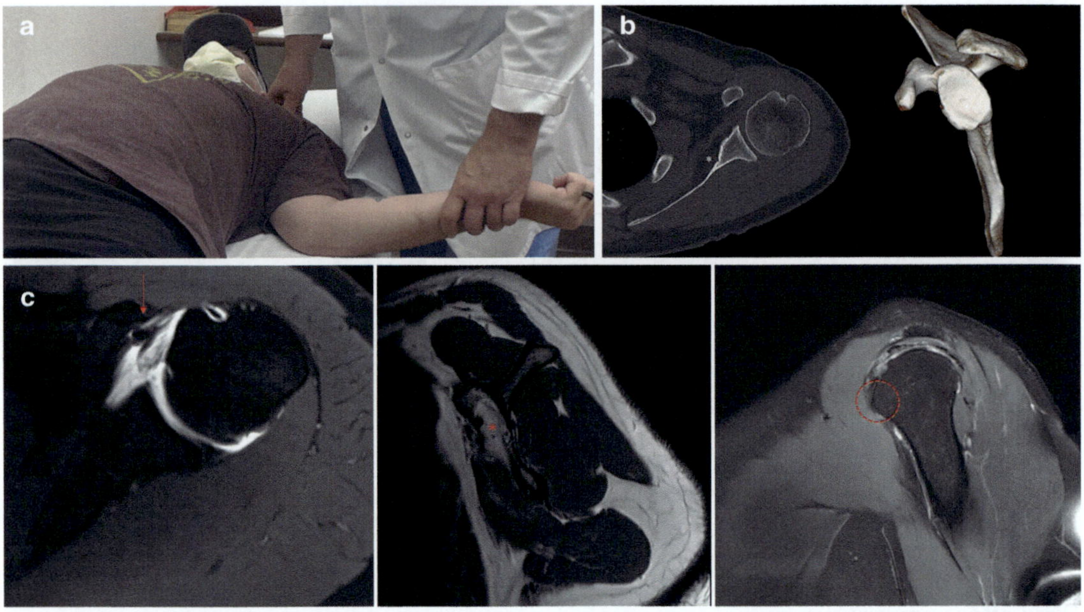

Fig. 36.4 Case example of subscapularis deficiency in a 39-year-old-male with a remote history of a left shoulder injury sustained 20 years prior while playing football and chief complaint of instability and weakness. (**a**) Clinical image obtained at the time of physical examination, revealing excessive passive external rotation of 90°. (**b**) Axial CT and 3D reconstruction revealing no signs of glenohumeral osteoarthritis or glenoid bone loss, with subscapularis fatty infiltration evident on axial CT reconstruction (asterisk). (**c**) Shoulder MRI evaluation of the subscapularis as described by Adams et al., revealing a retracted tear of the subscapularis (arrow) with a located LHBT on axial imaging, grade IV fatty degeneration of the subscapularis muscle belly (asterisk) on sagittal imaging, and a bare lesser tuberosity (circle) on sagittal imaging [1]

A thorough history should be taken to elucidate a clear understanding of the etiology and history of the diagnosis. Physical examination should include maneuvers to test subscapularis integrity, including passive external rotation (Fig. 36.4a), lift-off test, internal rotation lag sign, belly-press test, and bear-hug test, with comparison of the affected shoulder to the contralateral side [2]. The condition of the long head of the biceps tendon (LHBT; pain, pop-eye deformity) and the remainder of the rotator cuff should be assessed as well. Examination maneuvers for anterior instability should be performed cautiously, as the absence of the subscapularis may result in dislocation of the shoulder in the office. The hyperextension-internal rotation (HERI) test, or a gentle "surprise" test, are favored. When mild to moderate arthritis is noticed in conjunction with subscapularis insufficiency, the articular shear test may help discriminate whether articular joint degeneration is actually painful. Finally, in patients with prior surgery, the condition of the deltoid and axillary nerve should be assessed as well.

Imaging

Standard shoulder radiographs (anteroposterior views in internal and external rotation, axillary, and scapular Y views) should be obtained in all patients. These radiographs can be evaluated for a variety of pathologic findings, which include cystic changes in the tuberosities, subluxation of the glenohumeral joint, glenoid and humeral bone loss, and radiographic signs of glenohumeral osteoarthritis [3].

Ultrasound is a cost-effective imaging modality that can be utilized to evaluate the subscapularis, especially in patients with pre-existing metallic surgical implants that may cause image artifact on alternative advanced imaging modalities. One study reported high accuracy at detecting both full-thickness (92.3% sensitivity and 94.4% specificity) and partial-thickness (66.7% sensitivity and 93.5% specificity) rotator cuff tears [1]. Another benefit of ultrasound is that it allows for a dynamic and comparative evaluation of both shoulders. In addition, in shoulders with prior surgery where infection may need to be excluded, aspiration under ultrasound guidance can be valuable in diagnostic evaluation.

Computed tomography (CT) imaging is best utilized for evaluation of glenoid and humeral bone loss in the setting of glenohumeral instability. CT imaging can also be used to evaluate rotator cuff musculature for atrophy or fatty infiltration, which can be appreciated in cases of chronic subscapularis deficiency (white asterisk, Fig. 36.4b). In patients with contraindications for magnetic resonance imaging (MRI) or metallic objects known to create artifacts (e.g., multiple anchors, retained screws, arthroplasty), a CT arthrogram can delineate the condition of the rotator cuff quite well.

Shoulder MRI is a commonly utilized advanced imaging modality that is particularly useful for examination of the rotator cuff. Interestingly, MRI is not as reliable in the detection of subscapularis tears as it is for posterior superior cuff tears, especially for tears involving only the upper third [4]. However, MRI remains a useful imaging modality in evaluating subscapularis deficiency, as these tears typically involve a majority of the tendon footprint. In one study, the sensitivity and specificity of MRI in the detection of subscapularis tears when the tear involves over 50% of the cranial-caudal footprint have been reported to be 56% and 98%, respectively [4]. A stepwise approach for evaluating the subscapularis on MRI, described by Adams et al., can be utilized as an algorithm for subscapularis evaluation and improved diagnostic accuracy [5]. Adams et al. recommend four steps for evaluation, as shown in Fig. 36.4c, which they outline as follows: (1) the presence or absence of a subscapularis tear on axial imaging, (2) the presence or absence of LHBT subluxation on axial imaging, (3) the presence or absence of subscapularis atrophy on sagittal imaging, and (4) the presence or absence of subscapularis tear off of the lesser tuberosity on sagittal imaging [5]. Two or more positive findings in the stepwise approach outlined yielded a sensitivity of 73% and a specificity of 94% in the identification of subscapularis tears on MRI. Careful evaluation of the rotator cuff in the T1 parasagittal sequence is particularly useful to grade fatty infiltration; patients with subscapularis deficiency typically present with the majority of the subscapularis muscle belly replaced with fat.

Classification

The Lafosse classification for subscapularis tears, which considers both the tear size and degree of fatty degeneration, can be utilized to categorize the severity of subscapularis tears and guide surgical management. Lafosse Types I to IV represent repairable subscapularis tears. Lafosse Type V tears, which are characterized by complete subscapularis tears with advanced fatty degeneration and/or static anterior subluxation on advanced imaging studies, represent irreparable subscapularis tears, also known as "subscapularis deficiency" or "subscapularis insufficiency." These lesions are not amenable to primary repair and require surgical intervention with salvage reconstruction techniques [6].

Surgical Management

Surgical management of the unstable shoulder with subscapularis insufficiency represents a formidable challenge. This problem commonly affects younger patients with a desire to preserve shoulder motion and return to demanding activities, including sports. When recurrent glenohumeral instability is associated with extensive rotator cuff insufficiency, not only of the subscapularis but also of the posterosuperior rotator cuff, joint preservation is unpredictable, and *reverse arthroplasty* or *arthrodesis* are favored by most. The same is true for shoulders with not only instability and subscapularis deficiency, but also symptomatic advanced arthritis.

Provided the glenohumeral joint is not severely arthritic and the posterosuperior cuff is adequate, unstable shoulders with subscapularis deficiency require some sort of soft tissue reconstruction to compensate for the deficient subscapularis and anterior capsule. These soft tissue reconstructions may be beneficial, but they also require adequate bone structures. As such, *critical glenoid and humeral bone loss areas* need to be properly addressed when soft tissue reconstructions are attempted in the subscapularis-deficient shoulder. Soft tissue procedures that can be considered in these circumstances include *attempted subscapularis repair with augmentation*, *reconstruction of the anterior capsule*, and *tendon transfers*. Controversy remains regarding which of these procedures is best for a given shoulder, and currently, there is no widely accepted treatment algorithm, with shoulder pathology and surgeon preferences often guiding technique selection.

Subscapularis Reconstruction with Augmentation

Retracted rotator cuff tears with limited or no tendon stump can be treated by bridging the gap between the muscle belly and the tuberosities. Irreparable subscapularis tears with instability can be reconstructed using a tendon allograft. At our institution, the allograft of choice for this indication is the Achilles tendon. The wider aponeurotic portion of the Achilles can be draped and secured to the muscle belly of the subscapularis and the narrower calcaneal end secured to the lesser tuberosity. This technique is ideal for patients with a reasonable muscle belly and either severe retraction or a compromised tendon stump. This technique should be avoided in shoulders with advanced fatty infiltration of the subscapularis. To the best of our knowledge, the outcome of this technique has not been formally reported.

Anterior Capsular Reconstruction

Anterior capsular reconstruction has been utilized by many as a reconstructive technique to treat instability arising from subscapularis insufficiency. This technique introduces a static stabilizer to the anterior glenohumeral joint in hopes of reconstituting a functional glenohumeral capsular fulcrum and eliminating instability. Many techniques have been described, with variations in approach, allograft versus autograft selection, as well as graft orientation and fixation at the glenohumeral joint [7–11]. Outcomes following this type of reconstructive technique have shown success in restoring stability to the glenohumeral joint and relieving shoulder pain while typically resulting in some range of motion loss when compared to the normal contralateral extremity [7–9]. Due to varied surgical techniques and the relatively rare incidence of subscapularis deficiency, literature on long-term outcomes for this intervention is limited. Capsular reconstruction techniques do not restore internal rotation strength, as may be seen with tendon transfer techniques, and often utilize allografts, which are perceived by some as shortcomings of this reconstructive technique. Proponents of these techniques highlight the accelerated recovery, anatomic reconstruction, and improved cosmesis when compared to tendon transfer reconstructions.

Dynamic Muscle and Tendon Transfers

Surgical transfers of musculotendinous units can be utilized for the treatment of chronic subscapularis deficiency. Most commonly, these procedures are performed in stable shoulders with very limited information on the outcome in shoulders with combined shoulder instability and subscapularis deficiency.

Proponents of these techniques highlight the dynamic nature of the muscle-tendon unit, mimicking the function of the subscapularis in re-establishing the rotator cuff force couple to promote glenohumeral stability. Additionally, advocates also report improved internal rotation strength observed with these techniques when compared to capsular reconstruction. Many muscle-tendon units have been described as potential donors for this indication, including the pectoralis major, pectoralis minor, latissimus dorsi, and others [12]. To date, pectoralis major and latissimus dorsi tendon transfers have become the most commonly utilized reconstruction techniques in the treatment of subscapularis deficiency [12].

Pectoralis Major Tendon Transfer

Pectoralis major transfer for the treatment of subscapularis deficiency was first described by Wirth and Rockwood in 1997 [13] and Resch in 2000 [14]. Over the last two decades, it has become a popular technique with multiple variations described [14–16]. These variations include transfer of the entire pectoralis insertion, the upper half of the pectoralis, and the sternal head of the pectoralis with passage either superficial or deep to the conjoint tendon [13–16].

In all techniques, the pectoralis major tendon is identified and mobilized from the lateral ridge of the bicipital groove and transferred to the lesser tuberosity. During mobilization of the pectoralis major, care should be taken to protect the lateral pectoral nerve, which lies approximately 8 cm medial to its humeral insertion [16]. Placement of the tendon transfer superficial or deep to the conjoint tendon is based on surgeon's preference. One biomechanical study observed that pectoralis transfer deep to the conjoint tendon introduces a muscle tendon line of pull that more closely restores native glenohumeral joint kinematics [17]. However, sub-conjoint pectoralis transfer carries the additional risk of injury to the musculocutaneous nerve, and some authors have recommended only performing a partial transfer to minimize bulk between the conjoined tendon and the musculocutaneous nerve [14, 16]. Fixation of the pectoralis major to the prepared lesser tuberosity can be achieved with transosseous sutures or suture anchors.

Moroder et al. recently published on the long-term outcomes of pectoralis major transfer for the irreparable subscapularis tear [18]. The authors observed significant and sustained clinical improvement in pain scores and internal rotation at an average of 10 years postoperative follow-up, with a low rate of salvage with a reverse shoulder arthroplasty despite radiographic progression of cuff tear arthropathy in two-thirds of the cohort. In addition, a systematic review of eight studies evaluating pectoralis major transfers in 195 shoulders with subscapularis deficiency reported good overall outcomes [19]. Constant scores significantly improved following tendon transfer, and a trend in pain reduction following surgery was noted in all studies. Constant scores were noted to be significantly higher in patients who underwent sub-conjoint pectoralis major transfer when compared to patients with supra-conjoint pectoralis major transfer. Not unexpectedly, functional outcomes were less favorable in shoulders with pre-existing shoulder arthroplasty or massive rotator cuff tears when compared to isolated subscapularis deficiency [19].

Latissimus Dorsi Tendon Transfer

One potential drawback of transferring the pectoralis major for subscapularis deficiency is that the pectoralis major muscle is anterior to the chest wall; as such, active contraction of the pectoralis major tends to translate the humeral head anteriorly. This may not affect the overall outcome for patients with subscapularis deficiency and no anterior instability, but it may potentially worsen anterior instability if present preoperatively. This has been particularly problematic for subscapularis failure and anterior instability complicating anatomic shoulder arthroplasty [20].

Originating from the posterior chest wall, the latissimus dorsi exerts a force vector on the proximal humerus that is very similar to that of the subscapularis. As such, conceptually, the latissimus dorsi is a very appealing alternative to the pectoralis major, especially in shoulders with the combination of subscapularis insufficiency and instability. The feasibility of performing this procedure has been investigated in one cadaver study [21].

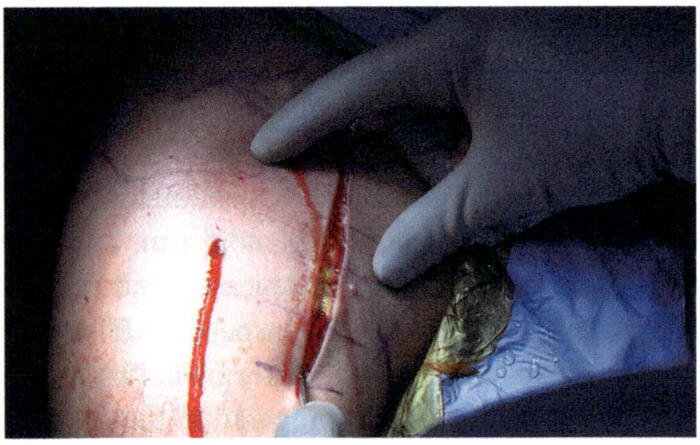

Fig. 37.3 Open incision made in the right shoulder with the patient in beach-chair position. The 12-cm longitudinal incision is made lateral to the coracoid

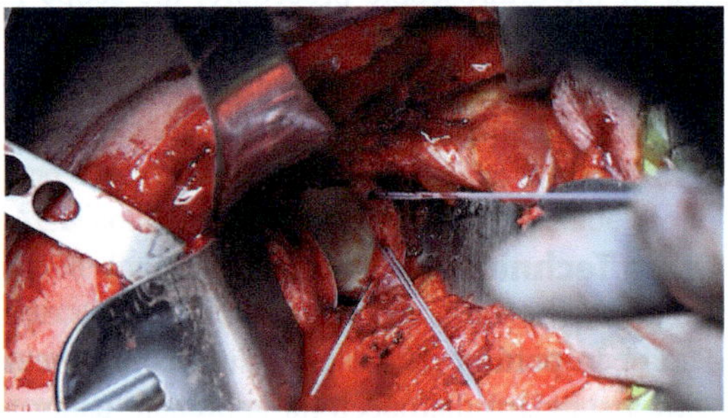

Fig. 37.4 Three preloaded 3-mm knotted anchors are placed into the anterior glenoid rim at the five, three, and one o'clock positions

glenoid rim at the five, three, and one o'clock positions (Fig. 37.4). As a technical pearl, the senior surgeon suggests starting with the inferior anchor placement.

Next, the arm is placed in 30 degrees of abduction, 30 degrees of forward flexion, and 30 degrees of external rotation, and the defect size is measured in the coronal and axial planes. A 3.5-mm-thick dermal allograft is prepared to match accordingly. The sutures from the suture anchors are then shuttled through the medial edge of the dermal allograft in a mattress configuration and secured onto the anterior glenoid rim (Fig. 37.5). An arthroscopic knot pusher can help facilitate securing the graft and sutures.

It should be noted that in contrast to the square-shaped supraspinatus tendon footprint, the footprint of the SSC tendon constitutes a trapezoidal shape. To respect this anatomical configuration and optimize the biomechanical load distribution, the superior-medial anchor is placed more medially than the inferior-medial anchor, resulting in a skewed double-row repair to completely cover the footprint. The senior surgeon suggests a superior to inferior bone bridge of

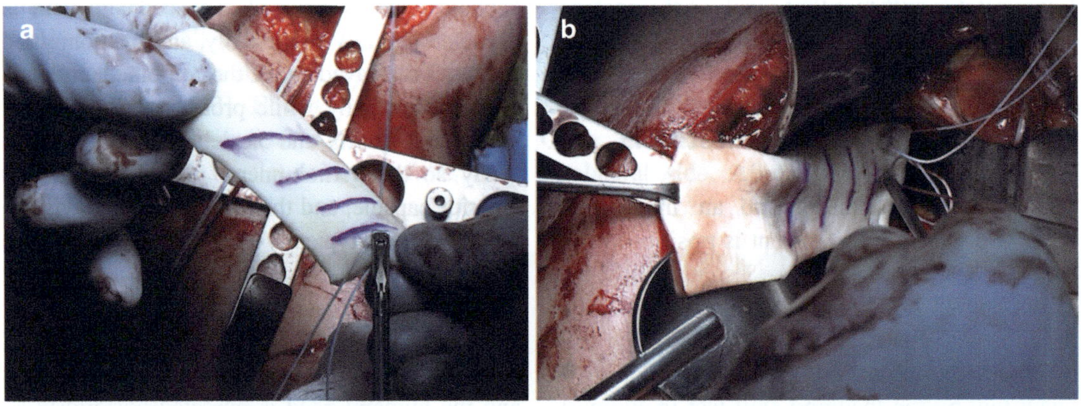

Fig. 37.5 A 3.5-mm dermal allograft is fixed with three suture anchors on the medial glenoid rim

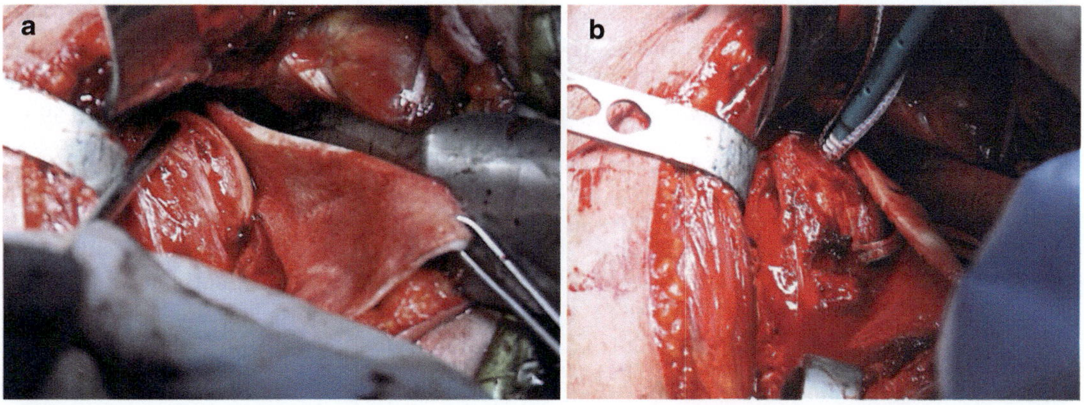

Fig. 37.6 Preparation of the medial tuberosity (**a**) and medial anchor positioning (**b**)

10 mm in the inferior-lateral direction between each medial anchor.

Next, the lesser tuberosity is prepared, again with a motorized shaver to enhance graft-to-bone healing (Fig. 37.6).

For the humeral-sided fixation, the senior surgeon prefers two preloaded medial and two unloaded lateral anchors in a double row bridging (SpeedBridge, Arthrex, Naples, Fl) configuration (Fig. 37.7). For this, an arthroscopic punch is used to create a medial bone socket 1–2 mm lateral to the articular margin. The suture tapes are shuttled through the lateral superior and inferior edges of the 3.5-mm dermal allograft. The allograft is secured on the humeral side, and with the help of the lateral humeral-sided row (15 mm to the medial row), compression is applied throughout the former SSC footprint. The upper border of the graft can be additionally secured to the leading edge of the supraspinatus tendon in a margin convergence technique. The remaining medial aspect of the rotator interval is typically left open. At the end of the surgery, a dynamic exam is performed intraoperatively to assess the stability and security of the repair.

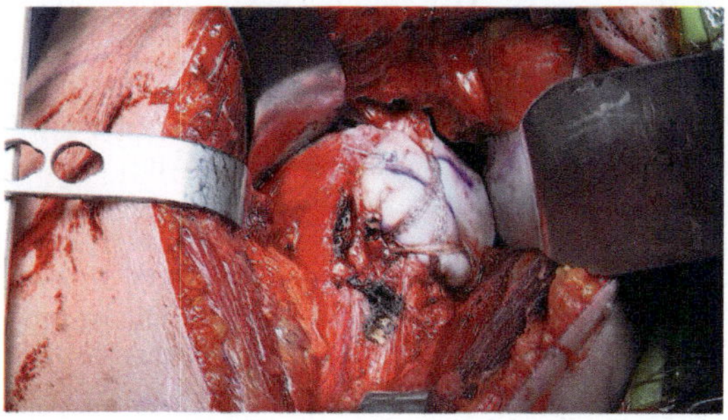

Fig. 37.7 Final view of the ACR reconstruction demonstrating a double-row bridging repair with two medial and two lateral anchors

Postoperative Protocol

Postoperatively, the patient is immobilized in a sling for 6 weeks. External rotation is limited to neutral rotation for 2 weeks and 30° through week six. The long head biceps tendon is always addressed in these procedures, most commonly with a biceps tenodesis using a suture anchor. In instances where the biceps is tenodesed, resisted elbow flexion is restricted for 6 weeks. Active glenohumeral range of motion is started at 6–8 weeks, with an estimated return to activity and sport at 5–6 months postoperatively (Table 37.1).

Table 37.1 Pearls and pitfalls

Pearls
Place arm in 30-30-30 position
Place the anchors from inferior to superior
Use an arthroscopic knot pusher
For precise preparation of the dermal allograft, utilization of a template or use of an arthroscopic ruler beforehand (arthroscopic measurement probe, 220 mm, 60°) is suggested. Use foil from a scalpel blade as a template to determine graft size
Plan to position the anchors on the lesser tuberosity SSC footprint to create maximum surface area for healing
Pitfalls
Wrong indication—Do not perform ACR if the supra and/or supra and infra are also torn!—Do not perform ACR if there is glenohumeral osteoarthritis (GHOA)
Graft tensioning—Make sure to appropriately position the arm BEFORE measuring
Measure twice, cut once!
Secure graft medially first, then laterally
Dog-ear formation during the medial row—It is recommended to start the medial fixation with the middle anchor and fix the inferior and superior edges of the graft with suture loops
Missing concomitant lesions—a diagnostic arthroscopy should be performed before starting the surgery
Failure of healing—Go slow with rehab. This is avascular allograft tissue. It needs time to revascularize and heal!
Postoperative stiffness—Gradually increased early passive range of motion and progression to active range of motion from week six

Conclusion/Future Outlook

Irreparable SSC deficiency with anterior instability is a rare condition with severe consequences for patients. Currently, the predominant treatment options include muscle transfers like the PM transfer, TM transfer, and the LD transfer. While moderate to high patient satisfaction has been reported for these procedures, overall failure rates of up to 12.9% and complication rates of approximately 15% have been reported [38]. Restoring static stability with grafts and bone block procedures is an approach that has been used for some time with success. More recently, ACR, which utilizes modern grafts and fixation, has simplified the procedure to restore static glenohumeral joint stability. This reproducible surgical technique has shown promising early results. In the senior surgeon's two-year follow-up study of seven patients (Lee, Millett et al.), the patients demonstrated a mean postoperative ASES score of 87.9 points (preoperative 59.9), SANE score of 79.8 points (preoperative 45), and QUICKDASH score of 10.2 points (preoperative 36.3) [16]. There were no intraoperative complications. One patient with a combined ACR and SCR received a reverse total shoulder arthroplasty after 6.8 months. Consequently, we do not advocate using this technique in larger tears that also disrupt the coronal plane force couple and involve the supraspinatus or the supraspinatus and infraspinatus [38].

In conclusion, ACR with a dermal allograft can be a viable salvage operation for irreparable SSC tears with instability due to the loss of the transverse force couple and static restraints. ACR has shown promising results with favorable clinical outcomes and low complication profiles, all while avoiding excessively distorting the anatomy in the event of future reconstructive or salvage procedures.

References

1. Inman VT, Saunders JB, Abbott LC. Observations of the function of the shoulder joint. 1944. Clin Orthop Relat Res. 1996;330:3–12.
2. Burkhart SS. Arthroscopic treatment of massive rotator cuff tears. Clinical results and biomechanical rationale. Clin Orthop Relat Res. 1991;267:45–56.
3. Burkhart SS. Fluoroscopic comparison of kinematic patterns in massive rotator cuff tears. A suspension bridge model. Clin Orthop Relat Res. 1992;284:144–52.
4. Keating JF, Waterworth P, Shaw-Dunn J, Crossan J. The relative strengths of the rotator cuff muscles. A cadaver study. J Bone Joint Surg Br. 1993;75(1):137–40.
5. Millett PJ, van der Meijden OA, Gaskill T. Surgical anatomy of the shoulder. Instr Course Lect. 2012;61:87–95.
6. Richards DP, Burkhart SS, Tehrany AM, Wirth MA. The subscapularis footprint: an anatomic description of its insertion site. Arthroscopy. 2007;23(3):251–4.
7. Pogorzelski J, Hussain ZB, Lebus GF, Fritz EM, Millett PJ. Anterior capsular reconstruction for irreparable subscapularis tears. Arthrosc Tech. 2017;6(4):e951–e8.

8. Bokor DJ, Hawkins RJ, Huckell GH, Angelo RL, Schickendantz MS. Results of nonoperative management of full-thickness tears of the rotator cuff. Clin Orthop Relat Res. 1993;294:103–10.
9. Neer CS 2nd, Craig EV, Fukuda H. Cuff-tear arthropathy. J Bone Joint Surg Am. 1983;65(9):1232–44.
10. Barth JR, Burkhart SS, De Beer JF. The bear-hug test: a new and sensitive test for diagnosing a subscapularis tear. Arthroscopy. 2006;22(10):1076–84.
11. Deutsch A, Altchek DW, Veltri DM, Potter HG, Warren RF. Traumatic tears of the subscapularis tendon. Clinical diagnosis, magnetic resonance imaging findings, and operative treatment. Am J Sports Med. 1997;25(1):13–22.
12. Lo IK, Burkhart SS. The etiology and assessment of subscapularis tendon tears: a case for subcoracoid impingement, the roller-wringer effect, and TUFF lesions of the subscapularis. Arthroscopy. 2003;19(10):1142–50.
13. Katthagen JC, Vap AR, Tahal DS, Horan MP, Millett PJ. Arthroscopic repair of isolated partial- and full-thickness upper third subscapularis tendon tears: minimum 2-year outcomes after single-anchor repair and biceps tenodesis. Arthroscopy. 2017;33(7):1286–93.
14. Pearce SS, Ruzbarsky JJ, Ernat JJ, Rakowski DR, Hanson JA, Millett PJ. Arthroscopic subcoracoid decompression, coracoplasty, and subscapularis repair for subscapularis tears in the setting of subcoracoid impingement. Arthrosc Tech. 2022;11(3):e333–e8.
15. Gerber C, Krushell RJ. Isolated rupture of the tendon of the subscapularis muscle. Clinical features in 16 cases. J Bone Joint Surg Br. 1991;73(3):389–94.
16. Lee S, Rakowski DR, Horan MP, Hanson JA, Ernat JJ, Millett PJ. Open anterior capsular reconstruction with a dermal allograft is a viable nonarthroplasty salvage procedure for irreparable subscapularis tears at a minimum 2-year follow-up. Arthrosc Sports Med Rehabil. 2022;4(4):e1291–e7.
17. Tokish JM, Decker MJ, Ellis HB, Torry MR, Hawkins RJ. The belly-press test for the physical examination of the subscapularis muscle: electromyographic validation and comparison to the lift-off test. J Shoulder Elb Surg. 2003;12(5):427–30.
18. Sakurai G, Ozaki J, Tomita Y, Kondo T, Tamai S. Incomplete tears of the subscapularis tendon associated with tears of the supraspinatus tendon: cadaveric and clinical studies. J Shoulder Elb Surg. 1998;7(5):510–5.
19. Frandsen JJ, Quinlan NJ, Smith KM, Lu CC, Chalmers PN, Tashjian RZ. Symptomatic rotator cuff tear progression: conservatively treated full- and partial-thickness tears continue to progress. Arthrosc Sports Med Rehabil. 2022;4(3):e1091–e6.
20. Keener JD, Galatz LM, Teefey SA, Middleton WD, Steger-May K, Stobbs-Cucchi G, et al. A prospective evaluation of survivorship of asymptomatic degenerative rotator cuff tears. J Bone Joint Surg Am. 2015;97(2):89–98.
21. Elhassan B, Ozbaydar M, Massimini D, Diller D, Higgins L, Warner JJ. Transfer of pectoralis major for the treatment of irreparable tears of subscapularis: does it work? J Bone Joint Surg Br. 2008;90(8):1059–65.
22. Zingg PO, Jost B, Sukthankar A, Buhler M, Pfirrmann CW, Gerber C. Clinical and structural outcomes of nonoperative management of massive rotator cuff tears. J Bone Joint Surg Am. 2007;89(9):1928–34.
23. Greenspoon JA, Petri M, Warth RJ, Millett PJ. Massive rotator cuff tears: pathomechanics, current treatment options, and clinical outcomes. J Shoulder Elb Surg. 2015;24(9):1493–505.
24. Dewing CB, Horan MP, Millett PJ. Two-year outcomes of open shoulder anterior capsular reconstruction for instability from severe capsular deficiency. Arthroscopy. 2012;28(1):43–51.
25. Elhassan BT, Wagner ER, Kany J. Latissimus dorsi transfer for irreparable subscapularis tear. J Shoulder Elb Surg. 2020;29(10):2128–34.
26. Jost B, Puskas GJ, Lustenberger A, Gerber C. Outcome of pectoralis major transfer for the treatment of irreparable subscapularis tears. J Bone Joint Surg Am. 2003;85(10):1944–51.
27. Moroder P, Schulz E, Mitterer M, Plachel F, Resch H, Lederer S. Long-term outcome after pectoralis major transfer for irreparable anterosuperior rotator cuff tears. J Bone Joint Surg Am. 2017;99(3):239–45.
28. Resch H, Povacz P, Ritter E, Matschi W. Transfer of the pectoralis major muscle for the treatment of irreparable rupture of the subscapularis tendon. J Bone Joint Surg Am. 2000;82(3):372–82.
29. Rogers JP, Kwapisz A, Tokish JM. Anterior capsule reconstruction for irreparable subscapularis tears. Arthrosc Tech. 2017;6(6):e2241–e7.
30. Shin JJ, Saccomanno MF, Cole BJ, Romeo AA, Nicholson GP, Verma NN. Pectoralis major transfer for treatment of irreparable subscapularis tear: a systematic review. Knee Surg Sports Traumatol Arthrosc. 2016;24(6):1951–60.
31. Gerber A, Clavert P, Millett PJ, Holovacs TF, Warner JJP. Split pectoralis major and teres major tendon transfers for reconstruction of irreparable tears of the subscapularis. Tech Shoulder Elbow Surg. 2004;5(1):5–12.
32. Ruiz-Iban MA, Murillo-Gonzalez JA, Diaz-Heredia J, Avila-Lafuente JL, Cuellar R. Pectoralis major transfer for subscapular deficiency: anatomical study of the relationship between the transferred muscle and the musculocutaneous nerve. Knee Surg Sports Traumatol Arthrosc. 2013;21(9):2177–83.
33. Moeckel BH, Altchek DW, Warren RF, Wickiewicz TL, Dines DM. Instability of the shoulder after arthroplasty. J Bone Joint Surg Am. 1993;75(4):492–7.
34. Mihata T, McGarry MH, Pirolo JM, Kinoshita M, Lee TQ. Superior capsule reconstruction to restore superior stability in irreparable rotator cuff tears: a biomechanical cadaveric study. Am J Sports Med. 2012;40(10):2248–55.
35. Komperda KW, Adamson GJ, Itami Y, McGarry MH, Kantor A, Lin CC, et al. Anterior capsule reconstruction versus pectoralis major transfer for irreparable subscapularis tears involving the ante-

can produce across the graft-glenoid interface is of utmost importance to study.

Future options will prioritize ease of insertion of the graft as well as the subsequent hardware for fixation for both arthroscopic and open techniques. They will continue to allow indirect (non-in-line) access to the anterior or posterior glenoid to avoid any potential injury to the anterior neurovascular structures. Lastly, they will conclusively prove that they can provide enough compressive strength to not compromise graft healing.

Graft Types

Autograft types currently available for glenoid reconstruction include coracoid (Latarjet), iliac crest, distal clavicle, and scapular spine. Allograft sources are largely distal tibia (fresh or frozen), talus, and frozen, pre-shaped, pre-drilled allograft cortical bone augmentation (Glenojet; Arthrosurface Inc., Franklin, MA). Due to difficulty in harvesting cadaveric scapulae, allograft glenoid is not routinely available, and other sources for allografts have not been routinely described.

Allografts are available with different types of preparation, which affect the viability of chondrocytes. Fresh (never frozen) allografts have viable chondrocytes. These grafts have a small window of time to be implanted, typically around 30 days from the time of harvest to implantation. These grafts are more expensive compared to frozen grafts and also cannot routinely be sent back to the graft companies or kept in the hospital if no longer needed. They are also typically harder to procure than a frozen graft. Frozen grafts, by comparison, are less expensive and easier to procure and can be retained if not needed in many cases. However, they do not have the benefit of live chondrocytes. Despite the theoretical advantage of live chondrocytes in fresh allografts, clinical studies have continued to demonstrate similar outcomes in patients despite the difference in bone graft use and allograft sources, which have performed very favorably even when compared to autograft [13].

Xenografts have a historical use in many different parts of the body, including shoulder surgery.

Equine grafts are being studied in Europe as they are very cost-effective; however, routine use of xenografts in glenoid reconstruction is not mainstream. Surgeons should continue to be aware of all graft options that are available in their region, as different countries have varying access to allograft types. Future work with grafts will prioritize a graft source that does not add significant morbidity from harvest if an autograft. Allograft or xenograft sources will need to be inexpensive, easily modifiable to fit the patient's anatomy and still produce reliable incorporation without resorption. The addition of a cartilaginous surface is a big advantage with grafts such as the distal tibia (Fig. 38.5) and, to a lesser degree, the distal clavicle, although fibrocartilage is seen to cover the surface of purely bony grafts such as the Latarjet on follow-up arthroscopy (Fig. 38.6). Concerns exist about bony healing with all types of allografts, especially frozen and prefabricated grafts. This is further complicated by the fact that resorption is known to occur even when autograft is utilized and is impacted by biology (adequate preparation of glenoid and graft surfaces) and biomechanics (adequate compression forces, extent or absence of glenoid bone loss) [14].

As the use of biologics continue to evolve in orthopaedic surgery, there is hope that the addition of an autograft biologic additive could improve the likelihood of incorporation if combined with a structural allograft. Despite the fact that injecting biologics is routinely performed by many surgeons, currently there is no concrete data that the addition of biologics (stem cells, platelet-rich plasma) improves graft incorporation or diminishes graft failure rates.

Prefabricated grafts that are ready to implant with already prepared holes are available as well. These grafts have extended shelf life and can be used without the time-consuming process of obtaining a fresh graft, which is intriguing; however, the literature is sparse with follow-up studies demonstrating incorporation. While not containing an actual articular surface, they have

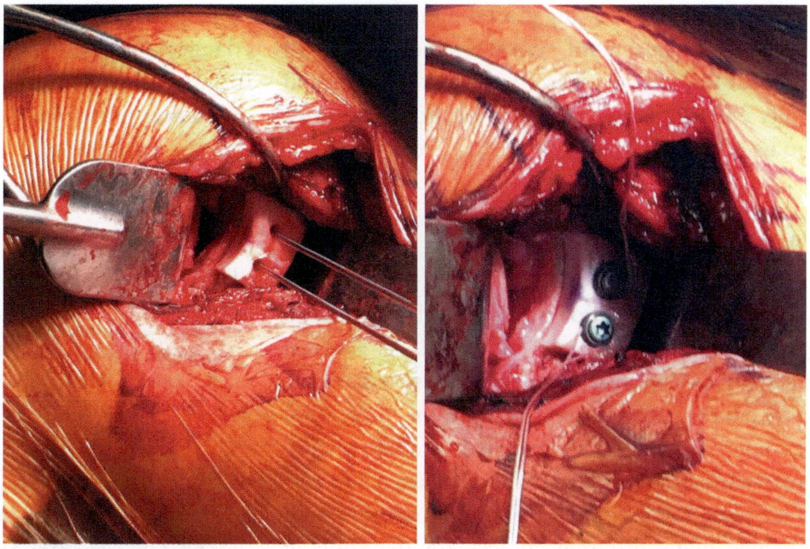

Fig. 38.5 Intraoperative image demonstrating glenoid reconstruction with osteoarticular allograft and near perfect fit of graft contour with native glenoid

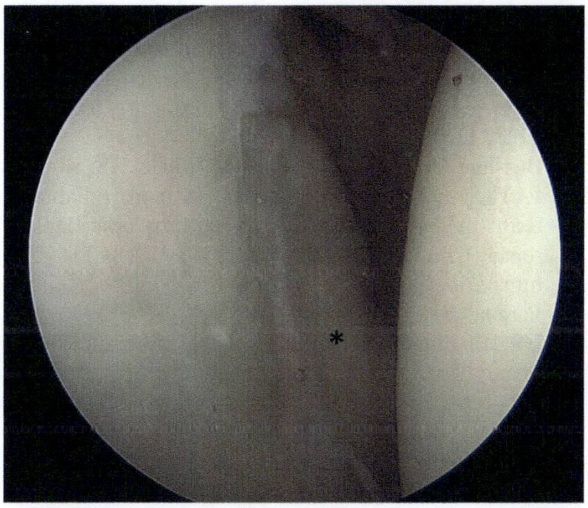

Fig. 38.6 Arthroscopic image of the anterior glenoid viewed from the posterior portal after a Latarjet demonstrating the fibrocartilage cover (*) of the coracoid graft

polished cortical bone so as not to cause any friction or irregularity with humerus articulation. Like many newer techniques, more long-term studies are needed to demonstrate bony integration and clinical results.

Patient-Specific Instrumentation

Patient-specific instrumentation is becoming increasingly popular in the field of arthroplasty, and custom guides to prepare the glenoid during a shoulder replacement are available from multiple companies to improve the accuracy of glenoid component placement [15, 16]. As 3D printing becomes progressively inexpensive and available, patient-specific instrumentation research in the field of glenoid bone is increasing [17]. Companies are now investigating the use of custom cutting guides to improve the ease of the coracoid osteotomy during a Latarjet, as well as custom drill guides to allow instrumentation of the glenoid. These advances will likely become available as an aid for surgeons as this technology becomes more cost-effective.

Many arthroplasty systems also allow the surgeon to plan their case in the preoperative setting using a 3D reconstructed scapula using the patient's CT scan. This part of the preoperative process allows surgeons the advantage of working through difficult planning concerns before they take the patient to the operating room. As many patients are already having CT scans as part of their preoperative work-up for instability, the future will undoubtedly facilitate the use of planning software to assist surgeons with preoperative planning of glenoid reconstruction cases. This would allow surgeons a view of the 3D anatomy and plan their coracoid osteotomy, determine the size of their graft, and allow them to plan the position of the graft on the glenoid. Software would allow the surgeons to visualize how varying graft dimensions would allow replication of normal anatomy with respect to glenoid surface area and contour, and may even influence the decision of which graft to use.

Authors' Final Note

Glenoid reconstruction surgery will continue to play a prominent role in the future. As surgical techniques continue to modernize, nonanatomic procedures will likely decrease in utilization compared to surgeries designed to anatomically reconstruct the native glenoid with respect to surface area and contour. Fixation options will include many different choices for the surgeon that allow the graft to be introduced through the rotator interval and avoid any splits in the subscapularis. They will allow the surgeon to use arthroscopic guides that can be drilled from posterior to anterior and not require in-line access to the anterior glenoid that metal screws require. These fixation options will allow rigid compression across the glenoid-graft interface that provides bony integration of the graft, but if hardware failure does occur, there will not be devastating damage to the joint. Graft sources that allow the surgeon to selectively reconstruct the necessary percentage of bone loss will be favored. Grafts will be easy to procure and to modify based on the specific needs of the patient, and will have a bearing surface that provides a smooth contour that does not lead to arthritic changes over time. Grafts will be inexpensive and provide reliable incorporation, either on their own or with the addition of a biologic additive. Software will exist that will allow surgeons the ability to "perform" these surgeries virtually before they get to the operating room and work out any difficult issues with graft preparation, location, or fixation. Custom guides will be available to assist the surgeon with creating a coracoid osteotomy or to better position the graft against the glenoid surface, as well as prepare the glenoid to receive the necessary fixation. Glenoid reconstruction surgery will remain a valuable surgery in the armamentarium of any surgeon who takes care of patients with glenohumeral instability, and future changes will continually improve the ease of performing this surgery as well as the clinical outcomes.

References

1. Shaha JS, Cook JB, Song DJ, Rowles DJ, Bottoni CR, Shaha SH, et al. Redefining "critical" bone loss in shoulder instability: functional outcomes worsen with "subcritical" bone loss. Am J Sports Med. 2015;43(7):1719–25. https://doi.org/10.1177/0363546515578250.
2. Moroder P, Damm P, Wierer G, Bohm E, Minkus M, Plachel F, et al. Challenging the current concept of critical glenoid bone loss in shoulder instability: does the size measurement really tell it all? Am J Sports Med. 2019;47(3):688–94. https://doi.org/10.1177/0363546518819102.
3. Min KS, Wake J, Cruz C, Miles R, Chan S, Shaha J, et al. Surgical treatment of shoulder instability in active-duty service members with subcritical glenoid bone loss - Bankart versus Latarjet. J Shoulder Elbow Surg. 2022; https://doi.org/10.1016/j.jse.2022.10.011.
4. Bessiere C, Trojani C, Carles M, Mehta SS, Boileau P. The open Latarjet procedure is more reliable in terms of shoulder stability than arthroscopic Bankart repair. Clin Orthop Relat Res. 2014;472(8):2345–51. https://doi.org/10.1007/s11999-014-3550-9.
5. Parada SA, Griffith MS, Shaw KA, Waterman BR, Eichinger JK, Li X, et al. Demographics and distal Tibial dimensions of suitable distal Tibial allografts for glenoid reconstruction. Arthroscopy. 2019;35(10):2788–94. https://doi.org/10.1016/j.arthro.2019.05.019.
6. Frank RM, Romeo AA, Richardson C, Sumner S, Verma NN, Cole BJ, et al. Outcomes of Latarjet versus distal tibia allograft for anterior shoulder instability repair: a matched cohort analysis. Am J Sports Med. 2018;46(5):1030–8. https://doi.org/10.1177/0363546517744203.
7. Provencher MT, Peebles LA, Aman ZS, Bernhardson AS, Murphy CP, Sanchez A, et al. Management of the failed Latarjet procedure: outcomes of revision surgery with fresh distal Tibial allograft. Am J Sports Med. 2019;47(12):2795–802. https://doi.org/10.1177/0363546519871896.
8. Moroder P, Schulz E, Wierer G, Auffarth A, Habermeyer P, Resch H, et al. Neer Award 2019: Latarjet procedure vs. iliac crest bone graft transfer for treatment of anterior shoulder instability with glenoid bone loss: a prospective randomized trial. J Shoulder Elb Surg. 2019;28(7):1298–307. https://doi.org/10.1016/j.jse.2019.03.035.
9. Dines JS, Dodson CC, McGarry MH, Oh JH, Altchek DW, Lee TQ. Contribution of osseous and muscu-

lar stabilizing effects with the Latarjet procedure for anterior instability without glenoid bone loss. J Shoulder Elb Surg. 2013;22(12):1689–94. https://doi.org/10.1016/j.jse.2013.02.014.
10. Balestro JC, Young A, Maccioni C, Walch G. Graft osteolysis and recurrent instability after the Latarjet procedure performed with bioabsorbable screw fixation. J Shoulder Elb Surg. 2015;24(5):711–8. https://doi.org/10.1016/j.jse.2014.07.014.
11. Weick JW, Kalia V, Pacheco E, Jacobson JA, Freehill MT. Osseous healing with nonrigid suture fixation in the arthroscopic Latarjet procedure. Orthop J Sports Med. 2020;8(11):2325967120964489. https://doi.org/10.1177/2325967120964489.
12. Kalogrianitis S, Tsouparopoulos V. Arthroscopic iliac crest bone block for reconstruction of the glenoid: a fixation technique using an adjustable-length loop cortical suspensory fixation device. Arthrosc Tech. 2016;5(6):e1197–e202. https://doi.org/10.1016/j.eats.2016.07.007.
13. Gilat R, Wong SE, Lavoie-Gagne O, Haunschild ED, Knapik DM, Fu MC, et al. Outcomes are comparable using free bone block autografts versus allografts for the management of anterior shoulder instability with glenoid bone loss: a systematic review and meta-analysis of "The Non-Latarjet". Knee Surg Sports Traumatol Arthrosc. 2021;29(7):2159–74. https://doi.org/10.1007/s00167-020-06194-z.
14. Di Giacomo G, Costantini A, de Gasperis N, De Vita A, Lin BK, Francone M, et al. Coracoid graft osteolysis after the Latarjet procedure for anteroinferior shoulder instability: a computed tomography scan study of twenty-six patients. J Shoulder Elb Surg. 2011;20(6):989–95. https://doi.org/10.1016/j.jse.2010.11.016.
15. Throckmorton TW, Gulotta LV, Bonnarens FO, Wright SA, Hartzell JL, Rozzi WB, et al. Patient-specific targeting guides compared with traditional instrumentation for glenoid component placement in shoulder arthroplasty: a multi-surgeon study in 70 arthritic cadaver specimens. J Shoulder Elb Surg. 2015;24(6):965–71. https://doi.org/10.1016/j.jse.2014.10.013.
16. Levins JG, Kukreja M, Paxton ES, Green A. Computer-assisted preoperative planning and patient-specific instrumentation for glenoid implants in shoulder arthroplasty. JBJS Rev. 2021;9(9) https://doi.org/10.2106/JBJS.RVW.20.00236.
17. John R, Wong I. Innovative approaches in the management of shoulder instability: current concept review. Curr Rev Musculoskelet Med. 2019;12(3):386–96. https://doi.org/10.1007/s12178-019-09569-z.

39 Epilogue: What the Future Holds—Controversies for the Next Edition

Rachel M. Frank and John M. Tokish

Shoulder instability remains both a satisfying and humbling condition to treat. As evidenced in the pages of this book, there have been great strides in multiple fields that have helped us arrive at the cutting edge of modern treatment. The emergence of the arthroscope has enabled a far less invasive approach but has required a redefined understanding of anatomy, as well as surgical instruments and implants more suited for minimally invasive techniques. Some would say that the pendulum has swung too far and lament the loss of the standard practice of open surgical approaches, which clearly have a role in instability treatment but are becoming a lost art.

As the pace of technology accelerates, it makes it increasingly difficult to fully evaluate a new technique or approach before it evolves into yet another technique. In this epilogue, we hope to look forward to what is just beyond the horizon and perhaps preview what is in store for the next generation of this book. Innovation will undoubtedly provide solutions to many of our current challenges but will also likely lead to new questions and challenges for the next generation of surgeons to pursue.

Questions for the next edition:

1. What will emerge as the ideal bone graft?

Several chapters in this book describe different approaches to restoring glenoid bone stock. All techniques have advantages and disadvantages. Autograft sources such as the coracoid, iliac crest, distal clavicle, and posterior acromion have the advantages of being readily available, logistically simple, and very cheap. The Latarjet (coracoid transfer), which includes the added potential benefit of the sling effect, would have to be considered the current gold standard. However, we are still defining just how important the sling effect is to the overall construct, with the biomechanical data showing definite advantages [1], but with clinical studies showing little difference between bone grafts with and without the attached conjoined tendon [2, 3]. Novel allograft options, including the distal tibial allograft (DTA), have emerged as an attractive alternative to autograft sources [4]. These options eliminate donor site morbidity and can be generally shaped to fit any size defect. The fresh DTA has the potential added benefit of being a true osteochondral transplant with fresh chondrocytes that may provide a joint preservation benefit in later years. The disadvantage of these grafts is their cost, logistical expense, and their resorption profile. Recent data

R. M. Frank
Orthopedic Surgery, University of Colorado Anschutz Medical Center, Denver, CO, USA

J. M. Tokish (✉)
Orthopedic Surgery, Mayo Clinic, Scottsdale, AZ, USA

© The Author(s), under exclusive license to Springer Nature Switzerland AG 2026
R. M. Frank, J. M. Tokish (eds.), *Management of Shoulder Instability*,
https://doi.org/10.1007/978-3-032-18089-6_39

shows that a frozen DTA performs as well as a fresh graft, at a fraction of the cost, and we do not know the long-term fate of the transplanted chondrocyte. If the fresh transplant prevents the progression to osteoarthritis, then the value proposition of the graft certainly increases, but the logistics and cost of this graft may limit its widespread adoption.

In Europe, xenograft is emerging as a potential option [5]. These grafts may provide a cheap, widely available, and effective graft of any size, but incorporation and longer-term remodeling are unknown at this time. Finally, manufactured implants may play a role in glenoid bone restoration, but the techniques are in their infancy, and much work remains to be done on fixation and long-term interaction between the implant and the host bone. Given that many of our instability patients are young, the ideal solution to glenoid bone loss must consider a shoulder that often has more than half a century to live, and thus, durability is another major consideration.

2. What will emerge as the critical measure and ideal treatment for the Hill-Sachs lesion?

The importance of bipolar bone loss was brought into focus with the emergence of Yamamoto and Etoi's glenoid track concept [6]. It should be noted that the relevance of the Hill-Sachs lesion has been recognized for much longer, as even Rowe in his 1978 paper [7] found that the Hill-Sachs lesion did affect results. But it was the landmark 2014 paper by DiGiacomo, Burkhart, and Itoi that brought bipolar bone loss into the consciousness of practicing surgeons [8]. Since then, attempts to address the Hill-Sachs lesion have become much more emphasized, most notably, at least in the United States, with the emergence of the *remplissage* technique. Many studies have reported its superior results to arthroscopic Bankart repair alone [9–12], but other authors have noted its higher rates of failure in revision cases, contact athletes, and patients with significant bone loss compared to Latarjet [13]. The threshold for adding a *remplissage* is getting lower and lower, and an excellent chapter in this text by Romeo et al. reviews the pertinent ways to measure and approach the lesion. There are lesions that are less amenable to a *remplissage*, such as those that occur when the initial dislocation is in adduction, as described by DiGiacomo et al. [14], or when the Hill-Sachs lesion is massive. In those cases, it remains to be seen whether a soft tissue approach is ideal or if larger bone grafting, osteochondral grafting, or even metal approaches will prove necessary.

3. Will we achieve consensus in the treatment of shoulder instability in the first time dislocator?

In 2018, the newly formed Neer Circle of the American Shoulder and Elbow Society set out to publish a consensus statement on the ideal treatment for the first time dislocator [15]. Over 2 years and three rounds of a Delphi process, over 162 scenarios were presented to a panel of experienced shoulder surgeons to determine where consensus would be on this condition. We learned that there was little agreement, even among experts. Of the 162 scenarios presented, only eight (5%) reached a 90% consensus for surgical intervention. Essentially, the patient had to be an athlete at the end of his or her season, have positive bone loss, and have positive apprehension on examination. In scenarios where none of those conditions were met, nonoperative consensus was achieved (14%). Such a low level of consensus reveals how much nuance and disagreement exist in this group of shoulder instability experts. There is data to suggest that multiple dislocations have a negative effect on bone loss and that the number of dislocations is a risk factor for failure [16], but other data suggests that in some populations, patients can return to their previous level of sport without surgical intervention [17]. This question remains controversial, but the immortal words of Champ Baker, former AOSSM president, are pertinent here: "I don't think you have to fix the patient after the first dislocation, but you should probably do it before the second."

4. How should we approach laxity in shoulder instability?

Hyperlaxity is a clear risk factor for failure of instability surgery [18]. Most surgeons understand this, yet there is little consensus on the appropriate treatment for it. Rotator interval closure was touted for such patients but has largely fallen out of favor [19, 20], due to inconsistent techniques and conflicting biomechanical evidence of efficacy. This remains a challenging issue for many reasons, including the lack of true diagnostic criteria and a tendency for the biology of these patients to return to baseline. Notably, laxity is not synonymous with pathology. In many athletes, hyperlaxity is a competitive advantage, and thus, a very narrow window exists between performance and disability. Differentiating between laxity and instability continues to be a challenge, and the degree to which a surgeon "corrects" the instability has yet to be conclusively determined.

5. What is the appropriate Management of the bony Bankart lesion?

Several chapters in this book offer excellent advice and technical guidance on addressing the bony Bankart lesion. But even herein, there is advice to either ignore it, incorporate it, or replace it. Direct comparison studies on this topic are lacking. Some studies suggest that failure rates are high, especially when bone fragments are small [21], while others show very good results and even bone hypertrophy with arthroscopic treatment [22]. In this book, Peter Millett beautifully illustrates his bony Bankart bridge technique, which has emerged as perhaps the most popular of incorporation techniques, and he has published excellent results on its outcomes [23]. Other authors have been more aggressive with the Latarjet in this setting, including Di Giacomo et al., who reported better results in patients treated with Latarjet vs. those patients who underwent arthroscopic bony Bankart repair with subcritical bone loss [24]. Other bone blocks are emerging as potential options here as well, and future studies will undoubtedly explore how to manage the native bone fragment in this setting.

6. How will the management of Posterior instability in the setting of the non-ideal glenoid evolve?

Arthroscopic posterior labral repair has proven a very successful approach to many patients with painful subluxations and posterior labral tears [25]. These results, however, have proven difficult to replicate in patients with significant glenoid changes such as retroversion and bone loss [26, 27]. Defining what is meant by too much retroversion or too much bone loss is a prolific topic currently. Provencher et al. provide an excellent chapter in this book that provides the reader with the very best current understanding of this condition, but as the authors themselves point out, our understanding of posterior instability lags compared to its anterior counterpart. We have much to learn about the role of the reverse Hill-Sachs lesion, as well as the ideal graft or role of glenoid osteotomy in the setting of deficient posterior bone.

In spite of these many controversies and unsolved challenges, one hopeful conclusion that we can draw is that while we do not yet have a complete solution to the problem of shoulder instability, we certainly are confused at a much deeper level than ever, and our understanding continues to evolve. The innovative and thoughtful approaches by the surgeons contributing to this text represent great hope in improving the treatment of patients with shoulder instability.

References

1. Yamamoto N, Muraki T, An KN, et al. The stabilizing mechanism of the Latarjet procedure: a cadaveric study. J Bone Joint Surg Am. 2013;95:1390–7.
2. Moroder P, Schulz E, Wierer G, et al. Neer Award 2019: Latarjet procedure vs. iliac crest bone graft transfer for treatment of anterior shoulder instability with glenoid bone loss: a prospective randomized trial. J Shoulder Elb Surg. 2019;28:1298–307.
3. Frank RM, Romeo AA, Richardson C, et al. Outcomes of Latarjet versus distal tibia allograft for anterior

shoulder instability repair: a matched cohort analysis. Am J Sports Med. 2018;46:1030–8.
4. Provencher MT, Frank RM, Golijanin P, et al. Distal tibia allograft glenoid reconstruction in recurrent anterior shoulder instability: clinical and radiographic outcomes. Arthroscopy. 2017;33:891–7.
5. Maiotti M, Massoni C. Arthroscopic xenograft with cerclage fixation: a method for glenoid bone loss reconstruction with cerclage fixation using a specific posterior guide. Arthrosc Tech. 2023;12:e1657–64.
6. Yamamoto N, Itoi E, Abe H, et al. Contact between the glenoid and the humeral head in abduction, external rotation, and horizontal extension: a new concept of glenoid track. J Shoulder Elb Surg. 2007;16:649–56.
7. Rowe CR, Patel D, Southmayd WW. The Bankart procedure: a long-term end-result study. J Bone Joint Surg Am. 1978;60:1–16.
8. Di Giacomo G, Itoi E, Burkhart SS. Evolving concept of bipolar bone loss and the Hill-Sachs lesion: from "engaging/non-engaging" lesion to "on-track/off-track" lesion. Arthroscopy. 2014;30:90–8.
9. Schrouff C, Verlaan L. Bankart repair with remplissage vs. Latarjet procedure on recurrence, postoperative pain scores, external rotation, and Rowe score in patients with a Hill-Sachs lesion. A systematic review. JSES Rev Rep Tech. 2023;3:461–8.
10. Camus D, Domos P, Berard E, Toulemonde J, Mansat P, Bonnevialle N. Isolated arthroscopic Bankart repair vs. Bankart repair with "remplissage" for anterior shoulder instability with engaging Hill-Sachs lesion: a meta-analysis. Orthop Traumatol Surg Res. 2018;104:803–9.
11. Cho NS, Yoo JH, Rhee YG. Management of an engaging Hill-Sachs lesion: arthroscopic remplissage with Bankart repair versus Latarjet procedure. Knee Surg Sports Traumatol Arthrosc. 2016;24:3793–800.
12. Grimberg J, Diop A, Bou Ghosn R, Lanari D, Canonne A, Maurel N. Bankart repair versus Bankart repair plus remplissage: an in vitro biomechanical comparative study. Knee Surg Sports Traumatol Arthrosc. 2016;24:374–80.
13. Yang JS, Mehran N, Mazzocca AD, Pearl ML, Chen VW, Arciero RA. Remplissage versus modified Latarjet for off-track Hill-Sachs lesions with subcritical glenoid bone loss. Am J Sports Med. 2018;46:1885–91.
14. Di Giacomo G, Golijanin P, Sanchez G, Provencher MT. Radiographic analysis of the Hill-Sachs lesion in anteroinferior shoulder instability after first-time dislocations. Arthroscopy. 2016;32:1509–14.
15. Tokish JM, Kuhn JE, Ayers GD, et al. Decision making in treatment after a first-time anterior glenohumeral dislocation: a Delphi approach by the Neer circle of the American shoulder and elbow surgeons. J Shoulder Elb Surg. 2020;29:2429–45.
16. Dickens JF, Slaven SE, Cameron KL, et al. Prospective evaluation of glenoid bone loss after first-time and recurrent anterior glenohumeral instability events. Am J Sport Med. 2019;47:1082–9.
17. Shanley E, Thigpen C, Brooks J, et al. Return to sport as an outcome measure for shoulder instability surprising findings in nonoperative management in a high school athlete population. Am J Sport Med. 2019;47:1062–7.
18. Balg F, Boileau P. The instability severity index score. J Bone Joint Surg Br. 2007;89b:1470–7.
19. Provencher MT, Peebles LA. Rotator interval closure of the shoulder continues to be a challenge in consensus on treatment. Arthroscopy. 2018;34:3109–11.
20. Maman E, Dolkart O, Kazum E, et al. Rotator interval closure has no additional effect on shoulder stability compared to Bankart repair alone. Arch Orthop Trauma Surg. 2017;137:673–7.
21. Nakagawa S, Ozaki R, Take Y, Mae T, Hayashida K. Bone fragment union and remodeling after arthroscopic bony Bankart repair for traumatic anterior shoulder instability with a glenoid defect: influence on postoperative recurrence of instability. Am J Sport Med. 2015;43:1438–47.
22. Kitayama S, Sugaya H, Takahashi N, et al. Clinical outcome and glenoid morphology after arthroscopic repair of chronic osseous Bankart lesions: a five to eight-year follow-up study. J Bone Joint Surg Am. 2015;97:1833–43.
23. Millett PJ, Horan MP, Martetschlager F. The "bony Bankart bridge" technique for restoration of anterior shoulder stability. Am J Sports Med. 2013;41:608–14.
24. Giacomo GD, Pugliese M, Peebles AM, Provencher MT. Bone fragment resorption and clinical outcomes of traumatic bony Bankart lesion treated with arthroscopic repair versus open Latarjet. Am J Sports Med. 2022;50:1336–43.
25. Bradley JP, Baker CL 3rd, Kline AJ, Armfield DR, Chhabra A. Arthroscopic capsulolabral reconstruction for posterior instability of the shoulder: a prospective study of 100 shoulders. Am J Sports Med. 2006;34:1061–71.
26. Hines A, Cook JB, Shaha JS, et al. Glenoid bone loss in posterior shoulder instability: prevalence and outcomes in arthroscopic treatment. Am J Sports Med. 2018;46:1053–7.
27. Testa EJ, van der List JP, Waterman BR, Caldwell PE 3rd, Parada SA, Owens BD. Management of bone loss in posterior glenohumeral shoulder instability: current concepts. JBJS Rev. 2024;12

Index

© The Editor(s) (if applicable) and The Author(s), under exclusive license to Springer Nature Switzerland AG 2026
R. M. Frank, J. M. Tokish (eds.), *Management of Shoulder Instability*,
https://doi.org/10.1007/978-3-032-18089-6

GPSR Compliance

The European Union's (EU) General Product Safety Regulation (GPSR) is a set of rules that requires consumer products to be safe and our obligations to ensure this.

If you have any concerns about our products, you can contact us on ProductSafety@springernature.com

In case Publisher is established outside the EU, the EU authorized representative is:

Springer Nature Customer Service Center GmbH
Europaplatz 3
69115 Heidelberg, Germany

Batch number: 10731393

Printed by Printforce, the Netherlands